The
Aged Person
and the
Nursing Process

Ann Gera Yurick, RN, PhD
Associate Professor of Nursing
University of Pittsburgh

Barbara Elliott Spier, BSN, MSN, NP
Assistant Professor of Nursing
University of Pittsburgh

Susanne S. Robb, RNC, PhD, FAAN
Associate Chief, Nursing Service for Research
Veterans Administration Medical Center
Pittsburgh (University Drive)

Nancy J. Ebert, BSN, MSN, NP
Assistant Professor of Nursing
University of Pittsburgh

with a contribution by
Margaret H. Magnussen, BSN, MPH, NP, CCNC
Assistant Chief, Nursing Service
Veterans Administration Medical Center
Assistant Professor (Adjunct)
College of Nursing
University of New Mexico
Albuquerque, New Mexico

The Aged Person and the Nursing Process

SECOND EDITION

APPLETON-CENTURY-CROFTS/Norwalk, Connecticut

0-8385-0083-8

Notice: The author(s) and publisher of this volume have taken care that the information and recommendations contained herein are accurate and compatible with the standards generally accepted at the time of publication.

84 85 86 87 88 89 / 10 9 8 7 6 5 4 3 2 1

Prentice-Hall International, Inc., London
Prentice-Hall of Australia, Pty. Ltd., Sydney
Prentice-Hall Canada, Inc.
Prentice-Hall of India Private Limited, New Delhi
Prentice-Hall of Japan, Inc., Tokyo
Prentice-Hall of Southeast Asia (Pte.) Ltd., Singapore
Whitehall Books Ltd., Wellington, New Zealand
Editora Prentice-Hall do Brasil Ltda., Rio de Janeiro

Library of Congress Cataloging in Publication Data
Main entry under title:

The Aged person and the nursing process.

   Includes index.
   1. Geriatric nursing.   2. Geriatric nursing—Social
aspects. I. Yurick, Ann Gera, 1935–   [DNLM:
1. Geriatric nursing. WY 152 A265]
RC954.A34 1984   610.73'65   84-281
ISBN 0-8385-0083-8

Design: Jean M. Sabato

Cartoons: Harry Trumbore

Photo Credits (Cover): Shawn Mertz/Pittsburgh, PA, woman with little girl and man and nurse on steps; Saul M. Weiss, Chief, Medical Media Service, University Drive, V.A. Medical Center, Pittsburgh, PA, man with dog.

Photo Credits (Part Openers): Eugene Mizikar, p. 1, p. 2, top right; Ed Spier/Murrysville, PA, p. 2, bottom right, p. 272, top right; Shawn Mertz, p. 273; Saul M. Weiss/Pittsburgh, PA, p. 2, bottom left, p. 3, and p. 272, bottom left.

PRINTED IN THE UNITED STATES OF AMERICA

To our aging and aged friends

Preface

Application of the nursing process to elderly people is the focus of this book's second edition. The emphasis is on promotion of health among the elderly, and includes an awareness of their environmental needs and support resources. In addition, nursing interventions are presented to maximize the health potential of the elderly person who experiences alterations in health. Realizing maximum health potential necessarily includes both the elements of safety and comfort. Consideration must also be directed toward psychologic, physiologic, and sociologic factors affecting health. The nurse's role can occur in any setting (community or institutional) and relationship (independent, quasi-independent, or dependent). Emphasis is placed on supporting the functional abilities of the elderly person.

This book was written primarily for use as a textbook by undergraduate nursing students. It is also intended to serve as a reference for nurses who work with the elderly in institutional (acute and extended care) and in community settings. Based on the expressed needs of these nurses, this edition considers some alterations in health that affect the functional ability of the elderly person. Interventions are directed toward optimizing functioning, providing comfort, and limiting disabilities associated with health alterations.

The book is divided into two parts. Part One provides information necessary to understand the elderly within the context of American society and the health care system. Nursing implications are incorporated throughout. The first chapter is an overview of the nursing process in relation to the aged person—especially the ways in which implementation of the process differs because of the target group to which it is applied. The description of today's elderly and their health status in Chapter 2 provides a base for the following chapters. Chapter 3 presents selected theories of aging and their relevance to the practice of nursing. The implications of nurses' behaviors on the health status of the elderly are presented in Chapter 4. Chapters 5 and 6 present the multitude of resources available for support of the elderly. Included is the nurse's role in assisting in the use of these resources. Part One of this book concludes with an overview of the developmental changes that confront the elderly.

Part Two focuses on the application of the nursing process to the adaptive experience of the aged person in order to increase the feeling of well-being. Included are developmental changes, cognition, sensory experiences, nutrition, elimination, activity, and body protection. This conceptual approach addresses the question of how to optimize the functioning of the elderly when alterations in health occur. The concluding chapter presents a discussion of the aged person who takes medications. Drugs as therapeutic interventions are integrated throughout the book as appropriate.

The collaborative role of the nurse as a member of the professional team concerned with the needs of the elderly permeates this book. Other nursing roles that are discussed include those of assessor, planner, advocate, teacher, holistic care provider, investigator of health related problems, and evaluator. As an advocate, the nurse presents the options while supporting the elderly person in making decisions. This book addresses these options. Ethnic, cultural, and minority group issues of the elderly are also addressed.

The many acute and chronic health problems to which the elderly are prone are not specifically emphasized in this book. There are many excellent references in which these are presented in detail. However, the specific functional needs of the elderly to maintain health or to regain health do receive emphatic treatment. Even though some techniques of physical assessment are included, to teach physical assessment is not the intent herein. Print resources and audiovisual materials are available to provide further direction in learning skills. The specific needs of the elderly during the assessment process, however, are included.

Throughout this book, the term *client,* rather than patient, is used to refer to the consumer of nursing services. *Patient* can connote one who waits without protest and who has no voice in the processes of health care received. The term *client* is more appropriate for one who is expected to participate actively in goal setting and health care decisions.

Nurse refers to a student preparing to become a registered nurse or to a graduate of a program leading to registered nurse licensure. *Nursing staff* refers to various levels of nursing personnel, including those (licensed practical/vocational nurses and nursing aides/assistants) who assist nurses in their work with the elderly.

The use of personal pronouns is not intended to imply sexual role discrimination. Throughout the book, "he" or "his" and "she" or "hers" are all used.

The popular long-term goal of gerontology is that people should remain physically and psychologically intact for as long as possible and then die without a long period of illness. The reality may well be the opposite; with increasing age, people may experience a protracted period of disability, with health and social services that keep them alive but keep them neither healthy nor happy. This is the specter that haunts nurses and other health professionals as they care for the elderly and makes them afraid of their own old age. The quality, not merely the quantity of life needs to be the overriding goal of nursing efforts involving the elderly lest our future as aged people be in jeopardy. Recognition of the needs and quality of life of the family members and/or other support people is included.

The authors of this book recognize the challenge confronting nurses who help to reshape society's beliefs about aging and the aged. Effective health promotion for elderly people is required for those who are old today and those of us who will be old tomorrow. Thus, the self-interest of each of us is appropriately directed toward improving the quality of life in old age.

Ann Gera Yurick
Susanne S. Robb
Barbara Elliott Spier
Nancy J. Ebert

Acknowledgments

The authors are grateful for the illustrations done by Harry Andrew Trumbore of Summit, New Jersey and New York City. He most generously gave of his time and talent to illustrate some of the concepts presented in this book.

We thank the staff at Appleton-Century-Crofts for the support and guidance they have provided throughout the preparation of this book. Marian Kalstein, Acquisitions Editor, and Kathleen Kelly, Production Editor, provided valuable assistance with this second edition. Karen Emilson Schroeder gave much support with the first edition.

The authors gratefully acknowledge the expertise of the nurse educators who reviewed the manuscript of this edition: Laurie Gunter, PhD, Pennsylvania State University; Kathy King, MS, University of Utah; Joyce Shoemaker, PhD, Temple University, and Leona Smolinski, PhD, Loyola University.

The nurse educators who offered valuable review assistance with the first edition were: Mary Adams, Janet Burge, Kathy Corso, Janet Gelein, Laurie Gunter, Mildred Hamner, Joyce Shoemaker, Ida Unsain, Thelma Wells, Gerry C. Whinnery, and Helen Wolff. Much gratitude is extended to these nurse educators and the nurse educators and students at the University of Pittsburgh whose suggestions have contributed to this book.

Contents

You Tell Me
I Am Getting Old

You tell me I am getting old
    I tell you that's not so:
The "house" I live in is worn out,
    and that, of course, I know.
It's been in use a long, long while;
    it's weathered many a gale;
I'm really not surprised you think
    it's getting somewhat frail.
The color changing on the roof,
    the windows getting dim . . .
My "house" is getting shaky,
    but my "house" isn't me.
My few short years can't make me old.
    I feel I'm in my youth . . .
You tell me I'm getting old?
    You just don't understand.
The dweller in my little "house"
    is young and bright and gay;
Just starting on a life
    to last throughout eternal day.
You only see the outside,
    which is all that most folks see.
You tell me I'm getting old?
    You've mixed my "house" with me!

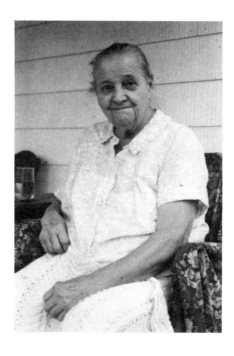

Source: Jednota Annual Furdek, 1978

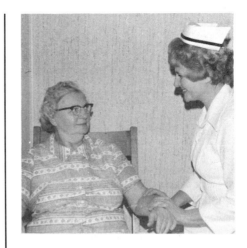

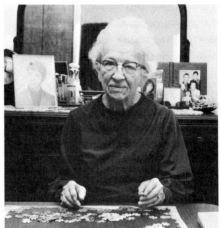

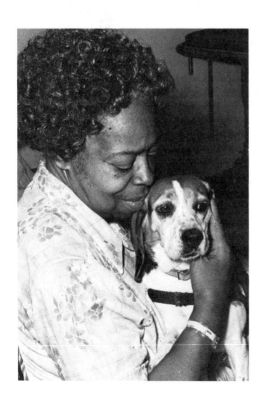

Part 1

The Aging Process and the Aged Person

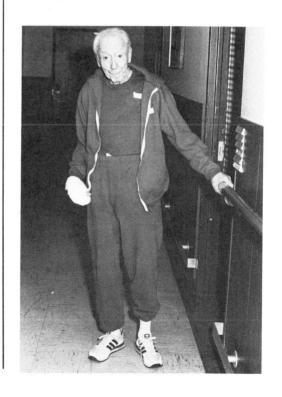

1

The Nursing Process and the Aged Person

Ann Gera Yurick

Reading this chapter will enable the individual to:

1. Know the steps of the nursing process
2. Relate the nursing process to the needs of elderly people
3. Recognize the individuality of minority and ethnic groups of elderly people
4. Recognize the special needs of elderly women
5. Recognize the importance of the nursing diagnosis in planning care with elderly people
6. Relate the work of the nurse to the multidisciplinary team effort to meet the needs of elderly people

Nurses have a major role in meeting the health needs of the rapidly increasing proportion of aged people throughout the world. Their focus in working with the elderly is to promote health. The nurse promotes quality of life for the elderly through health promotion and health protection. These goals have been identified as national health priorities (Benson and McDevitt, 1982). International health recommendations also have been made. The first worldwide conference on aging was organized and conducted by the United Nations in Vienna, Austria in 1982. Recommendations from this conference called for the prevention of illness and the promotion of wellness, the provision of primary care, the elevation of the quality of institutional care, the expansion and integration of services provided in the homes of families, the raising of nutrition levels, and the control of drugs, toxic substances, and environmental hazards (Tibbitts, 1983). The nurse is a vital practitioner in national as well as international health for elderly people.

The nurse can help the elderly person to understand the aging process and to distinguish the effects of aging from those of disease. A person is not ill simply because he or she is old, but because of illness. Major functional decline, especially if sudden, can usually be attributed to pathology rather than to aging. Illness can result from a lack of care directed toward prevention earlier in the person's lifespan (Pender, 1982). Severe physical and mental decline should not be accepted as being inevitable with age. The nurse can show people how to live so that health, vigor, and attractiveness persist into old age. Health practices to consider include maintenance of social support systems, control of the environment, exercise and physical fitness, nutrition and weight control, and stress management (Pender, 1982). The nurse must emphasize the fact that illness is more likely to occur in the elderly person who neglects the principles of healthful living. When illness does occur, the nurse helps the aged person through the recovery process involving the restoration and preservation of maximum functioning for that individual. If recovery is not a realistic goal, the nurse aids in the person's adjustment to health losses. Ultimately, the nurse may guide the elderly person through the dying process, the final stage of living. As a nurse works with the client, he or she uses the nursing process—a sequence of steps based upon a decision-making process. This process provides the organizing framework for this book.

This chapter examines the nursing process as it relates to health needs of aged persons. Important terms frequently used in connection with the process are defined. The nursing process is described with particular reference to how each step applies to the aged client. Finally, issues and differences inherent in nursing of the elderly person are explored.

The steps of the nursing process seldom take place in a clearly defined sequence. For example, intervention may be necessary before assessment is completed. The nurse may need to deal with an apparent health crisis before a comprehensive data base has been established. Such premature implementation often leads to evaluation without client-developed goals or outcome criteria. Evaluation, in turn, may show that further assessment is needed. Overlap in these steps is inevitable when a thinking nurse is working with a dynamic client.

DEFINITION OF TERMS

The *nursing process* emphasizes the use of decision-making with clients. It provides the nurse with a systematic approach to assist with the health goals of the elderly. This can include directing an elderly person's strengths toward health-generating behaviors. A series of decisions accompany the nursing process. First, the assets as well as the health needs of the aged client must be assessed. Next, the nurse plans and intervenes to assist with meeting these needs and promoting a feeling of well-being. Finally, the effectiveness of the care provided is evaluated. The client's behavioral outcomes are part of this evaluation. The goal of these steps is to enable the client to achieve a level of health consistent with the changes imposed by the aging process.

Gerontology is the study of the aging process in humans and animals. It is often subdivided into its biologic, sociologic, and psychologic aspects. *Geriatrics* is the term for the medical treatment of age-associated disease. *Nursing gerontology* refers to the scientific study

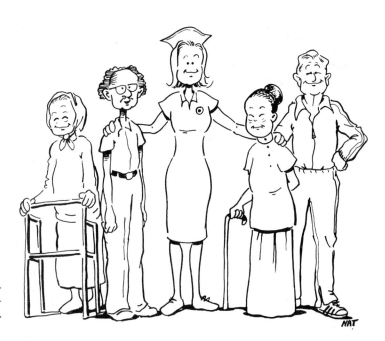

Figure 1.1. At its best, gerontologic nursing is a positive experience for everyone involved. (*Drawing by Harry Trumbore.*)

of the nursing care of the elderly. Nursing of the elderly is called *gerontologic* or *gerontic* nursing. The nurse who works with the elderly combines basic nursing knowledge and skills with specialized knowledge of aging.

The nursing process involves the steps of assessing, planning, intervening, and evaluating. Assessment is the process of collecting and analyzing data. These data are obtained by interviewing, observing, and examining the client. Data can also be obtained from other care-providers, family members, and/or significant others. In this case, "significant others" refers to people important to the elderly person, including relatives and nonrelatives. However, in this book the term is also used to include animals (pets) and plants that are valued by the client. The nursing assessment is an integral part of the client data base. When data from the assessment are summarized and arranged in an orderly way, the nurse has a base from which to arrive at nursing diagnoses.

The nursing history, obtained through a systematic interview of the client, provides further assessment data. Information about the client's past and present health is assembled. Gathering data for the nursing history is one way of using the nursing interview. This interview is goal-directed communication between the nurse and the client. In some cases, it involves other persons significant to the client. The nursing interview can even be a form of intervention when it is used in a therapeutic way.

Nursing planning is the process by which analysis of the data gathered is used to establish client-centered goals. A major part of this process is determining nursing diagnoses. Priorities are established in this planning process, which is directed toward promoting, protecting, and restoring the client's health, and may also include support while the person is dying. Nursing directives or nursing orders are derived from the planning process. These are actions the nurse performs to help the client meet goals. Health promotion is a major part of this nursing planning. Pender (1982) defines *health promotion* as activities directed toward

sustaining or increasing the level of well-being, self-actualization, and personal fulfillment of a given individual or group. The current health status of the client is maintained or there is movement toward a more desirable state of health. Pender (1982) defines *health protection* or *prevention* as the removal or avoidance of encumbrances to growth, maturation, fulfillment, and self-actualization throughout the life cycle. Among these encumbrances are personal illness, disturbances in interpersonal relationships, or social disruption. The emphasis is on guarding or defending the body from injury. Both health protection and health promotion are vital to the work of the nurse with elderly clients.

Nursing intervention or implementation is the action phase of the nursing process, in which the nurse carries out a plan of care with and on behalf of the client. To the greatest degree possible, the client and the client's significant others are encouraged to take active part in this intervention.

Evaluation is a review of client behavior change in response to nursing interventions. The degree to which the client maintains health-promoting behaviors previously established as criteria is a part of this evaluation. The responsibility assumed by the elderly person for personal wellness is part of this evaluation. Evaluation of outcomes is an important way to assure quality nursing care. Evaluation also contributes an overview of process effectiveness. On the basis of the evaluation, the nurse can act to correct deficiencies in care by gathering additional data or by changing plans and interventions. These changes are directed toward a more favorable outcome in the client's behavior. Each area of the nursing process is discussed in greater detail throughout this chapter. Application of this process to the aged person is presented in Chapters 8 through 17.

APPLYING THE PROCESS TO THE AGED PERSON

Nursing with the aged person is carried out in many kinds of settings, including the home, the institution, and the community. The milieu in which the nurse and other health professionals work with the elderly is changing and becoming more varied as new alternatives in living and leisure environments continue to become available to the elderly. Examples include day centers, specially planned high-rise apartment buildings, and senior centers. Many new kinds of workers are dealing with the elderly, directly influencing their knowledge, feelings, behaviors, and state of health. The nurse is a vital member of a professional team that works to promote health in the aged. The nurse has a direct impact on expanding home health service. This service helps to keep many elderly at home, preventing the need for institutionalization. An important role of the nurse is to help elderly persons to maintain their desired life-style. This even may be in opposition to the wishes of other health care providers who may encourage institutionalization of an elderly person especially when the person becomes more frail. The nurse needs to provide information to the elderly relating to alternatives as she promotes client decision-making. As the nurse contributes to the work of the health team, she promotes decision-making through the nursing process.

Significant Others

It is extremely important for the nurse to include the client's significant others in each phase of the nursing process. Some aged clients may no longer have any significant others living. In other cases, the significant other may not be easily identifiable or readily available. But the aged person is still a dynamic individual, with the capacity to form meaningful relationships with people and pets. The extended family may no longer be a major support system, and in its absence the elderly person may feel an intense need to be loved (Maslow, 1970). To be among people who care, and to have the chance to give love to another person or to a pet, can help meet this basic human need.

When the aged person does have family attachments, the nurse can help both client and family to maintain a positive family relationship. If life changes occur that call for assistance which family members cannot pro-

vide, the nurse must help relieve them of emotional obstacles, such as guilt, so that they feel free to ask for necessary aid. The degree to which families function as a support system for the elderly depends on patterns of family structure, interaction, norms, and expectations. These patterns vary according to ethnicity, socioeconomic status, sex, and age of the older person (Bengston, 1976).

The family is not always a viable alternative support system in meeting service needs of the aged member—housing, transportation, and health care. The nurse can support the family's efforts to further the aged person's own attempts to adjust when life changes do occur. Age-associated changes must be considered in each phase of the nursing process.

Individuality of the Aged Person

Old age is not necessarily a process of decline, and aging by itself does not mean illness, even though physical changes do occur. These physical changes can affect the psychosocial behavior of the elderly person, just as a psychosocial change, such as a change in living environment, can affect physical dimensions. Even though such changes can occur, to assume that they decrease the quality of life may decrease the effectiveness of nursing care. Through the nursing process, the nurse tries to preserve the client's individuality while assessing his or her health needs. This includes calling the client by the name he or she prefers. Seemingly endearing terms, such as "Granny" or "Grandpa," are inappropriate. They tend to place the aged person on a different level from the nurse, and may even imply that the client is senile. The inappropriate name also may relay a hidden message denigrating the value of the aged person's input within each phase of the nursing process. To take an example, consider the resentment expressed by an elderly resident of a nursing home. She pointed to a nurse, saying that she did not like this nurse because she called her "Emma" instead of using her last name. She continued by saying, "I am at least fifty years older than that nurse so I deserve to be called Mrs. R." Norms seem to be changing with regard to the name by which the health professional refers to the client.

However, it is still important to ask the client the preferred name. Mrs. R's objections to being called by her first name interfered with the relationship the nurse was trying to establish with her. Whatever her intentions, the nurse behaved in a manner that this client perceived as being disrespectful. All phases of the nursing process can be adversely affected by such a situation.

Little and Carnevali (1976) describe the nursing process as one that helps clients and their families to cope more effectively with demands of daily living and their desired lifestyle, in the face of actual or potential challenges to their health. In helping the elderly to meet their needs of daily living, the nurse should assess how the aged person views himself, and how he copes with life in a variety of settings. The wealth of the client's living experience, including values and sociocultural patterns, provides a broad base upon which the nurse can plan individualized care. Every elderly person faces certain changes of aging with which he or she must deal. The manner in which people cope with these changes can be different. Factors affecting the way in which an elderly person copes with change include the person's sex, socioeconomic background, family relationships, living situation, physical condition, and ethnicity (Gelfand, 1982). It is important to understand the significance of sociocultural patterns to the elderly person, particularly to those of minority and ethnic groups. Researchers are faced with defining the differences among ethnic groups and the degree to which these differences will continue to exist among future generations.

Minority and Ethnic Groups

Ethnic and minority group experiences have an impact on the elderly that must be considered by the nurse. While she learns to understand their needs, she must avoid making generalizations about elderly members of such groups. Although there is a need to be sensitive to the cultural beliefs and practices of ethnic groups, it is important to avoid overgeneralizations—simply being a member of a minority does not guarantee a particular belief or practice. Ethnic background should be used only as a *cue* to the nurse.

The immigration era provoked a degree of ethnic rivalry that still prevails among many of today's elderly people, many of whom were part of the immigration era. The white elderly who are in their eighties and nineties could have been part of the massive European migration to this country. When people age in a foreign culture, they either remain oriented to their original culture or else discard it entirely. Even when their orientation to the original culture is retained, they acquire some characteristics of the host culture (Pierce, 1978–79). The nurse must determine which characteristics of the original culture the elderly person wishes to retain. For example, the wish to observe dietary and religious customs may be more prominent. Nursing goals and interventions should take these values and beliefs into consideration. The way a person adapts to a new host culture is not determined solely by age and generation. Individual preferences must be considered even though shared culture, symbols, and rituals remain important to the individual. The problems encountered by the elderly are substantially similar, regardless of their ethnic backgrounds. However, the ability to retain ethnic group identification may provide support and comfort to the elderly person.

Members of some ethnic and racial groups may arrive at old age disadvantaged in terms of income, education, and access to health care. Social stratification reflects inequality in the distribution of power, privileges, and prestige. Many aged members of ethnic and minority groups have lived within a social context in which they experienced continual reminders of inequality (Bengston, 1976). Many members of ethnic and minority groups have been treated with disrespect. They may continue to be treated this way by some members of the health team. This may make some elderly persons reluctant to take part in the planning phase of the nursing process. Such a person may have had no experience in sharing in decision-making. The black and native American elderly, in particular, often have had little power, and generally have been told what to do. For them, it may be a new experience to express their needs and

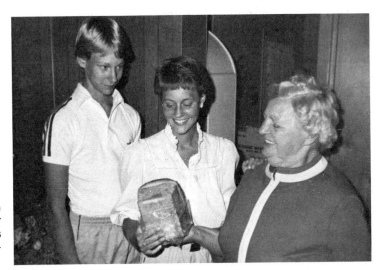

Figure 1.2. This elderly woman shares a loaf of bread with her grandchildren. The recipe was brought from Europe with her immigrant mother.

to help in the planning of programs (Newsome, 1977).

To provide adequate health care, there is a need for the nurse to have knowledge of and sensitivity to the values, myths, and life-styles of the black aged. Blacks comprise the fastest growing group of ethnic older persons (Gelfand, 1982). Carter (1982) asserts that age compounds the handicaps accrued to blacks from birth. Some aged black persons continue to have ambivalent feelings about being called "black" because of historic negative stereotypes. Carter (1982) reports that some elderly black persons continue to prefer "Negro" or "colored" for racial descriptions. A lifetime of inadequate and unequal medical care, housing, and jobs can result in feelings of lowered self-esteem in the elderly black person. The need to consider the degree of self-esteem of the elderly person has implications for the nurse and the client in all steps of the nursing process. There is a strong orientation toward religion and the church among the black elderly. They also tend to rely on strong family bonds. Ortega, Crutchfield, and Rushing (1983) reported that even though racial minorities suffer double jeopardy in terms of objective conditions such as income or housing, they tend to be at least as well off as older whites in terms of subjective well-being. Fre-

quency of contact with church-related friends was found to be the critical factor in accounting for race differences in well-being. For the elderly racial minority person, the church can serve as a pseudo-extended family.

In applying the nursing process, the nurse should be aware that some of the elderly—black persons, ethnic minorities who have immigrated to the United States from Europe, Spanish-speaking persons, Orientals, native Americans (Indians), and some white people—may not be able to read or write. They may say "my eyesight is poor" or that "I do not feel like doing that (reading or writing) today." They may give a variety of excuses for not reading or writing. Written messages or instructions from the nurse and health team may be misunderstood or neglected, and often must be supplemented with spoken instructions. Since some of these clients may not speak English, interpretation of verbal messages may present problems. Others may speak English but have trouble understanding it because of differences in intonation patterns, pronunciation, and sentence structure. The nurse should become familiar with the idioms and colloquial expressions used by the elderly with whom he or she works. An elderly person who does not understand the verbal or written message may nod in agreement to avoid further embarrassment. In other cases, the person may withdraw and avoid interaction with the health system.

Such avoidance of the health system also may be related to poverty levels. Home remedies and folk medicine may be an important therapy for some people. Examples include the use of herbs or the application of alcohol and copper to painful joints. An elderly person who is not familiar with agency services, rules, and regulations may go instead to family and friends for health-care advice. The Spanish-speaking elderly, for instance, tend to consult others outside the health-care system. Often they seek professional assistance only in crisis situations. This is also true of many elderly native Americans. There is a continuing lack of trust by elderly native Americans of any non-Indian who offers assistance (Newsome, 1977). The nurse working with these groups should aim for the goal of preventive health care.

Kinship ties are often more significant in minority settings with regard to the adjustment and morale of the aged. Elderly members of black families may be accustomed to group cohesiveness within an extended family living in the same household (Newsome, 1977). Among the Chinese, elderly persons are supported by kinship groups in which filial piety is an important virtue (Newsome, 1977). This concept requires the individual to respect, love and obey, support and care for his parents when they are in need. Filial piety, however, is becoming less important among younger Chinese. Continued examination of ethnicity and aging can focus on the basic elements that bind families together and the types of assistance and relationships between generations that are important in maintaining family units (Gelfand, 1982). Other questions to be answered include how members of various ethnic groups approach growing older, how they meet the changes associated with old age, what factors produce satisfaction in old age, and how the prospect of eventual death is viewed (Gelfand, 1982).

In applying the nursing process to the elderly, the nurse should take into consideration ethnic and minority differences, while remem-

bering that these alone cannot provide a full understanding of the client's health status. Variations occur in the aging process, across ethnic boundaries and within ethnic categories. Awareness of ethnic group experiences should not blind the nurse to the uniqueness of the individual client.

Elderly Women

The uniqueness of the needs of the elderly woman has gained increasing recognition through the Women's Movement. Ageism and sexism have affected the lives of many elderly women. The 1981 White House Conference on Aging included a committee called "Concerns of Older Women: Growing Numbers, Special Needs." A primary function of this group was to promote awareness of issues of older women.

The need to consider the unique needs of women is supported by the realization that women in the 65 and older age group are the fastest growing segment of the population. Three-fourths of all nursing home residents are women (Fackos, 1981). Although older women outnumber men, a major part of the present-day knowledge of the aging process is about the aging of men (Dunn and Linden, 1980). Because the experiences of infancy, childhood, adolescence, adulthood, and maturity are different for women and men, there is a need to consider the uniqueness of the present day circumstance in which women become old. As the nurse works with older women, assessment of the adequacy of finances for basic health needs is vital. The poverty rate for women is about 65 percent higher than it is for older men (Fackos, 1981). Older women have been described as the fastest growing poverty group in America.

Being old and a woman is a double disadvantage. Block, Davidson, and Grumbs (1981) report that elderly women are often considered inactive, unhealthy, asexual, and ineffective. The image of the elderly woman is likely to be portrayed as a kind of granny who spends time knitting in her rocking chair. However, older women are increasingly making their presence felt. In 1980, following the White House Mini-Conference on Aging, an advocacy group for midlife and older women was formed. This group, the Older Women's League (OWL), is working to change national policy and the image of older women. Members of the OWL staff are lobbying for Social Security, pension, and health-care reform. Even though the improvement for older women is dependent on general improvement of conditions for the elderly, a more significant consideration is the betterment of the place of women in society.

Attitudes of the Nurse Toward the Aged Person

Before nurses begin to work with aged clients, they should assess their own attitudes toward aging and the way in which these attitudes reflect the attitudes of society toward the aged person. A nurse who responds negatively to the elderly person—who may be seen as "bossy," "complaining," "gossipy," "helpless," or "a dirty old man"—should evaluate his or her own behavior to determine its role in eliciting or encouraging these responses. An elderly woman was seen standing in line at a store checkout counter. While she waited, she complained about the inefficiency of the store management and the employees. As she neared the counter, she said, "I know my complaining didn't make this line move faster, but it made me feel better to be able to complain." Complaining, therefore, gave this woman a sense of power.

Nurses should assess their personal and professional experiences with aged persons and their reactions to these experiences, including both satisfactions and frustrations. A nurse's personal experiences with aged family members, for example, may affect the attitudes she conveys to her aged clients. One nurse expressed an aversion to caring for the elderly based on memories of unpleasant days when her grandmother lived with her family. She saw this as a disruptive influence in her enjoyment of family life. However, this nurse did not perceive her 67-year-old mother as elderly.

The nurse's attitude toward personal aging may also affect the feeling she conveys to the aged client. If she is having difficulty accepting a new facial wrinkle or more gray hairs, her attitude toward the extensively wrinkled

skin of her elderly client may be altered. A nurse who sees only deficits in aging will find it difficult to recognize the resources of the elderly that enable them to maintain control over their own lives. In fact, her goal may be to fulfill an inner need to minister to the aged person, rather than to recognize the client's inner resources. Determining these resources is a significant aspect of the nursing assessment.

ASSESSMENT BASE

The nurse needs an assessment base that relates to aging and the inherent changes that can accompany it. These changes do not necessarily imply loss. The aging process can be viewed as a process of growth, even though losses do occur. The assessment base provided in Chapter 3 relates theories of aging to the biologic, psychologic, and sociologic changes that accompany it, and the interactions among these changes. For example, an understanding of biologic theories is necessary to determine the sensory changes that are discussed in the assessment base in Chapters 10–12.

To anticipate potential sensory changes, the nurse should plan to collect assessment data in such a way that these changes will not inhibit the data-gathering process. For example, since the elderly client tends to be sensitive to light glare, the nurse should conduct the interview in a glare-free area. Since glare can inhibit visual function, the elderly person who has a hearing loss may not be able to depend on the visual cues that help him interpret the auditory message. Hearing is thus affected because the elderly person cannot adequately see the nurse's face during the interview.

Problems of visual function can alter the accuracy of assessment data collected. For example, an elderly person may be asked to interpret written messages during the cognitive assessment. If poor vision interferes with accurate interpretation of the written message, this can lead to an inaccurate assessment of the client's cognitive function. The nurse need not perform a complete visual assessment of the elderly person before making adjustments for potential visual changes.

Hearing is still another consideration. The nurse should not raise her voice automatically when assessing an elderly person. This can actually alter the client's ability to hear. Hearing impairment in the elderly tends to begin with high-frequency tone loss. Speaking loudly may cause the pitch of the voice to be raised, thus making words with high frequency sounds even more difficult to hear. Awareness of these potential hearing changes tells the nurse how the voice should be modulated and that she should face the client while communicating. The elderly person's ability to hear during the assessment process can affect his response, and thus affect the accuracy of the data collected. Inaccurate assessment data, in turn, can alter goals and the plan of care.

ASSESSMENT

An assessment of the client is the initial step in the nursing process. The data thus obtained enable the nurse to plan with the client and significant others, and to determine priorities of care. Objectives of this assessment include identification of the client's assets and of the areas in which assistance or support services are needed. Kane and Kane (1981, p. 1) state that any strategy for altering the health status of the elderly person requires a technology for first assessing that health status and then detecting increments of progress. An important consideration in assessment is determining the characteristics of the elderly person that are to be altered. In making recommendations for the client's care, it is important to strive for the greatest accuracy possible. Kane and Kane (1981, pp. 9–10) indicate that a measurement instrument should document the problems that are most amenable to intervention and that would suggest a specific strategy. The decision of what to measure should be practical. The nurse should use assessment data already available since multiple requests for the same information can be disturbing as well as fati-

guing for the elderly person. Preventing repetition in data collection also is cost-effective.

Specific needs must be considered in the assessment of an elderly person. Even though these needs vary with the individual, the potential changes that can accompany aging should be considered. A knowledge of these potential changes, which are discussed in detail in the following chapters, can help the nurse decide which factors to assess. Because the physical, mental, and social well-being of an elderly person are interrelated, multidimensional assessment is indicated.

In this book the assessment categories for the aged person include environment, life changes, cognitive tasks, sensory perception, nutrition, elimination, activity, body protection, and medication consumption. Specific assessment questions relating to these areas are included in the following chapters. The nurse may use any assessment format that is systematic and complete. Nursing decisions relating to what information to collect about the client can be provided by the accepted conceptual framework in the nursing setting. Information collection should be logically related to one's view of nursing. Examples include Roger's life process model, Roy's adaptation model, Grubb's behavioral systems model, Orem's self-care agency model, Yura and Walsh's human needs model, and Neuman's stress model (Gordon, 1982). These models can give purpose and direction to the information collected in the nursing assessment.

A variety of assessment tools has been developed for use with elderly clients. Many of these tools provide client data for the multidisciplinary health team concerned with the needs of the elderly. Kane and Kane (1981) have done a comprehensive review of the state-of-the-art in assessing the elderly. They present assistance with the proper selection of an assessment tool. Instruments that have been standardized can assist with documentation of communication among health-care providers. Assessment tools can help with global planning for the elderly or with planning for an individual elderly person. Needs can be more accurately matched with resources. There is a need to reassess how people change. Services that people receive also change.

Functional Assessment

One type of assessment is the functional assessment. The functional assessment is a systematic, objective technique used to determine the levels at which the person is performing in a given environment. The client at risk can be identified. The fragility of the people in the support system is a factor to consider in assessment. Besides determining individual nursing needs, assessment of functional status can aid staff in institutional settings to determine the client assignment to appropriate levels and types of care and the adequacy and composition of staff needed for care. The ratio of nursing personnel to clients should be determined by the functional ability of the client.

Lawton (1971) developed a functional assessment that includes (1) physical health, (2) quality of self-maintenance, (3) quality of role activity, (4) intellectual status, (5) emotional status, (6) social activity, and (7) attitudes toward the world and self. Other examples of multidimensional measures of functional assessment include the Older American Resource Survey (OARS) and the Stockton Geriatric Rating Scale. The OARS can be used to assess individual functional status in relation to (1) social resources, (2) economic resources, (3) mental health, (4) physical health, and (5) activities of daily living. Activities of daily living usually include eating, mobility, grooming, dressing, and going to the toilet. Another assessment tool, the Lifestyle and Health Habits Assessment (Pender, 1982), is intended to help the nurse assist the client in the review of personal life-style in relation to impact on health. The areas assessed include (1) competence in self-care, (2) nutritional practices, (3) physical or recreational activity, (4) sleep patterns, (5) stress management, (6) self-actualization, (7) sense of purpose, (8) relationship with others, (9) environmental control, and (10) use of the health-care system. Pender (1982) reports that a review of life-style and health habits assists the client in systematically evaluating the extent to which personal behavior is supportive

of health. An additional area to assess is the person's source of health information.

Some assessment tools have been developed for use in long-term care to serve as guides to determine appropriate levels of care. One example is RAPIDS, which can be used to make decisions about whether a client is in the appropriate setting. This tool also can be used in utilization review (Kennedy, 1981). Another assessment tool to assist in the process of making effective long-term care decisions is the Long-Term Care Information System (LTCIS) Assessment Process. This comprehensive tool includes patient classification for long-term care and assessment information to determine what services are needed by the client (Falcone, 1981). Assessment, placement, and program planning are seen as interdependent. There is an increased emphasis on assessment measures that can better predict what health services are needed and how the quality and efficiency of the care provided can be improved. Hickey (1980) relates the emphasis on accurate assessment to those representing Medicare and Medicaid programs. Detailed and accurate information is needed to assess the quality of services, ensure their proper utilization, and develop the appropriate regulations, safeguards, and reimbursement rates.

Assessment of the elderly needs to be multidimensional and should be sensitive to small changes over time. It is necessary to be thorough and consistent in assessment. Assessment in an environment familiar to the elderly person is advisable. It is important for the nurse to have input in the development of a multidimensional assessment tool that is used to determine the elderly person's need for nursing service.

Because the time available for an assessment is usually limited, priorities must be established. One way to do this is to set up a screening assessment, designed to cover the factors in each area that are most likely to reveal problems. For example, the nurse may note the client's ability to read the headlines of a newspaper, or his or her ability to ambulate. If the screening assessment uncovers a problem, the nurse is expected to perform an "in-depth" assessment to determine the nature of the problem. This type of assessment can be time-consuming and tiring for both nurse and client, but the nurse can adjust the pace by returning on successive days, or by dividing the assessment into several segments over a 24-hour period. When an assessment must be paced, life-threatening details should be considered first. Next, the nurse should cover the areas most important to the client. Finally, the areas of greatest concern to the nurse should be considered. Throughout the process, the client should be told why the information is being sought, and how he may expect to benefit.

The quality of the assessment is important since key decisions are based on these data. A standardized assessment tool should help to insure validity of assessment. Careful assessment can enhance congruity between the needs of the elderly person and the amount and kind of care needed to achieve the desired outcomes for the elderly person. The process of assessment should make a difference for the client. Although a formal assessment tool that has been standardized is not included in this book, an assessment outline in each of the nursing process chapters includes key considerations in assessing the elderly person. An assessment guide is included in Appendix C.

Nursing History

The nursing history provides information on the health status of the elderly person and should reveal the client's ability to adapt to life stressors. Changes mean alterations in the aged person's capacity to adapt and compensate, and determination of this capacity is a part of the nursing assessment. Negative psychologic reactions to life changes often affect the way a client participates in the assessment and planning process. To encourage such participation, the nurse can have an elderly person relate meaningful life events, feelings about these events, and feelings about anticipation of such things as the birth of a grandchild or a long-awaited trip. The nurse does need to recognize that some elderly persons do not readily communicate verbally. More time may be needed to develop a relationship with these

people before a complete history can be obtained. There may be reluctance to divulge personal information. The elderly person may have difficulty understanding the reasons for collecting personal data. The relevance of these data to health promotion should be explained by the nurse.

The client also may tell about fears associated with the aging process—fear of loneliness or becoming unwanted, fear of becoming a burden on others, or fear of death. The elderly person may also describe feelings about the physical changes which accompany aging. Also significant is the way elderly persons view themselves, either as growing persons or as regressing persons. They may see the passing of years as losses or gains. They can tell of angry and happy feelings about people, places, or things. The way a client has responded to past crisis situations may alert the nurse to possible assistance that may be needed in the future. The aged person can tell about adjustments to daily living, how needs are met, or how much assistance he or she feels is necessary. Often clients' perceptions of their needs differ from the perceptions of the nurse in areas such as hygiene or eating patterns. Even though the elderly may become less independent, they should be seen as people who still have input on events affecting their lives, rather than helpless victims. A person who is made to feel significant and who has an opportunity to express feelings can experience a sense of power (Roberts, 1978). Thus, aged persons need to feel that they control the basic decisions affecting their lives, rather than having imposed upon them the values and decisions of others. Given the opportunity to make such decisions, they also need to know that their decisions will be recognized by others in the environment. The judgment that life is meaningful can be made only by the individual.

The opportunity for input can be rewarding to a client when the nurse recognizes the value of this input. The nurse should be aware that the client's input can provide important information about values and attitudes toward health. She should investigate the client's level of understanding optimal health care practices, including such things as diet, exercise, and rest. She should explore the client's knowledge of agencies concerned with health promotion, as well as curative and restorative services, and should assess the client's ability to use these services.

In obtaining these data through systematic history-taking, the nurse must consider any physical losses with which the aged client may be coping. These losses are often accompanied by dependency on supportive devices such as dentures, hearing aids, canes, walkers, wheelchairs, and braces. The elderly person's reaction to this dependency should be assessed, as well as his or her ability to use supportive devices efficiently. Changes in physical appearance also may be viewed as losses by the aged person. These changes can include slower movements and reaction times, postural changes, decreased strength and energy levels, gray hair or loss of hair, and wrinkling of the skin. It is important to assess the client's methods of adaptation and compensation to these changes.

When an elderly person's loss or change limits the amount of data the nurse can collect, secondary source input from significant others can add to the data available. Sometimes, the aged client is an "unreliable historian." Some old people, for a variety of reasons, are unable to recall information accurately, or in the detail required for assessment purposes. Too often, however, it is assumed automatically that old people are not as reliable as the written health care record previously compiled, a significant other, or the health professional's prior knowledge of old people.

The nurse should remember that the client (what he says and what he does) is the *only* primary, first-hand source of data. Other sources are secondary. Accepting a laboratory value from a medical record is one thing; accepting a verdict of confusion is quite another.

When an elderly client responds to a question in a way that seems inadequate or inappropriate, the nurse should consider what the client actually heard or saw. Sensory impairment is fairly commonplace among the elderly. The client's use of mind-altering drugs (seda-

tives, tranquilizers, analgesics) should be considered, and the individual's motivation to answer in a reliable manner should be evaluated. In short, the client who responds inappropriately to assessment questions requires more, not less, direct scrutiny by the nurse. The nurse should ask short and concise questions while ensuring that only one question is asked at a time. It is important to rephrase questions that are not understood.

The nurse is likely to encounter elderly clients who are unable to communicate. This problem places extra responsibility on the nurse to make use of other sources of data. Family members or significant others can add to the assessment even when the client can participate fully in providing data. When the nurse obtains assessment data from a family member in the presence of the elderly person, it is important to include the elderly person in the conversation as much as possible rather than talking about the person as if he or she were not present. The interpersonal relationships experienced by the client are often revealed by the input of significant others. Therefore, these data provide clues not only to the client's perceptions of himself, but to the way he is perceived by significant others. Other secondary sources include the health-care providers with whom the client has contact. This will vary with the client and his or her environment.

The elderly client may tend to get "off the subject" during any nurse–client discussion. This is often encountered during the health history. A tendency to engage in "life review" or reminiscence is common among old people and important to their psychosocial well-being. The nurse must balance the client's need to discuss "irrelevant" topics with her own need to collect "relevant" information. The nurse should be cautious in directing or focusing interview content, since much information divulged while discussing past events may be relevant to present nursing care. For example, discussion of past relationships with families and friends can identify support systems that continue to be maintained or that have been lost to the elderly person. On the other hand, the nurse who permits too much digression risks running out of time needed to acquire essential information.

The elderly client may be impatient with the many questions inherent in a nursing history. His impatience is often related to the scope of the assessment. Obviously, more questions must be asked to review 79 years than 42 and to cover actual or potential problem areas for an individual who is likely to experience multiple, interrelated health problems. Contributing to this impatience may be the client's disbelief in his or her own potential for being "helped." The myth that asserts that the elderly just get sick, sicker, and die is very pervasive. Still another reason for impatience may be the client's traditional orientation to the role of the nurse. Questions may be expected from a "male physician" but not from a "nurse."

Fear of health impairment or a feeling of malaise may also contribute to a wish to end the questioning and get on with the treatment. Possible guilt relating to noncompliance with prescribed therapy, such as medications, may inhibit the client's responses to the assessment interview. In the assessment, it is important to know what drugs have been taken as well as what drugs have been prescribed and not taken. In eliciting the latter information, the nurse needs to avoid a reprimanding attitude if adequate data are to be obtained regarding the elderly person's reasons for noncompliance with prescribed treatment.

To complete the nursing history, the nurse should include the client's habitual patterns of functioning, methods of communicating, thoughts and feelings, likes and dislikes, adaptation to the aging process as these affect his views of himself, relationships as a family member or significant other, use of time, sociocultural patterns of daily living, spiritual beliefs and values, ethnic beliefs and values, health beliefs and habits, and the elderly person's views of living and expectations of life. Feelings about one's anticipated death can be assessed also. This information can help to determine the course of action to follow if a crisis should arise. A dilemma that faces the gerontologic nurse is the degree of aggressive treatment to encourage versus allowing the elderly person to die (Olson, 1981).

Physical Assessment

Physical assessment of the elderly person adds valuable information to the client's data base. These objective data will help to provide information relating to the degree of congruence in the physical assessment data and the client's perception of health as obtained in the subjective health history. This examination should be done in a systematic way. Data are collected about the appearance and physical functioning of the aged person. The extensiveness of the nursing physical assessment depends upon the skill and preparation of the nurse. The nurse uses observation, listening, touch, and smell in gathering these data about physiologic functioning. Observation and listening provide data in such areas as general appearance, behavior, motor activity, and body language. Touch gives clues to skin temperature, perspiration, skin dryness, and muscle tension or relaxation. Much information can be gained by palpation. The use of palpation is dependent upon the skill of the nurse, but checking the pulse and examining the breast are types of palpation considered to be basic nursing skills. The nurse also utilizes physical assessment data obtained by the physician. Specific physical assessment techniques that can be used by the nurse are included in the assessment areas of the chapters concerning application of the nursing process. More complete physical assessment skills are demonstrated and discussed in books devoted entirely to this subject.

During the physical assessment of the elderly person, the nurse must use the knowledge base concerning potential physical changes of aging. For example, "normal" changes in the integument of the elderly include the graying and thinning of hair. The expected physical changes of aging are presented throughout the following chapters in the "assessment base" sections.

Cognitive Assessment

The nurse should be aware of the cognitive functioning of the elderly person. The nurse may utilize assessment data obtained by the psychologist, but tests which measure cognitive functioning must be analyzed with caution. With any test, it is vital to consider the norms established for the elderly population. The elderly person should not be evaluated according to norms established for a much younger population that has gone through the test-acculturation process. The results of the cognitive assessment can also be affected by physical changes. One example is the relationship between vision and mental functioning that was discovered in a study done at the Ebenezer Society (Snyder, Pyrek, and Smith, 1976). In collecting and using cognitive assessment data, the nurse must take care to avoid labeling the client as "confused" or "depressed." The assessment must be interrelated to determine reasons for behavior that the nurse considers inappropriate. If an elderly person is labeled as confused or depressed, the nurse may see no value in the assessment or planning process. Without assessment and planning, however, nursing actions only reinforce the depressed or confused state. The elderly client is then seen as a nonperson, or as a member of a group of nonpersons in an extended-care setting. The cognitive assessment is considered in greater detail in Chapter 8.

Environmental Assessment

Each elderly person must be considered in relation to his environment. The nurse has a major role in helping the elderly to live in the preferred environment as long as possible. When possible, the assessment data should include actual observation of the client's living environment. Environmental data gathered by the home health nurse should be conveyed to nurses in any other setting in which the elderly person may spend time. For example, the nurse who cares for an elderly person who is hospitalized needs to know about the person's environment when doing health teaching. The home health nurse can provide valuable data. Too often, communication goes from the nurse in the hospital setting to the home health nurse about orders for the client at home. However, the nurse in the hospital or nursing home needs to have information from the home health nurse about the client's living environment.

The environment of the elderly can affect their cognitive as well as their physical functioning. A review of research by Hiatt (1982) reveals the significance of environments to mental functioning of the elderly person. Environments that do not stimulate the senses or meet the mobility needs of older people may suppress competent behavior. Some impair-

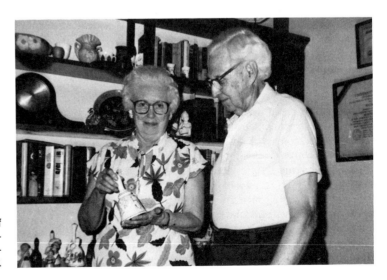

Figure 1.3. The significance of personal articles in the environment is demonstrated as this couple share a fiftieth anniversary gift.

ments of the elderly may relate to the living environment. The environment of the elderly can affect their cognitive as well as their physical functioning. This environment must be assessed in order to develop a realistic plan of care. Such a plan for an aged person in an extended-care setting will differ from a plan for an aged person in his home setting. The plan of care for an aged person living alone at home will also differ from a plan for an aged person who lives at home with family members or significant others. In assessing the living environment, the nurse should note the particular objects that are familiar to the client and that support his feelings of well-being. Such personal items may include family pictures, familiar furniture, handcrafted articles made by or for the client, gifts to the client, and religious articles.

The nurse must evaluate the way change in the living environment affects the aged person's personal boundaries. Perhaps the client has moved from a large house to a room that is shared with other elderly persons in a dependent-care setting. The nurse should assess the degree of territorial adjustment that the client has made to the new environment. Elderly people often tend to collect many small items, such as pictures and cards. The assessment must therefore include the client's feelings about such meaningful articles. If the nurse's value system does not include clutter in the environment, a conflict with the client may occur. The nurse should determine how free the aged person feels to decide what objects will be part of this environment. Personal objects tend to be especially scarce in the institutional setting. This may contribute to a loss of identity and more limited territorial boundaries. As a result of these losses depersonalization can occur. Part of the assessment should include a determination of the individual's response to intrusion of his territory by the staff and by other residents.

For the elderly person living in the home setting, the home should be assessed. This assessment also is important for the elderly person who plans to return home following a stay in an institutional setting. It is necessary to determine what barriers and facilitators for rehabilitation exist in the home. The design of the house, apartment, or room as well as the care of the living area should be considered. Assessment of the design of the living area should include the toilet and bathing facilities, the number and condition of stairs, water supply, cooking facilities, heating, lighting, and ventilation. Any environmental accident hazards should be noted, such as loose throw rugs or slippery floors in any part of the home. The size of the toilet facilities and the doorway leading to the toilet is of special importance for the elderly person who uses a wheelchair or a mobility aid such as a walker. In further assessing the bathroom, the bathtub and shower area should be examined for the availability of grips, rails, seats, and a nonslip surface. If the elderly person is in a communal living environment, the assessment should include the distance to the bathroom, the degree of privacy provided, as well as the number of persons using the toilet facilities. The support provided for the elderly person in the home setting should be assessed. This assessment should include the relationship between the elderly person and his relatives and friends as well as their willingness to help when this is needed. This relationship is especially significant if the elderly person is living in a relative's home. Included with this assessment is determining who does the cooking, shopping, and cleaning. It is necessary for the nurse to realize that an elderly person who is happy in his own home, even if unclean and untidy, may be better off than the same person who is clean and regimented but miserable (Caird and Judge, 1979).

The community to which the client belongs must also be assessed. This includes evaluation of community attitudes toward the elderly, as indicated by health maintenance, safety, and support services available. The nurse must determine what sort of community assistance is available to help the elderly cope with deficits and losses caused by aging and with crisis situations. Assessment of the adequacy of community services such as proximity to shopping, banking, pharmacy, post office, and the Social Security office (Rauckhorst,

Stokes, and Mezey, 1980). Accessibility to these services can promote the independence of the elderly person, especially if the person does not drive an automobile. For the elderly person who is able to walk to obtain these services, the availability of sidewalks, the condition of sidewalks, and safety provisions such as lights at crossings and the slope of the land terrain are important environmental considerations.

The availability, location, and condition of senior-citizen centers should be assessed. The community senior-citizen center that is located in an old building can be a barrier to the elderly. One example of this was observed in a senior center that was formerly a large two-story school building. The congregate meal was served on the first floor, where many of the major activities took place. The only bathrooms in the building, however, were on the second floor, requiring the elderly to maneuver steep, dimly lit stairs to reach them. Another senior-citizen meal center was in the musty, dark basement of a vacated store.

The nurse should use the sense of smell in the environmental assessment. Odors often provide clues about the environment and the way the client makes use of it. The nurse should investigate further to determine the source and causes of any odors. For example, the odor of decaying food may indicate that the aged person is hoarding food in his or her room in a dependent-care setting. A musty odor may mean that the client's diminished energy level hinders adequate cleaning of the environment, especially in the home setting. Mouth odors sometimes indicate mouth or gastrointestinal pathology. They can also result from altered hygiene habits or values. Finally, mouth odors may give clues to the client's eating habits. Other odors may show the elderly person's concern about appearance, as in the case of perfume or after-shave lotion. Hiatt (1982) suggests that assessment of the environment should focus on obtaining an environmental autobiography of the context within which the person is used to living.

Analysis of Assessment Data

The nursing assessment is a systematic technique for learning as much as possible about the client. Data do not need to be obtained at one time, nor by a single person. Limitations imposed by the environment, the client himself, and by anyone else providing input will determine the pacing of data collection. Even before the final analysis of the data collected, the nurse should analyze information as it is obtained. Often it will be necessary to intervene before the data base is complete. In such a situation, intervention is directed toward support of the client's basic needs. Intervention can take place while gathering assessment data. During the assessment, the nurse has an opportunity to indicate to the person how the areas being assessed relate to health.

The assessment should not duplicate information gathered by others in the health team, but should use data already collected. The nurse can also share significant data with other members of the multidisciplinary team. This helps to conserve the elderly client's energy levels and to provide more effective care built upon a broader data base. When a formal method is used for assessing an elderly person, the assessor must be aware of the client's problems with language, sensory reception, comprehension, attention, or motivation (Lawton, 1971). Information about such problems should thus be shared among the multidisciplinary team.

Any data collected by the nurse or another member of the multidisciplinary team that will assist the nurse in working with the elderly client should be included in the data analysis. The nurse summarizes and collates these data, groups similar data, and arranges everything in an orderly format that will enable him or her to draw conclusions (Yura and Walsh, 1983). With the elderly person, there is a strong possibility of the coexistence of physical, psychologic, nutritional, and social disturbances. An alteration in any one of these areas predisposes the person to a disturbance in the other areas.

Data collected should reflect assets as well as changes or losses of the elderly person. In analyzing such data, the nurse must evaluate the significance and extent of these assets and losses. The nurse should determine the impact of changes that have occurred in the client's life, and his or her attitude toward these changes, which may involve physiologic, psychologic, social, and environmental areas. For example, a behavioral problem may be created by environmental factors. An analysis of these changes can provide clues to how the elderly person's assets might lessen the negative impact of the losses.

The data collected should include the way in which the client planned for and is adapting to change. The supports available to the client to maintain health or to assist change must be evaluated. Aspects of the environment that affect the aged person's safety and health, as well as those which encourage expressions of his individuality and independence, should be considered. As Little and Carnevali (1976) define the nursing process, assessment is the collection of a data base which is used to interpret the situation by first forming tentative impressions, validating these impressions, and ruling out problems. Ruling out a problem indicates that the client was coping effectively in the specific area at the time the assessment was performed.

As the data are categorized and analyzed, the nurse makes a determination of needs. These include the needs recognized by the nurse and the health team as well as the wishes of the client. Occasionally there may be a difference of opinion on needs. For example, the nurse may decide that an elderly person's communication problems resulting from hearing loss are a priority need, since the client had difficulty hearing questions during an interview. On the other hand, the client may be far more concerned about how he or she will be able to pay a utility bill. Unless the client has a chance to define what is a priority need of the moment, neither nurse nor client will be able to establish realistic goals. In this case, the nurse should recognize that achieving more effective communication is not a priority for this client at this time. While she assists the client in dealing with the utility bill, however, the nurse can analyze the way the client copes with the hearing loss, and perhaps discover an immediate helping alternative while postponing consultation for a hearing aid. Understanding the elderly person is a key to acceptance of the person as an individual.

Nursing Diagnosis

After the data are analyzed, a nursing diagnosis can be made. The diagnosis is a conclusion reached by the nurse based on data gathered in the client assessment. The accuracy and completeness of the assessment data and data analysis affect the accuracy of the diagnosis. The process of diagnosing includes integrating physiologic, psychologic, interpersonal, social, economic, and religious information. Through the nursing diagnosis, existing or potential health problems that the nurse is qualified and licensed to treat are identified (Price, 1980). Nursing diagnosis statements can generally be classified as action, reaction, or interaction (Jones, 1979). Gleit and Tatro (1981) have defined nursing diagnosis for supporting a condition of good health for the healthy person. They see nursing diagnosis as the statement of an individual's response that is healthy or actually or potentially unhealthy and a response that independent nursing interventions can help to reinforce or strengthen in the direction of optimal health. This definition of nursing diagnosis recognizes the person's assets.

A system for classifying those health states or health problems diagnosed by nurses and treated by means of nursing interventions has been developed by National Conferences on Classification of Nursing Diagnoses. This conference group has been meeting every several years since 1973. However, the process of developing the nomenclature and applying nursing diagnoses continues to evolve. Part of this process involves testing the diagnoses in various settings to determine their adequacy. An example of a nursing diagnosis that has been challenged is "noncompliance" (Stanitis and Ryan, 1982). To some care providers compliance can suggest coercion to an expected client role and adherence to a treatment plan. Value issues and conflicts become involved with the attempt to develop an acceptable list of nursing diagnoses. Effort is continuing toward developing more clearly defined and more widely understood and accepted nursing diagnoses. As a prerequisite to planning care, it is important for the nurse to list nursing diagnoses derived from the analysis of assessment data, even though the recommended nomenclature continues to be tested clinically. The ultimate goal is to standardize labels to facilitate communication among nurses and between nurses and practitioners in related disciplines (Yura and Walsh, 1983). Nursing diagnoses will promote a greater degree of accountability of the nurse for the care planned and provided for the elderly client. The purpose of nursing diagnosis differs from that of the medical diagnosis. The nurse does not diagnose and treat an underlying pathologic process, even though he or she may draw on conclusions reached by the physician. For example, a medical diagnosis of congestive heart failure might require the nurse to work with impaired physical mobility related to dependent edema in the client's legs.

The nursing diagnosis is concerned with the needs and wishes of the client as he interacts with his environment. It is not concerned with the situation or problems faced by the nurse as she administers care. Her statement that an elderly person is "uncooperative" reflects problems the nurse is having. It is not a diagnosis of the patient's problem. This behavior may reflect the elderly person's difficulty in coping with changes or losses. The person described as uncooperative may have to cope with additional stress imposed by the behavior of the nurse who has so labeled him. Instead of labeling, it is imperative for the nurse to use the assessment data to determine which needs of the client are producing the observed behavior. In this way the elderly person can be helped to develop alternative ways of coping, or can be supported in his or her present way of coping. The assets of the client can give clues to alternative responses.

Perhaps the response labeled as uncooperative behavior is the client's way of protecting territorial rights. An elderly person may be labeled uncooperative because he or she screams after being left in a wheelchair for three hours, or complains that sleep is lost because a roommate snores loudly during the night. This label may be applied to the elderly person who questions medications, or refuses to take a medication because it is too difficult to swallow or because it causes dizziness, to the person who hoards food, or to the person

who prefers to remain in the quiet of his or her home rather than to attend a craft session or a bingo game at the senior-citizen center. The list of behaviors labeled as uncooperative by nurses and other health team members is extensive. This does not mean that the examples given here are the most desirable or health-promoting behaviors. However, attaching the label "uncooperative" rather than diagnosing hinders the formulation of client-centered goals directed toward behavior change.

The nursing goal is to help aged persons to identify and meet their health needs. The plan of care that is formulated according to this goal should incorporate individual factors that influence health needs. Emphasizing that the client must cooperate and conform is a controlling maneuver by the nurse, and it hinders attempts to have the client take part in the planning process.

PLANNING CARE

The nursing diagnoses based on the needs and assets of the aged client forms the foundation on which a plan of nursing intervention is built. Just as the client's input was used to obtain the assessment data, client input is important during formulation of the plan of care. This reinforces the value that the nurse places on the individual client as he or she utilizes the client's assets in planning to meet the client's needs. Formulating the plan should be viewed as a dynamic process that recognizes the constant change taking place in the client's internal and external environments. The elderly person must not be viewed as rigid or incapable of change. Planning with the elderly person should reduce the need for the person to make decisions while under stress. Adequate time for input on decision-making in the planning process should increase client satisfaction with the final decision. When an individual loses the ability to make choices and decisions about his life, a condition of "learned helplessness" can result (Seligman, 1975). Learned helplessness is characterized by depression, discontinuation of efforts to control outcomes, and inability to appreciate when one's actions have actually influenced outcomes. To avoid this condition, the nurse must include the elderly person in the care planning process. Nursing knowledge is utilized when the elderly person is helped with options from which to make decisions.

The input of other members of the health team is also important. Ideally, a plan of care would be formulated by all professional workers with the client, assisted by the client and significant others. When a total client plan is not available, nursing care planning requires collaborative efforts with other disciplines, as well as involvement of the client and family in decisions. The plan of care should reflect the sociocultural patterns and spiritual needs of the aged client.

Statement of Goals

A vital part of planning care is the statement of goals. Determination of goals involves the participation of the client, his family or significant others, and other health-team members. These goals are called client or nurse–client goals. Client participation in goal setting is a way to ensure a freely made decision and the client's acceptance of responsibility for action. The overall goal should include achievement of the highest level of health possible for the aged client.

In setting goals, an initial question to be considered relates to the desired outcomes of the client. An outcome is a valued health state, condition, or behavior exhibited by a client (Gordon, 1982). In goal statements, outcomes are projected and need to be measurable in order to guide decisions about care that has been provided. The nursing diagnosis describes the present health state of the client whereas the goal describes the desired health state. The nursing diagnosis is the necessary base for outcome projection. Expected outcomes relate to the changes that can be observed with the elderly client. The projected outcomes should list how the elderly person will look, feel, or act. Short-term goals contribute to the achievement of long-term goals. An example follows:

NURSING DIAGNOSIS:

Alterations in sleep pattern related to return home following hospitalization

LONG-TERM GOAL:

The client will reestablish sleep patterns to include eight hours of sleep during the night within the next two weeks.

SHORT-TERM OR CONTRIBUTORY GOALS:

The client will not need to go to the bathroom more than once each night by establishing a fluid intake schedule to reduce the amount of late evening fluids.

The client will eliminate a late afternoon nap after the first three days at home.

The client will walk a minimum of three blocks before dinner in the late afternoon after the first five days at home.

The client will perform relaxation exercises before bedtime by the end of the first week at home.

The client will discontinue the bedtime sedative medication after the first week at home.

A goal is a statement of a desired outcome to be attained within a predicted period of time, given the presenting situation and resources (Little and Carneveli, 1976).

Another example relates to a diagnosis of self-care deficits. If the elderly person's independence is to be supported, the goals must reflect ways in which the client can maintain independence appropriate to the environment. An independence goal for an elderly person living at home might involve moving to a bedroom on the first floor when hemiparesis limits climbing stairs. By comparison, an elderly person in any living environment might have a goal to maintain independence by learning to get out of bed to the wheelchair without assistance. The aged person needs to express his or her own idea of independence as he works with the nurse in setting goals. The nurse may see independence as the client's being able to manage hygiene needs without help. The client, however, may see being able to shave or brush his teeth and wash his face as being independent.

The attainment of any goal cannot be measured accurately if the expectations of the client and nurse differ. To state a goal "to maintain the client's independence" is not enough; the outcome criterion must also be included. Outcome criteria can be defined in terms of client changes with regard to the environment, community, friends, or family. One goal, relating to alterations in nutrition, may be to improve nutrition by having the main meal each day at the congregate meal center. Another goal could be to increase socialization by attending the community senior-citizen center each week. Including conditions under which the goals will be met gives further direction to the nursing actions. The use of the elderly person's assets and the support systems available to him should be reflected in the expected outcomes.

Goals should be stated so that they convey the intent of those dealing with the problem—the client, his family or significant others, and members of the nursing and health teams who are involved with the client. The clear and complete statement of the goal must reflect the nursing diagnosis. Nurse–client goals must give specific direction in guiding care.

Priority Setting
Goals should be ranked in order of priority, and nurse and client should try first to meet those which seem most urgent. Goals that seem to be less urgent or that will take longer to attain can be given lower priority. However, the client should help to determine these priorities. The advocacy role of the nurse includes the act of informing and supporting a person so that he can make the best decisions possible for himself (Kohnke, 1982). Goals should also be described within a realistic framework, taking into consideration what is achievable in terms of time, energy, motivation, and available resources. Analysis of the environmental assessment will determine whether goals set are attainable. This analysis should include the constraints or facilitators present, such as housing and finances.

Substandard housing, with inadequate heating and barriers to mobility such as steep, dimly lit stairways, can be a constraint. Moving to an environment with fewer such barriers, if income is adequate, may take priority over attempting to increase mobility in the present setting. Even though goals should relate to the promotion of the elderly person's independence, it is realistic to recognize that sometimes goals related to the comfort of the aged person during times of needed dependence take priority.

Nursing Directives
Nursing directives, interventions, or orders are actions the nurse plans to perform to help the client achieve goals which are part of the plan of care. The focus of a nursing directive is to individualize care. These directives define the nurse's accountability to the client and should specify who does what, where, when, how, how often, and for how long. A nursing directive must be dated and reviewed at regular intervals. Based on this review, the directive may be discontinued, renewed, or revised. The frequency of review is determined by the client's changing needs and by the policy of the setting in which he lives. In a long-term setting, for example, a monthly review of the nursing directives may be adequate. However, for a person who just has arrived at a long-term care setting, a daily review may be necessary for the first several weeks.

A nursing directive describes the process by which a goal outcome can be achieved. For example, consider the following goal—the client will maintain bowel elimination every one or two days. If this client is in a setting that permits daily contact with the nurse, the directive might be: Provide a 4-ounce glass of prune juice with breakfast each morning. If this client is in his home setting, the order might be: Teach the client the potential effect of juices, such as prune juice, on elimination patterns; or explain to the client the adverse physical and psychologic effects of long-term laxative ingestion. If this client lives in his home setting but is dependent on his wife for meal planning and preparation, the order might be: Teach both the client and his wife the potential effect of juices, such as prune juice, on elimination patterns. The nursing order should define the planned action as it relates to a content area at a specified time. The content area lists *what* the nurse will do to, with, and for the client. The time element indicates *when* the action occurs, *how frequently* it takes place, and *how long* it is to last. An example of this might be: Assist the client into a wheelchair that he can maneuver himself each day after lunch, from 12:30 P.M. until 4:00 P.M.

Nursing orders are recorded on the client's legal record and evidence must be provided for the number, type, and outcomes of nursing actions. With Problem Oriented Medical Records, the nurse would record by using a S-O-A-P or S-O-A-P-I-E format. This includes the subjective response of the client, the objective observations of the nurse, the assumption or assessment of the situation, and the plan for the problem. A description of the intervention and the evaluation of the outcome may also be included. With the establishment of problem-oriented records and recording systems, nurses need to recognize that nursing problems need to be recorded in terms compatible with nursing goals and interventions (Jones, 1979). Nursing diagnoses are recorded by nurses on the problem list (Gordon, 1982). Also, ongoing notes must be written so that progress toward goal attainment can be monitored. The format of the client record may vary with the setting, but the nurse is always responsible for documenting the nursing activity.

Standards of nursing care have been established for the elderly client. These include the (1) American Nurses Association Standards for Gerontological Nursing Practice, and (2) Program Guide Nursing Service: Standards and Educational Guidelines for Gerontological Nursing Practice of the Veterans Administration. These standards of care provide guidelines for nursing directives appropriate for the elderly person. The nursing directives are a part of the total plan of care.

Nursing Plan of Care

The nursing plan of care is a written plan, organized in a systematic way, that provides a central source of information for the nursing team. Other professional and nonprofessional personnel may have access to this plan, which is developed by the professional nurse. If the nurse does not understand the value of the plan of care, the plan she develops may not be effective. Since this plan takes time to develop, the nurse may use lack of time as a way of expressing lack of interest. If the nurse thinks of the elderly client in stereotypical terms, as an unchanging person taking up space in a long-term setting, the nurse may not believe that a plan of care is necessary. However, fail-

ure to assess and plan properly before intervening can lead to ineffective efforts which contribute little to quality care for the client.

INTERVENTION

Intervention is the action phase of the nursing process, during which the plan of care is carried out. The extent to which the client took part in this planning largely determines the degree to which he will participate in the interventions. The elderly person needs to participate in informed decision-making. As an advocate for the elderly person, the nurse needs to inform the client and then support the client in the decision that is made. The nurse must provide opportunity for the client to make his own decisions even when these decisions differ from the nurse's personal judgment. As part of intervention, there is a need to know how to support without assuming a defending or rescuing position. If the client is encouraged to be responsible in planning his or her care, the person may feel more freedom to accept or reject the care. If an elderly person can perform an activity slowly, this person should be encouraged to participate even though the nurse alone could administer the care much more quickly and efficiently. The long-term effect of client participation can save nursing time and satisfy the elderly person by promoting independence, and should therefore be encouraged. In the beginning, the client may be capable only of washing his or her face. Later, however, activity may be restored to the point where the client can take complete care of personal hygiene needs. If the person had not been given the original opportunity to wash his or her face, activity levels would have regressed instead of progressed.

Intervention should allow for the aged person to claim his or her own territory or living space within the environment. Maintaining the need for personal props, such as pictures or other objects, encourages a sense of personal and social identity (Roberts, 1978). Such props help continue familiarity with the environment and can assist in adaptation to environmental change. The impact of an unfamiliar environment, in which personal territory has not been claimed, can cause confusion, anxiety, and disorientation in the elderly person.

Participation in intervention enables the aged person to feel valued and significant. Too often the elderly are made to feel useless. The nurse should be aware of unconscious messages she conveys to the client as they implement the plan of care together. An avoidance approach can convey negative messages, increasing the elderly person's feelings of loss and expressions of anger. Just as the client is given the chance to take part in the planning of his or her care, the client needs the opportunity to choose alternatives as the plan is implemented. The opportunity to change approaches promotes a greater degree of sensitivity between the nurse and the aged person.

The client's financial status may be a constraint to implementation. This can be determined during the nursing assessment, if the client agrees to share this information. Many aged persons live on fixed incomes, and limited finances may be a problem with some approaches. For example, the cost of an activity that might be planned to avoid loneliness or hopelessness may be prohibitive to the client.

Hopelessness can result when an approach fails and no alternative approaches are available. However, the aged person can draw upon the energy of the hopeful nurse. The hopeful nurse helps the client look toward the future, if only on a daily basis or if only in hope for support during the dying process. The nurse may have to support the aged person's hope of dying in peace.

The family or significant others can take part in the client's care, but the nurse often must actively promote their participation. If the elderly person has many dependency needs, the family can be helped to meet these needs by direct aid from the nurse. She can also suggest alternative helpers to free the family for certain periods of time.

An individualized plan of care should provide guidelines for all members of the nursing team. As care proceeds, additional assessment data can be obtained to provide further guides for implementation of care in the future. In gathering additional data, the nurse may de- termine that the client is able to take greater part in his care. The aged person should be encouraged to become a more active participant when assessment data indicate readiness for this.

EVALUATION

Evaluation is concerned with the client's status or movement within a specified goal area. In evaluation, the nurse considers the effect of support offered and services provided as the client is helped to cope with problems of living or assisted with health generation. Evidence is needed to determine whether a goal has or has not been met, and what changes have occurred with the elderly person. Evaluative data should be collected in a prescribed consistent way that lends itself to quantitative and qualitative measurement. Units of measurement or qualifying terms should be indicated in the criteria, so that each nurse caring for the client will collect data in the same way. Reference to the nursing diagnosis is a necessary part of the evaluation.

The optimal frequency for reassessing or evaluating nursing care is often debated. Since change tends to be slow, one might argue for infrequent efforts. On the other hand, change also tends to be subtle, calling for frequent review. There is no certain answer to this debate. Whether the nurse reassesses or evaluates at frequent or infrequent intervals depends on the type of health problem, the goal established, and the intervention(s) utilized. If the goal is for the client to become more alert and the intervention is increased intake of vitamins and protein, evaluation time should probably be set at six to eight weeks in the future. If the intervention is a medication that affects memory or alters mood, the evaluation should be scheduled for three to four days in the future, since such drugs have the potential to cause adverse as well as therapeutic effects.

After evaluation, goals may have to be changed or eliminated, or new goals formulated. Goal changes have a direct effect on interventions. The establishment of alternative approaches in the plan of care gives greater latitude to implementation. The way the client responds and the way the nurse and family observe these responses are part of the evaluation data. Even though problems exist in the measurement of outcomes, outcome seems to be related to how much the client wants to participate, to try, to endure, to achieve, and to live, and to how much the elderly person is encouraged or permitted to participate. Nurses play a major role in supporting clients and their families to take an active part in goal-directed activities.

If client and family are encouraged to participate in assessment, goal-setting, planning, and implementation, their input in evaluating outcomes of care will be more valid. Negative as well as positive evaluation should be encouraged, as it can lead to a change in approaches that have been ineffective or a continuation of those that have been effective. The likelihood of client-centered goal attainment should increase as the client and family participate.

One increasingly significant aspect of evaluation is quality review. This is the collection of data that demonstrate the quality of care provided. Quality refers to effect of care on the health of the individual client. Quality assurance refers to measures directed toward assuring quality care. Instruments have been developed to measure the quality of nursing care. These instruments include approaches that evaluate the quality of care for elderly persons who are cared for over an extended period. Appraisal methods range from patient questionnaires to surveys of settings, patients, staff, and records (Plant, 1977). Reimbursement of medical costs by hospitalization insurance companies, Medicare, and Medicaid has given rise to an era of professional standards review organizations, health systems agencies, and utilization reviews. However, quality should not be confused with efficiency when outcomes are measured. Quality is concerned with outcome whereas efficiency is related to process of care. It has been suggested that control of costs for health care of the elderly may be promoted by providing payment based on the outcome of the elderly receiving care. With this,

reimbursement would be based on need for care and the degree of congruence of the outcome with the prognosis (Linn and Linn, 1980). Standardized quantitative methods of functional assessment can provide a component for treatment outcome and program evaluation.

The most desirable instrument for measuring quality care is one that benefits the client most by bothering him the least (Plant, 1977). Some assessment tools have been time-consuming and tiring to the elderly client. The patient appraisal and care evaluation (PACE) is directed toward evaluating the quality of care actually provided. PACE is a client-oriented approach that measures the achievement of time-limited goals. The basic features include a client history and assessment, master problem list, plan of care, and goal-achievement analysis. Using a multidisciplinary assessment form covering client behavior, activity preference, activities of daily living functioning, medical history, and discharge planning, the client is appraised periodically. This is done upon admission and at least annually after discharge. Another instrument is based on the concept of Patient Care Management System (PCMS). This management system is performed by an interdisciplinary care team using client assessment, care planning, and care evaluation (Chow, 1980). A review of literature indicates the need to develop valid and reliable instruments to measure the quality of care and the quality of life when extended care is needed in any setting. It is also necessary to concentrate on care processes as well as outcomes of care. Evaluation of the nursing process without documentation of the effect of nursing actions on specific client outcomes leaves the evaluator without an objective basis for administrative action. Evaluation of outcomes without determination of process leaves nursing vulnerable to the charge that some other process contributed to the result.

Bloch (1975) developed a framework that clarifies the need to work toward the goal of process–outcome evaluation. Nursing practice should be evaluated with respect to client outcomes by applying process as well as outcome measurement. In a process evaluation the activities performed by the care provider are judged. In outcome evaluation, a judgment is made about the achievement of client-oriented objectives. An evaluation that encompasses both process and outcome has the potential for an even greater impact on the quality of care.

Standards of practice are based on the present understanding of what nursing care should be. In efforts to improve quality of care, professional practice must be changed with the expectation that outcomes will change. It is the outcome of total care that is significant to the client. Change requires commitment and support in innovation and planning. It is a function of individual values, attitudes, sociocultural roles, and relationships (Felton, Frevert, Galligan, Neill, and Williams, 1976).

The following client history is presented to demonstrate the outcome of a goal set by an elderly client. Members of the health team were able to change their attitudes and support the client in meeting this goal.

Mrs. G, age 82, was brought to a primary care setting by her daughter. The problem Mrs. G presented was a lesion on her left great toe that did not heal. Mrs. G had not had a health evaluation for "years," but came to a healthcare facility at this time because of a limp noted by her daughter. Upon further investigation, her daughter discovered the lesion on her mother's toe. Mrs. G was hospitalized for treatment of a gangrenous toe. The recommended medical therapy was amputation of the left leg; but she refused this amputation and requested discharge to her home. The health-team members, including nurses, attempted to convince Mrs. G that she should have an amputation. Mrs. G replied that she was ready for death and that she wanted to die with both legs.

Mrs. G was discharged to her home and was followed by the home health team. Two daughters who lived nearby were able to participate in changing dressings on the affected toe. They also helped with the housekeeping activities while supporting their mother's independence in her home setting. The home health nurses instructed Mrs. G's daughters in techniques of caring for the affected toe. They listened as Mrs. G talked about her philosophy of life and her strong desire to remain in the home in which she had lived for fifty years.

The home health nurses were supportive of Mrs. G's daughters in the assistance they were giving their mother. Goals were established in collaboration with Mrs. G and her family. Because the recommended medical therapy was not accepted, alternative plans were formulated with the client and her family.

Mrs. G's problem was limited to the great toe and the two adjacent toes. She continued to hope that the lesions would heal, and maintained independence in daily activities with the aid of a walker. Even though she received assistance from her daughters in preparing meals, she was able to continue eating the foods that had always been familiar to her. Some of these were ethnic recipes which her daughters learned to prepare. It pleased Mrs. G to know that this preparation of ethnic foods would be carried on by her daughters. Although she was unable to attend church services, her priest made frequent visits to her home. She had religious articles nearby that had been important to her throughout her life, as well as pictures of her family. When the weather permitted, Mrs. G would sit on her porch to enjoy the outdoor views that were important and meaningful to her. She enjoyed visits from her grandchildren.

Eighteen months after the onset of her foot problem, Mrs. G developed an influenza infection. She told her daughters and the home health nurse that she was ready to die and wished to die in her own bed. She asked that she not be taken to the hospital if she was unable to communicate this verbally. Mrs. G was in bed for several days before she died. On the day of her death, her daughters and granddaughter were with her. Even though she could not speak, communication occurred through touch. She could also hear the spoken words of her family, and she responded by a squeeze of the person's hand. The home health nurse visited on the day of Mrs. G's death. Mrs. G seemed to convey anxiety at this time through increased restlessness, and the nurse reassured her that she would not be sent to the hospital. The home health nurse was in constant communication with the physician, who also visited Mrs. G in her home. The nurse was able to support Mrs. G's family in the decisions that they made with their mother. She recognized their grief and encouraged them to cry. Several hours after the nurse left the home, Mrs. G died in her own bed with her family at her side. She had attained a goal that she herself had established. Her funeral was as she requested. She was permitted to express these wishes while she was living her life in the way she wanted.

Evaluation of the process and the outcomes of Mrs. G's goals shows that quality of care did result as she was supported by the nurse during the living and dying process. The nurse functioned as a key person in the health team, and as a key person in the lives of Mrs. G and her family.

RECOMMENDED READINGS

Abdellah, F.G. Nursing care of the aged in the United States. Journal of Gerontological Nursing 7 (11):657–663, 1981. *The need for and strategies to advance the scope of nursing care of the elderly are presented.*

Benson, E.R., McDevitt, J.Q. Health promotion by nursing in care of the elderly. Nursing and Health Care 3(1):39–43, 1982. *Nursing's response to the challenge of improving the quality of life for the elderly is presented. Preventive health care services are stressed.*

Gelfand, D.E. Aging: The Ethnic Factor. Boston, Little, Brown, 1982. *A comprehensive look at the ethnic aged in the United States. Serving the ethnic aged population also is addressed.*

Gordon, M. Nursing Diagnosis: Process and Application. New York, McGraw-Hill, 1982. *The process of formulating nursing diagnoses is presented. The importance of nursing diagnoses is stressed.*

Hiatt, L.G. The environment as a participant in health care. The Journal of Long-Term Care Administration 10(1):1–17, 1982. *Realistic suggestions for arranging the physical and social environments in order to promote effective care giving for the elderly.*

Kane, R.A., Kane, R.L. The Rand Corporation: Assessing the Elderly. Lexington, MA, Lexington, 1981. *This comprehensive guide provides an analysis of available instruments for assessing the elderly.*

Mayers, M.G., Norby, R.B., Watson, A.B. Quality Assurance for Patient Care. New York, Appleton-Century-Crofts, 1977. *Emphasis is placed on the evaluation process. Evaluation is related to the im-*

plementation of Quality Assurance Programs in health care agencies.

Raukhorst, L.M., Stokes, S.A., Mezey, M.D. Community and home assessment. Journal of Gerontological Nursing. 6(6):319–327, 1980. *Detailed assessment considerations for the home as well as the community setting are presented. Safety concerns for the elderly are included.*

Yura, H., Walsh, M.B. The Nursing Process, 4th ed. Norwalk, CT, Appleton-Century-Crofts, 1983. *The nursing process as it applies throughout human developmental stages. Situations are presented to illustrate the application of the nursing process.*

REFERENCES CITED

Abdellah, F.G. Nursing care of the aged in the United States. Journal of Gerontological Nursing 7(11):657–663, 1981

Benson, E.R., McDevitt, J.Q: Health promotion by nursing in care of the elderly. Nursing and Health Care 3(1):39–43, 1982

Bengston, V.L. Families, support systems and ethnic groups: Patterns of contrast and congruence. Paper presented at the annual meeting of the Gerontological Society, New York, October 13, 1976

Bloch, D. Evaluation of nursing care in terms of process and outcome: Issues in research and quality assurance. Nursing Research 24:256, 1975

Block, M.R., Davidson, J.L., Grumbs, J.D. Women Over Forty: Visions and Realities. New York: Springer, 1981

Caird, F.I., Judge, T.G.: Assessment of the Elderly Patient, 2nd ed. Philadelphia, J.B. Lippincott, 1979

Carter, J.H. The Black Aged: Implications for Mental Health Care. Journal of American Geriatrics Society 30(1):67–70, 1982

Chow, R.K. Quality of care: A present and future challenge for all nurses. Journal of Gerontological Nursing 6(1):256–259, 1980

Dancy, J. The Black Elderly, a Guide for Practitioners. The Institute of Gerontology. The University of Michigan, Wayne State University, 1977

Dunn, T., Linden, R.R. Surviving the silence: Old women and the power of naming. Generations 4(4):4–5, 1980

Ernst, N.S. Functional assessment: Planning for service delivery. Generations. 5(3):21,41, 1981

Fackos, L. Older women. Perspectives on Aging 10(3):19–21, 1981

Falcone, A.R. Synopsis of Long-Term Care Information System Programs. Assessment Training Center, Cornell University Medical Center, Department of Public Health, New York, NY, 1981

Felton, G., Frevert, E., Galligan, K., Neill, M.K., Williams, K. Pathway to accountability: Implementation of a quality assurance program. Journal of Nursing Administration 6(1):20, 1976

Gelfand, D.E. Aging: The Ethnic Factor. Boston, Little, Brown, 1982

Gleit, C.J., Tatro, S. Nursing diagnoses for healthy individuals. Nursing and Health Care 2(8):456–457, 1981

Gordon, M. Nursing Diagnosis: Process and Application. New York, McGraw-Hill, 1982

Gray, J.N., Aldred, H. Care plans in long-term facilities. American Journal of Nursing 80(11): 2054–2057, 1980

Gunter, L., Miller, J.C.: Toward a nursing gerontology. Nursing Research 26:208, 1977

Harel, Z. Quality of care, congruence, and well-being among institutionalized aged. The Gerontologist 21(5):523–531, 1981

Hiatt, L.G. The environment as a participant in health care. The Journal of Long-Term Care Administration 10(1):1–17, 1982

Hickey, T. Health and Aging. Monterey, CA, Brooks/Cole, 1980

Jones, P.E. A terminology for nursing diagnoses. Advances in Nursing Science 2(1):65–71, 1979

Kane, R.A., Kane, R.L.: Assessing the Elderly: A Practical Guide to Measurement. Lexington, MA, D.C. Heath, 1981

Kennedy, C. Use of health assessment for placing patients for geropsychiatry. Journal of Gerontological Nursing 7(5):275–279, 1981

Kohnke, M.F. Advocacy, what is it? Nursing and Health 3(6):314–318, 1982

Lawton, M.P. The functional assessment of elderly people. Journal of the American Geriatric Society 19:465, 1971

Linn, M.W., Linn, B.S.: Qualities of institutional care that affect outcome. Aged Care and Services Review 2(3):1–12, 1980

Little, D, Carnevali, D.: Nursing Care Planning, 2nd ed. Philadelphia, Lippincott, 1976

Maslow, A: Motivation and Personality, 2nd ed. New York, Harper, 1970

Mayers, G.M., Norby, R.B., Watson, A.B. Quality Assurance for Patient Care: Nursing Perspectives. New York, Appleton-Century-Crofts, 1977

Millard, P.H., Smith, C.S. Personal belongings—a positive effect. The Gerontologist 21(1):85–90, 1981

Newsome, B.L. (ed): Insights on the Minority Elderly. The National Center on Black Aged, Inc. The Institute of Gerontology, University of the District of Columbia, 1977

Olson, J. To treat or to allow to die. Journal of Gerontological Nursing 7(3):141–147, 1981

Ortega, S.T., Crutchfield, R.D., Rushing, W.A. Race differences in elderly personal well-being: Friendship, family, and church. Research on Aging 5(1):101–118, 1983

Pender, N.J. Health Promotion in Nursing Practice. Norwalk, CT, Appleton-Century-Crofts, 1982

Pierce, R.C., Clark, M., Kaufman, S. Generation and ethnic identity: A topological analysis. International Journal of Aging and Human Development 9(1), 1978–1979

Price, M.R. Nursing diagnosis: Making a concept come alive. American Journal of Nursing 80(4):668–671, 1980

Plant, J. Various approaches proposed to assess quality in long-term care. Hospitals 51(17):93, 1977

Rauckhorst, L.M., Stokes, S.A., Mezey, M.D. Community and home assessment. Journal of Gerontological Nursing 6(6):319–327, 1980

Roberts, S. Behavioral Concepts and Nursing Throughout the Life Span. Englewood Cliffs, NJ, Prentice-Hall, 1978

Sarver, S.C., Howard, M. Planning a self-care unit in an inpatient setting. American Journal of Nursing 82(7):1112–1114, 1982

Seligman, E.E. Helplessness. San Franscisco, Freeman, 1975

Snyder, L.H., Pyrek, J., Smith K. Vision and mental function in the elderly. The Gerontologist 16:491, 1976

Stanitis, M.A., Ryan, J. Noncompliance, an unacceptable diagnosis? American Journal of Nursing 82(6):941–942, 1982

Taylor, R.B. (ed) Health Promotion: Principles and Clinical Applications. Norwalk, CT, Appleton-Century-Crofts, 1982

Tibbitts, C. Success: First world assembly on aging termed long-range success. Aging 337:2–5, 1983

Yura, H., Walsh, M.B. The Nursing Process, 4th ed. Norwalk, CT, Appleton-Century-Crofts, 1983

BIBLIOGRAPHY

Abbey, J.C. Thoughts on interdisciplinary approaches to nursing. Image 6(2):15, 1974

Anderson, C.A. Home or nursing home: Let the elderly patient decide. American Journal of Nursing 79(8):1448–1449, 1979

Aquilera, D.C. Stressors in late adulthood. Family and Community Health. 2(2):61–69, 1980

Beattie, B.L., Crashaw, M. Team approach to the problem-oriented record in a long-term care facility. Journal of the American Geriatrics Society 30(2):109–113, 1982

Beaudry, M.D., Ronning, P.L. Implementing a holistic model of geriatric nursing care. Concern 4(1):11, 1977

Berk, M.L., Bernstein, A.B. Regular source of care and the minority aged. Journal of the American Geriatrics Society 30(4):251–254, 1982

Binstock, R.H. The aged as scapegoat. The Gerontologist 23(2):136–143, 1983

Block, G.J., Nolan, J.W., Dempsey, M.K. Health Assessment for Professional Nursing, a Developmental Approach. New York, Appleton-Century-Crofts, 1981

Bower, F.L. The Process of Planning Nursing Care, 3rd ed. St. Louis, Mosby, 1982

Brubaker, B.H. Health Promotion: A linguistic analysis. Advances in Nursing Science 5(3):1–14, 1983

Caro, F.G. Objectives, standards, and evaluation in long-term care. Home Health Care Services Quarterly 2(1):5–26, 1981

Chow, R.K. Development of a patient appraisal and care evaluation for long-term care. Journal of Long-Term Care Administration 5(2):21, 1977

Cuellar, J.B., Stanford, E.P., Miller-Soule, D.I. Understanding Minority Aging: Perspectives and Sources. San Diego, University Center on Aging, College of Human Services, San Diego State University, 1982

Davis, A.J., Aroskar, M.A. Ethical Dilemmas and Nursing Practice, 2nd ed. Norwalk, CT, Appleton-Century-Crofts, 1983

Falcone, A.R. Using the long-term care information system for effective community care. Home Health Care Services Quarterly 2(1):83–97, 1981

Ferguson, V. Future directions in the nursing care of the aged. Journal of Gerontological Nursing 7(12):759–762, 1981

Frankfather, D.L., Smith, M.J., Caro, F.G. Family Care of the Elderly: Public Initiatives and Private Obligations. Lexington, MA, Lexington, 1981

Fulmer, T. The world assembly on aging. Journal of Gerontological Nursing 8(12):702–705, 1982

Gathers, P., Johnson, N., Magill, K., Mahoney, C. Geriatric Nursing Audit. Geriatric Nursing 2(3):195–198, 1981

Giele, J.Z. (ed.) Women in the Middle Years: Current Knowledge and Directions for Research Policy. New York, Wiley, 1982

Griffin, M. A holistic approach to the health care of an elderly client. Journal of Gerontological Nursing 6(4):193–196, 1980

Hartford, M.E., Parsons, R. Groups with relatives of dependent older adults. The Gerontologist 22(4):394–398, 1982

Hedrick, S.C., Katz, S., Stroad, M. Patient assessment in long-term care: Is there a common language. Aged Care and Services Review 2(4):3–19, 1980–1981

Holzberg, C.S. Ethnicity and aging: Anthropological perspectives on more than just the minority elderly. The Gerontologist 22(3):249–257, 1982

Janik, S.W., Wells, K.S. Multidimensional assessment of the elderly client: A training program for the development of a new specialist. Journal of Applied Gerontology 1:45–52, 1982

Johnson, F. Responses to territorial intrusion by nursing home residents. Advances in Nursing Science 1(4):21–34,1979

Knowles, L. Gerontological nursing 1982. International Journal of Nursing Studies 20(1):45–54, 1983

Kuhn, M., Sommers, T. Common concern: Blueprint for a new age. Geriatric Nursing 2(3):214–217, 1981

Lareau, L.S., Heumann, L.F. The inadequacy of needs assessments of the elderly. The Gerontologist 22(3):324–330, 1982

Lawton, M.P. A research and service oriented multilevel assessment instrument. Journal of Gerontology 37(1):91–99, 1982

Lindeman, C.A. Measuring quality of nursing care. Journal of Nursing Administration 6(5):7, 1976

Louis, M. Personal space boundary needs of elderly persons: An empirical study. Journal of Gerontological Nursing 7(7):395–400, 1981

Lunney, M. Nursing diagnosis: Refining the system. American Journal of Nursing 82(3):456–459, 1982

Manuel, R.C. Minority Aging: Sociological and Social Psychological Issues. Westport, CT, Greenwood, 1982

Marriner, A. The Nursing Process. A Scientific Approach to Nursing Care, 3rd ed. St. Louis, Mosby, 1983

Marriner, A. The research process in quality assurance. American Journal of Nursing 79(12): 2158–2159, 1979

Mayers, M.G. A Systematic Approach to the Nursing Care Plan, 3rd ed. Norwalk, CT, Appleton-Century-Crofts, 1983

Mezey, M., Rauckhorst, L.M., Stokes, S.A. The health history of the aged person. Journal of Gerontological Nursing 3(3):47, 1977

O'Neal, D.J. Promotion of health for the aged in the family. Journal of Gerontological Nursing 8(3):146–148, 1982

Oriol, W.E. Aging in all Nations: A special report on the United Nations World Assembly on Aging,

Including the Text of the International Action Program on Aging. Vienna, Austria, July 26 to August 6, 1982. Washington, D.C., National Council on the Aging, Inc., 1982

Pedrin, V., Brown, S. Sexism and ageism: Obstacles to health care for women. Generations 4(4):20–21, 1980

Rankin, N., Burggraf, V. Aging in the 80s. Journal of Gerontological Nursing 9(5):272–275, 1983

Register, J.C. Aging and race: A black-white comparative analysis. The Gerontologist 21(4):438–443, 1981

Rogers, C.J., Gallion, T.E. Characteristics of elderly Pueblo Indians in New Mexico. The Gerontologist 18:482, 1978

Sandiford, J.R. Nursing home ombudsman. Nursing and Health Care 2(9):492–495, 1981

Schaefer, J. The interrelatedness of decision making and the nursing process. American Journal of Nursing 74:1852, 1974

Snyder, P. Creating culturally supportive environments in long-term care institutions. The Journal of Long-Term Care Administration 10(1):19–28, 1982

Solomon, K. Social antecedents of learned helplessness in the health care setting. The Gerontologist 22(3):282–287, 1982

Sundeen, S.J., Stuart, G.W., Rankin, E., Cohen, S.P. Nurse-Client Interaction: Implementing the Nursing Process. St. Louis, Mosby, 1976

Tiger, L. Optimism, the biological roots of hope. Psychology Today 12(8):18, 1979

Tripp-Reimer, T. Retention of a folk healing practice (Matiasma) among four generations of urban Greek immigrants. Nursing Research 32(2):97–101, 1983

Wandelt, M.A., Phaneuf, M.C. Three instruments for measuring the quality of nursing care. Hospital Topics 30(8):20, 1972

2

The Elderly in the United States: Numbers, Proportions, Health Status, and Use of Health Services

Susanne S. Robb

Reading this chapter will enable the individual to:

1. Define the term "old"
2. Name three forces responsible for the current "gerontology boom"
3. Explain the meaning of the following statements:
   a. "The aged population is aging within itself"
   b. "Old age is primarily a woman's problem"
4. Distinguish between the terms "minority" and "ethnic"
5. List three states with the highest and lowest proportions of elderly people
6. Explain why national demographic trends cannot be used to decide local needs for nursing and other services
7. Compare and contrast the major functional impairments of elderly people in the community with those residing in institutional settings
8. Name the three leading causes of death
9. Describe the influences of each of the following factors on life expectancy:
   a. Life-style
   b. Marital status
   c. Living arrangements
   d. Educational attainment
   e. Financial situation
10. Identify where most older people receive medical services
11. Indicate two barriers that prevent elderly people from using preventive and promotional health services

This chapter considers demographic facts as they relate to elderly people, provides an indication of their health and disability status, and relates this information to furnishing nursing care. A great deal of demographic information is available. Although the facts are not always exactly the ones needed, organized according to specific requirements or easily located, nurses need to consider what is known in order to plan their services and programs. To survive in times of declining resources, programs must produce highly visible and valued results. Demonstration of such results is directly related to importance of needs addressed. To target service programs correctly, nurses must know the needs of the population they are serving.

Demography is the statistical study of human populations, especially with regard to size, density, distribution, and vital statistics. Basic demographic facts about elderly people are well established and widely known: the number of old people is increasing, old people constitute an increasing proportion of the total population, life expectancy is increasing, the elderly population is aging within itself, and the likelihood of disability increases with age. Figure 2.1 illustrates some of these trends. A widowed woman is the oldest member of a four generation family in which her daughter and son-in-law are also approaching old age.

The implications of these facts for provision of nursing services would seem obvious. If nursing services were provided in relation to needs for those services, then elderly people would receive more health care provided by nurses than children receive. For a variety of reasons, however, nurses have not directed a proportionate share of their attention to el-

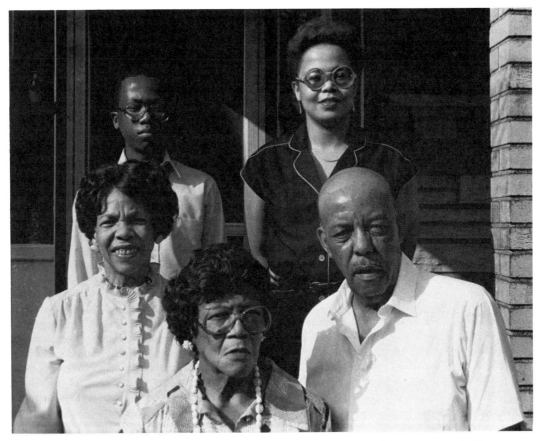

Figure 2.1. This multigeneration family demonstrates the long-lived older woman and children in the middle who are themselves old. *(Photograph by Shawn Mertz, Pittsburgh, PA.)*

derly people. The "graying of America" has raised a number of major issues for the nursing profession. These issues can be posed as questions. Does care of the elderly constitute a specialty? What modifications in roles and programs (administrative, clinical, educational, and research) are required to enable nurses to address the health needs of elderly people? What proportion of nurses should be trained to care for the elderly? Is a nonmedical model more appropriate for structuring delivery of nursing services to the elderly? How should assessment, planning, intervention, and evaluation be altered to accommodate the health-related needs of old people? What research is needed to provide a scientific basis for nursing care of the aged? How can nurses most easily apply what they already know about the elderly?

SOCIODEMOGRAPHIC TRENDS AND HEALTH IMPLICATIONS

The Meaning of "Old"

"Old age" does not begin on some specific date. Each of us is constantly and continually aging from the moment we are conceived. Changes from day to day are so slight as to be imperceptible, but they accumulate. Variations in the rate and timing of major aging events cause differences between people in any age group; the elderly are no exception. Thus, use of a single factor, such as chronologic age, is a restricted basis from which to define "older persons," determine their health status, and evaluate needs for services.

The concept of age is best viewed in relation to several perspectives. Social age, psychologic age, and functional age have all been identified as useful perspectives for reviewing the concept (Hindricks, 1978).

Some gerontologists (Atchley, 1980) believe that a definition of "old person" should be based on a life-cycle criterion rather than on chronologic age. Economic convenience, however, has encouraged use of a chronologic definition. The important point to remember is that the older population is not a single homogeneous group, and its characteristics vary within the age range of 55 and over. This population is sometimes categorized according to age group: the older population (55 or 60 and over); the elderly (65 and over); the aged (75 and over); and the extreme aged (85 and over). Some authorities distinguish between the young-old (60 to 74), the middle-old (75 to 84), and the old-old (85 and over) (Brody, 1980, p. 63). The phase of life called "old age" is longer (20 to 30 years or more) than the phases of childhood and adolescence combined. Distinctions between age groups within the elderly population will be increasingly recognized in the future as research provides a basis for making them.

Origins of the "Gerontology Boom"

A population increases or decreases in size and changes in composition as a result of three basic demographic processes: fertility, mortality, and immigration. *Fertility* refers to those factors that affect births; *mortality* includes factors that affect death and dying; and *immigration* is defined as those factors that influence residential movement into and out of a population. The present aging of the U.S. population has occurred as a result of two of these factors—declining fertility and declining mortality (Fingerhut and Rosenberg, 1981, p. 15). The last high level of immigration occurred before World War I and the impact has already been realized. During the first half of the century, the major factor was declining fertility. Women born at the start of the 1900s had an average of two to three children each, compared to four children each for the group of women whose childbearing years ended just before the turn of the century (Fingerhut and Rosenberg, 1982). During this same period, mortality declines oc-

curred for younger people. The net effect was an increase in the numbers of younger people in the population. During the second half of the century, mortality declines occurred across all age groups while fertility rates remained at a replacement-level. This change resulted in a larger elderly population than would have occurred if mortality declines had continued only for younger people.

In terms of the future, the size of the elderly population, until about 2025, has been determined already by past trends in fertility (for example, the "baby boom" of the mid 1940s through the late 1950s and the decreased number of births after the early 1960s). Further changes in the size of the elderly population after 2025 will probably result mainly from changes in mortality patterns in this population.

Numbers

The number of elderly people in the United States has been increasing steadily since 1900, when slightly more than 3 million people were 65 years of age or older. In 1980 there were more than 22.5 million elderly, representing an 8.3 percent increase since 1900 compared to increases of only 3.8 percent for persons aged 40 to 64 (a 25-year range), 3.0 percent for people aged 20–39 (a 20-year range), and 2.7 percent for the group aged 19 or fewer years (a 20-year range). Fertility is regarded as responsible for the present large numbers of old people. The number of people who reach 65 in a given year depends heavily on the number of births 65 years earlier. Large birth cohorts (groups) born at the turn of the century resulted in large numbers of elderly people approximately 65 years later. The postwar "baby boom," from the late 1940s through the 1950s, is expected to create a "gerontology boom" in the years 2010 to 2020.

Mortality factors have also contributed to the gerontology boom. Mortality is subject to less variation than fertility, and has steadily removed fewer people from the groups born each year. Death rates, especially among infants and children, have been reduced by advances in medicine, sanitation, and employment practices. Thus, more people have been able to survive to age 65. In 1978, approximately 73 percent of the newborn were expected to reach age 65, in contrast to 47 percent of those born in 1900.

The third major factor influencing increases in the elderly population was the influx of large numbers of immigrants before World War I. Immigration has been less important in the growth of elderly populations since 1960 and is expected to be a minor factor in the future.

Population projections for the aged have rested heavily on anticipated fertility rates. Despite periodic upward revisions, the number of aged persons for given future dates has been consistently underestimated. These underestimates appear to be due to inadequate consideration of mortality trends in the older ages (Myers, 1978). Although the projected numbers may be low, the United States, as indicated in Figure 2.2, can expect an increase in the number of elderly people at least through the year 2050 with 36.8 million elderly predicted by 1990 and 67.0 million by 2050 (Brotman, 1982b).

A sharp drop in the amount and rate of increase of the population 65 and over is expected, beginning in 1990. This decrease should last for about two decades, and will reflect the decline in births during the 1920–1930 and 1930–1940 decades. Births during the postwar "baby boom" from 1945 to 1959 will ultimately influence the size of the elderly population. Between 2010 and 2020, the number of persons 65 and over will increase dramatically. After about 2020, the rapid drop in the size of birth groups during the 1960s will lead to a very gradual increase in the number of persons 65 and over.

Proportions

As they increase in numbers, elderly people also represent a steadily increasing share of the total U.S. population. This proportion is affected by changes in the numbers of people in other age categories. Basically, this increase is more attributable to declining fertility than to lower death rates. In 1900, about 4 percent of the nation's 76 million people were 65 years old or over. In the first decade of the 20th century, high fertility and immigration of young adults limited the proportion of elderly, despite

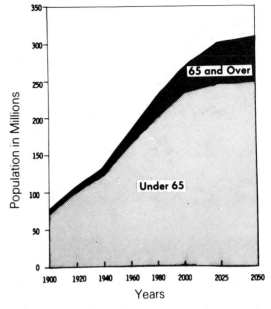

Figure 2.2. Numbers of people in the United States aged 65 and over and under age 65, 1900 through 1980, and projected to 2050 under middle series fertility assumptions.

1. Fertility rates below "zero population growth; net population loss after 2050." Slight increase from 1.83 births per woman in 1980 to 1.96 in 2000 and decrease to 1.90 in 2050.
2. Life expectancy at birth to increase:

	1981	2005	2050
Male	70.7	73.3	75.1
Female	78.3	81.3	81.6

3. Net immigration constant at 450,000 per year (Brotman, 1982b).

(U. S. Bureau of the Census. Census of the Population, 1970, Vol 1, Characteristics of the Population, Part 1, United States Summary, Section 1, 1973, p 276. U. S. Bureau of the Census. Age, sex, race, and Spanish origin of the population by regions, divisions, and states: 1980. 1980 Census of the Population, PC 80-51-1, 1981, p 3. Brotman, H.B. Unpublished data from the U. S. Census Bureau, November, 1982b.)

increases in numbers of old people. By 1940, the number of elderly had tripled, but they still made up only 6.8 percent of the total population. At this point fertility rates had declined,

TABLE 2.1 PERCENT OF PEOPLE AGED 65 YEARS AND
OVER, 1900–1980, AND PROJECTIONS UNDER
MIDDLE SERIES FERTILITY ASSUMPTIONS,* 1990–2050

Year	Percent	Year	Percent
1900	4.1	1990	12.7
1910	4.3		
1920	4.7	1995	13.1
1930	5.5		
1940	6.8	2000	13.1
1950	8.2		
1960	9.2	2025	19.5
1970	9.9		
1980	11.2	2050	21.7

*See caption to Figure 2.2 for assumptions. (U. S. Bureau of
the Census. Census of the Population, 1970, Vol. 1, Characteristics of the Population, Part 1, United States Summary,
Section 1, 1973, p. 276. U. S. Bureau of the Census. Age, sex,
race, and Spanish origin of the population by regions, divisions, and states, 1980. 1980 Census of the Population, PC
80-S1-1, 1981, p. 3. Brotman, H. B. Unpublished data from
the U. S. Census Bureau, November, 1982b.)

but decreases in infant and child mortality kept
the proportion of elderly small. By 1970, low
fertility, low immigration, and the affect of large
numbers of births at the turn of the century
(cohort effect) combined to cause a large increase in the proportion of the elderly in the
United States. In 1970, 9.9 percent of Americans were elderly. The percentage of the pop-

ulation 65 years of age and over, as recorded
at 10-year intervals from 1900 to 1980 and as
projected to 2050, is as indicated in Table 2.1.

Projections of an increase in proportion of
elderly are based upon assumptions that low
fertility will continue, immigration will be
constant, and mortality will continue to decline at the present rate. If women continue to
average slightly under two children each, the
population of elderly should increase to about
12.7 percent by 1990. When the postwar baby
boom cohort of the late 1940s and early 1950s
reaches 65, between 2010 and 2020, this proportion will increase dramatically. By 2025,
the elderly could make up a fairly constant 19
percent of the population (Brotman, 1982b).

Age Composition
Within the age group 65 years and over, the
proportion of people aged 65 to 74 is decreasing
and the proportion of those aged 75 and over
is increasing. This trend is expected to continue at least until the end of the century. People aged 75 and over made up 27 percent of the
population 65 years and over in 1900, and 39
percent by 1980. They are expected to comprise
45 percent by 2000. In other words, the elderly
population is aging within itself. This situation
is presented in Figure 2.3, with steadily in-

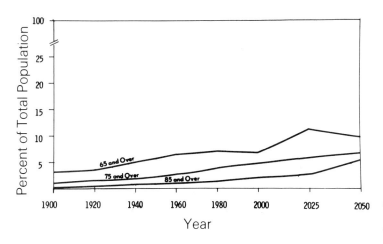

Figure 2.3. Percent of the total
population in the older age
groups, 1900 through 1980, and
projected from 2000 through 2050
based upon below zero population growth, net immigration
constant at 450,000 per year, and
a slightly declining death rate.
(U.S. Bureau of the Census. Census of the Population, 1970. Vol
1, Characteristics of the Population, Part 1, United States Summary, Section 1, 1973, p 276. U.S.
Bureau of the Census. Age, sex,
race, and Spanish origin of the
population by regions, divisions,
and states, 1980. 1980 Census of
the Population, PC 80-S1-1, 1981,
p 3. Brotman, H.B. Unpublished
data from the U.S. Census Bureau, November, 1982b.)

creasing percentages of people aged 75 and 85 years and over from 1900 through 2050. This trend is primarily due to the large numbers of people born in the late nineteenth and early twentieth centuries who have now moved into advanced old age. It is also the result of modern improvements in health care that enabled a large proportion of these birth cohorts to survive. A high proportion of people 75 and over has important implications for the delivery of health care. The prevalence of chronic diseases and functional impairments, as well as the utilization of health services, increases dramatically starting at about this age.

Racial Composition

Compared to whites, of whom 12.2 percent were 65 years or older in 1980, smaller percentages of other racial groups were 65 years or older: blacks, 7.9%; Asian and Pacific islanders, 6.1%; American Indians, Eskimos, and Aleutians, 5.3%; and people of Spanish origin,* 4.9%. These differences probably resulted from higher infant death rates for nonwhites and whites of Spanish origin in the past, which limited the proportion of those born that survived to old age, and a higher fertility rate, which increased the percentage of the young. Substantial differences were noted in the age composition of different racial groups and persons of Spanish origin. Whites were the oldest population group, with a median age of 31.3 years, followed by Asian and Pacific islanders, 28.6 years; blacks, 24.9 years; persons of Spanish origin, 23.2 years; and American Indians, Eskimos, and Aleuts combined, 23.0 years (U.S. Bureau of the Census, 1981).

By 2000, the Census Bureau projects over 3 million blacks 65 years and over, which, if borne out, will increase the older black population to 11.2 percent of the total black population. In comparison, the same projection will

---

* "Persons of Spanish origins" may be of any race but have their origins in Mexico, Cuba, Puerto Rico, Spain, or the Spanish-speaking countries of Central or South America. These individuals were also counted in the 1980 Census by racial groups, usually as white, black, or "other" (U.S. Bureau of the Census, 1981).

increase the older white population to only 12.9 percent of the total white population (U.S. Bureau of the Census, 1973). The black elderly population will thus increase by 43 percent between 1980 and 2000, or 25 percent more than the elderly white population over that same time span. Similar comparisons cannot be made for other minority groups because projections have not included groups other than "blacks" or "blacks and other races." However, comparisons made for American Indians, people of Spanish origin, Chinese, Japanese, Filipinos, and Koreans, between 1970 and 1978 in all cases, and across the years 1900, 1930, 1973, and 1978 for some groups, indicated the proportion of persons aged 65 years and older was increasing within each minority group (Jackson, 1980).

Health implications of being a minority group (black, American Indian, Eskimo, and so forth) within a minority group (the elderly) are not clear. There are several conceptional problems with gerontologic literature about the minority elderly. "Minority" and "ethnic" are not synonyms. A minority group is defined more in relation to numeric and class status within the total society. A *minority* is a group of people who differ from others in some characteristics and are often subjected to differential and unequal treatment and who therefore regard themselves as objects of discrimination (Wirth, 1945). An *ethnic*, or a *cultural* group is defined by similar beliefs and norms derived from shared history, common place of origin, language, dress, food preferences, and participation in voluntary clubs and associations.

Ethnicity is an ideology that supports pursuit of major values not shared by others in the sociopolitical arena. An ethnic ideology is representative of group attitudes that differ on the ultimate values (or goals and ends) of the system. The group wishes to be left alone (preferably with enough resources) to pursue its own ends (Aronson, 1976, pp. 14–15). Although *class* ideologies tend not to challenge dominant values in a society, ethnic ideologies tend to reflect cultural norms not shared by others in society. As an example, an individual who is forced to retire from gainful employment may find this exclusion from the larger society less traumatic if ethnic affiliations are maintained.

The first problem that occurs frequently in the literature is that social class imperatives and ethnic or cultural imperatives are treated as equivalent. Certainly position in class structure influences peoples' beliefs, behaviors, and adjustment to aging processes. However, social class position is largely determined by the larger society and is not unique to specific ethnic groups. That is, problems of being unemployed, uneducated, ill, and inadequately housed place the same pressures on Navaho Indian, Mandarin Chinese, and Lebanese people. The response of each of these ethnic groups to these social class–related problems may well vary according to the characteristics (values, traditions, self-concepts, customary life-styles, and so forth) that define their respective cultures or ethnicities.

A second common problem is to treat various members of ethnic groups as if they were culturally homogeneous (Holzberg, 1982, p. 251). In reality, ethnic groups may be quite diverse, having come from different regions in their countries of origin, at different times, and having been exposed to different experiences within this society. Assumptions of homogeneity may be used by some people to avoid providing services to elderly people. For example, although popular sociologic theory assumes that aged Chicanos can find support required to maintain themselves within their extended families, in reality, the extended family is only a myth. Urbanization has forced the breakup of Chicano families along with families in general. The role of elderly Chicanos has thus been undermined, leaving them with service needs similar to the larger elderly population (Waldonardo, 1979, p. 213).

To the extent that ethnicity actually operates as a mediator in solving some problems inherent in the aging process, problems such as normlessness, ambiguity, and identity loss, ethnicity should not be ignored (Holzberg, 1982, p. 253). To the extent that threats to health or actual health impairments can be linked to specific ethnic or racial groups, ethnicity and race become important phenomena to consider

when providing nursing services for elderly people. However, such associations remain to be established. In gathering information about the impact of ethnicity and racial identity on aging, nurses and others need to be careful not to confound "ethnic" or "racial" with "minority" or make assumptions about individuals based on their group affiliations.

Sex Composition

As a result of the unexplained longer, and more rapidly increasing life expectancy for women as compared to men, most older people are women: 15.2 million women and 10.3 million men were aged 65 years and older in 1980. Death rates are lower for females than for males at every age, including fetuses. Although there are 105 male babies born for every 100 female babies, the numbers at the same age are even by the end of the teen years and then females outnumber males in steadily increasing numbers thereafter. For every 100 women aged 65 and over, there were only 68 men; for every 100 women aged 75 and over, there were only 55 men and for every 100 women aged 85 and over there were only 44 men, in 1980 (U.S. Bureau of the Census, 1981). As little as 50 years ago, the numbers of elderly females and males was approximately equal. After 1930, females began living longer as infectious disease deaths and maternal mortality decreased. These trends have been the same, although less dramatic, for blacks as for whites. These figures are reported in Table 2.2.

The discrepancy between proportions of elderly women and men is expected to increase as numbers increase among the old-old, an age group where women especially outnumber men. This fact has significant health policy implications because age 75 and older is the time when disability due to chronic disease tends to increase, prompting greater reliance on social supports and economic resources. Old-old women tend to be widowed, live alone, and have less money than old-old men. These considerations have prompted gerontologists to acknowledge old age as primarily a women's problem (Krucoff, 1980; Hess, 1982).

TABLE 2.2 MEN AGED 65 YEARS AND OVER PER 100 WOMEN 65 YEARS
AND OVER, BY AGE AND RACE: 1900 TO 2000

Age and Race	1900	1930	1960	1970	1980	2000
Total 65 and over						
Over 65	102.0	100.4	82.6	72.2	67.6	67.7
Over 75	96.2	91.9	75.2	64.0	55.3	53.3
White						
Over 65	101.9	100.1	82.1	71.6	67.1	67.7
Over 75	97.1	92.0	74.3	63.2	54.5	53.3
Black						
Over 65	102.9	105.7	90.1	79.8	68.2	70.7
Over 75	89.6	89.6	87.6	74.7	60.3	62.8

(U. S. Bureau of the Census. Age, sex, race, and Spanish origin of the population
by regions, divisions and states, 1980. 1980 Census of the Population, PC 80-S1-
1, 1981, p. 3. U. S. Bureau of the Census. Projections of the population of the United
States: 1977–2050. Current Population Reports, Series P25, No. 704, 1977, p. 70.

Considerable advocacy needs to be done by nurses and others to change the economic picture for older women. Most of the institutions that provide retirement income, including social security, fail to recognize the contribution of women within the home or their interrupted work in the outside labor force because of years devoted to child care. Women who began formal employment at a late age due to divorce or widowhood often fail to qualify for the minimum number of years required to receive pensions. Among the aged in 1980 women were heavily overrepresented among the poor, with 19 percent having cash incomes below the official poverty level ($4,954 for an older couple household or $3,941 for an older individual living alone). Black women were among the poorest of the poor, with 43 percent living in households with incomes below the poverty level (Brotman, 1981, p. 4).

The importance of social support as a mechanism to enhance health has been underestimated. Social support seems to buffer the effects of stressors that enhance disease susceptibility (Cobb, 1976; Backus and Dudley, 1977; Moss, 1977; Blazer, 1982). The absence of social supports also appears to increase individual susceptibility to various pathologic conditions (McMiller and Ingham, 1976; Holmes, 1954). In the interests of promoting health, nurses need to make elderly clients aware of the value of social support and to use counseling or training techniques to help elderly clients learn and practice socially supportive behaviors (Gelein, 1980).

Research is required as part of the effort to help more men live longer. Such research will need to consider female–male differences in psychologic makeup as well as psychosocial differences that can be identified as sex-linked. Mortality statistics for women will receive close scrutiny as women enter the work force in greater numbers, and thus expose themselves to many of the stresses and hazards that have been blamed for causing or contributing to premature death in men.

Location

The elderly population tends to be distributed among the states in the same general pattern as the total population, except for slightly larger concentrations of elderly people in some of the larger states. Elderly people are more heavily concentrated in the Northeast and Northcentral regions than in the South and West. Within states, the proportion of elderly ranges from a high of 17.3 in Florida and 13.7 in Arkansas, to a low of 2.9 in Alaska, 7.5 in Utah, and 7.9 in Hawaii (Brotman, 1982, p. 44). These percentages are included in the complete list provided in Table 2.3.

TABLE 2.3 STATES BY PERCENT OF POPULATION AGED 65 AND OVER, 1980

Percent of Population 65 and over	States
17.3	Florida
13.7	Arkansas
13.4	Rhode Island
13.3	Iowa
13.2	Missouri, South Dakota
13.1	Nebraska
13.0	Kansas
12.9	Pennsylvania
12.7	Massachusetts
12.5	Maine
12.4	Oklahoma
12.3	New York, North Dakota
12.2	West Virginia
12.0	Wisconsin
11.8	Minnesota
11.7	Connecticut, New Jersey
11.6	District of Columbia
11.5	Mississippi, Oregon
11.4	Vermont
11.3	Tennessee, Arizona, Alabama
11.2	Kentucky, New Hampshire
11.0	Illinois
10.8	Ohio
10.7	Montana, Indiana
10.4	Washington
10.2	California, North Carolina
10.0	Delaware
9.9	Idaho
9.8	Michigan
9.6	Louisiana, Texas
9.5	Georgia
9.4	Maryland, Virginia
9.2	South Carolina
8.9	New Mexico
8.6	Colorado
8.2	Nevada
8.0	Wyoming
7.9	Hawaii
7.5	Utah
2.9	Alaska

(Brotman, H. B. Every Ninth American (1982 edition). Washington D.C., U. S. Government Printing Office, 1982, p. 44.)

Geographic mobility of the elderly has been examined in terms of general mobility that considers movers between states, within states, and within local communities (Brotman, 1982a).

Movers between states tend to be younger, married, in good physical health, and economically stable. The move is often to retirement communities or rural settings, in search of recreation, a temperate climate, or satisfaction associated with returning to the state of birth (Wiseman, 1980; Biggar, 1980). Intrastate moves are usually motivated by a need to be close to children or other significant people. People who move within a state also tend to be financially comfortable although beginning to experience declines in their physical resources (Aday and Miles, 1982). Unlike in the other two types of moves, people who move locally are often forced to relocate to find assistance in dealing with poor health and low financial resources (Lawton, Kleban, and Carlson, 1973). Aging-in-place has, since 1950, represented the single most important factor in growth of the percentage of population 65 years and over for both metropolitan and nonmetropolitan areas (Lichter et al., 1981). People simply grow older where they live, without moving. Particularly in metropolitan areas, the effect of net migration of elderly people has been minimal, at least through 1975. In nonmetropolitan areas, elderly net migration has shown a substantial increase between 1950–60 and 1970–75. However, similar immigration of younger people has almost entirely offset the elderly effect so the change in the elderly percentage in nonmetropolitan areas has been minimal (Lichter et al., 1981). In examining the migration phenomenon, a second study found that a majority of elderly people exchange similar settings, moving either within metropolitan areas or within nonmetropolitan areas. Among the minority of elderly whose moves were to a different environment, a majority tended to move from metropolitan to nonmetropolitan areas. Within states, similar movement by younger people offset the net increase in nonmetropolitan areas. Across states, however, migration of elderly people into nonmetropolitan areas resulted in an actual increase in the proportion of elderly people (Longino, 1982).

In societies like the United States, with low fertility and mortality rates, migration is the main means of population redistribution.

The implication of this redistribution for service delivery relates directly to the service needs of the particular population. It is felt that elderly people (1) have a greater impact on consumption demands than on labor market pressure, (2) increase demands for housing, public safety, and transportation, and (3) present substantial needs for health-care resources. Actually, these assumptions cannot be used to plan local or regional programs without considering attributes specific to elderly people in the geographic area of interest. If an area, state or local, receives immigrants with characteristics that indicate a healthier and more active group of elders, or loses residents who are older and more economically and residentially dependent, then migration benefits the state. When the opposite pattern prevails, migration does not benefit the state.

Assessments of health service needs of elderly people depend not only on their numbers, including the size and patterns of geographic distribution, but on their demographic and socioeconomic characteristics. For example, a study comparing elderly migrants to Florida versus California found that both migrant groups were economically advantaged. However, key differences emerged in respect to demographic and residential characteristics. Florida attracted more married couples and white people who owned their own homes and lived independently. California attracted more widows who lived with children and other relatives (Longino and Biggar, 1982). Nurse-planners need to know numbers and proportions of elderly people who are (1) below the poverty level and (2) over age 75 years in order to decide the extent to which nursing services should be directed toward secondary and tertiary prevention as opposed to primary prevention. This same information can help educators plan the extent to which gerontologic nursing needs to be included in curricula and permit researchers to justify problems chosen for studies. Graduate nurses can use information about geographically specific service needs to decide the state and local area in which they want to practice nursing, depending on their preference for and knowledge of gerontologic nursing.

HEALTH STATUS OF THE ELDERLY

This section defines the health status of elderly people by considering the following indicators of health: global ratings of self-assessed health, chronic conditions and functional impairments, and death. Factors commonly associated with variations in health status are discussed: social support (marital status and living arrangements), educational attainment, and economic status.

Health can be defined holistically as the "actualization of human potential through purposeful self-initiated behavior, satisfying relationships with others, and competent personal care" (Pender, 1982, p. 39), although health is a concept that still requires clarification. Health indicators selected for this section were not chosen to support an alternative definition of health as the "absence of disease." Rather these indicators were chosen because they are the traditional methods used to define and measure the level of health within populations. As such, they are understood by large segments of society. Indication of other components of health such as "engagement in purposeful, self-initiated behavior," and "satisfying relationships with others" was not possible because these concepts have not been precisely defined to permit accurate measurement. Some indication of how elderly people fare in respect to their relationships with others, as well as their work and leisure pursuits, is provided in chapters that follow.

The aged who are apparently well are not necessarily free of health-related problems. The aged who are ill are to some degree healthy, or they would not be alive. Nursing's concern with health relates to helping people to help themselves toward attainable health. That is, nursing practice is the diagnosis and treatment of human responses to actual or potential health problems (American Nurses' Association, 1980). The kinds of activities involved in such practice are aggressive health promotion, early detection of signs, symptoms, or risks of disease, and provision of indicated treatment. Insofar as the nursing profession can continue to develop the skills to support people in healthful lifetime behavior patterns, nurses may be instrumental in improving the quality of health among the elderly population. The goal of such an effort is to ensure that the thrill of living does not end before life itself.

Self-Assessed Health Status

Utility of self-assessed health has been questioned in terms of both the right of individuals to judge for themselves and the accuracy of the decisions made (Weiss and Lord, 1980). Some people believe a "health definer," usually a physician, is required to define normal health and that disagreement between these two parties signifies aberrant behavior on the part of the individual (Twaddle, 1974). Other people believe an individual's self-assessment of health can be as important as physician-defined medical status in predicting general emotional state and behavior (Maddox and Douglas, 1973).

Most elderly people, aged 65 years and older, regard themselves as healthy. Table 2.4 presents self-health ratings of 1836 noninstitutionalized elderly Americans surveyed in 1981. Over half (56 percent) of this group rated their health as good or excellent. Poor health was reported by only 13 percent and was somewhat more common among women than men (15 versus 11 percent) and among older age

groups: 17 percent for people aged 80 years and older; 15 percent, 70–79 years; and 9 percent, 65–69 years. However, in each sex and age category, a majority of older people viewed their health positively, as being good or excellent (National Council on the Aging, 1981, pp. 136–137).

Examination of self-rated health by race, however, revealed a decidedly different picture. Majorities of elderly blacks (63 percent) and Hispanics (62 percent) regarded their health as "only fair" or "poor."

Results from this National Council on the Aging study were similar to those from the 1979 household interview sample survey conducted by the National Center for Health Statistics, in which 68 percent of the older persons reported their health as good or excellent and only 9 percent reported their health as poor. Minority group members, residents of the South, residents of nonmetropolitan areas, and people with low incomes were more likely to report their health as poor (Brotman, 1980; 1982a).

Differences observed in self-assessed health between white and minority elderly Americans, as well as males and females, are supported by other measures of health status, such as life expectancy and mortality statistics, and serve to highlight differences in access to health support resources.

TABLE 2.4 SELF-RATED PERSONAL HEALTH STATUS BY NONINSTITUTIONALIZED PEOPLE AGED 65 YEARS AND OLDER, 1981

Demographic Characteristic	Number	Health Status (Percent Distribution)				
		Excellent	Good	Only Fair	Poor	Not Sure
Age group						
65+	1836	17	39	30	13	*
65–69	675	21	43	27	9	*
70–79	844	15	37	32	15	*
80+	317	14	37	31	17	1
Sex						
Female	1050	17	37	31	15	*
Male	786	18	42	29	11	*
Race/Minority						
White	1345	18	41	29	12	*
Black	274	11	25	42	21	*
Hispanic	190	10	28	41	21	*

*Less than 0.5%. (National Council on the Aging. Aging in the Eighties: America in Transition. Washington, D.C., National Council on Aging, 1981, p. 137.)

Chronic Conditions and Functional Impairments

Aging does not cause any specific disease, but certain illnesses, especially chronic ones, are more prevalent among elderly people. Acute illnesses (lasting less than three months) are less common among the elderly than the total population. For the individual, the major inconvenience of health problems is limitation of abilities to do things, that is to see, hear, speak, walk, think clearly, and control elimination, to name a few of the abilities people rely upon to perform social roles or obligations.

Nurses and elderly clients alike are more immediately concerned about the impact of chronic conditions on functional status. Chronic conditions are those that last three months or more. Only 14 percent of the noninstitutionalized elderly can claim to be free of chronic illnesses (Soldo, 1980; Brotman, 1980). The most frequently reported chronic conditions among noninstitutionalized elderly people in 1979 were arthritis (44 percent), hypertension (39 percent), hearing impairment (28 percent), heart conditions (27 percent), and vision impairments and arteriosclerosis (each about 12 percent) (Brotman, 1982a, p. 12). The 1975 U.S. Federal Commission on Chronic Illness estimated a rate of 4402 chronic diseases per 1000 people aged 65 years or older, compared with a rate of 407 chronic diseases per 1000 people under 16 years of age (Jette and Branch, 1981, p. 1211).

However, chronic illness does not always lead to functional disability. Data collected from noninstitutionalized elderly people in the Framingham study (2635 people interviewed) were compared with data from other large sample surveys that examined similar disabilities: Branch's 1976 Massachusetts Elders survey (1623 elderly people) (Branch, 1977) and the 1979 National Health Interview Survey (23,343 elderly people) (National Center for Health Statistics, 1982). If the measure "inability to do heavy housework" from the first two studies is considered comparable to "limited in" or "unable to carry on major activity" such as housework or other work, the measure used in the third study, then the functional

impairment rates were 36 percent in the Framingham study, 43 percent in Branch's study, and 39 percent in the National Health Interview Survey. From a positive perspective, between 57 and 64 percent of elderly people were able to carry on their major activity.

Examination of the ability of elderly people living in the community to perform selected activities of daily living from three different studies produced remarkably consistent results. The Framingham Study, 1976–1978 (Jette and Branch, 1981), the National Health Interview Survey, 1977 (unpublished), and Massachusetts Elders Study, 1976 (Branch, 1977) found that 95 to 99 percent of the respondents could walk, at least within their homes, 94 to 98 percent could bathe independently, 96 to 99 percent could dress themselves, and 98 to 99 percent could eat without assistance. Thus, noninstitutionalized elderly people are not necessarily bothered by physical disabilities, despite their having chronic diseases. In fact, evidence indicates that a majority of these elderly enjoy substantial physical ability.

This picture does change for the worse as people approach and go beyond 85 years of age. The 1977 National Health Interview Survey found the percent of elderly people needing assistance to move about increased from 10.5 for those aged 65–74 years to 71.8 for those aged 85 years and older; need for help with bathing increased from 2.1 to 15.1 percent; dressing from 1.5 to 9.5 percent; toileting from 0.9 to 6.7 percent; and eating from 0.5 to 3.9 percent. These results may be found in Table 2.5.

Prevalence rates for functional disabilities increase markedly in the nursing home population compared with the noninstitutionalized elderly population. Table 2.6 compares these rates for selected activities of daily living. In the community in 1977, 80.9 percent of people aged 65 years and older were independent in terms of mobility compared with only 30.8 percent of the predominantly elderly population in nursing homes. The same comparison was 96.2 versus 11.4 percent for bathing; 97.4 versus 28.3 for dressing; 98.6 versus 54.8 percent for toileting, and 99.2 versus 66.4 percent for eating.

TABLE 2.5 PERCENT OF ELDERLY PEOPLE NEEDING HELP WITH SELECTED ACTIVITIES OF DAILY LIVING BECAUSE OF A DISABILITY OR HEALTH PROBLEM, UNITED STATES, 1977

Functional Disability	Noninstitutionalized Elderly People			
	65 + Years	65–74 Years	75–84 Years	85 + Years
	Total Number of Persons in Thousands			
	22,666	14,259	6652	1355
	Percent Distribution			
Help Needed:				
Moving About	19.1	10.5	26.3	71.8
Help needed outside neighborhood	(8.4)	(4.6)	(12.0)	(30.6)
Help needed in neighborhood	(6.0)	(3.1)	(8.3)	(24.4)
Help needed inside house	(2.6)	(1.4)	(3.4)	(10.8)
Confined to bed	(2.1)	(1.4)	(2.6)	(6.0)
Bathing	3.8	2.1	5.3	15.1
Dressing	2.6	1.5	3.6	9.5
Toileting	1.4	0.9	1.6	6.7
Eating	0.8	0.5	0.9	3.9
No Help Needed:				
Moving about	80.9	89.5	73.7	28.2
Bathing	96.2	97.9	94.7	84.9
Dressing	97.4	98.5	96.4	90.5
Toileting	98.6	99.1	98.4	93.3
Eating	99.2	99.5	99.1	96.1

(Unpublished data from the National Health Interview Survey, National Center for Health Statistics, 1977. National Center for Health Statistics. A comparison of nursing home residents and discharges from the 1977 National Nursing Home Survey: United States, 1978, p. 4. Brotman, H. B. Every Ninth American. In Developments in Aging: 1979. A Report of the Special Committee on Aging, United States Senate. Washington, D.C., U. S. Government Printing Office, 1980, p. 12.)

Table 2.7 presents data comparing vision, hearing, and speech impairments between elderly people in the community and those in nursing homes. Rates of vision and hearing impairments derived from self-reports are lower than those derived from objective measurements. Objective testing used in the Health and Nutrition Examination Survey revealed that 66.8 percent of people aged 65 to 74 years failed to meet the speech reception test criterion (National Center for Health Statistics, 1980, p. 2) and that the potential for people to see at the 20/20 level was only 32.9 percent with correction (National Center for Health Statistics, 1978, p. 12). The discrepancies in subjectively versus objectively assessed vision and hearing status support a need for objective testing to determine how well older people see and hear.

Old age as such is not a disease, but even experts sometimes have difficulty distinguishing changes that come with normal aging and that are not reversible from changes that occur as a result of disease and that can be reversed. Normal aging may involve change (increases or decreases) or stability. Nurses and others who work with elderly people tend to expect decreases and increases but overlook stability. For example, hematocrit values do not change in old age (Kannel and Gordon, 1974).

If the laboratory report for an 88-year-old woman showed a hematocrit value of 36 percent, a nurse expecting decline might plan with the client for energy conservation as a means of coping with associated complaints of fatigue. Further assessment to determine cause for the "normal" value would not be considered necessary.

TABLE 2.6 COMPARISON OF ELDERLY PEOPLE NEEDING HELP WITH SELECTED ACTIVITIES OF DAILY LIVING BETWEEN COMMUNITY AND NURSING HOME SETTINGS, UNITED STATES, 1977

Functional Disability	Noninstitutionalized, 65 Years and Over (1977 National Health Interview Survey)	Institutionalized, 65 Years and Over (1977 National Nursing Home Survey)
	Total Number of Persons in Thousands	
	22,666	1126
	Percent Distribution	
Mobility		
Independent	80.9	30.8
Requires assistance	17.0	63.8
Bedfast	2.1	5.2
Bathing		
Independent	96.2	11.4
Requires assistance	3.8	88.6
Dressing		
Independent	97.4	28.3
Requires assistance	2.6	71.7
Toileting		
Independent	98.6	45.2
Requires assistance or does not use toilet	1.4	54.8
Eating		
Independent	99.2	66.4
Requires assistance	0.8	33.6

(Unpublished data from the National Health Interview Survey, National Center for Health Statistics, 1977. National Center for Health Statistics. Characteristics of nursing home residents, health status, and care received: National Nursing Home Survey, United States, May–December, 1977, 1981, p. 64. Brotman, H. B. Every Ninth American. In Developments in Aging: 1979. A Report of the Special Committee on Aging, United States Senate. Washington, D.C., U. S. Government Printing Office, 1980, p. 12.)

TABLE 2.7 COMPARISON OF PEOPLE AGED 65 YEARS AND OVER WITH VISION, HEARING, AND COMMUNICATION IMPAIRMENTS—COMMUNITY (1980) VERSUS NURSING HOME (1977)

Functional Disability	Nursing Home Residents* 1977 (1,126,000)	Community Residents† 1980 (Rate per 1000)
Vision impairment	30.6%	12.2%
Hearing impairment	29.7%	28.3%
Speech impairment	21.4%	1.5%

*National Nursing Home Survey, 1977 (based on staff reports).
†Unpublished data from the National Household Interview Survey, 1980 (based on self-reports). (Unpublished data from the National Health Interview Survey, National Center for Health Statistics, 1980. National Center for Health Statistics. Characteristics of nursing home residents, health status, and care received: National Nursing Home Survey, United States, May–December, 1977, 1981, pp. 17, 63. U. S. Bureau of the Census. Age, sex, race, and Spanish origin of the population by regions, divisions, and states, 1980, 1981, p. 3.)

A second bias involves the assumption that normality means harmlessness. For example, systolic blood pressure values increase with advancing age. However, research might reveal that people who experience the greatest elevations are more likely to experience transient ischemic attacks or cerebrovascular accidents. Advancing age is a risk factor for both disease and death (Hickey, 1980; Rowe, 1981).

Only a comparatively small proportion of noninstitutionalized elderly people have sufficient social disability to require extensive public assistance or support. Social disability has been defined as "limitation in or inability to perform social roles or obligations" (Branch and Jette, 1981, p. 1202). Examples of social roles or obligations include maintaining an income and performing household chores required to ensure food, clothing, and shelter. Comparisons among results of three large sample surveys yielded remarkably similar conclusions about social disability among noninstitutionalized elderly people. The studies compared were the 1976 Massachusetts Elders Survey (Branch, 1977), the University of Delaware Study (Barnekov, 1980), and the Framingham Disability Study (Branch and Jette, 1981). These results, compared in Table 2.8, indicated that from 64–79 percent of elderly people, residing in the community, were self-sufficient in terms of transportation; 70–86 percent were able to manage housekeeping

chores without apparent problems; 67–70 percent were able to meet their own needs for social interaction; 79–86 percent were able to prepare food without assistance; and 76–91 percent needed no help to shop for groceries. Even in the area of transportation, where the smallest percentages (64 and 69 percent) in two of the studies were able to meet their own needs and the highest level of unmet need was noted (4 and 7 percent) in two of the three studies, a majority of the noninstitutionalized elderly people were self-sufficient.

Although social disability increased with advancing age, members of even the oldest age group living in the community did not display an overwhelming amount of unmet social need. Table 2.9 indicates that in the oldest of three groups, aged 75–84 years, a majority of elderly people were able to meet their own needs in the five areas of potential social disability considered. In each of three age groups, females were less likely than males to have their needs met.

Death

The medical model assumes all death is caused by disease and if there were no disease, there would be no death (Fries, 1981). Discussions of death among elderly people are fused with discussions of illnesses as causes of death. Planning for elderly people is largely directed

TABLE 2.8 COMPARISON OF PERCENTAGE OF SOCIAL DISABILITY ESTIMATES FOR PEOPLE AGED 65 YEARS AND OLDER FROM THREE LARGE-SAMPLE SURVEYS: FRAMINGHAM DISABILITY STUDY (FDS), MASSACHUSETTS ELDERS STUDY (MASS.), AND UNIVERSITY OF DELAWARE STUDY (DEL.)

Social Area	Need Met No Apparent Problem			Potential Problem			Need Unmet Current Problem		
	FDS	Mass.	Del.	FDS	Mass.	Del.	FDS	Mass.	Del.
Housekeeping	74	86	70	23	12	20	3	2	10
Transportation	79	69	64	16	24	28	4	7	8
Social interaction	68	70	67	31	27	31	2	2	2
Food preparation	84	86	79	17	13	21	*	*	1
Grocery shopping	91	86	76	9	13	20	*	1	3

*Percent greater than zero but less than 0.5 percent. (Branch, L. G., Jette, A. M. The Framingham disability study, I: Social disability among the aging. American Journal of Public Health 71(11):1207, 1981. Copyright 1981 by the American Public Health Association. Reprinted by permission.)

TABLE 2.9 PERCENT OF NONINSTITUTIONALIZED ELDERLY PEOPLE, BY SEX, WITH SOCIAL NEEDS MET/NO APPARENT PROBLEMS IN FIVE NEED AREAS

| Age Groups | Area of Potential Social Disability | | | | |
	Housekeeping	Transportation	Social Interaction	Food Preparation	Grocery Shopping
Total					
55–64	80	86	71	72	93
65–74	79	86	70	82	95
75–84	64	67	64	86	83
55–64					
Female	73	81	72	71	94
Male	89	90	69	74	92
65–74					
Female	72	83	70	78	95
Male	90	91	69	88	95
75–84					
Female	56	59	62	84	79
Male	79	80	68	89	89

(Branch, L. G., Jette, A. M. The Framingham disability study, I: Social disability among the aging. American Journal of Public Health 71(11):1205–1206, 1981. Copyright 1981 by the American Public Health Association. Reprinted by permission.)

by the assumption that old age is a period of decremental function and disability that leads to escalating requirements for expensive medical care and social support. Examination of trends in morbidity* and mortality† curves suggests that the medical model is not correct and the gloomy view of old age the model inspires will not come to pass. Adult vigor may extend far into a fixed lifespan so that first infirmities, if they occur at all, occur near the end of life.

The length of life (longevity) is fixed but the average length of life (life expectancy) is increasing. Length of life concerns the question, "How long could a person live if . . . (there were no disease; if the person tried hard enough)?" If immortality were possible, some people could reasonably be expected to have avoided disease and lived much longer than expected. Information from studies of people with documented birth dates indicates that people do not live on and on. To illustrate, ad-

equate data on the number of centenarians have been available in England since 1837; over this time, despite a great change in average life expectancy, there has been no detectable change in the number of people living longer than 100 years or in the maximum age of people dying in a given year (Comfort, 1979, pp. 81–86). In Sweden, where careful studies of centenarians are conducted, not one has exceeded 110 years of age. The greatest documented age in the world was recorded in Japan—114 years of age (McWhirter, 1980). Approximately 1 in 10,000 people in developed countries lives beyond 100 years of age (Fries, 1981, p. 106). There has been no satisfactory evidence that any society enjoys exceptional longevity. The *Guinness Book of World Records* reports the correlation between the claimed density of centenarians in a country and the regional illiteracy rate as 0.83 (McWhirter, 1980). Theoretic reasons for limited longevity are considered under biologic theories of aging in Chapter 3.

Life expectancy concerns the question, "How many of the years theoretically available to me, can I expect to actually live?" More people live the number of years they are expected to live than ever before. Life expectancy has

---

* Morbidity refers to the incidence of illness within a population.
† Mortality refers to the incidence of death within a population.

increased steadily since the turn of the century. Mortality refers to the incidence of death within a population. The nation's mortality rate declined during the 1900s from 17 per 1000 population to less than 9 per 1000 in recent years (Soldo, 1980, p. 15). During the first half of the century, mortality decline was concentrated at the younger ages, resulting in a relative increase in the number of young people in the population. During the second half of the century, decreases in mortality occurred for people of all ages, resulting in a larger elderly population than would have occurred if declines had remained entirely at the younger years (Fingerhut and Rosenberg, 1982, p. 15).

A person born in 1900 could expect to live to age 47.3 years on the average; a person born in 1978, could live to age 73 years on the average—a gain of 26 years. A person who had reached age 65 in 1900 could expect, on the average, to live another 11.9 years; a person who reached age 65 in 1978 could expect, on the average, to live another 16.1 years—a gain of only 4.2 years. A steady rise in life expectancy from the early years of the century changed to a relative plateau after 1950. In 1970, the rate of improvement picked up again when the gain was 2.4 years, almost as much improvement as occurred between 1950 and 1970 (Soldo, 1980, p. 15). These mortality figures reflect progress in the elimination of premature death. A dramatic fall in deaths from infectious diseases and a modest decline in diseases of early infancy influenced the decline during the first half of the century. For people aged 40 years and older, life expectancy has increased little and for people aged 75 years and older, the improvement is barely noticeable. However, the decline in deaths that began in 1970 benefited people in the older age groups and has been attributed to steady declines in death from cardiovascular diseases (Myers, 1978). These life expectancy figures for people at various ages are presented in Figure 2.4.*

_____

* Figure 2.4 presents a paradox. If the lines were extrapolated into the future, at some point in the twenty-first century, the average life expectancy as projected at birth would exceed the average age of death as projected at age 75 (Fries, 1981, p. 107).

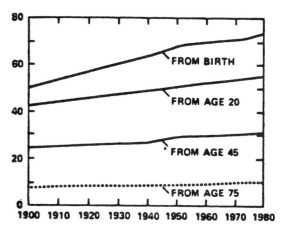

Figure 2.4. Life expectancy trends in the United States. Life expectancy at birth has increased by 26 years and life expectancy at 75 (broken line) by only 3 years. The slope decreases as the lifespan is neared. *(Fries, J.F. Aging, natural death, and the compression of morbidity. In Somers, A.R., Fabian, D.R., (eds.). The Geriatric Imperative. New York, Appleton-Century-Crofts, 1981, p 107. Copyright 1981 by Appleton-Century-Crofts. Reprinted by permission.)*

The net effect of changes in mortality/life expectancy rates has been to make sequential survival curves throughout the century more rectangular to reflect an increasingly sharp downslope to the natural lifespan. Figure 2.5 shows the ideal, rectangular survival curve that would occur if all premature death were eliminated and the progress made toward that ideal curve between 1900 and 1980 were maintained. A normal biologic distribution (without trauma) suggests that under ideal societal conditions, mean age at death is about 85 years.

At all ages, men have shorter life expectancies than women. A woman aged 65 years in 1978 could expect to live 18 more years (on the average) compared to a man in the same year and of the same age who could expect to live 14 more years (Soldo, 1980, p. 16). Taken from birth, the difference in life expectancy between the sexes is greater. A woman born in 1978 could expect to live 77.2 years, on the average, while a man could expect to live 69.5 years—a difference of 7.7 years. This difference in life expectancy has increased steadily since the turn of the century. In 1900, the difference in life expectancy at age 65 was 0.7 years (12.2

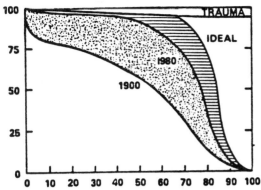

Figure 2.5. The increasingly rectangular survival curve. About 80 percent (stippled area) of the difference between the 1900 curve and the ideal curve (stippled area plus hatched area) had been eliminated by 1980. Trauma is the dominant cause of death in early life. *(Fries, J.F. Aging, natural death, and the compression of morbidity. In Somers, A.R., Fabian, D.R., (eds.). The Geriatric Imperative. New York, Appleton-Century-Crofts, 1981, p 108. Copyright 1981 by Appleton-Century-Crofts. Reprinted by permission.)*

1973). Chronic illness is now responsible for over 70 percent of all deaths and for an even higher percent of cases of total disability (Brotman, 1982a). Heart disease, cancer, and cerebrovascular accidents accounted for three-fourths of the deaths of the elderly in 1978, as they did in 1965. However, during this period the death rate for older people from heart disease dropped 18 percent; the death rate from cerebrovascular accidents dropped 33 percent, but the rate of death from cancer increased 11 percent. These declines in death rates are largely responsible for the recent increases in life expectancy in the upper ages (Brotman, 1982a. pp. 14–15). Figure 2.6 illustrates the relative impact of various causes of death among people aged 65 years and older.

Arteriosclerosis (including coronary heart

years for women versus 11.5 years for men). In 1950, the difference was 2.2 years (15 years for women versus 12.8 years for men). In 1978, the difference was 3.9 years (18.0 years for women versus 14.1 for men).

At all but the extremes of old age, non-whites have fewer years remaining to them than whites. A 65-year-old white woman in 1978 could expect to live to age 83.4, 4.4 years longer than either a white or nonwhite man and 2.3 years more than a nonwhite woman. Table 2.10 presents shifts in life expectancies for the sexes and races from birth and from age 65 for selected years.

The leading causes of death have shifted from acute to chronic illnesses. In the early 1900s mortality was largely due to acute, usually infectious disease. Tuberculosis, acute rheumatic fever, smallpox, diphtheria, tetanus, poliomyelitis, and pneumococcal pneumonia were the main causes of death (National Center for Health Statistics, 1978). The decline in these diseases can be attributed to a number of factors: improved nutrition, water sterilization, less crowded living arrangements, immunization, and specific antibiotics (Ashley,

TABLE 2.10 CHANGES IN LIFE EXPECTANCIES AT BIRTH AND AT AGE 65, BY RACE AND SEX, FOR SELECTED YEARS

Age, Sex, and Race	1900*	1950	1978†
	Life Expectancy at Birth		
Total	47.3	68.2	73.3
Men	46.3	65.6	69.5
Women	48.3	71.1	77.2
White	47.6	69.1	74.0
Men	46.6	66.5	70.2
Women	48.7	72.2	77.8
Nonwhite	33.0	60.8	69.2
Men	32.5	59.1	65.0
Women	33.5	62.9	73.6
	Life Expectancy at Age 65		
Total	11.9	13.9	16.1
Men	11.5	12.8	14.1
Women	12.2	15.0	18.0
White	—	—	16.4
Men	11.5	12.8	14.0
Women	12.2	15.1	18.4
Nonwhite	—	—	16.1
Men	10.4	12.5	14.0
Women	11.4	14.5	16.1

*Death registration area only.
†Excludes deaths of U. S. nonresidents. *(From Soldo, B. J., America's elderly in the 1980s. Population Bulletin 35(4):16, 1980.)*

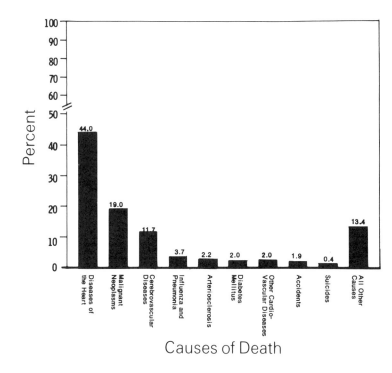

Figure 2.6. Major causes of death for people 65 years and older, 1978. (Brotman, H. *Every Ninth American* (1982 Edition). Washington, D.C., U.S. Government Printing Office, 1982, p. 15.)

disease and cerebrovascular disease), arthritis, adult-onset diabetes, chronic obstructive pulmonary disease, cancer, and cirrhosis are widespread health problems that probably originate early in life and develop insidiously. The likelihood of their occurrence increases with age. These problems can be considered to involve gradual loss of organ reserves with slow progression occurring below a clinical threshold. When and if the clinical threshold is reached, the process becomes clinically evident, progresses, and usually ends in disability or death. If this assumption is true, chronic diseases may be effectively approached using a strategy of "postponement" rather than cure. If the rate of progression is decreased, then the date of passage through a clinical threshold is delayed; if delayed long enough, the symptomatic threshold may not be crossed during a lifetime and the disease can be considered "prevented" (Fries, 1981, p. 110). Postponement of chronic illness will result in a more rectangular morbidity as well as mortality curve. Implications of these trends for society and for health-care delivery are profound.

By implication, the practical focus on health improvement over the next decades must be on chronic instead of acute disease, on morbidity not mortality, on quality of life rather than its duration, and on postponement rather than cure. The complex nature of the major diseases calls attention to multifactorial influences on outcome, in particular, social and psychologic factors. Outcome is related to choice; assumption of personal responsibility, education for making decisions about personal health, and ability to encourage self-care are clearly essential to changing health behaviors (Fries, 1981, p. 112).

In the years to come, the elderly population may follow this essentially healthy model, "in which life is physically, emotionally, and intellectually vigorous until shortly before its close, when . . . everything comes apart at once and repair is impossible" (Fries, 1981, p. 114). Alternatively, elderly people may become a larger and more disabled population as more people live to be very old and require expensive care. The course followed may depend on how able people are to postpone chronic illnesses by changing their life-styles. Premature organ dysfunction, whether of muscle, heart, lung, or joint, is beginning to be viewed as caused by disease of the part, not overuse. If loss of reserve function represents aging in some way, then exercising an organ presents a strategy for modifying the aging process. Nurses, with skills in teaching and motivating clients, may indeed emerge as the professionals most able to help clients change life-styles to promote health. Appendix A of this book contains a longevity quiz that nurses may wish to use themselves and with their clients to estimate life expectancy.

When elderly people die and under what conditions has not been adequately documented. For example, do the elderly die at home or in institutions? Do they die alone? Are they physically comfortable as they die? Are they asleep or awake? The National Institute on Aging identified location of death and related events as priority areas for study in 1982 (National Institute on Aging, 1982). Thus, results of research may eventually permit accurate description of this neglected area of the death experience.

Associated Factors
Ability to manage changes in health that come with old age depends heavily on whether or not people are married, their living arrangements, educational attainment, and financial situation.

Life-Style
Improving the quality of life for the old and the old-old is a complex task. Although it may be disappointing to learn that a pill or a surgical procedure will not provide a solution, the answer probably does not lie in improving the health-care system. "Life styles—including pollution exposure, exercise patterns, nutrition, smoking behavior, alcohol consumption—can have a greater impact on health than the health care system itself" (National Council on the Aging, 1978, p. 102). Additional evidence for this proposition was provided by Miller and Stokes (1978). Community characteristics, such as income, education, occupation, and residence (urban or rural), were found to have a greater impact on health status (mortality) than

the prevailing health-care resources. In addition, mortality rates tended to be lower in areas where nurses were relatively more concentrated as compared to physicians, and higher where the opposite relationship existed (Miller and Stokes, 1978). A second study used physiologic measurements to assess the effects of medical care resources on health status. Results were consistent with the view that medical resources have less of an impact on an individual's health than the individual does (or does not do) for himself (Newhouse and Freidlander, 1979).

The amount of choice people have about their health in old age is increasing constantly as people exert control over health-related factors such as diet, exercise, weight control, responses to stress, and habits concerning alcohol, tobacco, and drugs.

A positive relationship has been found between good health practices and good physical health (Billoc and Breslow, 1972) as well as lower age-specific mortality rates (Breslow and Enstrom, 1980). The health practices, evaluated in these studies, conducted in 1965 in Alameda County, California, and reassessed in the 1977 National Health Interview Survey (National Center for Health Statistics, 1980) were as follows: (1) averaging 7–8 hours of sleep per night, (2) eating breakfast almost every day, (3) seldom, if ever, eating snacks, (4) controlling body weight to within 5 percent under and 19.9 percent over the desirable standard weight if male or not weighing more than 9.9 percent over the desirable standard weight, if female; (5) exercising by (a) engaging in active sports, (b) swimming, (c) taking long walks, (d) gardening, or (e) doing physical exercises; (6) limiting alcohol consumption to less than five drinks at one sitting, and (7) never having smoked cigarettes. In the 1965 survey, persons who reported six or seven of these health practices had better health status and lived longer than persons reporting less than four of them. In the 1977 survey, substantial majorities of elderly people were found to eat breakfast daily (36 percent), engage in more or at least the same amount of activity as other persons their age (85 percent), never drink or drink only occasionally (82 percent), and smoke no longer or to have never smoked (83 percent). Many of these health practices are included in the longevity quiz contained in Appendix A of this book.

Marital Status

In 1980, most older men were married (7.3 million, or 76 percent) while most older women were widowed (7.1 million, or 51 percent) (U.S. Senate Special Committee on Aging, 1982, p. 13). Marrying a younger person is more socially acceptable for men than for women. About 35 percent of men aged 65 years or older have wives who are under 65 years of age (Brotman, 1982a, p. 22), whereas few women aged 65 or older have husbands who are under 65 years of age. In addition, elderly men have a large number of single women in their own age group to marry while, elderly women have few potential mates to choose from in their own age group.

Living Arrangements

The vast majority of elderly people live in the community and most of these people live in family households (with spouse or another relative). Women and the old-old, however, are more likely than men or the young-old to be living alone or with a nonrelative. In 1980, 83 percent of older men but only 57 percent of the older women lived in a family setting. Four out of every 10 older women lived alone or with nonrelatives compared to less than two out of every 10 older men. Living arrangements of the elderly population residing in the community are detailed in Table 2.11.

Contrary to widespread beliefs among the lay public, only about 1 in 20 of all elderly people and 1 in 11 of the 75-year and older age groups reside in institutions at any one time. The institutionalized elderly are disproportionately older, white, female, and unmarried compared to the community-based elderly population (Soldo, 1980, p. 26).

Educational Attainment

Educational levels have increased over time as each succeeding generation has had an opportunity to receive more education than its predecessor. Thus, as each group with more years of schooling reaches old age and the oldest age group dies, the median educational level increases. From 1970 to 1979, the median educational attainment of the elderly population

TABLE 2.11 LIVING ARRANGEMENTS OF THE 65 YEAR AND OLDER, NONINSTITUTIONAL POPULATION, 1980

Age and Living Arrangements	Male		Female	
	Number*	Percent	Number*	Percent
65+:				
Total	9783	100.0	13,960	100.0
Living with spouse	7389	75.5	5311	38.0
Living with other relative	727	7.4	2660	19.1
Living alone or with nonrelative	1667	17.0	5989	42.9
65–74:				
Total	6549	100.0	8549	100.0
Living with spouse	5199	79.4	4114	48.1
Living with other relative	426	6.5	1243	14.5
Living alone or with nonrelative	924	14.1	3192	37.3
75+:				
Total	3234	100.0	5411	100.0
Living with spouse	2190	67.7	1197	22.1
Living with other relative	301	9.3	1417	26.2
Living alone or with nonrelative	743	23.0	2797	51.7

*Numbers in thousands. (Brotman, H. Every Ninth American (1982 Edition). Washington, D.C., U. S. Government Printing Office, 1982a, p. 27.)

increased by more than one year. In 1978, about half the population under age 65 had at least a high school education compared to only a third of those people aged 65 or older (Soldo, 1980, p. 19). About 9 percent of elderly people were "functionally illiterate," having had less than five years of schooling, while about 8 percent were college graduates (Brotman, 1982a, p. 26).

Comparatively low levels of education do handicap elderly people. Poorly educated people experience difficulty locating service and benefit programs as well as coping with the paperwork and bureaucratic structure inherent in such programs. The association between better health status and greater educational attainment (Miller and Stokes, 1978) suggests that poorly educated people may be less able to recognize deviations in health status, engage in health-promoting behaviors such as adequate nutrition or exercise, and select appropriate intervention for health problems. With retirement, poorly educated people are limited in their activities because they tend not to enjoy intellectually stimulating pursuits that require reading and writing abilities and they may be physically unable to pursue activities that require physical strength, coordination, and endurance.

Financial Situation
Reductions in income after retirement are not offset by relative decreases in expenditures. Retirees must still pay for basic necessities. Families headed by older people spend more of their income than younger families on food, housing, and health care (Soldo, 1980, p. 23).

Elderly people are heavily dependent on third party payment for health-care costs. Only 5 percent of the elderly say they have no coverage at all for these costs (National Council on the Aging, 1981, p. 151). Comparison of direct out-of-pocket, insurance, and philanthropic sources on a per capita basis for the years 1966 and 1977 indicates that the direct costs borne by elderly people increased from $237 to $462 but that the percent of the total health bill that these dollars represented declined from 51 to 32 percent (Brotman, 1982a, p. 11).

The major implication of the positive, direct association between income levels and health status is that when people of any age, the elderly included, do not have enough money for basic necessities, health and medical expenditures tend to be reduced or avoided. Slightly more than one in two of retired Americans think they cannot "make ends meet, or just manage to get by" (National Council on the Aging, 1981, p. 71). "Inflation, high costs of living, high prices" and "poor/failing health, illness, sickness" were ranked equally by the elderly as their greatest problems (National Council on the Aging, 1981).

Eighty-six percent of people aged 65 years and over use private physicians for most of their medical care. However, 39 percent of people aged 65 and over indicated in the 1980 survey conducted by the National Council on the Aging (1981) that they should have seen a physician but did not because of the costs. People of all ages avoid seeing physicians in steadily increasing percentages as their incomes decline. This trend holds for the elderly and is particularly pronounced for blacks and Hispanics.

USE OF HEALTH AND MEDICAL SERVICES

In the three major types of medical-care services—physician visits, short-stay hospitalization, and long-term institutionalization—the elderly have higher utilization rates than the younger population but lower rates than might be expected on the basis of their health problems. Available utilization figures tend to be low in the first two types of medical services, since most surveys do not include those people who reside in institutions or who have died but may have used services during the survey period.

Physician Visits
Elderly people visit physicians only slightly more often than younger people, despite the greater frequency of chronic illness and disability found among this age group. Of all physician visits in the United States in 1980, the

elderly accounted for 17.5 percent. The average number of physician visits that year was 2.7 for people of all ages; people aged 65 years and older averaged 4.2 visits (National Center for Health Statistics, 1982). These results from the National Ambulatory Care Survey are similar to those from the 1980 Household Survey of the Noninstitutional Population in which people of all ages reported 4.8 physician "contacts" (telephone, hospital outpatient department or emergency room, or office/clinic setting) per year compared to 6.4 contacts for people aged 65 years and older (Brotman, 1982a, p. 14). In the latter survey, 74.9 percent of the total population had seen a physician during the past year compared with 79.4 percent of the elderly. However, the elderly also stay away from physicians. Of the total population, 3.7 percent had not seen a physician during the previous 5 years or more, compared to 6.1 percent of the elderly population.

Dental visits reported by the elderly are less frequent than those reported for the total population: 1.4 and 1.7 visits per person per year, respectively. Reports of intervals since the last dental visit show that the elderly tend to see dentists far less often than the general population. At intervals from under 6 months through 1 year the elderly were less likely to have seen a dentist and from 2 through 5 years or more, the elderly were more likely to have seen a dentist. These results from the 1980 Household Interview Survey of Noninstitutionalized Persons (Brotman, 1982a) are similar to those found from the 1976–78 surveys that found 39.9 percent of the elderly had visited a dentist at least once during the past 2 years compared to 63.8 percent of people of all ages (Foster, Machlin, and Kleinman, 1982). Examinations conducted between 1971 and 1974 revealed that of people aged 65–74 years, 60 percent had lost at least half of their permanent teeth and 75 percent of this group (45 percent of the total population aged 65–74 years) had lost all of their permanent teeth. Within this population, about 76 percent with some or all of their teeth needed dental care (Kelly and Harvey, 1979). In the population aged 65 years and over, as is true for other age groups, people who are poor, black, and residents of nonmet-

ropolitan areas report lower utilization of dental services (Foster, Machlin, and Kleinman, 1982). These effects of income, race, and residence on dental visits for elderly people during 1976–78 are summarized in Table 2.12. Periodontal disease refers to a variety of conditions of the supporting structures of the teeth. The prevalence of periodontal disease is associated with growing older, being male, and being black. In a survey reported in 1979, of the 54 percent of the population aged 65–74 years who had their natural teeth, 28 percent needed periodontal treatment (National Center for Health Statistics, 1978). In summary, differences in dental service utilization patterns suggest that removal of structural barriers related to the supply of dentists in nonmetropolitan areas and the cost of dental services would improve access to dental services for elderly people. In addition, client beliefs about the importance of dental care for people with few or no teeth need to be evaluated as a possible deterrent to seeking dental services.

Short-Stay Hospitalization

In 1980, the average length of stay in a short-stay hospital for persons with one or more hospital stays was 7.6 for all ages and 10.0 for people aged 65 and over. Averaging people with hospital stays with the vast majority of people without hospital stays, the average number of hospital days was as follows by age group: 1.9 days for ages 55–64; 3.2 days for ages 65–74; and 6.0 days for people aged 75 and over. Stated positively, in 1980, 90 percent of the elderly population was not hospitalized compared to 92 percent of the total population. Thus, the majority of elderly people do not require hospitalization during the course of any single year. However, the rate of hospitalization, the number of days of hospitalization per 1000 people, and the average length of stay per client all increase with advancing age (National Center for Health Statistics, 1982, pp. 163–165). Support for these trends is presented in Table 2.13. As might be expected, men have a higher rate of hospitalization after age 65 years and more days of care per person than women (National Center for Health Statistics, 1982, pp. 163–165). The reason for the comparatively higher rate

TABLE 2.12 PERSONS 65 YEARS OF AGE AND OVER WITH AT LEAST ONE DENTAL VISIT DURING THE PAST 2 YEARS, ACCORDING TO LOCATION OF RESIDENCE, RACE, AND FAMILY INCOME LEVEL, UNITED STATES 1976–78*

Race and Family Income Level	Total	Location of Residence	
		Metropolitan	Nonmetropolitan
All Races		Percent of Population	
All incomes†	39.9	43.4	34.0
Below poverty	23.4	26.5	20.3
100–150 percent poverty	31.6	33.3	28.8
150–300 percent poverty	49.6	51.5	46.8
Above 200 percent poverty	57.1	59.1	52.1
White			
All incomes†	41.2	45.2	34.8
Below poverty	23.5	27.3	20.1
100–150 percent poverty	32.0	34.2	28.8
150–200 percent poverty	40.1	42.0	37.1
Above 200 percent poverty	57.9	60.4	52.3
Black			
All incomes†	26.4	27.6	23.5
Below poverty	22.6	23.4	21.3
100–150 percent poverty	26.0	24.7	29.1
150–200 percent poverty	31.9	34.1	22.6
Above 200 percent poverty	35.6	35.6	35.7

*Data from 1976, 1977, and 1978 were combined. Family income was categorized to approximate the official poverty income level adjusted for family size; for example, poverty was defined at $7000 for a family of 4 and $4000 for a family of 2. †Includes respondents who did not report income (9 percent of all interviewees).
(Division of Health Interview Statistics, National Center for Health Statistics: Data from the National Health Interview Surveys 1976, 1977, 1978, reported by J.E. Foster, S.R. Machlin, and J.C. Kleinman, Use of dental services. In National Center for Health Services Research. Health, United States 1981 (DHHS Publication No. (PHS) 82-1232). Washington, D.C., U. S. Government Printing Office, 1982.)

TABLE 2.13 DISCHARGES FROM AND DAYS OF CARE IN NONFEDERAL SHORT-STAY HOSPITALS PER 1000 POPULATION ACCORDING TO AGE AND SEX, 1979.

	All Ages	Under 15 Years	15–44 Years	45–64 Years	65 Years and Over
Discharges per 1000 population					
Both Sexes	162.8	—	—	—	—
Males	—	80.3	97.1	193.2	410.5
Females	—	64.7	213.0	199.0	373.6
Days of care per 1000 population					
Both Sexes	1158.2	—	—	—	—
Males	—	352.4	616.5	1562.7	4287.1
Females	—	275.5	10,009.0	1642.3	4109.1

(Data from the National Hospital Discharge survey, 1979, reported in National Center for Health Statistics. Health, United States, 1981 (DHHS Publication No. (PHS) 82-1232). Washington, D.C., U. S. Government Printing Office, 1982, pp. 163–165.)

of hospitalization for men in their later years probably relates to the greater prevalence of heart disease and malignant neoplasms in men. Standard treatments of these conditions tend to be offered in hospitals. The leading "first listed" diagnoses for people aged 65 and over are diseases of the heart, malignant neoplasms, and cerebrovascular disease. The leading kinds of surgery for men are prostatectomies and biopsies and for women are biopsies and extraction of lenses. Table 2.14 lists the leading "first diagnoses" and surgical categories, discharges, and days of care per 1000 population for both sexes aged 65 and over.

Long-Stay Institutionalization

Three out of four Americans are correct when they say they will not enter a nursing home in their old age. For many years, the 4 to 5 percent of elderly people in nursing homes was assumed to represent the total chance of institutionalization after age 65. This has been revised to between 6 and 25 percent (Kastenbaum and Candy, 1973; Wershow, 1976; Pal-

more, 1976; Ingram and Barry, 1977; Kastenbaum, 1983; McConnel, 1983; Rosenberg and Short, 1983). Five percent represents the number of nursing home beds available; 6 to 25 percent is the proportion of people 65 years and over who can expect to spend some time in nursing homes before they die. In a 20-year study of 207 normal elderly people, factors related to total chances of institutionalization were grouped into those associated with need and those indicating better access to institutions (Palmore, 1976). Single individuals living alone and without children were most likely to need institutionalization. Thus, significant others seem important to the avoidance of institutionalization. In terms of access, white people with adequate incomes were more likely to enter institutions than either blacks or people with lower incomes. Greater access by whites could not be explained entirely on the basis of higher income, that is, race was definitely a factor. Possibly blacks experience discrimination in trying to enter institutions, or perhaps they use noninstitutional support systems to a

TABLE 2.14 FIRST-LISTED DIAGNOSES AND LEADING SURGICAL CATEGORIES, ASSOCIATED DISCHARGES, AND DAYS OF CARE FOR MALES AND FEMALES AGED 65 AND OVER, 1979

	Male		Female	
	Discharges	Days of Care	Discharge	Days of Care
First-Listed Diagnoses				
Diseases of the heart	77.9	792.1	65.1	695.1
Malignant neoplasms	48.6	621.2	31.1	429.4
Cerebrovascular disease	24.4	307.6	23.2	299.2
Fracture	—	—	21.3	348.8
Hyperplasia of prostate	16.5	172.4	—	—
Eye diseases and conditions	—	—	17.1	70.7
Pneumonia	13.5	146.0	—	—
Rheumatoid and osteoarthritis			8.8	112.1
Leading Surgical Categories				
Prostatectomy	218.0	22.6	—	—
Biopsy	217.0	22.6	222.0	16.1
Extraction of lens	108.0	11.2	198.0	14.4
Reduction of fracture with fixation	—	—	116.0	8.4
Repair of inguinal hernia	112.0	11.6	—	—

(Data from the National Hospital Discharge Survey, 1979, reported in National Center for Health Statistics. Health, United States, 1981 (DHHS Publication No. (PHS) 82-1232). Washington, D.C., U.S. Government Printing Office, 1982, pp. 163–165, 170–171.)

greater extent than whites. Usually old people in institutions are financially disadvantaged. This study indicated that the chance of institutionalization was lower for the financially disadvantaged. This paradox is believed to exist because financial adequacy provides greater access to institutions, while institutionalization depletes financial resources (Palmore, 1976).

The 1977 National Nursing Home Survey (National Center for Health Statistics, 1979) indicated that 86 percent of the 1,303,100 nursing home residents were 75 years of age or older: 16 percent were aged 65–74; 36 percent were aged 75–84; 31 percent were aged 85–94; and 3.4 percent were 95 years and over. These percentages are compared in Figure 2.7.

The percent of the total elderly population in institutions increases sharply with advancing age, from 4.8 percent of the total population aged 65 and over, to 10.3 percent of people aged 75 and over, and 21.6 percent of people aged 85 and over. However, the *total chance* of institutionalization does not increase with advancing age. Younger elderly people have a lower annual risk of institutionalization but more years ahead, while older elderly people have a greater annual risk with fewer years ahead.

There is no particular type of person who is either more likely to remain in the community or to seek institutionalization (Tobin and Lieberman, 1976). The critical change that seems to make the difference between those who seek institutionalization and the larger number who do not is related to the sudden or gradual loss of social supports, and the individual's subsequent conclusion that he can no longer manage independently in the community.

Health Protection and Promotional Services

Health has been defined by a variety of criteria that include physiologic processes, feelings, and capacity to function (Pender, 1982, p. 39). The primary goal of *health protection services* is the removal or avoidance of encumbrances to growth, maturation, fulfillment, and self-actualization throughout the life cycle (Pender, 1982, p. 41). Three levels of prevention are traditionally defined in public health:

1. Primary prevention—activities directed toward decreasing the probability of encoun-

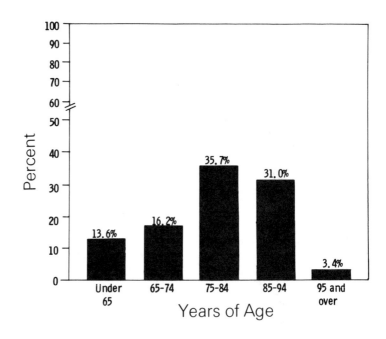

Figure 2.7. Percentages of nursing home residents by age groups, 1977. *(National Center for Health Statistics. The National Nursing Home Survey: 1977 Summary for the United States, Series 13, No. 43 (DHEW Publication No. (PHS) 79-1794). Washington, D.C., U.S. Government Printing Office, 1979, p. 29.)*

tering illness, including active protection of the body against unnecessary stressors (Pender, 1982, p. 42).

2. Secondary prevention—activities directed toward early diagnoses and prompt intervention to halt pathologic processes and thus shorten their duration and severity, permitting the individual to regain normal function as quickly as possible.

3. Tertiary prevention—activities to restore the individual to an optimum level of functioning within the limits imposed by disability.

Emphasis in health protection is on guarding or defending the individual from health threats or injuries (Pender, 1982, p. 42). In contrast, *health promotional services* are directed toward sustaining or increasing the individual's or group's level of well-being, self-actualization, and fulfillment. Movement in health promotion is toward a positively weighted state of increased health and well-being through growth, maturation, and expression of inherent and acquired human potential (Pender, 1982, p. 65).

Using these definitions, clearly identified services do not exist to promote health among elderly people. Like people of any age, elderly people can learn health-promoting behaviors from conversations with others or from mass media. In terms of health protection, programs and services for the elderly have been severely restricted by (1) incomplete knowledge of health-care measures to prevent chronic disease and (2) lack of third-party payment for preventive care. For example, it is common knowledge that elderly people are prone to falls, with the consequent fractures restricting physical mobility and contributing eventually to long-term institutional placement or death. Still, most elderly people who fall once are not assessed in depth to discover the reason and thus possibly prevent a recurrence. Health professionals do not have the time (or are not paid) to use the falls algorithm developed by Tideiskarr (1980). As a second example, consider "relocation trauma." Research has indicated what kinds of elderly people are at risk (those who are physically ill, depressed, confused, disoriented, and moving involuntarily). Studies have also

revealed the steps to be taken to effectively reduce or prevent the problem (opportunity for choice, individualized preparation, premove orientation to the new location, and participation in the decision-making process). However, this information is seldom found in the written procedures and protocols used by health professionals.

In part, because preventive health measures are seldom used with elderly people, research demonstrating the effectiveness of this care is lacking. A computer search of medical and health literature from August 1972 to August 1982 revealed only 33 research-based studies. A mere 13 of the 33 used control versus experimental group designs. Eight of these 13 studies contained enough information to permit secondary analysis. The results indicated a highly positive response to preventive intervention regardless of whether the intervention was psychologically or physiologically related. Preventive interventions considered fell in the areas of screening, exercise, client education, nutrition, primary care, and psychosocial support and guidance (Wilson, Simson, and McCaughey, 1982). An important epidemiologic study conducted by Breslow (1979) found that people who practiced positive health behavior extended their lifespans by over 10 years.

Based on numbers, these healthy aged people represent appropriate targets for health protective and promotional nursing services. Based on money, however, the frail, ill, and dependent aged people, who reside in institutions and comprise only 5 percent of the aged population, receive a disproportionate share of nursing services. In times of economic constraint, political expediency requires that nurses be equally involved with both aged populations in an effort to shift resources from after-the-fact-of-illness secondary and tertiary prevention to primary prevention.

UNITED STATES ELDERLY IN WORLD PERSPECTIVE

Population projections indicate that the entire world is experiencing an increase in the absolute and relative size of the aging population.

In 1950, the number of aged in the world was 190 million; in 1970, 290 million. By 1985, it is estimated that the aged population will be 405 million; by 2000, this will reach 585 million (an increase of 450 percent in the last 50 years). The 1985 population of 405 million elderly people (8.2 percent of the total world population of all ages) will continue to be distributed in all countries. However, because of varying health and social conditions, the elderly population is expected to continue to be greater in the more developed regions (North America, Japan, Europe, Australia, New Zealand, and U.S.S.R.) (16 percent) than in the less developed regions (Africa, Latin America, China and other East Asia, South Asia, Melanesia, Micronesia, and Polynesia) (6 percent) (Aragon, 1981).

In general, the likelihood of surviving into old age is directly related to improvements in patterns of rational and regional standards of living that, in turn, have been related to the adoption of a wage economy, industrialization, urbanization, and emergence of an organized system of social welfare programs and services. Virtually all large countries have, or are developing, income transfer plans to provide for the social welfare needs of their aging populations. These patterns of social welfare planning reflect universal trends prompted by weakened family ties, an increasingly female, over-65 population, and a mobile work force not tied to economic responsibilities for aged or disabled family members (Estes, 1980).

Social and economic problems persist despite social service programs in more developed countries. "Except in Japan where multigenerational family living is still common, many of the elderly in urbanized, industrialized countries end up living and interacting mainly with others of their own age, cut off from meaningful social roles and activities" (Soldo, 1980, p. 43).

Nurses may want to advocate adoption of solutions to health and social problems that have proven effective in other countries with social and economic structures similar to ours. For example, Sweden trains rural postal workers to monitor the elderly on their routes, provide temporary help, and to report findings to a district coordinating service agency (Soldo, 1980).

CONCLUSION

Generally speaking, increased longevity is a reflection of better, not poorer, health. This increase stands as one of the great achievements of the twentieth century. The information presented in this chapter supports the conclusion that the number and proportion of elderly people have increased dramatically, and will continue to do so in the foreseeable future. Smaller proportions of blacks, people of Spanish origin, and men of all racial and ethnic groups reach old age than whites and women. The majority of elderly people are functionally healthy and live in community settings with little or no dependence on the health-care system. People who will be old in the future will be survivors of a different generation than the elderly of today or yesterday. The elderly of the future will have different attitudes toward society and toward their roles and rights in that society. Therefore, professionals who deal with the aged should realize that traditional images of the aged may no longer be valid. Not only do individuals age differently, but generations also grow old differently. The dramatically rising number of old people lends increasing urgency to the need for information about promoting and maintaining health in this group. These conclusions have given rise to a number of questions and issues, many of which are discussed in the chapters that follow.

RECOMMENDED READINGS

Bytheway, W. R. Demographic statistics and old age ideology. Aging and Society 1(3):347–364, 1981. *An analysis of descriptions of retirement, found in popular books, that indicates how statistics are presented and interpreted to reflect a certain set of beliefs about old age—a set of beliefs that fails to recognize the relationship between old age and death. The article serves to warn readers to question assumptions inherent in statistical portraits of the elderly.*
Every Ninth American is the title of articles and

reports prepared annually by H.B. Brotman, consultant to congressional committees on aging. These reports are occasionally published in gerontologic journals, and sometimes are available from the committee chairperson. *A comprehensive compilation of basic information about the elderly related to demography, income, employment, health, housing, transportation, and crime. Useful primarily as a reference rather than cover-to-cover reading.*

Health Data Advisory Committee. Health data inventory, FY 1982, A report from the Health Data Advisory Committee to the Secretary, Department of Health and Human Services. Washington, D.C., U.S. Government Printing Office, 1982. *A reference that lists a brief description of each project or system, the name of a contact person, the purpose of data collection, and implementation status for FY 1982. If this report continues to be published annually, the information may be useful to nurses planning health services.*

National Clearing House on Aging. Inventory of Federal Statistics Programs Relating to Older Persons (DHEW Publication No. (OHDS) 79-20291). Washington, D.C., U.S. Government Printing Office, 1979. *Although this is an older reference, the report lists and describes the purpose, sample, frequency, and dissemination plans for a number of ongoing surveys that are national in scope and include age-related data.*

Population Bulletin, published six issues to a volume, and available from the Population Reference Bureau, 1337 Connecticut Avenue N.W., Washington, D.C. 20036. Occasionally an entire issue relates to the elderly. An example of such an issue is Soldo BJ: America's elderly in the 1980s 35(4):1–50, 1980. *The Soldo (1980) reference is a statistical overview of the elderly completed before 1980 census data were available. Topics include demography, death and illness, quality of life, help for the elderly, initiatives for change, and aging in international perspective. Useful as a reference rather than cover-to-cover reading.*

Research on Aging 3(4):371–501, 1981. *A special issue devoted to the presentation of investigations that describe and, in part, indicate directions for the use of some of the larger data sets collected under federal government sponsorship. These articles were based on papers that were presented at the Conference on Demographic and Health Information for Aging Research: Resources and Needs, held by the Epidemiology, Demography, and Biometry Program of the National Institute on Aging (NIA), National Institutes of Health, on June 25–27, 1979. Content indicates both sources and limitations of the data discussed. This reference is recommended for nurses interested in doing research or planning involving large segments of the population.*

Schecter I, Oriol W: 1982–3 Chartbook of Federal Programs in Aging. Bethesda, MD, Care Reports, 1982. *A reference for locating data sources with age-related components. Presumably this reference will be revised annually. The list is also summarized in the newsletter, Aging Research and Training News (50):4–6, 1982. The listing provides the name of the age-related data source and the address and telephone number of the source's best contact person.*

REFERENCES CITED

Aday, R.H., Miles, L.A. Long-term implications of rural migration of the elderly: Implications for research. The Gerontologist 22(3):331–336, 1982

American Nurses' Association. Nursing: A Social Policy Statement. Kansas City, MO, The American Nurses Association, 1980, p. 11

Aragon, J.G. Perspectives of the aged in the world demography. Aging and Leisure Living 4(4):6–9, 1981

Aronson, D.R. Ethnicity as a cultural system: An introductory essay. In Henry, F. (ed.), Ethnicity in the Americas. The Hague: Mouton, 1976

Ashley, J.A. This I believe about power in nursing. Nursing Outlook 21(10):637–641, 1973

Atchley, R.S. Social Forces in Later Life, 3rd ed. Belmont, CA, Wadsworth, 1980

Backus, F.I., Dudley, D.L. Observations of psychosocial factors and their relationship to organic disease. In Lipowski, Z.J., Lipsitt, D.R., Whybrow, P.C. (eds.), Psychosomatic Medicine. New York, Oxford University Press, 1977

Barnekov, T.K. An Assessment of the Social Service Needs of the Elderly in Group Subsidized Housing. Newark, DE, College of Urban Affairs and Public Policy, University of Delaware, 1980

Belloc, N.B., Breslow, L. Relationship of physical health status and health practices. Preventive Medicine 1(3):409–421, 1972

Biggar, J.C. Reassessing elderly sunbelt migration. Research on Aging 2(2):172–190, 1980

Blazer, D.G. Social support and mortality in an elderly community population. American Journal of Epidemiology 115(5):684–694, 1982

Branch, L.G. Understanding the Health and Social Service Needs of People over Age 65. Cambridge, MA, Center for Survey Research of the University of Massachusetts and the Joint Center for Urban Studies of MIT and Harvard University, 1977

Branch, L.G., Jette, A.M. The Framingham disability study I: Social disability among the aging. American Journal of Public Health 71(11): 1202–1210, 1981

Breslow, L. A Positive Strategy for the Nation's Health. Proceedings of the National Health Forum, New York, National Health Council, 1979

Breslow, L., Enstrom, J.E. Persistence of health habits and their relationship to mortality. Preventive Medicine 9:469–483, 1980

Brody, S.J. The graying of America. Hospitals 54(10):63–66, 123, 1980

Brotman, H. Every Ninth American. In Developments in Aging: 1979. A Report of the Special Committee on Aging, United States Senate. Washington, D.C., U.S. Government Printing Office, 1980

Brotman, H.B. Every Ninth American. An unpublished report prepared for the Special Committee on Aging, United States Senate, Washington, D.C., 1981

Brotman, H.B. Every Ninth American, 1982 Edition: An Analysis for the Chairman of the U.S. House of Representatives Select Committee on Aging. Washington, D.C., U.S. Government Printing Office, 1982a

Brotman, H.B. Unpublished data from the U.S. Census Bureau, November, 1982b

Cobb, S. Social support as a mediator of life stress. Psychosomatic Medicine 38(5):300–314, 1976

Comfort, A. The Biology of Senescence, 3rd ed. New York, Elswur Science, 1979

Estes, R.J. International trends in aging. Center for the Study of Aging Newsletter 3(2):1–2, 1980

Fingerhut, L.A., Rosenberg, H.M. Mortality among the elderly. In National Center for Health Services Research. Health, United States 1981 (DHHS Publication No. (PHS) 82-1232). Washington, D.C., U.S. Government Printing Office, 1982

Foster, J.E., Machlin, S.R., Kleinman, J.C. Use of dental services. In National Center for Health Statistics. Health, United States, 1981 (DHHS Publication No. (PHS) 82-1232). Washington, D.C., U.S. Government Printing Office, 1982

Fries, J.F. Aging, natural death, and the compression of morbidity. In Somers, A.R., Fabian, D.R. (eds.), The Geriatric Imperative. New York, Appleton-Century-Crofts, 1981

Gelein, J.L. The aged American female. Journal of Gerontological Nursing 6(2):69–73, 1980

Hassenplug, L.W. Personal perspectives on aging and nursing. Journal of Gerontological Nursing 8(1):23–29, 1982

Hess, B. Research in gerontology: State of the art. Gerontology News 3, May 1982

Hickey, T. Health and Aging. Monterey, CA, Brooks/Cole, 1980

Hindricks, J. (ed.). Being and Becoming Old. New York, Baywood, 1978

Holmes, T. Multidiscipline study of tuberculosis. In Sparer P.J. (ed.), Personality, Stress and Tuberculosis. New York, International Press, 1954

Holzberg, C.S. Ethnicity and aging: Anthropological perspectives on more than just the minority elderly. The Gerontologist 22(3):249–257, 1982

Jackson, J.J. Minorities and Aging. Belmont, CA, Wadsworth, 1980

Jette, A.M., Branch, L.G. The Framingham disability study II. Physical disability among the aging. American Journal of Public Health 71(11): 1211–1216, 1981

Ingram, D.K., Barry, J.R. National statistics on deaths in nursing homes: Interpretations and implications. The Gerontologist 17(4):303–308, 1977

Kannel, W.B., Gordon, T. (eds.). The Framingham Study (DHEW Publication No. (NIH) 74-478). Washington, D.C., U.S. Government Printing Office, 1974

Kastenbaum, R. The 4% fallacy: R.I.P. International Journal of Aging and Human Development 17(1):71–74, 1983

Kastenbaum, R.S., Candy, S. The four percent fallacy: A methodological and empirical critique of extended care facility program statistics. Aging and Human Development 4(1):15–21, 1973

Kelly, J., Harvey, C. Basic data on dental examination findings of persons 1–74 years, United States, 1971–74. Vital and Health Statistics Series 11, No. 214 (DHEW Publication No. (PHS) 79-1662). Washington, D.C., U.S. Government Printing Office, 1982

Krucoff, C. Coping: The plight of women in a graying America. The Washington Post B5, May 6, 1980

Lawton, M.P., Kleban, M.H., Carlson, D.A. The inner city resident: To move or not to move. The Gerontologist 13(4):443–448, 1973

Lichter, D.T., Fuguitt, G.V., Heaton, T.B., Clifford, W.B. Components of change in the residential concentration of the elderly population: 1950–1975. Journal of Gerontology 36(4):480–489, 1981

Longino, C.F. Changing aged nonmetropolitan migration patterns, 1955 to 1960 and 1965 to 1970. Journal of Gerontology 37(2):228–234, 1982

Longino, C.F., Biggar, J.C. The impact of population redistribution on service delivery. The Gerontologist 22(2):153–159, 1982

Maddox, G.L., Douglass, E.B. Self-assessment of health: A longitudinal study of elderly subjects.

Journal of Health and Social Behavior 14:87–93, 1973

Maldonado, D. Aging in the Chicano context. In Gelfand, D.E., Kutzik, A.J. (eds.), Ethnicity and Aging: Theory Research and Policy. New York, Springer, 1979

McConnel, C.E. A note on methodological fallacies in the "X90 fallacy" literature. International Journal of Aging and Human Development 17(1):57–69, 1983

McMiller, C., Ingham, J.D. Friends, confidants and symptoms. Social Psychiatry, 11:51–58, 1976

McWhirter, N. Guinness Book of World Records. New York, Bartan, 1980

Miller, M.K., Stokes, C.S. Health status, health resources, and consolidated structural parameters, implications for health care policy. Journal of Health and Social Behavior 19(3):263–279, 1978

Moss, G.E. Biosocial resonation: A conceptual model of the links between social behavior and physical illness. In Lipowski, Z.J., Lipsitt, D.R., Whybrow, P.C. (eds.), Psychosomatic Medicine. New York, Oxford University Press, 1977

Myers, G.C. Cross-national trends in mortality rates among the elderly. The Gerontologist 18(5): 441–448, 1978

National Center for Health Statistics Basic data on hearing levels of adults 25–74 years, United States, 1971–75. Vital and Health Statistics, Series 11, Number 215 (DHEW Publication No. (PHS) 80-1663). Washington, D.C., U.S. Government Printing Office, 1980

National Center for Health Statistics. Health practices among adults: United States, 1977. Advance Data from Vital and Health Statistics, No. 64. Washington, D.C., U.S. Department of Health and Human Services, Public Health Service, Office of Health Research Statistics, and Technology, 1980

National Center for Health Statistics. Health, United States, 1978 (DHEW Publication No. (PHS) 78-1232). Washington, D.C., U.S. Government Printing Office, 1978

National Center for Health Services Research. Health, United States, 1981 (DHHS Publication No. (PHS) 82-1232). Washington, D.C., U.S. Government Printing Office, 1982

National Center for Health Statistics: The national nursing home survey: 1977 summary for the United States. Vital and Health Statistics, Series 13, Number 43 (DHEW Publication No. (PHS) 79-1794). Washington, D.C., U.S. Government Printing Office, 1979

National Center for Health Statistics. Refraction status and motility defects of persons 4–74 years,

United States, 1971–1972. Vital and Health Statistics, Series 11, Number 206 (U.S. D.H.E.W. Publication No. (PHS) 78-1654). Washington, D.C., U.S. Government Printing Office, 1978

National Center for Health Statistics. 1980 Summary: National Ambulatory Medical Care Survey. Advance Data from Vital and Health Statistics, No. 77. Washington, D.C., U.S. Department of Health and Human Services, Public Health Service, Office of Health Research, Statistics, and Technology, 1982

National Council on the Aging. Aging in the Eighties: America in Transition. Washington, D.C., National Council on the Aging, 1981

National Council on the Aging. Fact Book on Aging: A Profile of America's Older Population. Washington, D.C., National Council on the Aging, 1978

National Institute on Aging. Survey of the Last Days of Life. A request for proposal, NIH-AG-82-20, March 15, 1982

Newhouse, J.P., Friedlander, L.J. The relationship between medical resources and measures of health: Some additional evidence. The Journal of Human Resources 15(2):200–218, 1979

Palmore, E. Total chance of institutionalization among the aged. The Gerontologist 16(6):504–507, 1976

Pender, N.J. Health Promotion in Nursing Practice. Norwalk, CT, Appleton-Century-Crofts, 1982

Rosenberg, E., Short, C. Issues of institutionalization: Five percent fallacies and terminal care. International Journal of Aging and Human Development 17(1):43–55, 1983

Rowe, J.W. Research in geriatrics and gerontology. In Somers, A.R., Fabian, D.R. (eds.). The Geriatric Imperative. New York, Appleton-Century-Crofts, 1981

Soldo, G.J. America's elderly in the 1980's. Population Bulletin 35(4):1–48, 1980

Tideiskarr, R. Is Falling Preventable in the Elderly? A paper presented at the 33rd Annual Scientific Meeting of the Gerontology Society of America, San Diego, CA, November 21–25, 1980

Tobin, S.S., Lieberman, M.A. Last Home for the Aged: Critical Implications for Institutionalization. San Francisco, CA, Jossey Bass, 1976

Twaddle, A.C. The concept of health status. Social Science Medicine 8(1):29–38, 1974

U.S. Bureau of the Census. Age, sex, race, and Spanish origin of the population by regions, divisions, and status: 1980. Supplementary Reports: 1980 Census of Population, 1982, PC 80-S1-1. Washington, D.C., Superintendent of Documents, 1981

U.S. Bureau of the Census of the population, 1970, Vol 1. Characteristics of the population Part I,

United States Summary, Section 1. Washington, D.C., U.S. Government Printing Office, 1973

U.S. Bureau of the Census. Projections of the population of the United States, 1972–2050. Current Population Reports Series P-25, No. 704. Washington, D.C., U.S. Government Printing Office, 1973

U.S. Senate Special Committee on Aging. Developments in Aging, 1981, Vol 1. Washington, D.C., U.S. Government Printing Office, 1982

Weiss, B., Lord, G.L. Inaccurate Health Status Perception in the Aged. Unpublished manuscript, Hahneman Medical College, 1981

Wershow, H.J. The four percent fallacy: Some further evidence and policy implications. The Gerontologist 16(1):52–55, 1976

Wilson, L.B., Simson, S., McCaughey, K. The Status of Preventive Care for the Aged: A Meta-Analysis. A paper presented at the 35th Annual Scientific Meeting of the Gerontological Society of America, Boston, MA, November 1982

Wirth, L. The problem of minority groups. In Linton, R. (ed.). The Science of Man in the World Crisis. New York, Columbia University Press, 1945

Wiseman, R.F. Why older people move: Theoretical issues. Research on Aging: 2(2):141–154, 1980

3

Theory in Aging and Theory-Related Issues

Susanne S. Robb

Reading this chapter will enable the individual to:

1. Define aging generally and in terms of social, psychologic, functional, and biologic aspects
2. List three barriers to theory development in aging
3. Reply to questions frequently asked about aging:
   a. What makes people grow old?
   b. What biophysiologic changes are normal in old age?
   c. What actions can people take if they want to live longer?
4. Describe the concerns of psychologic theories of aging
5. Identify examples from nursing practice that suggest a nurse is influenced by one or the other of the three major sociologic perspectives
6. Discuss at least one problem associated with a functional versus a chronological definition of aging
7. List ways nurses can provide opportunities for clients to feel competent
8. Indicate why considering the elderly as a group in need of special attention may not benefit the elderly
9. Name the advantages and disadvantages of gerontologic nursing as a speciality area
10. Report two strategies for discovering problems that nurses might want to study and that relate to elderly people
11. List priority problem areas that nurses need to study in order to improve the quality of life for elderly people

The human quest for eternal youth has taken many forms, from searching for the fountain of youth to freezing corpses for rejuvenation at some future date. Today, most people who wish to discover the causes of aging channel their interest into research and theory development in the field of gerontology.

Any theoretician who tries to explain the phenomenon of human aging faces a formidable challenge (see Fig. 3.1). Aging is associated with increased losses and unique gains, continuity of individual personality and diversity as a group, and responsiveness to both genetic and environmental influences—factors that seem hard to reconcile within a theoretical framework. Innumerable theories, models, and concepts from a variety of disciplines have been used to explain aspects of aging. Many more will probably be applied before a unified theory of aging evolves.

For the most part, nurses are concerned with human responses to actual or potential health problems that are manifested by whole people as integrated behaviors rather than with parts or subdivisions of people. Nurses also have more use for information that is specific and sufficiently verified through research to provide direction for nursing practice, as opposed to propositions that may be interesting but lack empirical support. Consistent with these assumptions, this chapter emphasizes psychosociologic over biophysiologic theories of aging. Readers are advised that few of the theories formulated and tested thus far provide clear direction for nursing action in the sense of "if this, then do this, and this will occur."

The fact that theories fail to provide specific direction for nursing practice does not mean

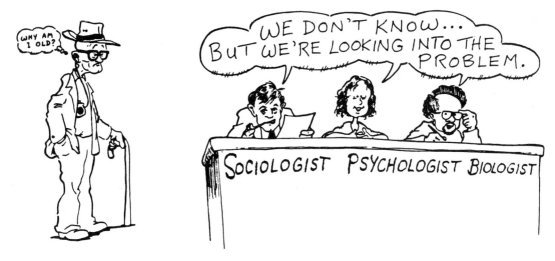

Figure 3.1. Gerontologists are still searching for answers to the big question. (*Drawing by Harry Trumbore*)

nurses have no need to know about them. Knowingly or unknowingly, and regardless of how well developed theories are, nurses use them in their practice. For example, many nurses are influenced by the biomedical model that prevails in service settings without realizing that the model represents a number of untested assumptions and has serious limitations. The biomedical perspective individualizes and medicalizes old age and overlooks relationships between socioeconomic status, the economy, and health (Estes, Swan, and Gerard, 1982). Thus "senility" is assumed to be caused by some physiologic or structural factor within the body and not by the social creation of dependency through forced role loss, economic dependence, and isolation. Age-related priorities of the major federal research institutes dictate study of hypothesized biologic and physiologic sources of decline with age in the eventual hope of curing the disease called "old age." Nurses who do not realize they are operating on the basis of the biomedical, or any other theoretical, stance cannot examine that theory critically. Also, theories related to aging consider questions that clients may pose to nurses. In responding, nurses need to distinguish between information that is well supported by research and assumptions and propositions that require further testing. At present, there is very little a nurse can tell a client about biophysiologic, psychologic, or sociologic aging that the client could not refute by reading other references in a good library.

AGING DEFINED

Aging refers to the "regular behavioral changes that occur in mature genetically representative organisms living under representative environmental conditions as they advance in chronologic age" (Birren and Renner, 1977, p. 4). Alternatively, aging has been defined according to the interests of the scientists. "*Social age* refers to the roles and social habits of an individual with respect to other members of a society" (Birren and Renner, 1977, italics added). The focus of inquiry is whether the individual behaves younger or older than his chronologic age. *Psychologic age* can be defined as the adaptive responses the individual makes to changing environmental demands, in comparison to the average (Birren and Renner, 1977, p. 5). Closely related to psychologic age is the concept of *functional age,* the individual's level of capacities for behaving in a specific society compared to others of the same age (Birren and

Renner, 1977). *Biologic age* is an estimate of the individual's present status with respect to his potential lifespan (Birren and Renner, 1977). Determination of biologic age usually involves evaluation of the functional capacities of vital organ systems. Thus, a 70-year-old woman may be judged to have the heart of a 50-year-old. The first definition of aging has the advantages of not suggesting a specific cause for the aging phenomenon or a judgment as to the purpose of the process: incremental (toward growth and gain) or decremental (toward diminishment and loss).

Each human being may be viewed as an organism that happens, and as an event which extends in space and time. Figure 3.2 presents this conceptual view of aging. Aging can be viewed vertically with respect to several levels—molecule, cell, organ, individual, group, and society. It can also be viewed horizontally in relation to three attributes:

1. Being may be equivalent to structure (anatomic, biochemical).
2. Behaving may be equivalent to function (physiologic and behavioral).
3. Becoming may refer either to development or progress.

The aging phenomenon is studied to discover why the lifespan is finite, and to determine what interventions are possible. At present, no single theory explains the many events related to aging. These include molecular and cellular occurrences, physiologic and psychologic changes in individuals, and social factors associated with interaction within and between different age groups. Just as many diseases are multicaused, aging is a complex phenomenon that may require different explanations for different facets of the process (Shock, 1977). Present evidence indicates that biologic mechanisms are no more fundamental to the aging process than are psychologic or sociologic mechanisms (Shock, 1977, p. 103). Thus, research must proceed at all levels, from molecular to societal. The causes of aging may be different depending on whether the question concerns how long people live, what changes in mental abilities occur, or how social behavior changes with advancing age.

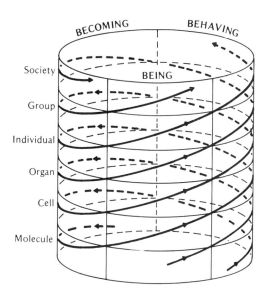

Figure 3.2. Diagram illustrating the triad of major attributes of all systems: being, behaving, and becoming. The spiraling lines show the ascent through the levels of organization. *(Gerard, R.W., Aging and organization. In Birren, J.E. (ed.). Handbook of Aging and the Individual. Chicago, IL, The University of Chicago Press, 1959. Copyright 1959 by the University of Chicago. Reprinted by permission.)*

THE CURRENT STATUS OF THEORY DEVELOPMENT IN AGING

No general theory of aging exists presently, and the few that have been proposed are quite narrow or specific in character. Thus, there is no complete answer to the question "Why does man grow old?" There exists only a collection of concepts and hypotheses proposed to explain limited aspects of how people behave as they progress through their lifespan.

A theory is an internally consistent set of interrelated concepts, definitions, and propositions that present a systematic view of phenomena by specifying relations among variables (concepts) (Kerlinger, 1973). The purpose of a theory is to (1) describe, (2) explain, (3) predict, and, ultimately, (4) control phenomena. Theory is useful for both the scientist and the practitioner because it organizes observations into some logical relationship. Policy-makers and practitioners, however, rely on theories to guide programs and practices. These individuals need theories that say, "if this, and this, and this occurs, then that will surely follow," in order to select correct plans of action. Some people believe that a theory has been developed only when events can be predicted, based on testing and application of theoretical statements (Chinn and Jacobs, 1978).

Theories in gerontology, at present, do not meet criteria of prediction and control. They can only be called "theories of aging" with the understanding that the term is being used loosely. Some more appropriate labels might be "conceptual frameworks," "theoretical formulations," or "theories of the middle range." A conceptual framework is a set of statements that provides descriptions and explanations of phenomena, or that has undeveloped or untested potential for prediction and control (Chinn and Jacobs, 1978, p. 2).

Theory development in aging has been impeded by several factors. First, the science of gerontology is new compared to most other sciences. The number of publications in psychologic gerontology did not begin to rise consistently until the 1930s (Riegel, 1977, p. 93). The first book that might be called a social-psychologic investigation of aging appeared two decades later (Havighurst and Albrecht, 1953). Widespread study of the biology and physiology of aging could not begin until significant communicable disease control and other scientific developments permitted large numbers of people to reach old age.

Second, a sufficiently large and empirically tested body of facts about social, psychologic, and biologic processes in aging has not yet accumulated. Few studies involving the elderly are beyond criticism. Gerontologists often suspect that their results would be different if they had had a different sample, or had worded their questions differently, or, perhaps, if they had asked different questions. Old people may be more diverse than any other age group after their lifetimes of individual experiences with race, religion, social class, education, and occupation. Instruments may not account for this variation. Measurement instruments age as

people do, and tend not to be widely applicable across age or cultural groups. Findings from studies have often been restricted to American society or similar societies. Cross-national studies have been relatively rare, as have investigations of minority groups within American society.

Third, research, especially psychosocial research, is extremely expensive and time-consuming. A generation of human beings changes more slowly than a generation of laboratory rats. Illness and death interrupt the many years of observation required to identify human change over time. Thus a unified theory of aging does not exist at the present time. In fact, given the problems listed above, a grand theory that ties together all facets of the aging phenomenon and permits control is unlikely to be developed in the near future. This does not mean that a complete answer to the questions of why and how aging occurs will not be found, however, or that present explanations are not relevant to gerontologists.

THE AGING PHENOMENON FROM MAJOR PERSPECTIVES

Three points of view have organized studies of the aging process, based upon the dependent variables being studied: (1) biologic, (2) psychologic, and (3) sociologic. The latter two perspectives have been combined under the heading "Psychosocial Views" because the various theories tend to overlap or interrelate very closely.

Biologic Views
Biologic theory tries to explain the physiologic process and structural alterations in living organisms that determine developmental changes, longevity, and death. The term "senescence" has been used by some biologists to describe biologic aging, although it is not widely used (Birren and Renner, 1977).* No system prop-

---

* Senescence should not be confused with senility, an archaic term once used to describe mental impairments believed to be the result of aging.

erty persists indefinitely in time. "Given any system, and any characteristic property of that system, there is only a finite time interval during which the property persists" (Schimke and Agniel, 1983, p. 41). Thus, the study of senescence involves attempts to understand how and why biologic processes cause the property of living to be time-limited in organisms.

The aging process manifests itself in three rather obvious ways. One of these is the way in which the individual and society interrelate. The other two are probably based on changes within the body (Atchley, 1977). The first is deterioration in the major organs and systems of the body. Lungs, kidneys, heart, nervous system, liver, and digestive system all decline in function as the organism ages. The second factor is the loss of ability to resist disease.

Numerous theories of biologic aspects of aging have been formulated, and many of these have been tested. None, however, has produced an effective explanation of the various aging processes (Reff and Schneider, 1982; Schimke and Agniel, 1983). At least one expert (Adelman, 1980) has refused to define the term "biologic aging" because too many questions remain unanswered. For example, does biologic aging mean that specific populations have finite maximal life years that can differ enormously from one population to another? Do all members of a given population eventually undergo a progressive decline in their capability for physiologic performance as time passes? Do these fundamental features of aging populations relate to each other? Do mechanisms reponsible for the biology of aging reside in all cells in a particular organism or only a specific cell population? Is there one or are there several mechanisms that are responsible for the wide variety of changes in elderly people? The maximal lifespan of certain species may correlate with (1) the capability for repair of a specific type of desoxyribonucleic acid (DNA) damage (Hart and Setlow, 1974), (2) the resistance of DNA to chemically caused mutagenesis (Schwartz, 1975), and (3) the probability for reproduction and survival of specific cell populations grown in culture (Hayflick, 1981).

Once factors that are reliably associated with aging have been described, another series of questions must be answered. In what cell populations will such factors originate? What specific molecular event causes a specific factor to occur? What is the developmental course of this factor? At what age in the lifespan of the animal is this factor first apparent?

The question of greatest interest to nurses is how biologic factors associated with the aging process relate to health and longevity and what actions can people take to minimize or avoid deleterious consequences of these factors. Given that present theories do not provide answers to this question, what does the nurse need to know about biologic aging theories and how might the nurse use this information? Nurses require some idea about biologic explanations that researchers are considering in order to respond to such questions as, "What causes people to grow old?" "How much of what I can or cannot do is normal in old age?" and "What can I do to live longer?"

Regardless of biologic level considered, the familiar "nature versus nurture" debate provides two "causes" for aging. The first view holds that aging is an involuntary process that operates cumulatively over time to modify cells, tissues, and fluids. This process is based upon genetic factors operating within the individual (endogenously). Basic metabolic processes of the cells produce waste products such as lipofuscin, or "age pigment," that accumulate until they reach a critical level and cause a decrease in functioning. This perspective is sometimes called the waste, or wear-and-tear, theory. In this view, life itself implies aging as an inherent part of growth and development. Biologic age can thus be determined by the amount of metabolic waste accumulated.

The second view maintains that alterations throughout the lifespan are due to a host of external factors—infections, toxins, traumas, radiation, nutritional disturbances, depletion of fixed energy stores or materials, or other inadequacies—that cause degenerative changes and impairments. This view considers such exogenous factors as "accidents" that bring about changes. These changes sometimes take the form of chromosomal mutations in the gametes and somatic cells. More mutations are presumed to have occurred in older organisms, increasing the likelihood of structural or functional defects.

Both major theoretical perspectives of biologic aging emphasize loss and decline. This emphasis has biased investigation away from aging as an adaptive process. The elderly display declines in mobility, energy, strength, and stress tolerance, alterations in neurologic, immune, and cardiovascular status; and modifications of cognition and affect. However, aged individuals are still capable of love, thought, exercise, sleep, ingestion, excretion, etc. Given more time, the elderly can learn new tasks, integrate information, or cope with new situations as effectively as young people.

What Causes People to Grow Old?
No one knows what causes people to grow old but possible reasons are being studied. One way of organizing biologic theories is according to the level of biologic function studied. Senescence and death occur at every level of biologic organization: cell, tissue, organ, organ system, and organism levels (Schimke and Agniel, 1983).

Molecular Aging Theories. Molecular aging theories usually postulate that aging results when inappropriate information is provided for normal cell function from the cell nucleus. Thus, these theories are sometimes called the error theories (Finch, 1979). The basic genetic information in cells is coded in desoxyribonucleic acid (DNA). When DNA is replicated, histone and other regulatory molecules are arranged on newly produced DNA in such a way as to insure that daughter cells either reproduce the parent cell or are suitably modified for the next stage of differentiation (Sinex, 1977). Four ways that expression of information might be altered to produce aging effects include (Sinex, 1977):

1. Changes in the base pairs or coding of DNA due to:
   a. coding errors in replication (more reproductions of cells yield more errors),
   b. point mutation (as cells age, chemical changes occur), and
   c. chromosome aberrations (strands of DNA are broken, lost or joined incorrectly).

2. Increases in levels of error in:
   a. Ribonucleic acid (RNA) synthesis (messenger RNA has a longer half-life in adult organs)
   b. charges in transfer RNA (transfer RNA carries inappropriate amino acids to protect cells from errors in transfer RNA), and
   c. protein synthesis (proteins are improperly constructed because of errors in DNA and RNA).

3. Deterioration in the arrangement of basic control elements in chromatin such as:
   a. histone,
   b. nonhistone protein,
   c. RNA.
   Overall, the effect is to make chromatin a less favorable substrate for DNA and RNA synthesis.

4. Expression of a normal program of aging that includes aging as a final step:
   a. aging as the result of a well-ordered program operating without error, and
   b. aging as a result of defects in the control of a genetic program.

Molecular error theories inspired considerable research on the fidelity of protein synthesis as a function of age. Results have been mixed, with some supporting and some not supporting the theory. The theory is difficult to test and the gap is large between showing the plausibility of transcriptive errors and demonstrating the biologic importance of the phenomenon (Sacher, 1980, p. 15).

Cellular Aging Theories. Normal human embryonic fibroblasts, when cultured outside the body (in vitro), undergo a limited (finite) number of doublings, approximately 50, and then die. The decline period of proliferation has been labeled the Phase III phenomenon and interpreted as a sign that senescence occurs at the cellular level (Hayflick, 1980). Studies using other human tissue supported results found with embryo tissue: human liver tissue (LeGuilly et al., 1973), skin (Schneider and Mitsui, 1976), and arterial smooth muscle (Bierman, 1978).

The focus of study has shifted from which human cells are lost to why cells are lost. Two leading possibilities are (1) programmed cell aging, that is, aging processes that are under some degree of genetic control or (2) some other obligation on the part of cells, such as responding to an "aging pacemaker" located somewhere in the body and in which no genetic control is observable (Sacher, 1980). Substantial evidence has been gathered to indicate that loss of all doubling capacity is not due to an accumulation of errors in enzymes or other proteins (for example, Wright and Hayflick, 1975a, 1975b; Goldstein and Csullog, 1977). Genetic control, in this case, has been proposed as a process in which cells stop or are prevented from exchanging genetic information and, "left to their own devices" undergo a process of senescence (Hayflick, 1980). The "aging pacemaker" notion proposes a single organ or tissue as responsible for limiting cell proliferation or otherwise starting a process of senescence in all body cells. The thymus and its dependent tissues has been proposed as a possible pacemaker or biologic clock (Burnet, 1970a, 1970b).

Thus, what is known about cellular aging is simply that normal human (and other species') cells have a finite capacity for reproduction. However, Hayflick (1980), a leading researcher in the area of cell biology, doubts this finite limit is ever reached by cells living within the body. He suggests that most of the functional losses that occur in cells occur before ability to reproduce is lost. Thus cell death is not the reason why cells, and by implication, the entire body, shows signs of aging.

Physiologic Theories. Theories at the tissue and organ level move outside of molecules and cell contents and behavior to deal with interrelationships between different organ systems during aging. Immunologic aging and neuroendocrine controls are two mechanisms that have been studied to explain age-related changes in tissue and organ function (Schimke and Agniel, 1983). Support for the proposition that immunologic function regulates genetic control of longevity has been found in at least three areas. Older women have more of a histocompatibility determinant (HLA-B8) that has been associated with impaired lymphocyte functions, increased autoimmune reactivity, and

shortened survival (Greenberg and Yunis, 1977). People over 80 years old with poor delayed skin responses to antigens had a death rate three times as high as that for age-matched controls (Roberts-Thompson et al., 1974). Two environmental modifications have altered immune reactivity and examined the effect on lifespan. Caloric restriction without malnutrition has been found to consistently prolong lifespan of rats (McCay, Cronell, and Maynard, 1935) and mice (Walford, Meredith, and Cheney, 1977). Lifespan has also been prolonged by reducing body temperature in fish. However, attempts to lower temperature in animals that regulate their own temperature (homeotherms) have not been successful (Liu and Walford, 1972). The immune system is thought to be controlled by the thymus, which, in turn, may be controlled by the pituitary.

An example of neuroendocrine control exists in the ovarian–pituitary–brain relationship, the neuroendocrine axes about which the most is known (Finch, 1977). Ovaries transplanted from old to young rats start to ovulate again while ovaries transplanted from young to old rats stop ovulating (Peng and Huang, 1972). Selected drugs such as catecholamine antagonists act on the hypothalamus to reactivate ovarian cycles in old rats (Huang and Meites, 1975). These results suggest the possibility that changes in some brain cells could serve as pacemakers of aging (Finch, 1979).

How Much of What I Can or Cannot Do Is Normal in Old Age?

The question concerning functional abilities can be answered on the basis of what changes are normal in old age and what changes are not normal and, thus, relate to disease processes. Strehler (1962) identified criteria that are useful in distinguishing senescence from other biologic processes. First, for a process to be considered characteristic of senescence, it must be universal; it must eventually occur in all people. An example is the decline in the effectiveness of the immune system, which is universal. However, the onset and rate of decline vary considerably from one person to another. The second criterion is that the changes that constitute senescence must come from within the organism. Changes caused by outside factors, such as radiation, are not true causes, since they can be modified. The third criterion states that the processes occur gradually rather than suddenly. This rules out accidents as causes of senescence. Finally, the changes that characterize senescence must have a deleterious effect on the organism, in that function declines and mortality increases. Probably, senescence reflects several processes. Biologic aging appears to occur at different rates in different people. Thus, older people vary widely with regard to the signs and symptoms of senescence.

Nurses who want to know what is biologically normal in aging can consider changes at any level of biologic structure from molecules to entire organisms. For example, Hayflick prepared convenient charts of changes and supporting references that indicated 63 properties that increase, 55 properties that decrease, and 50 properties that do not change as human cells approach the end of their lifespan in laboratory cultures (Hayflick, 1980, pp. 30–38).

What Can I Do to Live Longer?

An answer to clients' questions about what actions might be taken to enable them to live longer can be developed by considering both results of experimental laboratory research and descriptive studies of long-lived people.

Three methods, all supported by extensive laboratory research, have been shown to extend the human lifespan: (1) lower caloric intake, (2) fewer hours of sleep, and (3) reduced basal metabolic rates (Hayflick, 1981). Studies begun by McKay and associates (McKay, Crowell, and Maynard, 1935), and confirmed by many others, including Walford and colleagues (Walford et al., 1974; Walford, 1981), clearly indicate that rats fed diets that contain all essential nutrients, but are very low in calories, experience longevity that is increased by as much as 50 percent. The effects are greatest when caloric restriction diets begin when animals are very young. Each of the developmental stages—infancy, puberty, maturity, adulthood, and aging—occur later than usual and thus, the total lifespan is increased. Research in this area has shifted from documenting the effect of food restriction to discovering the mechanism involved and learning whether effects occur in mammals other than laboratory rodents (Masoro, 1981).

The interesting point about calorie reduction as a strategy to permit longer life is that no one has chosen to use the strategy, not even the biologists who are closest to the data (Hayflick, 1981, p. 39). Assuming the method is reasonably well-known, effective, and not dangerous, the only conclusion is that people prefer a life of quality rather than quantity.

Sleep researchers indicate that no negative health effects have been observed in people who make moderate reductions in the amount of time they spend asleep (Hayflick, 1981, p. 40). If people applied this information over the present life-span, they would enjoy an increase in waking time of over 2 years. This extension is equivalent to the gain that would be realized if cancer were halted as a cause of death.

Basal metabolic rate can be reduced most practically by living in environments where temperatures are cool but not low enough to cause shivering. An alternative method would use drugs to inhibit the sympathetic nervous system and produce a twilight sleep for a period of up to 10 years. This approach would add 5 years to the human life-span (Hayflick, 1981). However, sleeping for 10 years earlier in life to gain 5 years at the end seems like a bad risk. Living in cooler environments is a far more feasible method for reducing the basal metabolic rate.

Studies of long-lived people provide clues about actions people can take to increase their own chances of living out their expected lifespans. A considerable amount of research on longevity has been conducted at Duke University (Palmore, 1980). Predictors of longevity can be sorted into two categories: (1) behavioral predictors that lend themselves to control by individuals and (2) less modifiable predictors. More easily controllable predictors are diet, exercise, smoking, work, marital activity, and social involvement. Less easily controlled predictors are heredity, sex, race, intelligence, and socioeconomic status.

Diet. Simply stated, too much or too little food reduces longevity. The First Longitudinal Study at Duke revealed that the 10 percent of participants with the lowest and the 10 percent with the highest weight/height ratios had substantially more illness and less longevity than the middle 80 percent (Palmore, 1980).

Exercise. Older people who are more active and get more exercise tend to live longer than those who are less active. The extent to which lack of exercise and obesity are interrelated is not clear (Palmore, 1980).

Smoking. The association between smoking and greater mortality has been well supported. People who give up smoking live longer than those who continue to smoke (Palmore, 1980). However, some other factor than smoking per se may explain why nonsmokers live longer. For example, nonsmokers may have different personalities or be more generally conscientious about promoting their health.

Work/Retirement. Retired people have a higher mortality rate than those who continue to work (Palmore, 1980). The extent to which retirement forced by failing health and ability to find satisfaction in "work substitute" activities influence this association is not clear.

Marriage. Among elderly people, married people have lower mortality rates than unmarried people (Palmore, 1980). Patterns of mortality for never-married versus widowed people are reversed between the two sexes, with never-married women less at risk of dying than widowed women. Reasons for this phenomenon are not known.

Social Activity. Moderate to strong positive correlations have been found between the number of social activities engaged in by old people and greater longevity (Palmore, 1980). What is not clear is the extent to which better health acts to influence greater social activity and longevity.

Heredity. The general association between longevity of parents and offspring has been demonstrated in many studies. The Duke studies, however, found that this association disappeared once people reached age 60. This finding suggests longevity among old people is mostly the result of environmental and life-style differences, many of which can be changed (Palmore, 1980).

Sex. Women tend to live longer than men. However, the extent to which this tendency relates to sex-linked differences as opposed to life-style differences such as less hazardous occupations, less cigarette smoking, and more careful driving remains to be determined (Palmore, 1980). If life-style differences can be shown to be responsible for enabling women to live longer, then sex as such will cease to be associated with longevity.

Race. Blacks have greater mortality than whites up to age 75. This difference probably relates to differences in life-style and socioeconomic status. After age 75, similar longevity between the two races was thought to occur because only the fittest survived. Recent evidence suggests the phenomenon may occur because blacks exaggerate their ages in the absence of documentation of their true birth dates (Rosenwaike, 1982).

Socioeconomic Status. Education and income are strong predictors of longevity. For example, an analysis of 864 elderly people in Durham, NC used a Longevity Quotient (LQ) to assess several health and socioeconomic factors for their predictive power and relative importance to longevity (Palmore and Stone, 1973). The Longevity Quotient is the observed number of years survived after an initial interview, divided by the expected number of years based upon actuarial tables. An LQ of 1.0 means that a person lived as long as expected. An LQ of 1.5 means that the individual survived 50 percent longer than expected. Physical mobility, education, occupation, and continued employment were found to be significant predictors of longevity, and mobility was the strongest of these. However, the three socioeconomic status variables accounted for two-thirds of the explained variance in longevity (Palmore and

Stone, 1973, p. 88). Higher intelligence or better mental function has been associated with
greater longevity. However, there are several
alternative explanations for this association.
Better mental function may result from better
health. Greater intelligence may simply be the
factor that leads to more education (Palmore,
1980).

Considering results of research that produced extensions of longevity as well as research that identified factors common to people
who had already lived beyond their life expectancy, nurses may reply to clients' questions
about actions to promote longevity. Motivated
clients can be told to reduce what they eat in
terms of calories, but not essential nutrients, and
live in cool environments to add years.
People can sleep less to at least increase waking time during the years available. Maintaining a life-style characterized by physical
activity, meaningful use of time, non-smoking,
marriage, education, and wealth may enable
individuals to avoid losing years that would
otherwise be available to them. Longevity-as-
sociated factors have been used to develop a
quiz that nurses may wish to share so that
clients can assess their longevity potential. This
quiz may be found in Appendix A.

Psychosocial Views

Psychologic Theories of Aging

Theories of psychologic aging are concerned
with behavior changes within and between individuals (Baltes and Willis, 1977, p. 148). The
boundaries that define the area of psychologic
aging are vague and subject to dispute. Figure
3.3 indicates the lack of agreement as to the
domain of psychologic theory. Traditional systems are still considered, along with more contemporary orientations and a variety of behavior areas extending from the cellular to
societal levels. Because the subject matter is
so diffuse, most of the concepts and theories
listed in Figure 3.3 will not be discussed. Those
wishing to obtain information about these concepts are advised to consult current references
on the topic of interest such as "memory," "personality," or "learning." In reviewing material
about these topics, nurses need to remember
that the theories are incomplete, imprecise, and
limited in scope.

In trying to develop theories to explain
behavior changes involving elderly people, target classes of behavior require identification
and appropriate ways to describe those behaviors must be determined. Psychologic aging has

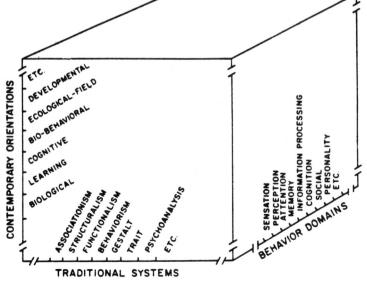

Figure 3.3. An illustration of the
lack of agreement regarding the
domain of psychologic theory.
*(Baltes, P.B., Willis, S.L. Toward
psychological theories of aging
and development. In Birren, J.F.,
Schaie, K.W., (eds.). Handbook of
the Psychology of Aging. New
York, Van Nostrand Reinhold,
1977. Copyright 1977 by Litton
Educational Publishing, Inc. Reprinted by permission.)*

been described through the following propositions (Baltes and Willis, 1977, pp. 135–139):

1. The term "aging" suggests a process and change. Nothing in the term aging implies that aging equals deterioration or decline. Nor does the term aging suggest that chronologic age can serve to explain aging behavior.
2. The nature of behavioral change at any stage of the lifespan can take many forms in reference to directionality (incremental or decremental), range (number of behavior domains), or intensity (marked or minimal changes).
3. Of all behaviors, those that may be labeled as developmental or aging-related are those that appear with regularity in a certain sequence after the reproductive period (during maturity).
4. Behavior-change processes are usually viewed in terms of the individual (intraindividual change) and differences between individuals (interindividual changes).
5. Behavior change patterns are viewed as incremental (↑), decremental (↓), or curvilinear (ˆ). The form and direction of change is based upon whether quantitative (more or less of some characteristic) or structural (different kinds of characteristics or different relations among characteristics) change is being considered.

   Those who wish to explain why individuals behave as they do must consider how variables relate to each other to account for change within and between individuals. Issues of importance in trying to explain psychologic aging include the following (Baltes and Willis, 1977, pp. 139-141):

1. Behavior may change as a result of one or several factors. Scientists tend to believe that there is no single cause for behavior changes in the elderly.
2. The methods used to study long-term behavior change may need to differ from those used to study short-term behavior change.
3. Decisions as to what is adequate evidence to explain behavior change in the elderly may be related to the theoretical viewpoint of those making the decisions. For example,

a personologist may be satisfied with predictive statements of the behavior–behavior type such as Erikson's* stage of integrity follows the stage of generativity; an ethologist would focus on evolutionary survival characteristics and organism–environment interactions as acceptable forms of explanation.
4. Factors that explain behavior change may be placed on a time-continuum that ranges from concurrent to historic. To illustrate, loss of short-term memory could be explained by a reduction of sensory input (the concurrent explanation) or by an absence of selected educational experiences in childhood (the historic explanation).
5. Factors that explain behavior may change from one developmental life phase to another. For example, intellectual function in a young adult may be more closely related to school experiences while intellectual functioning in a middle-aged adult may relate more closely to some physiologic or cellular change.

   Both biologic and environmental factors are believed to influence behavior change processes. Studies of a variety of behavioral processes indicate that movement "toward slowness, less behavior, less acquisition, less performance, and greater dependence" may not be a fair description of true changes, but rather a reflection of the theoretical orientation of the researcher (Baltes and Willis, 1977, p. 138). *Indeed, the less the individual is able to show competence or the ability to function in his environment, the more important the environment may be in shaping his behavior.* Nurses who work with the elderly have recognized the importance of environment as an influence on behavior by implementing programs to enhance short-term memory. Other nurses have experimented with audio tape recordings made by significant others as a tool for increasing re-

---

* Erikson (1959), a psychoanalytical theorist, proposed "eight stages of man," of which the last three cover periods after adolescence: intimacy versus isolation, generativity versus stagnation, and ego integrity versus despair. Each stage represents a crisis for an expanding ego. The resolution of each ego crisis determines the future development of the personality.

sponsiveness in the elderly. Persistent beliefs that the elderly can learn, be active, and remain independent have motivated nurses to continue rehabilitative efforts long after other members of the health team have lost hope for behavioral change in certain elderly clients.

Despite the large number of systems, orientations, and behavior domains implicated, psychologic theories of aging are often considered to include only theories of personality development. Personality has been defined as the enduring dimensions or distinctive characteristics of the individual (Staub, 1980). Personality does not have the inevitably declining characteristics of physiologically linked processes such as memory, perception, sensation, or cognition. Developmental theory seeks to discover the higher, more differentiated, growth processes that occur with aging. Characteristics of this optimization model have been summarized (Danish and D'Augelli, 1980):

1. Statements about desirable goals or end-states of behavior.
2. Focus on sequential change and conditions that lead to growth.
3. Emphasis on techniques of optimization.
4. Consideration of the individual as an integrative biopsychosocial unit.
5. A view of development occurring in a changing biocultural context.

The psychosocial model of ego development formulated by Erickson (1959, 1961) is probably the most well-known example of lifespan development theory. Other theories considered include those developed by Neugarten (1968; 1973), Clark and Anderson (1967), Buhler (1935) and Buhler and Massarik (1968), Emmerich (1968), Loevinger (1966; 1976); Maslow (1971), Havighurst (1975), Vaillant (1977), Gould (1978), Levinson (1978), Runyan (1980), and Ryff and Heinke (1981).

Each of these theories proposes a series of phases people pass through or tasks to perform over the life cycle, including the later years. Each theory regards old age as an inevitably different sequence in the life cycle, with its unique characteristics and challenges. The "inevitability" is caused by the physical changes associated with biologic aging. Physical changes, environmental factors, and facts of individual history act as forces to compel a progressive unfolding of the personality.

Lifespan developmental theories have been severely criticized because of their association with stage theory (Baltes, 1979; Brim and Kagan, 1980). Stage theory originated in a biologic growth theory of development and is considered to represent an inflexible course that is unidirectional, irreversible, hierarchical, invariant, and universal. Culture, individual differences, and environment are not included as influences in stage theory (Ryff, 1982, p. 12). Some of this criticism has been unfairly applied. For example, Emmerich (1968) clarified Erikson's theory to indicate that psychosocial crises do occur in a fixed developmental order but that each crisis can be resolved in one of two ways. These differing outcomes incorporate individual differences. More recently, researchers of adult personality (for example, Havighurst, 1975; Schaie and Parham, 1976; and Thomae, 1980) have rejected the proposition of a universal unidirectional pattern of development during the aging process, as was hypothesized by Erikson (1959) or Cumming and Henry (1961).

Developmental theories have also been faulted for establishing unrealistic standards of selflessness, contentment, and introspection. If attained, these standards would effectively place elderly people on "pedestals" and remove them from the power arena (Haymes, 1979).

Theories of adult personality development have had great face appeal. The challenge is to define the concepts (for example, "ego integrity" or "executive processes") in such a way that they can be validly and reliably measured and the theories they represent can be tested.

Sociologic Theories of Aging

Theory development related to sociologic aspects of aging has focused largely on ways the elderly adapt during later life (the individual's perspective). A second focus has been on environmental influences on the adaptive process and outcomes and the status elderly people hold as a group compared to other age groups in this society and to the elderly in other societies (the societal perspective). Sociologic theory formulations exist in crude form as blends of interesting concepts that have not necessarily been clearly defined or translated into statements of interrelationships.

Because of their assumptions, limitations, and lack of research-based support, individual social theories of aging cannot be used prescriptively to direct nursing practice. However, considered as a group, these theories suggest three broad theoretical perspectives that describe possible relationships involving elderly people and the larger society. Nurses may recognize these perspectives as influencing the way they practice and the kinds of policies they support. These theoretical perspectives are abandonment, liberation, and solidarity. These perspectives ask, respectively, (1) Do we abandon our elderly people? (2) Do we free elderly people from burdens of the middle years, especially those imposed by work? and (3) Do we need elderly people?

To illustrate these three perspectives, selected individual and societal level theories of sociologic aging that have been more widely discussed in the literature have been described and critiqued in order to identify major assumptions and limitations of each framework. Finally, implications of the three broad theoretical perspectives for practice, policy formation, and research have been discussed.

The Individual's Perspective. This first group of sociologic theories considers the broad question, "What do old people need to do in terms of relating to other people in order to be successful?" Theoretical formulations that attempt to answer this question include "disengagement theory," "activity theory," and "continuity theory."*

1. DISENGAGEMENT THEORY. Disengagement theory was the first theory to take into account some of the facts of development during the latter stages of normal aging and the only theory developed specifically for the elderly. Cumming and Henry (1961) challenged the assumption that people must be fully integrated socially throughout their lifetimes in order to maintain a sense of well-being. Their observations can be summarized in four propositions (Cumming, 1975, p. 188):

1. The life space of an individual decreases with age, in that he interacts with a narrower variety of role partners and spends a smaller proportion of time in social interaction. This proposition was later elaborated to highlight the importance of key life roles of work and family.
2. The individual anticipates this change and participates in the process by changing preferences, moving on a scale of interpersonal rewards from role connected to more individualized interactions.
3. The individual's preference for personal rewards becomes more individualized and expressive, and less role connected, as he grows older and thus his style of interaction changes.
4. If the individual has relinquished obligatory roles, and if he has become more individualized and expressive, which is to say less normative and confronting, then he is unlikely either to seek out or to be sought out for new obligatory roles. This is the same as saying that once started, disengagement has a momentum of its own. As the aging individual gives up obligatory roles, he gains freedom and loses centrality.

The disengagement perspective has had an unfortunate history, involving considerable misapplication. Presented in brief, tentative form in 1960 (Cumming et al., 1960), the theory was elaborated upon and modified in the book, *Growing Old* (Cumming and Henry, 1961), modified and contradicted in part by Henry (1964) and again modified by Cumming (1975). Cumming herself described the theory as "poorly operationalized and largely untested" (1975, p. 4).

---

* Other, less often mentioned formulations, include "minority group theory" (Breen, 1960; Barron, 1961; Palmore, 1978); "subculture theory" (Rose, 1962; Rose and Peterson, 1965; Longino, McClelland, and Peterson, 1980); "exchange theory" (Homans, 1974; Dowd, 1980); "normative socialization" (Rosow, 1974; Marshall, 1978–79); "interactionist theory" (Spence, 1975; Marshall, 1978–79); "socioenvironmental theory" (Gubrium, 1972); and "unitary man" (Rogers, 1970; 1980).

Disengagement theory has been attacked on three essential assumptions: (1) withdrawal from society is functional (beneficial) for both the individual (energy is conserved to permit preparation for death) and society (younger people fill roles left vacant by older people), (2) the process is universal and inevitable (everyone disengages sooner or later), and (3) differences in personality are not important. In disputing disengagement theory, the bulk of research-based evidence supports the conclusion that "engaged" individuals are more likely than "unengaged" people to express satisfaction with their situations. Support for an active life-style can be found in studies by Bengston, Chiriboga, and Keller, 1969; Havighurst et al., 1969; and Knapp, 1977). This finding does not imply that all individuals desire a level of contact consistent with engagement levels of their middle years. What is important, however, is the degree of agreement between actual and desired participation.

The agreement of universality is not supportable against cross-cultural evidence. Investigations conducted in other countries have revealed mutually satisfactory work arrangements that permit people past the age of 100 years to participate in hard, daily toil (Leaf, 1973).

In disregarding personality differences, disengagement theory runs counter to the belief of developmental theorists who regard personality as the pivotal dimension in describing patterns of aging and in predicting relationships between level of social role activity and life satisfaction (Neugarten, Havighurst, and Tobin, 1968).

Perhaps Cumming and Henry ought to have ignored questions of what *should be* and pursued the questions of what *is* the normal aging process. The false impression that disengagement was an alternative model to activity theory (which proposes a constantly expanding life-space) might then have been avoided. A person who assumes fewer obligatory roles or interactions within society may still remain active, traveling around the country, playing golf, cultivating his garden, or sitting in a chair, reading a book. The phenomenon of disengagement may become more pronounced in the old-old group than the young-old group. In other words, one should see disengagement more clearly as people continue to age. Most people aged 90 are less active or involved in activities than they were at age 65.

2. ACTIVITY THEORY. The roots of activity theory have been traced to studies reported by Cavan et al. (1949) and Havighurst and Albrecht (1953). This theory was considerably revised, ending in the formulations of Lemon, Bengston, and Peterson (1972). Activity theory asserts a positive relationship between individuals' levels of participation in social activities and their life satisfaction and that the greater the role loss, the lower the life satisfaction (Lemon et al., 1972). Central concepts used in activity theory are activity, role supports, self-concept, role change, and life satisfaction.

Activity is "any regularized or patterned action or pursuit that is regarded as beyond routine physical or personal maintenance" (Lemon et al., 1972, p. 513). Three separate types of activities are (1) informal activity on a personal or intimate level with friends and neighbors, (2) formal activity such as participation in voluntary associations and societies, and (3) solitary activity such as leisure pursuits, maintenance of household, and gardening. These activities are arranged on a continuum from most to least important for providing role support and, in turn, reinforcing self-concept.

Role support is defined as the expressed support accorded to an individual by his audience for his claims concerning his role identity (McCall and Simmons, 1966).

Self-concept refers to the individual's view of himself as he thinks of being and acting in a given situation. (Kinch, 1963; McCall and Simmons, 1966).

Role loss is defined as an "alteration in the set of behavior patterns expected of an individual by virtue of the loss of some status position within a given social structure," such as the transition from work to retirement (Lemon, et al., 1972, p. 513).

Life satisfaction is "the degree to which one is presently content or pleased with his general life situation" (Lemon, et al., 1972, p. 513).

Relationships among these central concepts can be as follows:

> Activity provides various role supports necessary for reaffirming one's self-concept. The more intimate and the more frequent the activity, the more reinforcing and the more specific will be the role supports. Role supports are necessary for the maintenance of a positive self-concept which, in turn, is associated with high life satisfaction.
>
> In order to more fully explain the relationship between activity and life satisfaction, the concept of role change is utilized for analyzing conditions that further specify increases and decreases in this relationship. The presence of a role loss should diminish the magnitude of the relationship, but the direction of the relationship should remain positive. (Lemon, Bengtson, and Peterson, 1972, p. 515)

Propositions relating activity to life satisfaction were stated as a series of postulates and theorems (Lemon, et al., 1972, p. 515):

P1. The greater the role loss, the less the activity one is likely to engage in.
P2. The greater the activity, the more role support one is likely to receive.
P3. The more role support one receives, the more positive one's self-concept is likely to be.
P4. The more positive one's self-concept, the greater one's life satisfaction is likely to be.

There are three first-order theorems that can be deduced from these postulates:

T1. The greater the role loss, the less role support one is likely to receive.
T2. The greater the activity, the more positive one's self-concept is likely to be.
T3. The greater the role support, the greater one's life satisfaction is likely to be.

Two second-order theorems can then be deduced from combining the above:

T4. The greater the role loss, the less the positive self-concept.

T5. The greater the activity, the greater one's life satisfaction.

Finally, one third-order theorem can be deduced:

T6. The greater the role loss, the lower the life satisfaction.

Except for the inevitable changes in biology and in health, older people are the same as middle aged people, with essentially the same psychologic and social needs (Havighurst, 1968); this suggests that the need for social activity is shared by all people. Thus, there is a natural tendency for elderly people to seek associations with others and to participate in group affairs, although these needs can be blocked by social norms such as mandatory retirement or by physical decline. When these forces act to constrict self-enhancing activities and interests, the individuals affected experience a crisis in self-esteem, leading to a negative self-image and alienation from the environment (Maddox and Eisdorfer, 1962).

Major assumptions of activity theory are that elderly people have the same needs as middle aged people and that activities common to the middle years are of equal value to those available in the older years. The first assumption disregards personality and other changes associated with normal aging that may serve to alter activity needs. The second assumption fails to consider that the meaning of vocational, professional, and fraternal associations of the middle years may not be readily replaced by the gardening, sport, and craft activities available to elderly people (Gubrium, 1973). Activity theory does not deal with the impacts of biologic changes and health problems, reduced income due to retirement, environmental barriers such as inadequate transportation, and institutional failures to provide activity options for residents. Preparation for death was not considered in this theory. The theory reflects a middle class bias in calling for elderly people to substitute roles and activities for those that are lost. Continuation or replacement is usually easier for people who have had the luxury of developing alternative interests early in life and may have retired electively.

When Lemon and others (1972) tested some of the propositions of activity theory, they found that only social activity with friends (not neighbors or relatives) was related to life satisfaction among a sample of individuals in a retirement community. Propositions that the greater the frequency of activity, the greater one's life satisfaction and that the greater the role loss, the lower the life satisfaction were not substantiated by the results.

3. CONTINUITY THEORY. The concept of continuity was offered as a more realistic and less elaborate explanation of the aging process and as an explanation of why neither disengagement nor activity theories seem to apply. The term, continuity, generally refers to "connectedness" of one's present to one's past. One explanation of continuity is offered by Atchley (1977):

> The continuity approach to individual aging assumes that in the process of becoming adults, individuals develop habits, commitments, preferences, and a host of other dispositions that become a part of their personalities. As the individuals grow older, they are predisposed toward maintaining continuity in habits, associations, preferences, and so on. Unlike the activity theory, the continuity theory does not assume that lost roles need to be replaced.
>
> In this context, *continuity* means that the individual's reaction to aging can be explained by examining the complex interrelationships among biologic and psychosocial changes; the person's habits, preferences, and associations; situational opportunities for continuity; and actual experience. The lifelong experience thus creates certain predispositions that individuals will maintain if at all possible. At all phases of the life course, these predispositions constantly evolve from interactions among personal preferences, biologic and psychologic capabilities, situational opportunities, and experience. Change is thus an adaptive process involving interaction among all of these elements (Atchley, 1977, p. 27).

In applying continuity theory to elderly people and their social roles, two central questions need to be addressed: (1) What factors account for an older person's success or failure in maintaining social roles in old age? and (2) Why do older people desire continuity in some

instances and not in others? Two general sets of factors affect continuity of social roles: (1) individual characteristics such as psychologic motivation, socioeconomic status, personality, health, and so forth and (2) societal characteristics such as flexibility/restrictiveness, age grading, and age stereotypes. These factors have been used to develop three propositions to answer the two central questions posed above (Covey, 1981, pp. 630–631):

1. As the person's resources and abilities increase, the ability to continue in social roles increases.
2. As the restrictiveness of the social structure declines, the ability of older people to maintain and continue desired social roles increases.
3. People with the most rewarding and desirable social roles, i.e., higher socioeconomic status roles, are unlikely to want to surrender these roles.

According to these propositions, "successful" aging depends on whether the balance rests in the individual's favor, implying he or she can perform any desired social role, or in favor of the social structure where the individual's options are dictated and restricted by role.

Studies that observed the same people over a number of years and used objective personality measures have provided evidence in support of predominant stability or consistency of personality throughout adulthood (Costa and McCrae, 1977, 1978; Douglas and Arenberg, 1978; Siegler, George and Okun, 1979; Costa, McCrae, and Arenberg, 1980). Thus challenges that arise in the later years should bring out responses very similar to those used during middle age. Individuals may accept losses or make substitutions, depending on previous responses in similar situations. Old age is not seen as a separate period of life, but as a continuation of some patterns set earlier, especially coping strategies of acting, thinking, and feeling. Implicit in this theory is the notion that continuity is positively related to successful aging. The more people can do what they have always done, the higher their morale will be.

Continuity theory implies a certain degree

of rigidity in the individual's social behavior. The amount of determinism or "fixedness" has not been decided. Do people who appear to make free choices and change radically do so because their personalities and life-style preprogrammed them to behave in this way? Or are changes in later life more consistent with the sociologic concept of "career," which implies change with relatedness or cohesiveness of phases with each other?

The idea that successful adjustment to old age is based upon a continuity of life patterns is rapidly emerging as one of the most promising theories in social gerontology (Bultena, 1969; Guttmann, 1979; Myerhoff, 1978; Holzberg, 1982). Continuity theory considers factors not included in other theories and thus addresses the common features of old age while allowing for individual variation.

One criticism of continuity theory is that it is too broad to be much value because it does consider multiple variables. "To observe that older people are content in a variety of settings, doing and thinking a variety of things, is merely to confirm the diversity of human existence" (Fox, 1981–82, p. 113). Diversity cannot, however, be assumed to be the same as continuity. Continuity has been defined variously as "stability," "persistence," "life-style," and "personality." A term that is not clearly defined cannot be translated into measures that permit systematic testing.

Fox (1981–82) examined evidence to decide whether continuity was, in fact, associated with adaptation and whether more continuity was better than less continuity. The strongest support for the notion that continuity is adaptive was evidence of the cumulative negative effects of life events. People who experience a great number of life changes within a year appear to be more prone to physical illness than are others (Holmes and Rahe, 1967). However, perceived control over the event(s)—foreknowledge and preplanning, prior expectation, and personal integration—can buffer the effect of a particular life event (Nuckolls, Cassel, and Kaplan, 1972; Cassel, 1974).

When continuity consists of clinging to old ways of thinking and behaving, people may be less able to develop a rewarding life-style in old age. For example, parents with high expectations of care and attention from children experience low morale (Kerckhoff, 1966; Seelback and Sauer, 1977). Retirees who try to function in retirement as they did in their work roles experience increased feelings of job deprivation (Simpson and McKinney, 1966). Women who refuse to give up parental roles experience more depression (Bart, 1971).

After considering available evidence, Fox (1981–82) proposed an ideal level of continuity that allows for initiation of change as well as response to change. This position is adaptive because people experience both connectedness with the past and present ability to control their lives. The extremes are not adaptive. At one extreme, people cling to past values and behaviors and are therefore unable to deal with life in the present. At the other extreme, people find so much of their world altered that they lose touch with their past.

Fox, however, cautions that continuity requires careful definition at both the conceptual and operational levels to permit hypotheses like the optimum level proposition to be tested. In the meantime, "continuity, as either descriptor of the aging process or facilitator of adaptation, is a variable whose potential and limitations are still uncharted" (Fox, 1981–82, p. 113).

The Society's Perspective. A second group of sociologic theories address the question, "What does society need to do with elderly people in order for society to be successful?" Theoretical formulations that relate to this question are the "modernization perspective" (Cowgill and Holmes, 1972), "intergenerational linkage theory" (Bengtson and Cutler, 1976), "structural–functional theory" (Bengtson and Dowd, 1980–81), the "world-we-have-lost perspective" (Laslett, 1976), and "solidarity theory" (Baum and Baum, 1980).

1. MODERNIZATION PERSPECTIVE. The modernization perspective holds that the distribution of resources and esteem to elderly persons in a given society is negatively related to the development of technology and occupational specialization, in short, to modernization (Cowgill and Holmes, 1972). Application

of exchange theory to observations of the fate of people in preindustrial and industrial societies yielded twenty-two general propositions that show why modern societies have comparatively less use for their older people and why becoming old in modern society must amount to suffering from relative status deprivation. For example, preindustrial societies had few social roles and little difference between social roles so that what was learned in one role applied to others. Role structures were stable so people could learn by experience. An oral, rather than a mechanical, tradition meant that experience and knowledge were shared by speaking and remembering rather than by writing. Thus, the elderly could continue to function in their roles and were useful to society because they possessed greater amounts of the knowledge and skills that were needed by everyone (Baum and Baum, 1980).

The modernization perspective was modified somewhat by Palmore and Manton (1974) to suggest that as societies move beyond the rapid modernization stage, discrepancies between the status of the elderly and the nonelderly decrease. Thus, the short- and long-range outcomes of modernization may be different for elderly people.

2. INTERGENERATIONAL LINKAGE. Differences between age groups has long been a popular concern, as evidenced by discussions of the "generation gap" and what people think they will be like when they are old. Intergenerational linkage theory is one of the most general in social gerontology, with its attention to differences and similarities in the formative experiences of successive generations and their relations with each other. At present, this perspective does not offer conclusions about whether we abandon, liberate, or need old people (Baum and Baum, 1980). Instead, this perspective provides a way of examining relations between generations. In examining differences between generations, intergenerational linkage theory considers three elements: (1) changes over time that result from maturing or aging (maturation effect), (2) changes created by historic or period events (period effect), and (3) contrasts that last throughout the lifespan of

a particular age group, often called "cohort" or "generational" effects (cohort effect).

A hypothetical example may help to explain how each of these factors operates. Mr. Smith, age 85, belongs to a club comprised of 150 elderly people, all over age 70. Club members associate primarily with each other, complain about other segments of society, and refuse to become involved in "politics." In short, this group appears disgruntled and alienated. If a maturation effect were responsible, the behavior would be explained as the result of the group's passing through this particular "time of life"; moreover, the next generation to reach their 70s and 80s would be expected to demonstrate this behavior as well. The conclusion would be that people become alienated as they grow older. If a period effect was responsible, the behavior would be due to some specific event that was happening at the same time, such as a threat to abolish retirement benefits for people who are presently retired. The conclusion might be that old people are alienated today because they resent the proposal to deprive them of an income. If a cohort effect explained the behavior, some event that occurred earlier in life for the group would be blamed for the behavior. The conclusion might be that old people are alienated today because they are the same group that lost all of their money during the Great Depression and have been alienated ever since that time.

Bengtson and Cutler (1976), who have done a number of studies of intergenerational relations, caution that all three hypotheses must be considered in a single study before any conclusion can be drawn as to which is the most appropriate. By studying relationships between generations to discover patterns of cooperation or conflict, issue by issue, and the outcomes that occur, analytic methods and concepts will develop to permit better prediction about the role of elderly people in the evolution of society (Bengtson and Cutler, 1976).

3. STRUCTURAL–FUNCTIONAL THEORY. The central proposition of the structural–functional orientation is that there exists functional and structural requirements related to the on-

going operation of any system. Societies award status to individuals according to how useful they are to the total society. In terms of a specific institution, the family, the dependent, nonfunctional position of "unwed adolescent" becomes, in turn, a "spouse," "parent of lastborn," "firstborn launched," "lastborn launched," and "grandparent," a series of functions that are alternately less, more, and less necessary for maintenance of the society. Individuals also perform in several institutions (such as family and economic) at once. Old age is commonly a time when people lose functional positions in major institutions: economically, old people lose functions as producers and consumers; in the family, old people cease procreating; and in major organizations like churches and fraternal associations, old people may retire from strategic positions. In summary, structural–functional theory holds that age seems curvilinearly related to functional status in the larger society, with young and old people contributing less of what society needs to survive than people in their middle years. Interaction between the individual and others in society occurs because (1) normative expectations require that interaction be maintained or (2) the interaction fulfills some socially required need (Bengtson and Dowd, 1980–81). Thus, interaction between old people and the rest of society depends on normative expectations.

4. THE WORLD-WE-HAVE-LOST PERSPECTIVE. Peter Laslett (1976) offered the idea that regardless of how society should relate to its elderly in the present, resurrection of strategies used in the past would probably not benefit the elderly. Four propositions served to summarize beliefs about the present and past that supported the notion that the past was better:

1. There has been a *before* and an *after* in the matter of aging. Before and after are sometimes distinguished on *chronologic* grounds associated with the transition from an agrarian to an industrial society and sometimes on *geographic* grounds referring to the nonindustrial and societies in the present world.

2. In the *before* the aged fared very well in that they were entitled to and received respect and a fair share of material goods; in the *after,* the aged fare very badly since they are rejected as worthless and are accorded little in terms of prestige or material goods.

3. In the *before* the aged had prescribed and valued roles to fill as workers until death, as grandparents in multigenerational households and as transmitters and symbols of the culture. In the *after,* these roles are no longer necessary and even become obstacles to the attainment of a "modern" way of life.

4. In the *before,* no aging relatives should have had to live alone or without adequate company, or perhaps worst of all, in an institution. In the *after,* the extended kin groups or households give way to the family consisting of an adult male and female and possibly a few children. Old people live with each other, if they can, or live alone, or enter institutions. The duties of significant others consist of economic assistance and visiting rather than permanent alteration of the family configuration (Laslett, 1976, pp. 89–91).

The unifying thread of these propositions is the idea that a *before* exists in the past and an *after* exists today. The transition from the past to the present is associated with a deep sense of loss. The aged were greatly deprived, and society as a whole was impoverished by its failure to consider them. Laslett calls these views *the world-we-have-lost syndrome,* in which present deficiencies are believed to result from the destruction of an ideal society at some time in the past (Laslett, 1976, p. 91). Using data from a careful review of historic materials from several different countries, he refutes the four propositions entirely.

The idea of a single transition is too simple. In theory, as economic development occurred, traditional society became modern, and a large portion of the population became old. Actually, at least in the United States and Great Britain, large increases in the numbers of elderly occurred much later. Role changes caused by movement from an agrarian to an industrial society may not have been as devastating as supposed. Retirement has proven to be desirable for most retirees, and old people have filled roles ranging from "satisfied senior citizen, free to pursue individual interests" to "second career." The notion that old people had an ideal domestic situation in the *before* may be more myth than fact.

The *after* picture is also less devastating than has been portrayed. The problems of old people who sought welfare services led observers to believe that their situation represented the norm. Upon closer examination, however, this view must be questioned. The elderly as a group are not economically deprived, psychologically alienated, or disabled by illness. They are overrepresented among persons with incomes below the poverty level, but these poor elderly are not the majority of the elderly. Examination of their life histories shows that many led marginal economic existences all their lives (Maddox, 1973).

The elderly retain basic legal rights and participate in political processes in a manner similar to other adults. Most old people live in private residences and maintain relationships with kin of different generations. Thus, age in itself does not appear to determine the degree of social integration. "Even if age, or age related characteristics such as illness or poverty, were demonstrably an impediment to integration within a given society, one would still need to explore the transience and modifiability of such a finding" (Maddox and Wiley, 1976, p. 15).

An alternative in the "world-we-have-lost" notion suggests that the position of the elderly in our present social structure is historically novel (Comfort, 1975; Laslett, 1976). If, indeed, the aged represent a problem to be solved, the problem is a new one. In the past, never did so many live to be so old. Many who are old today never expected to live so long. The elderly are finding roles to fill and are struggling to retain a fair share of material goods and services. Young people today have a chance to plan and prepare for old age. Efforts to define a social status for old people might proceed more smoothly if the idea of a lost utopia were allowed to fade (Laslett, 1976, p. 96).

5. SOLIDARITY THEORY. Movement from an agrarian society to a modern industrial society has increased the number of stages in life from three (infancy, adulthood, and old age) (Aries, 1962) to at least eight (infancy, childhood, adolescence, young adulthood, middle adulthood, young-old age, old age, and old-old age). An increase in age periods in the organization of social life has more potential for intergenerational conflict and raises the question of how a solid society is possible at all with an extensive division of labor.

Solidarity occurs in society because of peoples' experiences within their families. People enter their families not by their own choice but by their parents' choice. This is why children are simply given basic rights while obligations remain less clear. Family solidarity is the model of true human belonging. "Home is where they have to take you in" (Baum and Baum, 1980, p. 32). In a modern society, resolution of the problem of how special interests can get along requires application of basic kinship loyalties (ascribed rights and diffuse obligations) to non-kinship relationships. As a precondition to transferring kinship loyalties, Eisenstadt proposed that:

> The solidarity of a modern society demands the effective symbolization of the supremacy of collective over individual goals even where, and especially when, purely individualist value patterns prevail. Any integrative mechanism must reflect such primacy. (Eisenstadt 1971, p. 47)

This problem of how special interest groups can get along with each other at a given time has been termed the problem of synchronic solidarity.

A related problem concerns how identities can be shared from generation to generation. This second concern has been termed the problem of diachronic solidarity. Diachronic solidarity is "a social identity shared with successive generations, that always connects the younger with the older in a perpetual chain of community lasting through time, indefinitely" (Baum and Baum, 1980, p. 8).

The precondition that makes production of a shared sense of identity between successive generations necessary has been phrased to parallel that for transferring kinship loyalties (Baum and Baum, 1980, p. 23):

> The solidarity of a modern society demands also the effective symbolization of the supremacy of continuity over change in citizenship identities and their attendant rights and obligations even, and especially, under conditions of high rates of perceived social change.

Any stabilizing mechanism must reflect such primacy. The social rights of old age are a symbol of continuity to which people can cling while they experience the effects of life in a dynamic and changing society. Fulfilling an obligation to its old people lets the rest of society feel the sense of loyalty and belonging that is necessary for collective well-being.

To determine the fate of elderly people in modern societies, Baum and Baum (1980) examined several aspects of old age within industrial societies: economics, retirement, politics, family life, dying, and bereavement and death. They concluded the modern fate of being old is "a fourfold experience of (1) diachronic solidarity in economic or material care, (2) diachronic solidarity in political bonds of citizenship, (3) abandonment in the area of spiritual care, and (4) death as a liberation from the uncertainties inherent in the human condition" (Baum and Baum, 1980, p. 237).

Compared to the elderly who lived before the rise of industrialism, old people in modern societies are far more prosperous. However, if old age income is compared to incomes earned by people in their middle years or by older people in their years right before retirement, old age income certainly amounts to relative deprivation. The United States stands alone among modern societies in abandoning almost one-fourth of its elderly to economic misery through inadequate provisions for income and health services. No other country abandons this large a proportion of its elderly to relative poverty.

Using American facts and figures, Baum and Baum (1980) found "strong cross-generational support for retirement as an earned end phase in the human life cycle" (p. 239). Considering political support within the United States, the United Kingdom, and Sweden, in none of the three countries could the political support for social security systems be attributed to age-based lobbies. Support clearly came from people in other age categories. In addition, elderly people were reelected repeatedly to public office. This finding may reflect a preference for the generalist. An older person has lived longer and, therefore, has seen and experienced more than younger people.

Other evidence in support of diachronic solidarity was found in commitment to material care for old parents by their children. "Children, often near old age themselves, hardly ever shirk responsibility to care for their parents when failing health turns the latter into creatures dependent on their own offspring" (Baum and Baum, 1980, p. 245). However, the care provided tends to be material in nature and focused on physical well-being.

Abandonment in the area of spiritual care occurs when old people are visibly dying and when widows experience acute grief. For the most part, elderly parents live apart from their children while both parties exchange affection and caring. This relationship has been labeled, "intimacy at a distance." When failing health and growing incapacities indicate a terminal illness and a lengthy period of suffering for old people, this is the phase when old people are abandoned. "Dying is not a well-regulated status in modern society" (Baum and Baum, 1980, p. 250). Many people die in general hospitals where neither staff nor visitors know how to feel, how to share emotions, or what to say to the dying. The widow in bereavement experiences the same abandonment. Although grief is obviously "normal," the role does not tell others how to behave. Thus attempts to share the burden and otherwise help often fail.

The subjective experience of death appears to represent joyous liberation from life for most old people. Liberation in this instance refers to the uncertainty of ever finding comprehensive meaning in human life. Reports of the near dead in several societies, including North America and Western Europe, indicate that death implies finding a solution that eludes people in life. That is, death is a release from human existence as doubters (Baum and Baum, 1980, pp. 251–252).

Implications for Nursing Practice

The descriptions given previously should lead the nurse to realize that the capacities to prolong life or to maintain life satisfaction when confronted by physical, psychologic, and social changes in old age are phenomena that require further study. Empirical evidence supporting any single position is scant. Perhaps by close examination of elderly clients—who they are, how they appear, and what they want—nurses will contribute to more precise definitions of biopsychosocial aspects of aging and old age.

The main reason that nurses require knowledge of biologic theories of aging is to respond to clients' questions. At best, psychosocial theories suggest three possible relationships between our society and its elderly people: (1) abandonment, (2) liberation, and (3) solidarity. Nurses may find, if they examine their clinical practice, beliefs about social policies, and concerns about research, that they are influenced more by one of these perspectives than the other.

Abandonment

Do we abandon old people? This perspective is based on the idea that preindustrial societies needed old people, but modern societies do not need them. Thus, old people represent a social problem and stand as a group outside of society as a whole.

Support for the abandonment perspective can be found in a number of the social theories of aging previously reviewed. Disengagement theory suggests the elderly need to step aside and prepare for death. Subculture theory would have elderly people reengaging within their own age groups. Activity theory emphasizes giving up some activities according to the wishes of others. Developmental theory tends to place elderly people on a pedestal, apart and different from other people. Minority group theory indicates that the elderly are different from the larger society and there is nothing they can do to change the situation.

Implications for Practice, Policy, and Research. The abandonment perspective prescribes either no interventions or interventions that aid withdrawal of the individual and society from each other. Thus, a nurse who worked with elderly people would not consider their withdrawal as evidence of depression (Archbold, 1981). Confusion would not be regarded as a strategy to enable survival in a hostile environment. This practitioner might discourage elderly people from participating in decisions that affect their lives, teach elderly people how to die, and encourage reminiscence and life review.

The abandonment-oriented nurse would make assumptions about older clients based on their ages alone, without regard for their abilities to function. Consistent mention of age in shift reports given in health-care facilities provides evidence of an abandonment perspective.

This nurse would be surprised by clients' hostility and make every effort to control their behavior without considering its purpose. Indeed, the abandonment perspective discourages comprehensive and detailed client assessments. Research into the aging process and associated problems is regarded as a waste of money and effort.

Elderly clients would not be preferred because they represent the fate that awaits the practitioner who attains his or her life expectancy. When given a choice, the practitioner will devote more attention to clients in younger age groups. The abandonment-oriented nurse would not question institutional care being provided at only a minimum level and with very limited resources.

In terms of social policies, the abandonment perspective prescribes measures that separate elderly people from the rest of society and provide them with the fewest resources. The abandonment-oriented practitioner would therefore favor separate housing and treatment facilities for the elderly, mandatory retirement, and minimal economic support from social security or other income transfer programs. This practitioner would be opposed to new programs for elderly people and inclusion of elderly people in decision-making groups such as resident councils and health service re-source allocation organizations.

Liberation

Do we liberate older people from the bureaucratic cage of adult life? A liberation perspective assumes that old age is a time of opportunity when people are freed of the need to work (Baum and Baum, 1980) and confronted by a unique period of life that they need to control or master (Marshall, 1978–79). When younger people are elderly, they too will enjoy the many social rights that presently accrue to old people.

Support for this perspective can be found in the same theories that inspired the notion of abandonment. Disengagement theory says that the individual gains a sense of freedom by relinquishing obligatory roles, implying freedom to make choices. Activity theory suggests that elderly people need to be involved in some pursuit that has meaning for them. Subculture theory postulates that elderly people have work to do to become a political force. Developmental theory indicates specific tasks to be accomplished to enable personality growth.

Implications for Practice, Policy, and Research. The nurse who regards old age as an opportunity would probably assist older clients to find meaning in their health impairments, encourage preparation for old age as a strategy to ensure optimum functioning, promote participation in a variety of activities, and insist that clients make decisions on matters of concern to them. This same nurse might not accept client refusals to be active or make decisions and, thus, provoke open conflict or anxiety. Clients might not receive much support from this nurse when they try to prepare for death.

Detailed and thorough assessment is needed to deal with seemingly unresolvable health impairments such as urinary incontinence and memory losses. Research to explain the aging process and evaluate potential solutions to health problems frequently experienced by elderly people is considered essential.

Policies favored by the liberation-oriented nurse would include income transfer adequate to enable elderly people to be satisfied with their lives, optimum quality health care, age-integrated housing, and non-institutional solutions to health and social care problems. Although these policies might cost this nurse more than their alternatives, the cost would be rationalized as an investment that will be repaid when the nurse is old.

Solidarity

Is there a sense of trust between successive generations based on self-perpetuating obligations to care? The central assumption of solidarity is that continuity is more important than change in a modern society. The elderly are necessary because they can serve as a symbol of continuity if they retain their social rights. By maintaining social rights for old people, the entire society can feel a sense of loyalty and belonging that resists all change (Baum and Baum, 1980, p. 33). The solidarity perspective rests on the "live and let live" principle.

Continuity theory provides support for this concept by saying people are primarily the same people they were in their younger years. Socioenvironmental theory indicates that satisfaction in later years is achieved in the same manner as in earlier years, through balance between individual resources and societal demands. The unitary man perspective also suggests that old age is a progression in time or continuation. Both socioenvironmental and unitary man perspectives consider the environment to be an important force influencing the fate of individuals.

Implications for Practice, Policy, and Research. Nurses who incorporate a solidarity perspective in their practice consider environments and individual attributes of their clients as equally important. Assessments reflect this belief by considering the lighting, size of print, and amount of distraction as possible reasons why a client cannot read. An extensive history to discover habits, preferences, and associations developed in earlier years becomes critical to planning care. Care planning needs to be highly individualized and diversified. Nursing care is given in such a way that clients do not lose in the exchange. Opportunities are deliberately provided for clients to exert control. Clients are not blamed for their behaviors when they are powerless to change environmental forces that influence their actions.

Primary care becomes increasingly important when aging is viewed from a solidarity perspective. Problems associated with aging may have started years before, suggesting that emphasis should be placed on prevention efforts in younger years (Vander Zyl, 1979, p. 47).

In terms of policy, nurses who adopt a solidarity perspective would not be in favor of treating the elderly as a special group. These nurses would not support special tax incentives, reduced bus fares, mandatory retirement, age-segregated housing, or designation of gerontology/geriatrics as an area of specialization for health professionals. Solidarity adherents would be in favor of measures to improve health care for people of all ages such as reducing air and water pollution, labeling of food additives, and providing written information about drugs when they are dispensed.

The solidarity perspective would probably influence nurses to favor basic research on the aging process but not applied research to test interventions specific to older people. Research based on the notion of solidarity as continuity will use a longitudinal approach to permit comparison of people with themselves as they age and to enable analysis of the relationships between life-style and personality variables. Nurses in family health and/or long-term care practice have the opportunity to conduct longitudinal studies.

PERVASIVE THEORETIC ISSUES IN GERONTOLOGY

In gerontology today, there are numerous theoretic issues. The next section of this chapter describes those that are frequently mentioned in the literature, identifying those that are particularly relevant to nursing practice.

A Functional Versus a Chronologic Definition of Aging

Defining "old person" is difficult. Aging, whether viewed as a "controlled or random process, determined by genes, environment, or accumulated trauma and pathology, affects a wide variety of biological, psychological, and sociological processes, and all of these can be roughly indexed by chronological age" (Costa and McCrae, 1980, p. 23). Chronologic age refers to calendar-clock age. However, a wide range of individual differences exist in performance of age-associated functions. A popular saying acknowledges this diversity by saying people are as young as they feel. Daily experience suggests that chronologic age is not an adequate definition of an old person. As long as people feel well and are able to maintain a life-style that suits them, they tend to regard others but not themselves as "old." The phrase, "My, how she's aged" may describe a 30-year-old experiencing considerable stress just as aptly as the phrase, "He doesn't look his age," may describe an 80-year-old who is relatively independent in life-style.

Functional age has been suggested as an accurate, practical alternative to chronologic age. Functional age would be decided by combining measures of variety of normal aging changes such as concentration, body flexibility, heart recovery rate, and visual acuity into a single numerical value that would represent the individual's overall functional age. Functional age as a basis for making decisions about people has been particularly popular with policy-makers concerned with adverse effects of mandatory retirement. A single measure of people's ability to function would provide a fairer basis for retirement than chronologic age.

However, enthusiasm for a functional definition of aging declined when researchers matched functional age predictors against chronologic age and found that chronologic age was the better predictor (Costa and McCrae, 1980). The problem with a functional criterion was that it disregarded too much of what was known about the aging process and about the sources of variation in measures of specific biologic and psychosocial variables.

If a single mechanism of aging were responsible for all the characteristic changes seen with age, then the concept of functional age would probably prove useful. But aging results from a variety of normally independent sequences of events: the accumulation of trauma, the random decay of genetic transmitters, genetically programmed functional changes, disease processes, and all the complex interactions of these factors in varying systems of the body. All these processes share in common only one thing: they take time. And the best measure of the time they take is chronologic age (Costa and McCrae, 1980, p. 44).

For the time being at least, chronologic age needs to continue to be used as a variable in research and practice but with the understanding that age, defined as clock-calendar time, really does not explain why age-related changes occur or indicate how a specific individual functions.

Conclusions made on the basis of chronologic age alone constitute the practice of "ageism." Remembering this, the nurse should recognize and take steps to eliminate ageism. A popular story in health-care circles describes a 91-year-old gentleman who began to experience tenderness, edema, and some decreased range of motion in his left knee. He voiced his complaint to a health-care provider who responded, "Well, John, what do you expect at age 91?" John replied, "Well, I expect you ought to be able to do something for me. After all, my right knee is 91 years old too!"

In health-care settings, descriptions of clients often start, "A 60-year-old white male. . . ." Age is given top priority as a summary statistic. For children, whose physical and psychosocial development is closely linked to chronologic age, this practice may be justified. However, the older a person gets, the less his chronologic age reveals who and what that individual is.

In addition to witnessing and correcting ageism, the nurse should realize that he or she may become a victim of ageism at two career points. At the start of professional practice, the nurse may be "too young" to be regarded as knowledgeable. Upon entering the fifth and sixth decades of life, the nurse may be viewed as "out of touch" with current practices and information. Mandatory retirement may force the nurse to stop working, regardless of competence, while physicians practice into their seventh and eighth decades. Eventually, age may come to be viewed as an excuse, not a reason, for the phenomena associated with growing old.

Length of Life Versus Quality of Life

Humans are probably the only animals who are aware of their own mortality and who translate concern about death into concern about aging. For the future of the species, which is more advantageous: a slow or rapid turnover of generations? Regardless of the answer, gerontologists will probably continue to study aging and achieve increases in individual longevity, as a result. If the cause and cure of aging are ultimately discovered, it must be decided whether to apply these findings. Would application provide individuals with 20 years of progressive disability and institutional confinement, or with 20 years of option-filled, satisfying living? This question is important to nurses who work with the elderly, particularly in institutional settings where the major problems of old age are magnified. Nurses face the challenge of finding ways to increase options for the elderly. Figure 3.4 serves to illustrate this challenge.

"On the whole, social scientists have failed to provide consistent and concise definitions of quality of life" (George and Bearon, 1980, p. 1). The problem is that definitions of quality of life depend on personal or group values and different people value different things. Quality of life for elderly people in long-term care facilities has been defined by identifying environmental features necessary to support quality of life. Such an environment (1) provides for personal space, (2) is stable, (3) encourages and permits, but does not force, choice, (4) supports failing faculties without fostering dependence, (5) allows personal recognition of individual interests through the provision of recreational, educational, vocational, and spiritual activities, (6) encourages and permits aged

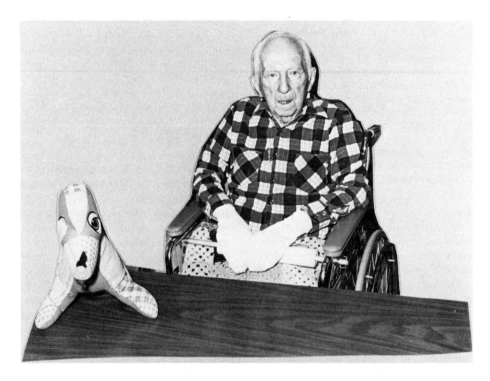

Figure 3.4. "Life goes on after the thrill of living is gone." *(Line from the song, "Jack and Diane," produced by Polygram Corporation, 1982. Copyright 1982 by Riva Music. Reprinted with permission. Photograph by Henry Lockhart, University Drive VA Medical Center, Pittsburgh, PA. Copyright 1983 by Slack, Incorporated. Reprinted by permission.)*

people to maintain contacts with families and communities, and (7) assures personal security and safety (Engquist, Davis, and Bryce, 1979, p. 97). These factors are probably equally relevant for elderly people who live at home. One element that is common to most definitions of quality of life is control/decision making/choice/option selection. At least one study has found that when one of two similar groups of elderly people was given the opportunity to make choices, that group experienced less mortality than the group that did not have the opportunity (Quality and Length of Life, 1980).

Competence has been suggested by Bengtson (1973) as a one-word summary of what health professionals hope to enhance in older individuals. Nurses do a reasonably adequate job of encouraging competence among the el-

derly, by helping old people cope with situations in their external environment through referrals to social agencies and in their internal environment by teaching clients about health and how to maintain or regain it. However, the profession does not do as well in helping people to be competent if competence is defined as coping and making personal choices about life-style. For example, old persons sometimes wish to remain in their own homes, but court orders are obtained to institutionalize them by persons concerned about their "safety," "competence," or "financial responsibility." An elderly woman sustained a fractured humerus en route to delivering money to her brother. The physician insisted that she be hospitalized, but the woman insisted on an outpatient cast application so she could be on her way. While the physician shouted his disapproval and threatened to admit her to a psychiatric hospital, the nurses let the woman fight her battle without support. Reassurance that she had a right to refuse treatment would have helped her to feel less alone.

At times nurses may be reluctant to assist a client achieve competence. When health-related goals a client sets do not match the nurse's views of appropriate health practices, those goals may not be accepted. Conflict thus exists between the individual's right to make decisions about this way of life and the health professional's mandate to improve the client's health status. To the extent that the nurse "wins," the client's competence as a controller of his world is diminished. Competence in an old person may also be undermined when nurses suggest reliance on professional services rather than on amateur helpers such as family or friends.

Competence and control are important concepts in gerontologic nursing. The following guides for nursing action may assist the nurse to reinforce client competence and control. To allow clients to have more influence over their worlds:

1. Offer clients a chance to make decisions only when the nurse is prepared to abide by the decision
2. Keep in mind that the health professional's role is to offer factual information in a comprehensive fashion so that the client can make an informed decision. The obligation to inform does not extend to coercion or deprogramming
3. Accept a client's right to decide in favor of unhealthful practices, such as eating the wrong foods; the consequences may be mentally or socially rewarding
4. Support clients' reliance on laypeople rather than professionals for essential services and assist amateurs to provide appropriate assistance through teaching programs, especially when professionals lack a proven approach to resolution of the client's problem(s)

In letting clients do as they choose, the nurse may have to relinquish some power and efficiency and possibly accept a feeling of helplessness. But consider the gains in competence for those who might then run their own congregate-living homes through a board of residents, or who might determine the extent of services to be provided by health professionals.

The Aged as a Problem: Legitimate or Contrived?

Old age is simply one of several phases in life. "That a society (including the old themselves) should perceive its aging population as a problem is a problem" (Wilson, 1973, p. 486). When the elderly are viewed as a problem, they and society both lose. Society loses because this view does not consider the meaning of life, and does not recognize that human beings are of value in themselves. Problems that affect all age groups are dismissed as peculiar to a small proportion of the population. Fears of nonproductivity, diminishment, and death, coupled with worship of youth and activism, are problems for all people, not just the elderly!

The elderly lose because when old people are viewed as a problem, they may be regarded as having an "illness" that needs to be "cured." This attitude leads to consequences that may not be in the best interests of the elderly. Emphasis on achieving a cure for problems without solutions contributes to a very depressing, passive view of the aging experience. Nurses serve the elderly with professional care and skill and, in so doing, collude with a system that deprives old people of their worth (Wilson, 1973). Nurses tend to use skills appropriate to *cure* (the physician's task) over and above skills appropriate to the *care* of people (the nurse's task).

In allocating money and personnel, society itself prefers curing to caring. Professional nurses have supported this preference by failing to fulfill their essential role in caring for the elderly. Clinical practice positions in nursing homes and day-care centers are filled by nonprofessional nursing personnel or by other professionals (social workers, physical and recreational therapists, and health educators). Professional nurses, meanwhile, cling to acute-care settings dominated by complex gadgetry, or prefer to assist physicians in identifying and managing clients' illness.

One prevalent myth asserts that institutionalized elderly people simply require good custodial care—the type provided by non-skilled workers trained in residential care with a gift for homemaking. "When you cure illness you don't end up with health; you have simply not got illness. Health is concerned with different factors such as personal sense of identity and worth, freedom to be yourself, social participation, and a sense of purpose" (Wilson, 1973). Care of the elderly directed toward hygiene and housekeeping needs produces well-scrubbed, well-fed, and well-housed animals. If nurses are to provide human care, they must regard old people as individuals with human needs and potentials. Anyone can provide adequate care to animals; professional nurses are needed for appropriate care of the elderly. Old people need the services of nurses who can (1) restore the individual's control over his situation, (2) help people make maximum use of minimum physical resources, and (3) emphasize the significance of life in the face of impending death.

In providing this care, the nurse should be aware that caring can be a way of keeping the elderly from assuming a valued and powerful place in this society. In the past, deviates were banned, imprisoned, or destroyed. Today, "deviates" such as psychotics, criminals, and the elderly receive care and treatment. If society decrees that once achievement ends, so does worth, and therefore refuses to allow old people the chance to learn work, share wisdom, or enjoy sex, then society itself creates the problems the elderly now face.

Lipman and Slater (1977) proposed that buildings housing the elderly with health professionals working under the same roof should be constructed in such a way as to *minimize* caring impulses while *maximizing* rights and options of the elderly residents. Comfort (1975) believes that in the future old people will be better protected against the myth of a dependent, valueless old age, more militant, and a "lot less willing to have laid on them the sort of garbage which is laid on the old today"

(Comfort, 1975, pp. 11–12). In the meantime, nurses caring for the elderly should be aware that their efforts toward caring may be detrimental. They must try to restore in the elderly their sense of worth and freedom.

Is Gerontologic Nursing Special?

Is gerontologic nursing special merely because the elderly belong to a certain age group? This question is related to the issue of the elderly as a problem. Typically, elderly people are regarded as victims of disabling physical defects, failing mentalities, loneliness, and poverty. Therefore, they represent a "social problem." The fact that many people of other ages have these problems and most elderly do not is completely ignored.

In view of the recent thrust to define gerontology, and particularly gerontologic nursing, as a specialty, nurses should consider who really benefits by this trend. The elderly gain to the extent that resources are more readily available for those individuals who do need help. Study of problems associated with highly dependent clients is stimulated, and if solutions are found, the elderly may benefit. However, old people may also lose from being designated as a specialty group for health care. "Expected problems" tend to receive attention, while other problems that bother the client may be disregarded.

Physical segregation of the old may inhibit their contacts with potentially supportive people of other ages. The stigma of belonging to a "problem" group may contribute to loss of self-esteem. Classifying the elderly as a separate group may draw attention away from the contribution nursing can make to promoting health in old age through care during the earlier years. By segregating the elderly sick in remote locations, administrative economy is achieved, but at the expense of the client. The health professional benefits because specialty practice tends to carry more prestige than general practice.

Nursing care of the elderly is very complex at the present time. However, this complexity is not related to the age of the clients. Factors that are difficult for the gerontologic nurse include:

1. Working in isolation, at some distance from qualified support from other members of the health team
2. Working with clients who suffer from problems related to multiple pathologies
3. A relative and sometimes increasing lack of human and material resources

Nurses who care for other "problem" groups—the mentally retarded, the mentally ill, the substance abusers—also face one or more of these difficulties.

The elderly need comprehensive care, with emphasis on prevention, rehabilitation, and the promotion of maximum independence—in other words, the same sort of care required by clients of all ages, nursed in a variety of settings. Perhaps a better focus for a new specialty area in nursing might be care of disabled people who are highly dependent on nursing service, rather than a focus on age, which appears to be largely irrelevant.

On the other hand, the need for a gerontologic specialty might be supported by the fact that many age-related changes (such as normal body temperature, hemoglobin and hematocrit levels, immune response potential, socialization patterns, and cognitive processes) have been identified. These facts tend to indicate that the elderly as a group are indeed different from other age groups, and thus require specialized health services from specially prepared professionals. The trend toward gerontologic nursing as a specialty seems to be based more upon political considerations than upon consideration of the characteristics common to all old people and unique to the age group. The intent of nursing is to provide care that fits the aims and needs of individual clients. Thus, nurses should exercise caution in accepting a specialty that may not be in the best interests of those that specialty serves.

Setting aside the issue of whether gerontologic nursing should be a specialty, the profession has consistently moved to support such a designation. Havighurst (1971) divided applied gerontology into two fields. *Medical gerontology* includes treatment and prevention of disease and disability, as well as preservation of energy in the elderly. *Social gerontology*

encompasses financial support, housing and living arrangements, and self-esteem supports for old people. Gunter and Miller (1977) have defined nursing gerontology as a third applied field which aims to:

1. Provide health promotion, maintenance, and rehabilitation for the elderly in general as well as support for the terminally ill
2. Improve care and services to old people regardless of setting (home or institution)
3. Educate nursing personnel in the delivery of health services to the elderly
4. Conduct research related to the provision of direct care to the elderly

The body of knowledge applied in the field of nursing gerontology is derived both from nursing research and from research conducted within other disciplines. Findings from the sciences of sociology, psychology, and biology have been used, as well as findings from the areas of social work, psychiatry, and medicine. "*Gerontologic nursing* is concerned with assessment of the health needs of older adults, planning and implementing health care to meet these needs and evaluating the effectiveness of such care" (American Nurses' Association, 1976, p. 3).

Theory as a Guide for Nursing Practice

Since the 1960s the nursing profession has exhibited an intense interest in developing conceptual frameworks, theoretical frameworks, and models to direct nursing practice. In some cases this preoccupation has resulted in "a disastrous marriage between unrelated and incongruent ideas. In others, the model bears no relation whatsoever to the work undertaken. It merely sits there looking embarrassingly conspicuous" (Downs, 1982, p. 259). Present theories of aging are vague, general, broad, and difficult to test. Rather than spending their limited resources to develop these theories, nurses need to study practice-relevant problems and thereby generate precise knowledge that may eventually support more specific theories of aging.

The theories of greatest use to nurses are called "practice theories" (Jacox, 1974). Such theories describe, explain, and predict events with enough certainty to permit control of outcomes. Practice theories say, "If this happens, then that always happens." For example, one practice theory useful to nurses asserts that a person in poor nutritional status who remains in a fixed position for an extended period of time will develop integumentary breakdown. Nurses control events (nutritional status, body position over time) to achieve a desired outcome (intact integument).

One method for identifying important problems in long-term care is the Delphi survey. The Delphi technique is a method of eliciting and refining group judgments. Its primary rationale is the adage, "Two heads are better than one." The procedures have three features: (1) anonymous response (opinions of the group members are obtained by formal questionnaire), (2) interaction and controlled feedback (interaction is affected by a systematic exercise conducted in several rounds with carefully controlled feedback between each round), and (3) statistical group response (the group opinion is defined as an appropriate aggregate of individual opinions on the final round (Dalkey, 1969). One Delphi survey was conducted in over 90 nursing homes and home health agencies in South East Florida (Brower and Christ, 1982). Results indicated that study of the following areas would be extremely important for client welfare:

1. Decubitus ulcers (prevention, formation, and treatment)
2. Coping mechanisms used by clients and families to manage care after discharge
3. Measures to increase physician interest in geriatrics
4. Age differences in responses to medications
5. Methods to improve gerontologic preparation of nursing personnel (students and staff)
6. Urinary tract infections (epidemiology and treatment)
7. Eating patterns and preferences of older adults
8. Means to improve physician follow-up of clients
9. Effective strategies to improve nurse-physician communication

10. Strategies for attracting and retaining knowledgeable and interested staff (Brower and Christ, 1982)

This list indicates that practicing nurses in long-term care are still more concerned with their one dependent function of implementing physician-ordered assessment and intervention than with their four independent functions that involve teaching and consultation along with other helping actions. (Items 3, 4, 8 and 9 are concerned with physicians and the physician's responsibilities.) However, if research is to be relevant to nursing practice, that research must involve studies of concerns shared by nurses and their clients. If this survey had included clients, as well as nurses, such shared concerns might have provided more valuable direction for studies by nurses.

A second strategy for selecting problems in need of study is to determine their monetary costs. The odds are good that support for research will be the most readily available to study those problems that cost our society the most money.

Scientific writing in the field of gerontology contains many suggestions about areas/problems that require study. For example, a prestigious planning panel completed work on "A National Plan for Research on Aging: Toward an Independent Old Age." The plan was a revision of one mandated by Congress with the creation of the National Institute on Aging. Highlights of research recommendations were published in *Aging Research and Training News* (Schecter, 1982, p. 4):

RESEARCH

Basic Mechanisms of Aging
Emphasis on genetic research, including research in molecular genetics to explore possible structural and functional alterations in DNA that might play a role in determining longevity; develop a variety of markers of aging processes; establish centers of excellence to test methods, study populations, or develop animal models.

Clinical Manifestations of Aging
Top priority to later-life dementia disorders, particularly Alzheimer's disease, including de-

termination of constitutional, genetic, and environmental factors (e.g., toxins or infections), diagnostic procedures, animal models of histopathologic changes, significance of increased aluminum and other trace elements found in the brains of patients with Alzheimer's disease.

Interactions Between Older People and Society

Emphasis on societal context of old age and the interactions of older people and social institutions, especially (a) longevity differences among population subgroups; (b) family and other institutions supporting older persons; and (c) work and retirement.

Increasing Productivity Among Older People

Conduct field trials to apply research findings on increasing productive activity of older persons, including paid work, unpaid mutual help and self-care.

In using lists of researchable areas developed by other disciplines, nurses need to decide whether the problems identified are relevant to the work of nurses, that is, implementation of the nursing process.

Care must be taken by nurses doing research and developing theory, to avoid a split that is common across disciplines. Very few nursing educators and researchers have recent, direct, practical experience in trying to meet the needs of elderly people, while very few nursing service personnel who care for elderly people have any formal training in gerontology. This dilemma is illustrated by a conversation that was overheard at a gerontology conference. ". . . the service provider accused the researcher of only being interested in aging rats, to which the researcher replied that the provider had no concern with what was true" (Knight, 1982, p. 229).

CONCLUSION

Given the past lack of solid evidence as to how people age and what can be done to help them adapt to the process, gerontologic nurses have had to rely too often on unreliable information

as a basis for action. Personal values, convictions, and untested inferences have been substituted for critical evaluation of alternative ideas. Nurses should be careful not to let past impressions of gerontologic research govern future usage. Verified information with implications for nursing practices is accumulating daily. Efforts must be made to speed the translation of research findings into practice. Studies of nursing care of the elderly have demonstrated that problems such as incontinence, memory loss, and immobility can be alleviated, or at least controlled. At the same time, each nursing project, program, and service provided to the elderly needs to be framed within a research design to evaluate the outcomes. Results will contribute to the base of verified information needed to support nursing practice with elderly clients. Whether the nurse is engaged in applying, verifying, or testing theoretical propositions, she is obligated to share findings through written materials or conferences, so that evolution of theory relevant to nursing care of the elderly may proceed.

RECOMMENDED READINGS

Archbold, P.G. Ethical issues in the selection of a theoretical framework for gerontological nursing research. Journal of Gerontological Nursing 7(7):408–411, 1981. *An analysis of several of the psychosocial gerontological theories in terms of the ethical and political consequences of their use by nurses.*

Baum, M., Baum, R.C. Growing Old: A Societal Perspective. Englewood Cliffs, NJ, Prentice Hall, 1980. *A review of many social theories of old age that presents three theoretical perspectives: abandonment, liberation, and dichronic solidarity.*

Fawcett, J. A framework for analysis and evaluation of conceptual models of nursing. Nurse Educator 5(6):10–14, 1980. *Defines and describes a framework for analysis and evaluation appropriate for nursing models.*

Hardy, M.E. Theories: Components, development, evaluation. Nursing Research 23(2):100–106, 1974. *A relatively jargon-free, comprehensible, article about material some nursing students find difficult. The roles of concepts, statements of relationship, and models in theory development are examined. Criteria for evaluating theories are outlined and the tentative nature of theories is discussed.*

Hayflick, L. Cell aging. In Eisdorfer, C. (ed.). Annual Review of Gerontology and Geriatrics. New York, Springer, 1980. *A review of selected areas of cytogerontology that had not been covered in previous reviews and also lists sources of other reviews. The tables that list properties of cells that increase, decrease, and do not change as cells approach the end of their vitro life span provides a model nurses might use in summarizing physiological and structural changes of aging.*

Reff, M.E., Schneider, E.L. Biological Markers of Aging. (NIH Publication No. 82-2221). Washington, D.C., U.S. Department of Health and Human Services, National Institutes of Health, Public Health Service, 1982. *Reports proceedings of a conference of nonlethal biological markers of physiological aging. Discovering of mechanisms that underlie human aging is a prerequisite to controlling those mechanisms through intervention. The book contains two sections: one on laboratory rodents and one on human studies.*

Schimke, R.T. (ed.). Biological Mechanisms in Aging. (NIH Publication No. 81-2194). Washington, D.C., U.S. Department of Health and Human Services, Public Health Service, National Institutes of Health, 1981. *A 726-page report of a conference sponsored by the NIH to address the question: What constitutes biological aging? Mechanisms of aging are considered from the standpoint of systems analysis, DNA structure, protein synthesis, and post-translational modification of proteins, immune, and neuroendocrine systems.*

REFERENCES CITED

Adelman, R.C. Definition of biological aging. In Haynes, S.G., Feinleib, M. (eds.). Second Conference on the Epidemiology of Aging. (NIH Publication No. 80-969). Washington, D.C., U.S. Government Printing Office, 1980

American Nurses' Association. Standards of Gerontological Nursing Practice. Kansas City, MO, American Nurses Association, 1976

Archbold, P.G. Ethical issues in the selection of a theoretical framework for gerontological nursing research. Journal of Gerontological Nursing 7(7):408–411, 1981

Aries, P. Centuries of Childhood. New York, Knopf, 1962

Atchley, R.C. The Social Forces in Later Life. Belmont, CA, Wadsworth, 1977

Baltes, P.B. Life-span developmental psychology: Some converging observations on history and theory. In Baltes, P.B., Brim, Jr., O.G. (eds.) Life-span Development and Behavior (Vol. 2). New York, Academic Press, 1979

Baltes, P.B., Willis, S.L. Toward psychological theories of aging and development. In Birren, J.E., Schaie, K.W., (eds). Handbook of the Psychology of Aging. New York, Van Nostrand Reinhold, 1977

Barron, M. The Aging American. New York, Cromwell, 1961

Bart, P. Depression in middle aged women. In Gornick, V., Moran, B. (eds), Women in Sexist Society. New York, New American Library, 1971

Baum, M., Baum, R.C. Growing Old: A Societal Perspective. Englewood Cliffs, NJ, Prentice Hall, 1980

Bengtson, V., Chiriboga, D., Keller, A.W. Occupational differences in retirement: Patterns of life-outlook and role activity among Chicago teachers and steelworkers. In Havigurst, R.J., Neugarten, B.L., Munnichs, J.M.A., Thomae, H., (eds.). Adjustment to Retirement: A Cross-national Study. Netherlands, Van Gorkum, 1969

Bengtson, V.L., Cutler, N.E. Generations and intergenerational relations: Perspectives on age groups and social change. In Binstock, R.H., Shanas, E. (eds.). Handbook of Aging and the Social Sciences. New York, Van Nostrand Reinhold, 1976

Bengtson, V.L., Dowd, J.J. Sociological functionalism, exchange theory, and life-cycle analysis: A call for more explicit theoretical bridges. International Journal of Aging and Human Development 12(1):55–73, 1980–81

Bierman, E.L. The effect of donor age on the in vitro lifespan of cultured human arterial smooth-muscle cells. In Vitro 14(3):951–955, 1978

Birren, J.E., Renner, V.J. Research on the psychology of aging: Principles and experimentation. In Birren, J.E., Schaie, K.W. (eds.). Handbook of the Psychology of Aging. New York, Van Nostrand Reinhold, 1977

Breen, L. The aging individual. In Tibbitts, C. (ed.). Handbook of Social Gerontology. Chicago, IL, The University of Chicago Press, 1980

Brim, O.G., Jr., Kagan, J. (eds.). Constancy and Change in Human Development. Cambridge, MA, Harvard University Press, 1980

Brower, H.T., Christ, M.A. A Delphi Study of Research Priorities for Long Term Care Nursing. Paper presented at the 35th Annual Scientific Meeting of the Gerontological Society of America, Boston, MA, November, 1982

Buhler, C. The curve of life as studied in biographies. Journal of Applied Psychology 19(6):405–409, 1935

Buhler, C., Massarik, F. (eds.). The Course of Human Life. New York, Springer, 1968

Bultena, G.L. Life continuity and morale in old age. The Gerontologist 9(3):251–253, 1969

Burnet, F.M. Immunological Surveillance. New York, Pergamon, 1970a

Burnet, F.M. An immunological approach to aging. Lancet 2(6):358–360, 1970b

Cassel, J. Psychosocial processes and stress: A theoretical formulation. International Journal of Health Services 4(5):474–482, 1974

Cavan, R.S., Burgess, E.W., Havighurst, R.J., Goldhammer, H. Personal Adjustments in Old Age. Chicago, IL, Science Research Associates, 1949

Chinn, P.L., Jacobs, M.K. A model for theory development in nursing. Advances in Nursing Science 1(1):1–11, 1978

Clark, M., Anderson, B.G. Culture and Aging. New York, Charles C. Thomas, 1967

Comfort, A. Prescribing the role of oldness often defies the realities of oldness. The Center Magazine 8(2):11–12, 1975

Costa, P.T., McCrae, R.R. Age differences in personality structure revisited: Studies in validity, stability, and change. Aging and Human Development 8(6):261–275, 1977

Costa, P.T., McCrae, R.R. Functional age: A conceptual and empirical critique. In Haynes, S.G. (ed.). Second Conference on the Epidemiology of Aging (NIH Publication No. 80-969). Washington, D.C., U.S. Government Printing Office, 1980

Costa, P.T., McCrae, R.R. Objective personality assessment. In Storandt, M., Siegler, I.C., Elias, M.F. (eds.). The Clinical Psychology of Aging. New York, Plenum, 1978

Costa, P.T., McCrea, R.R., Arenberg, D. Enduring dispositions in adult males. Journal of Personality and Social Psychology 38(5):793–800, 1980

Covey, H.C. A reconceptualization of continuity theory: Some preliminary thoughts. The Gerontologist, 21(6):628–633, 1981

Cowgill, D.O., Holmes, L.D. (eds.). Aging and Modernization. New York, Appleton-Century-Crofts, 1972

Cumming, E. Engagement with an old theory. International Journal of Aging and Human Development 6(3):187–191, 1975

Cumming, E. Further thoughts on the theory of disengagement. International Journal 15(4):377–393, 1963

Cumming, E., Dean, L.R., Newell, D.S., McCaffery, I. Disengagement: Alternative theory of aging. Sociometry 23(3):23–35. 1960

Cumming, E., Henry, W.E. Growing Old. New York, Basic, 1961

Dalkey, N. The Delphi Method: An Experimental Study of Group Opinion. Santa Monica, CA, Rand Corporation, RM-5888-PR, 1969

Danish, S.J., D'Augelli, A.R. Promoting competence and enhancing development through life development intervention. In Boyd, L.A., Rosen, J.C. (eds.). Primary Prevention of Pathology. Hanover, NY, University Press of New England, 1980, Vol 4

Douglas, K., Arenberg, D. Age changes, cohort differences, and cultural change on the Guilford-Zimmerman Temperament Survey. Journal of Gerontology 33(5):737–747, 1978

Dowd, J.J. Exchange rates and old people. Journal of Gerontology 35(4):596–602, 1980

Downs, F.S. A theoretical question. Editorial. Nursing Research 31(5):259, 1982

Emmerich, W. Personality development and concepts of structure. Child Development 39(6):671–690, 1968

Eisenstadt, S.N. Social Differentiation and Stratification. Glenview, IL, Scott, Foresman, Inc. 1971

Engquist, C.L., Davis, J.E., Bryce, R.H. Can quality of life be evaluated? Hospitals 53(9):97–100, 1979

Erikson, E. Childhood and Society, 2nd ed. New York, Norton, 1963

Erikson, E. Identity and the Life Cycle. New York, International Universities Press, 1959

Estes, C.L., Swan, J.H., Gerard, L.E. Dominant and competing paradigms in gerontology: Towards a political economy of ageing. Ageing and Society 2(2):151–164, 1982

Finch, C.E. Neuroendocrine and autonomic aspects of aging. In Finch, C.E., Hayflick, L. (eds.). Handbook of the Biology of Aging. New York, Van Nostrand Reinhold, 1977

Finch, C.E. Perspectives in biomedical research on aging. In Goldstein, K.K., Salisbury, P.A., Davison, W.P. (eds.). Aging: Research and Perspectives: A Briefing for the Press. New York, Columbia University, Graduate School of Journalism, 1979

Fox, J.H. Perspectives on the continuity perspective. International Aging and Human Development 14(2):97–115, 1981–82

George, L.K., Bearon, L.B. Quality of Life in Older Persons: Meaning and Measurement. New York, Human Sciences Press, 1980

Gerard, R.W. Aging and organization. In Birren, J.E. (ed), Handbook of Aging and the Individual. Chicago, IL, University of Chicago Press, 1959

Goldstein, S., Csullog, G.W. Macromolecular synthesis in human fibroblasts at 37° and 42° C during aging in vitro. Mechanisms of Aging and Development 6(7):185–195, 1977

Gould, R.L. Transformations. New York, Simon and Schuster, 1978

Greenberg, L.J., Yunis, E.J. Genetic control of autoimmune disease and immune responsiveness and the relationship to aging. In Harrison, D (ed.). Genetic Effects on Aging. New York, The National Foundation–March of Dimes, 1977

Grubrium, J. The Myth of the Golden Years. Springfield, IL, Charles C. Thomas, 1973

Gubrium, J.F. Toward a socioenvironmental theory of aging. The Gerontologist 12(5):281–284, 1972

Gunter, L.M., Miller, J.C. Toward a nursing gerontology. Nursing Research 26(3):208–221, 1977

Guttmann, D. Use of informal and formal supports by white ethnic aged. In Gelfand, D.E., Kutzik, A.J. (eds.). Ethnicity and Aging: Theory Research and Policy. New York, Springer, 1979

Hart, R.W., Setlow, R.B. Direct evidence that pyrimidine dimers in DNA result in neoplastic transformation. In Hanawalt, P.C., Setlow, R.B. (eds.). Molecular Mechanisms for Repair of DNA, Part B. New York, Plenum Press, 1974.

Havighurst, R.J. Life Style Transitions Related to Personality After Age Fifty. Paper presented at the International Society for Study of Behavioral Development Symposium, Kibbutz Kiryat Anavim, Israel, 1975

Havighurst, R.J., Munnichs, J.M.A., Neugarten, B.L., Thomas, H. (eds.). Adjustment to Retirement. Assen, Netherlands, Van Gorcum and Company, 1969.

Havighurst, R.J. Personality and patterns of aging. The Gerontologist 8(3):20–23, 1968

Havighurst, R.J., Abrecht, R. Older People. New York, Longmans, Green, 1953

Hayflick, L. Cell aging. In Eisdorfer, C. (ed.). Annual Review of Gerontology and Geriatrics. New York, Springer, 1980, Vol 1

Hayflick, L. Prospects for increasing human longevity. In Johnston, P. (ed.). Perspectives on Aging. Cambridge, MA, Ballinger, 1981

Haymes, H.J. Theories of aging and the older professional: An argument for continued environment. Aging and Leisure Living 2(9):15–20, 1979

Henry, W. The theory of intrinsic disengagement. In Hansen, P.F. (ed.). Age with a Future. Philadelphia, PA, Davis, 1964

Holmes, T.H., Rahe, R.H. The social readjustment rating scale. Journal of Psychosomatic Research 11(6):213–218, 1967

Holzberg, C.S. Ethnicity and aging: Anthropological perspectives on more than just the minority elderly. The Gerontologist 22(3):249–257, 1982

Homans, G.C. Social Behavior: Its Elementary Forms, rev ed. New York, Harcourt, Brace, Jovanovich, 1974

Huang, H.H., Meites, J. Reproductive capacity of aging female rats. Neuroendocrinology 17(4):289–295, 1975

Jacox, A. Theory construction in nursing: An overview. Nursing Research 23(1):4–13, 1974

Kerckhoff, A.C. Family patterns and morale in retirement. In Simpson, I.H., McKinney, J. (eds.).

Social Aspects of Aging. Durham, NC, Duke University Press, 1966

Kerlinger, F.N. Foundations of Behavioral Research. New York, Hold, Rinehart, and Winston, 1973

Kinch, J.W. A formalized theory of self-concept. American Journal of Sociology 68(5):481–486, 1963

Knapp, M.R.J. The activity theory of aging: An examination of the English context. The Gerontologist 17(6):553–559, 1977

Knight, B. To the editor (letter). The Gerontologist 22(3):229–230, 1982

Leaf, A. Search for the oldest people. National Geographic 143(5):92–119, 1973

Laslett, P. Societal development and aging. In Binstock, R.H., Shanas, E. (eds.). Handbook of Aging and the Social Sciences. New York, Van Nostrand Reinhold, 1976. pp 87–116

LeGuilly, Y., Simon, M., Lenoir, P., Bourel, M. Long term culture of human adult liver cells: Morphological changes related to in vitro senescence and effect of donor's age on growth potential. Gerontologia 19(5):303–313, 1973

Lemon, B.W., Bengtson, V.L., Peterson, J.A. An exploration of the activity theory of aging: Activity types and life satisfaction among in-movers to a retirement community. Journal of Gerontology, 27(4):511–523, 1972

Levinson, D.J. The Seasons of a Man's Life. New York, Knopf, 1978

Lipman, A., Slater, R. Homes for old people: Toward a positive environment. The Gerontologist 17(3):146–156, 1977

Liu, R.K., Walford, R.L. The effect of lowered body temperature on lifespan and immune and nonimmune processes. Gerontologia 18(3):363–366, 1972

Loevinger, J. The meaning and measurement of ego development. American Psychologist 21(2):195–206, 1966

Loevinger, J. Ego Development. San Francisco, CA, Jossey-Bass, 1976

Longino, C.F., McClelland, K.A., Peterson, W.A. The aged subculture hypothesis: Social integration, gerontophilia, and self-conception. Journal of Gerontology 35(5):758–767, 1980

Maddox, G.L. Themes and issues in sociological theories of human aging. In Brantyl, V.M., Brown, M.L. (eds.). Readings in Gerontology. St. Louis, MO, Mosby, 1973

Maddox, G., Eisdorfer, C. Some correlates of activity and morale among the elderly. Social Forces 41(7):254–260, 1962

Maddox, G.L., Wiley, J. Scope, concepts, and methods in the study of aging. In Binstock, R.H.,

Shanas, E (eds.). Handbook of Aging and the Social Sciences. New York, Van Nostrand Reinhold, 1976

Marshall, V.W. No exit: A symbolic interactionist perspective on aging. International Journal of Aging and Human Development 9(4):345–358, 1978–79

Maslow, A.H. The Farther Reaches of Human Nature. New York, Viking 1971

Masoro, E.J. Nutritional intervention in the aging process. In Johnson, P.W. (ed.). Perspectives on Aging. Cambridge, MA, Ballinger, 1981

McCall, G.J., Simmons, J.L. Identities and Interactions. New York, Free Press, 1966

McCay, C.M., Cronell, M.F., Maynard, L.A. The effect of retarded growth upon the length of lifespan and upon the ultimate body size. Journal of Nutrition 10(4):63, 1935

Myerhoff, B. Number Our Days. New York, Dutton, 1978

Neugarten, B.L. The awareness of middle age. In Neugarten, B.L. (ed.). Middle Age and Aging. Chicago, IL, University of Chicago Press, 1968

Neugarten, B.L. Personality change in the late life: A developmental perspective. In Eisdorfer, C., Lawton, M.P. (eds.). The Psychology of Adult Development and Aging. Washington, D.C., American Psychological Association, 1973

Neugarten, B.L., Havigurst, R.J., Tobin, S.S. Personality patterns and aging. In Neugarten, B.L. (ed.). Middle Age and Aging. Chicago, IL, University of Chicago Press, 1968

Nuckolls, K., Cassel, J., Kaplan, H. Psychological assets, life crises, and the prognosis of pregnancy. American Journal of Epidemiology 95(6):431–441, 1972

Palmore, E. Are the aged a minority group? Journal of the American Geriatrics Society 26(5):214–217, 1978

Palmore, E. Predictors of longevity. In Haynes, S.G., Feinleib, M. Second Conference on the Epidemiology of Aging (NIH Publication No 80-969). Washington, D.C., U.S. Government Printing Office, 1980

Palmore, E.B., Manton, K. Ageism compared to racism and sexism. Journal of Gerontology 38(4):353–369, 1973

Palmore, E.B., Stone, V. Predictors of longevity: A follow-up of the aged in Chapel Hill. The Gerontologist 13(4):88–90, 1973

Peng, M., Huang, H. Aging of hypothalamic–pituitary–ovarian function in the rat. Fertility and Sterility 23(4):535–542, 1972

Quality and Length of Life. Notable Notes 6(8):1, 1980

Reff, M.E., Schneider, E.L. Biological Markers of Aging (NIH Publication No. 82-2221). Bethesda, MD, U.S. Department of Health and Human Services, National Institutes of Health, Public Health Service, 1982

Riegel, K.F. History of psychological gerontology. In Birren, J.E., Schaie, K.W. (eds.). Handbook of the Psychology of Aging. New York, Van Nostrand Reinhold, 1977.

Roberts-Thomson, I.C., Whittingham, S., Youngchaiyud, U., MacKay, I.R. Aging, immune response, and mortality. Lancet 2(6):368–370, 1974

Rogers, M.E. Nursing: A science of unitary man. In Riehl, J.P., Roy, C. (eds.). Conceptual Models for Nursing Practice. New York, Appleton-Century-Crofts, 1980

Rogers, M.E. Theoretical Basis of Nursing. Philadelphia, PA, Davis, 1970

Rosenwaike, I. Accuracy of death certificate ages for the extreme aged. Center for the Study of Aging Newsletter 4(3):7, 1982

Rose, A.M. The subculture of the aging: A topic for sociological research. The Gerontologist 2(3):123–127, 1962

Rose, A.M., Peterson, W.A. (eds.). Older People and Their Social World. Philadelphia, PA, Davis, 1965

Rosow, I. Socialization to Old Age. Berkeley, CA, University of California Press, 1974

Runyan, W.M. A stage-state analysis of the life course. Journal of Personality and Social Psychology 38(3):951–962, 1980

Ryff, C.D., Heincke, S.G. The Subjective Organization of Personality in Adulthood and Aging. Paper presented at the Society for Research in Child Development Meetings, Boston, MA, April, 1981

Sacher, G.A. Theory in gerontology, part I. In Eisdorfer, C. (ed.). Annual Review of Gerontology and Geriatrics. New York, Springer, 1980, Vol 1

Schaie, K.W., Parham, I.A. Stability of adult personality traits. Facts or fable? Journal of Personality and Social Psychology 34(1):146–158, 1976

Schecter, I. (ed.). NIA plan for development of aging research and training completed. Aging Research and Training News 51:3–6 1982

Schimke, R.T., Angiel, M. Biological mechanisms in aging: Summary of conference proceedings. Journal of the American Geriatrics Society, 31(1):40–44, 1983

Schnider, E.L., Mitsui, Y. The relationship between the vitro cellular aging and in vivo human aging. Proceedings of the National Academy of Science, U.S.A. 73(7):3584–3588, 1976

Schwartz, A.G. Correlation between species lifespan and capacity to activate 7, 12-dimethylbenz-d-anthracane to a form mutagenic to a mammalian cell. Experimental Cell Research 44(5):445–457, 1975

Seelback, W., Sauer, W. Filial responsibility expectations among aged parents. The Gerontologist 17(6):492–499, 1977

Shock, N.W. Biological theories of aging. In Birren, J.E., Schaie, K.W. (eds.). Handbook of the Psychology of Aging. New York, Van Nostrand Reinhold, 1977

Siegler, I.C., George, L.K., Okun, M.A. Cross-sequential analysis of adult personality. Developmental Psychology 15(3):350–351, 1979

Simpson, I.H., McKinney, J. (eds.). Social Aspects of Aging. Durham, NC, Duke University Press, 1966

Sinex, F.M. The molecular genetics of aging. In Finch, C.E., Hayflick, L. (eds.). Handbook of the Biology of Aging. New York, Van Nostrand Reinhold, 1977

Spence, D.L. The meaning of engagement. International Journal of Aging and Human Development 6(3):193–198, 1975

Staub, E. The nature and study of human personality. In Staub, E. (ed.). Personality: Basic Aspects and Current Research. Englewood Cliffs, NJ, Prentice Hall, 1980

Strehler, B.L. Time, Cells, and Aging. New York, Academic, 1962

Thomae, H. Personality and adjustment to aging. In Birren, J.E., Sloane, B. (eds.). Handbook on Mental Health and Aging. Englewood Cliffs, NJ, Prentice Hall, 1980

Vaillant, G.E. Adoption to Life. Boston, MA, Little, Brown, 1977

Vander Zyl, S. Psychosocial theories of aging: Activity, disengagement, and continuity. Journal of Gerontological Nursing 5(3):45–48, 1979

Walford, R.L. Immunology and the Fountain of Youth. Paper presented at the 34th Annual Scientic Meeting of the Gerontological Society of America, Toronto, Ontario, November 8–12, 1981

Walford, R.L., Kiu, R.K., Delima-Berbasse, M., Mathis, M., Smith, G.S. Long-term dietary restriction and immune function in mice: Response to sheep red blood cells and to mitogenic agents. Mechanisms of Aging and Development 2(3): 447–454, 1974

Walford, R.L., Meredith, P.J., Cheney, K.E. Immunoengineering: Prospects for correction of age-related immunodeficiency states. In Makinodan, T., Yunis, E. (ed.). Immunology and Aging. New York, Plenum, 1977

Wilson, M. The problem for society. Nursing Times 69(13:2), 486–488, 1973

Wright, W.E., Hayflick, L. Use of biochemical lesions for selection of human cells with hybrid cytoplasms. Proceedings of the National Academy of Science, U.S.A. 72(10):1812–1816, 1975

4

Behavior in the Environment of the Aged

Susanne S. Robb

Reading this chapter will enable the individual to:

1. List two reasons why attitude studies that use existing instruments are not likely to produce useful information
2. Distinguish between the terms belief, attitude, behavioral intention, and behavior
3. Describe the importance of "correspondence" in identifying relationships between attitudes and behaviors
4. List at least four suggestions to follow in discovering attitudes toward old people
5. Identify at least three attributes of elderly people that may elicit negative responses from nursing personnel
6. Name two or more obstacles to studying nurses' behaviors directed toward old people
7. Describe an example of each of the following actions a nurse might take to improve the quality of nursing care provided to an elderly client: (a) recognizing potential function, (b) obtaining a detailed history, (c) making wide and detailed assessments, (d) using himself/herself, and (e) electing to work with a predominantly elderly population
8. List problems nurses are likely to encounter when they attempt to change clients' behavior in clinical settings
9. Identify two strategies for changing nurses' behaviors toward elderly clients
10. Explain why behaviors are more important than attitudes in the environment of the aged

The elderly in modern industrial societies tend to be subject to many forms of discrimination. They have often been short-changed in terms of services, goods, and opportunities. "The purified image of themselves that society offers the aged is that of a white-haired and venerable sage, rich in experience, planing high above the common state of mankind: if they vary from this, then they fall below it. The counterpart of the first image is that of the old fool in his dotage, a laughing stock for children. In any case, either by their virtue or by their degradation they stand outside humanity" (de Beauvoir, 1972, p. 11). Our society tends to hold negative attitudes about aging and the aged. This has been considered the major factor responsible for the self-images older persons have of themselves and of the conditions and circumstances in which they live. Much effort has been directed toward determining the attitudes of health professionals toward the elderly, on the assumption that there is a direct relationship between attitude and the kind of service provided. Actually, the question of how people in general view the elderly remains unanswered and open for further study. Infrequent efforts to demonstrate a consistent predictive relationship between attitudes and behavior have resulted in very limited success.

This chapter will focus on behavior, including the nature of, measurement of, and potential for changing nurses' behavior toward the elderly (Fig. 4.1). First, however, the uncertain influence of attitudes on behavior will be explored. This background material is presented to assist nurses in evaluating the adequacy of attitude and/or behavior studies involving the elderly. Insufficient attention to issues of definition and measurement has, in the past, contributed to a largely contradictory and confusing picture of nursing and societal attitudes and their relationship to behavior toward the elderly.

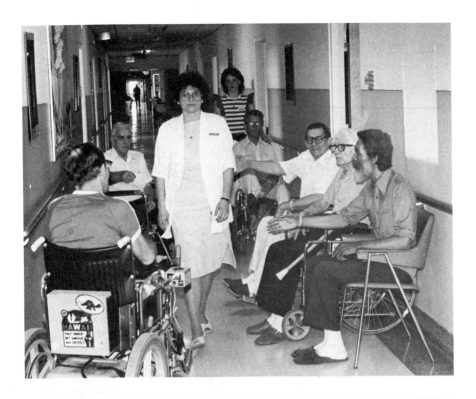

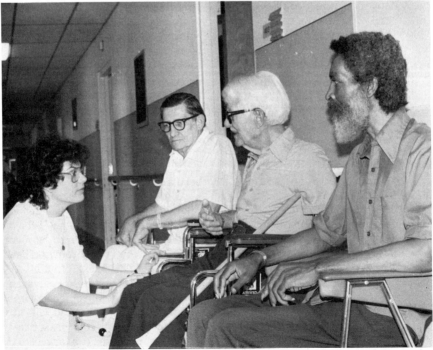

Figure 4.1. Nurses' behaviors mean more than their feelings; that is, actions speak louder than words! *(Photographs by Shawn Mertz, Pittsburgh, PA.)*

ATTITUDES

Clinical situations occur daily that raise questions about the interplay between the behaviors and the atttitudes of both the client and the health professional. As a prerequisite for being hired to work in the Valley View nursing home, nurses are asked to complete a 35-item inventory that measures attitude toward the elderly. The employer, however, is uncertain whether this inventory can predict actual nursing performance, so nurses are hired regardless of their scores and their subsequent nursing behaviors are evaluated. Thus far, results indicate that the nurses' general performance is only slightly related to attitude score, and nurse turnover is unrelated to score. This raises several questions about the relationship between attitude and behavior. Is there a consistent and predictive relationship between attitude and behavior? Does the way in which attitudes and behaviors are measured influence the likelihood of discovering a relationship? Are there other factors, aside from attitude, that may influence behavior? Is a written test the best way to identify attitudes? Is there overemphasis on the importance of attitudes?

A nurse in a long-term care facility returned to work after attending a continuing education program that emphasized the importance of providing accurate and consistent cues to people with memory impairment. Mr. K, a client who had apparently forgotten that he had been shaved an hour earlier, approached this nurse and requested his shaver. The nurse handed him the telephone receiver (apparently a long-standing practice that had become an automatic response to Mr. K's repetitious requests for a shaver). Mr. K began to "shave." Another nurse came along and, seeing this inappropriate use of the telephone, replaced the receiver on the cradle saying very firmly, "Mr. K, that is a telephone, not a shaver!"

The first nurse had scored high on a post-program test, and had been overheard to say that the program had given him many new ideas to be implemented in clinical practice. However, his behavior toward Mr. K did not support his voiced attitude. This prompts some additional questions about attitudes and be-

haviors. Which is more important, the nurse's beliefs, or attitudes, or the nurse's behavior toward the client? What elements, in addition to attitudes, influence behavior? To what extent does the client influence or provoke certain behaviors and attitudes on the part of the nurse? To what extent does the nurse influence or provoke certain behaviors and attitudes on the part of the client?

The Uncertain Influences of Attitudes on Behavior

A great deal of literature and a large number of measurement approaches have focused on the phenomenon variously referred to as "perceptions," "feelings," "beliefs," "attitudes," and "stereotypes" about or toward old people or old age (McTavish, 1982, p. 533). The reason for this marked interest is that emotional states are thought to be responsible for society's behavior toward its elderly people, and this behavior, in turn, affects the well-being of elderly people. The assumption is that the more positive the feelings people hold regarding old people, the more satisfying life will be for old people.

Toward Better Prediction with Fishbein's Conceptual Framework

The time has come for nurses to move beyond their preoccupation with attitudes and concern themselves, instead, with behavior toward the elderly. Rationale for this recommendation is provided by Fishbein's view of relationships involving attitudes and behavior. This conceptual framework includes four distinct components: (1) beliefs (cognitions), (2) attitudes or feelings (affect), (3) behavioral intentions (conative intentions), and (4) actual behaviors (conation) (Fishbein and Ajzen, 1975, p. 12).*

---

* Other concepts that have been used in the attitude area belong under one or the other of these categories. For example, concepts like "attraction," "value," "sentiment," "valence," and "utility" imply evaluation in terms of the two extremes of good and bad and thus may be considered as part of the category of "attitude." Similarly, "opinion," "information," "knowledge," "fact," and "stereotype" may all be viewed as beliefs held by an individual. Other terms

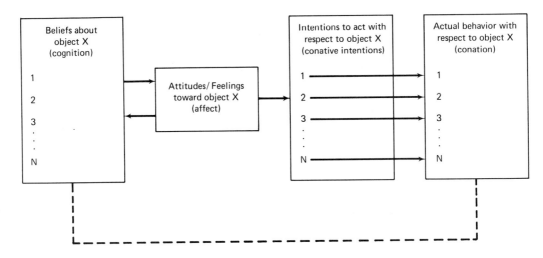

Figure 4.2. Schematic presentation of conceptual framework relating beliefs, attitudes, intentions and behaviors with respect to a given object. *(Adapted from Fishbein, M., Ajzen, I. Belief, Attitude, Intention, and Behavior. Reading, MA, Addison-Wesley, 1975. Copyright 1975 by the Addison-Wesley Publishing Co., Inc. Reprinted by permission.)*

A belief represents the verifiable information or facts a person has about an object. Specifically, a belief links an object to some attribute, such as "large," "wise," "poor," and so forth. An attribute can be any object, trait, property, quality, characteristic, outcome, or event (Fishbein and Ajzen, 1975, p. 12). An attitude refers to a person's favorable or unfavorable evaluation of an object. An attitude measure places an individual on a continuum according to his feeling for or against an object. Behavioral intentions simply refer to a person's commitment to perform various behaviors. Behavioral intentions are measured by linking a person to action that has yet to be performed in terms of how likely he or she is to perform act(s). Behavior is defined as overt actions taken by an individual that are studied in their own right. Verbal responses are also instances of overt behaviors in that they are observable actions. Frequently, however, verbalizations are not used as behaviors but instead are used to

infer beliefs, attitudes, or intentions (Fishbein and Ajzen, 1975, pp. 12–13). Failure to distinguish each of these concepts from the others has been one of the problems that has hindered demonstration of strong attitude–behavior relationships.

These four concepts relate to each other in a sequence diagrammed in Figure 4.2. Beliefs cause attitudes to be fixed somewhere on a continuum that extends from negative to positive. Attitudes, in turn, cause individuals to develop intentions to behave in a certain way. Behavioral intentions then cause individuals to actually perform certain behaviors or acts.

The central proposition in this conceptual framework is that the strength of an attitude–behavior relationship depends in large part on the degree of correspondence between attitudinal and behavioral entities. Correspondence is defined in terms of four elements that apply to *both* attitudes and behaviors: (1) the action, (2) the target at which the action is directed, (3) the context within which the action is performed, and (4) the time at which the action is performed (Ajzen and Fishbein, 1977, p. 889). A given action or behavior is always performed with respect to a given tar-

such as "prejudice," "morale," and "image" are defined so broadly that they may relate to all three categories. "Thus, a person may hold prejudicial beliefs, attitudes, and intentions" (Fishbein and Ajzen, 1975, p. 13).

get, within a given context, and at a given point in time. Examples of each of these elements are listed below:

Targets	Actions
Old people (person)	Supporting
Aging (process)	Assessing, testing, measuring
Old age (state)	Receiving
Contexts	**Times**
Clinic (public condition)	4:00 P.M. (immediate)
Home (private condition)	Tomorrow (future)
Convention (public condition)	August (future)

To predict a strong relationship between an attitude and a behavior, it is necessary to measure the individual's evaluation of, or attitude toward, performing that action with respect to a given target, within a given context, and at a given point in time. Alternatively, if prediction of a general behavior pattern is the goal, such as discrimination toward old people, the behavioral criterion should involve observation of different discriminatory behaviors toward old people within a variety of contexts at a variety of times. Under these circumstances, a general measure of attitude toward old people will correlate highly with the behavioral measure (Ajzen and Fishbein, 1972, p. 913).

The meaning of correspondence is presented in Figure 4.3. If correspondence exists between at least the target and the action elements of the measures used, strong relationships between attitude and behavior will be observed. That is, a general measure of attitude toward old people will correlate highly with general behavior toward old people, just as a specific measure of attitude toward old people will correlate highly with a specific measure of behavior toward old people. If the elements of time and context are also specified in both measures, the relationship will be even stronger. In addition, when trying to predict single acts/behaviors toward the target, behavior/action is more important than the attitude toward the target.

To illustrate, the nurse's behavior of measuring Mr. H's near and far visual acuities in the examining room of the gerontology clinic next Tuesday, at 10:00 A.M. will be more accurately predicted by asking that nurse to evaluate "measuring Mr. H's near and far visual acuity in the examining room, next Tuesday, at 10:00 A.M.," than by asking the nurse to evaluate "measuring Mr. H's vision." Prediction of whether a night nurse in a nursing home will observe and record urinary incontinence for 7 consecutive days on 10 elderly clients at 30-minute intervals and attend to those clients who are wet, is likely to be of interest to persons assessing urinary incontinence. To predict this behavior successfully, the night nurse needs to evaluate "observing and recording urinary incontinence for 7 consecutive days on 10 elderly clients at 30-minute intervals and cleaning up those clients who are wet." This same nurse's evaluation of "improving the quality of life for elderly people" is likely to have little correspondence with his or her performing the behavior of interest.

Alternatively, a general measure of nurses'

Attitude Measure Toward Target X	Behavioral Measure Toward Target X	
	Single Criterion/Action (Specific)	Multiple Criteria/Actions (General)
Single Criterion/Action (Specific)	High correlation (strong relationship)	Low correlation (weak relationship)
Multiple Criterion/Actions (General)	Low correlation (weak relationship)	High correlation (strong relationship)

Figure 4.3. When correspondence occurs between attitudes and behavior measures, strong relationships (high correlations between scores) tend to be observed.

attitudes toward improving the quality of life for old people will be highly correlated with a behavior measure that includes many different actions nurses might take in different settings at various times to make life better for old people. This same general attitude measure will not necessarily, however, be highly correlated with any single item on that behavior measure.

Attempts to change behavior by changing attitude must also consider the degree of correspondence between the behavior to be changed and the attitude toward which the influence attempt is directed. For example, nursing staff at the Peaceful Nursing Home have been successful in requesting physicians to order sedation for elderly residents who wander about or call out repeatedly during the night. Presenting an educational program about the harmful effects of sedation on elderly people in an attempt to change staff attitudes from favorable to unfavorable toward using sedation with elderly people is not likely to change the behavior. If the educational effort involves measuring the extent to which nurses who attended the program changed their feelings with regard to sedating elderly people, the results would probably support the educator's faith in the program. However, "demonstration of attitude change is insufficient evidence for one's ability to change behavior; only behaviors that correspond to the attitude are likely to change as a result of revisions in attitude" (Ajzen and Fishbein, 1977, p. 914). In this situation, the attitude that needs to change is probably "feeling about having night routines interrupted," rather than "feeling toward sedation in the elderly." The context is also important. An attitude held in a classroom may not be sufficient to motivate related behavior under the pressures that prevail on a busy clinical unit.

Finally, high correspondence between attitude and behavior measures will ensure strong relationships only to the extent that each measure is appropriate to the concept concerned. For example, attitude measures should contain only items that serve to indicate where the individual's feelings, with respect to a target object and action, fall on a bipolar evaluative dimension such as good–bad, for–against, or positive–negative. Attitude measures should not assess beliefs (knowledge) or behavioral intentions (likelihood of acting). Similarly, behavioral measures consist of one or more observable acts performed by the individual and somehow recorded by the invesigator. Behavioral acts include implementing a fire drill procedure, attending a meeting, feeding a paralyzed client, eating a balanced meal, and so forth. The less effort an action requires, the more the behavior becomes little more than an evaluation of the target. When this situation occurs, measurement of the attitude toward the target usually permits satisfactory prediction of behavior toward the target. To illustrate, the behavior of the nurse handing Mr. G his cigarettes when he asks for them and the nurse is near the drawer where cigarettes are kept is easily performed. Learning the nurse's attitude toward this action and target (handing cigarettes to Mr. G) would probably predict the nurse's behavior. On the other hand, teaching Mr. G the floor plan of the nursing home is a behavior that is more difficult to perform. Discovering the nurse's attitude in this instance would probably not predict the nurse's actual performance of that behavior.

Sometimes an individual's intention to perform the behavior(s) under consideration or self-report of behavior is substituted for direct observation. These "behavioroid" measures are acceptable behavioral criteria only when a direct measure of the behavior(s) of interest is difficult or impossible to obtain. Unfortunately, the fact that direct behavioral observation requires time, and thus money, and threatens people being observed, discourages direct measurement of behavior.

According to the conceptual framework and supportive evidence accumulated by Fishbein and associates (Fishbein and Ajzen, 1975), findings concerning the relation between attitude and behavior only appear to be inconsistent. A person's attitude has a consistently strong relation with his or her behavior when it is directed at the same target and when it involves the same action (Ajzen and Fishbein, 1977, p. 912). The following propositions need to be applied in studying attitudes and behaviors:

1. Intention to perform a given behavior is a more certain predictor of how an individual will behave than his or her beliefs about or attitude toward the behavior. If a nurse wants to know how someone will behave, the nurse needs to ask how that person intends to behave or better, observe the person's behavior unobtrusively.
2. General measures of beliefs or attitudes are only useful in predicting general—not, single, specific—behavioral intentions or behaviors. If a nurse-administrator wanted to know if the nurse she is about to hire will remain employed as a gerontologic clinical specialist, the administrator would have a better chance of predicting the behavior by asking the nurse. "Do you intend to fill the gerontologic clinical specialist position for at least 1 year?" than by administering an attitude-about-old people scale.

Attitude Instruments Used by Nurses in the Past

Instruments chosen by nurses in two or more studies to measure perceptions of old people have included the "Attitudes Toward Old People" scale (Tuckman and Lorge, 1953; Axelrod and Eisdorfer, 1961; Eisdorfer, 1966),* "Attitudes Toward Old People Scale" (Kogan, 1961),† "Opinions About People" (Ontario Welfare Council, Section on Aging, 1971; Hickey, Bragg, Rakowski, and Hultsch, 1978–79),‡ and the "Facts on Aging" quizzes (Palmore, 1977; 1981).§

These instruments are described as measuring "perceptions" because some assess concepts other than "attitudes," as previously defined. These instruments represent only a small proportion of the number available. Three of the four have serious deficiencies that mean the instruments require restructuring and fur-

ther testing. Therefore before using them to seriously evaluate perception measures, or spending time reviewing those listed above in greater detail, readers are advised to consult the following comprehensive instrument complications or reviews:

- Mangen, D.J., Peterson, W.A. Research Instruments in Social Gerontology, Vol. 1, Clinical and Social Psychology, Minneapolis, MN, University of Minnesota Press, 1982
  Chapter 12. "Perceptions of Old People," by D.G. McTavish, pp. 533–621.
  Chapter 11. "Life-Phase Analysis," by G.O. Hagestad, pp. 463–532.
  Chapter 10. "Subjective Age Identification," by N.E. Cutler, pp. 437–461.
- Eisdorfer, C., (ed.). Annual Review of Gerontology and Geriatrics, New York, Vol. 1, Springer, 1980.
  Chapter 13. "Attitudes toward Old Age and Elderly Persons," by N.S. Lutsky, pp. 287–336.

The nursing profession, along with other health professions, has treated what is only an assumption—that attitudes predict behavior—as fact. The truth is that:

1. It is still not certain that attitudes about any person, place, or thing, including old people and old age, indicate anything meaningful about human actions toward those target objects (Lutsky, 1980, p. 314).
2. It is clear that existing measures of attitudes, perceptions, or whatever term one chooses to call the phenomenon, do not measure anything worth measuring (Lutsky, 1980; McTavish, 1982; Palmore, 1982).

In selecting from existing instruments, nurses need to evaluate carefully instrument inadequacies in terms of both psychometric development* and conceptional grounding. Nurses

* Nurse-users: Campbell, 1971; Gunter, 1971; Kayser and Minnigerode, 1975; Burge, 1976; Wilhite and Johnson, 1976; Hart, Freel, and Crowell, 1976; Chamberland, Rawls, Powell, and Roberts, 1978; Meyer, Hassanein, and Bahr, 1980; and Tollet and Adamson, 1982.
† Nurse-users: Futrell, 1975; Heller and Walsh, 1976; Hatton, 1977; Taylor and Harned, 1978; Dye, 1979; Robb, 1979; and Brower, 1981.
‡ Nurse-users: Brower, 1979; and Devine, 1980.
§ Nurse-users: Weeks, 1979; and Devine, 1980.

* Psychometric properties refer to measurement devices' abilities to measure (1) what they were intended to measure, as opposed to some other concept, (2) in a consistent manner, (3) from one time to another, and (4) with reasonable sensitivity to changes in the target phenomenon. Thus an attitude-toward-old-people measure needs to measure attitude/feeling and not beliefs/attitude, behavioral

need to fulfill their obligation, as users of these instruments, to contribute to the continual improvement of assessment of the instrument's properties by reporting results of internal consistency, stability, dimensionality, and external correlation pattern analyses (Mangen and Peterson, 1982, pp. 15–16).

Future Directions in Attitude Measurement

Given the limitations of instruments nurses have chosen to measure attitudes, the question occurs, "How should attitudes be measured?" As can be seen in Figure 4.4, the question is not a simple one. The suggestions listed below are believed to be of particular importance to nurses seeking to use studies of attitudes to justify changes in clinical practices, educational programs, and policy formulation:

1. Beliefs and attitudes are distinctly different phenomena and should not be confused. Claims of having studied attitudes should not be made if it is knowledge or information that has been assessed (Kilty and Feld, 1976; Fishbein and Ajzen, 1975; Ajzen and Fishbein, 1977; Kogan, 1979).
2. Directions provided by Martin Fishbein and associates (Fishbein and Ajzen, 1975; Ajzen and Fishbein, 1977) need to be followed to demonstrate correspondence between attitude and behavior measures (Robb, 1980; Schmidt, 1981).
3. Limitations inherent in written, scaled/limited response option instruments require consideration. These procedures demand that respondents think in terms of fixed categories rather than employ the terms and dimensions they might ordinarily use. Re-

---

intentions or actual behaviors instead of attitude, and not "illness," "poverty," or "physical appearance" instead of "old people." This instrument needs to measure a person's attitude so the score stays the same from day to day as long as the person's attitude does not change, but to yield a change in score when the person's attitude does, in fact, change. The measure needs to produce scores that vary systematically to indicate very favorable and very unfavorable attitudes held by different people, and all degrees of favorability between these extremes.

spondents quickly figure out what is expected of them and respond on the basis of (a) researcher expectations (rather than their own expectations) and (b) social desirability concerns (socially acceptable responses, rather than socially deviant responses) (Green, 1981). Open-ended instruments are required to learn the richness and subtlety of a person's beliefs and attitudes about old people (Kogan, 1979). Items such as, "The thing I like best about old people is . . ." and "The thing I like least about old people is . . . ," from the Golde-Kogan Sentence-Completion Assessment (Golde and Kogan, 1959) might elicit responses more highly predictive of the nature of social interaction with old people than responses to generalized scales.

4. Distinctions between attitudes toward old people (person), aging (process), and old age (state) need to be recognized in selecting a target object (Bader, 1980).
5. When the target is the person, it must be remembered that responses are dependent on how the person is described. For example, responses have been found to vary between a generally defined target ("old people") and a specific target ("a healthy 70-year-old, male, marathon runner"), and between a stereotypically described specific person ("a 72-year-old female who leaves home only to purchase food and complains bitterly about her arthritis and the burdens she places on her family") versus an atypically described specific person ("a 72-year-old female who walks 3 miles each day and speaks enthusiastically about her travel plans") (Greenshields, Roberts, and Stewart, 1980; Green, 1981). To assume that age alone produces impressions about individuals is not realistic. Other individual attributes, such as sex, physical appearance, race, and social class, certainly combine to produce an overall impression of any individual.
6. While there is substantial evidence indicating that attitudes are multidimensional constructs (Eisdorfer and Altrocci, 1961; Hicks, Rogers, and Shemberg, 1976; Kilty

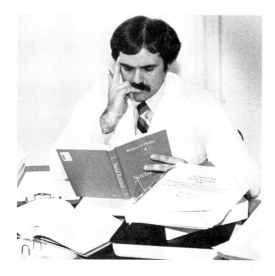 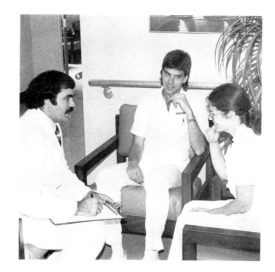

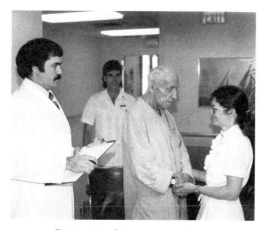 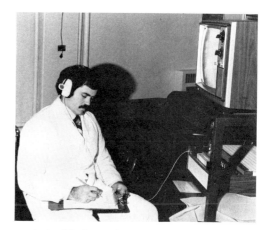

Figure 4.4. Discovering attitudes is not an easy task. *(Photographs by Shawn Mertz, Pittsburgh, PA.)*

and Feld, 1976; Richardson and Cunningham, 1978; Hickey, Bragg, Rakowski, and Hultsch, 1978–79; Holtzman, Beck, and Kerber, 1979; Wingard, 1980, Kafer, Rakowski, Lachman, and Hickey, 1980), the majority of attitude measures yield single scores instead of subscores that reflect various component factors. Component scores are important to consider because some of these scores may correlate more highly with or predict more adequately to other variables.

7. Finally, nurses might even ask themselves whether attitudes that can be measured and then presumably changed by some intervention (an educational program or direct

clinical experience) are of sufficient strength, relevance, or durability to be worth trying to assess and change in the first place (Bader, 1980).

The following instruments are recommended simply because they have been developed to measure either general beliefs/knowledge or general attitudes/feelings but not both. The "Facts on Aging Quiz" (Palmore, 1977; 1981) assesses beliefs/knowledge. Dr. Susan Whitbourne was in the process of developing separate belief and attitude scales (Whitbourne, Wheeler, and Sperbeck, 1980). However, Whitbourne and colleagues found little variation in attitude scores within most samples encountered. She concluded, "it is far more useful but also more difficult to measure actual behaviors" (Whitbourne, 1983). Items that comprise the evaluative factors of the following instruments* could be used appropriately to measure attitudes toward elderly people: (1) the Eisdorfer–Altrocchi Semantic Differential (Eisdorfer and Altrocchi, 1961), (2) the Kogan–Wallach Semantic Differential (Kogan and Wallach, 1961), and (3) the Rosencranz–McNevin Attitudes toward the Aged (Rosencranz and McNevin, 1969). Selected items from the Golde–Kogan Sentence Completion Assessment (Golde and Kogan, 1959) could be administered and reliable qualitative scoring categories constructed to yield an attitude score. Each of these instruments is most accessible in the instrument compilation, *Research Instruments in Social Gerontology, Volume 1, Clinical and Social Psychology* (Mangen and Peterson, 1982).

BEHAVIORS

A reciprocal relationship seems to exist between client behaviors and nurse behaviors, as suggested in Figure 4.5. Results from two studies support this reciprocity. In the first, elderly

people who received attending behavior from a nurse had higher performance ratings on a mental status test than elderly people who did not receive attending behavior. Attending behavior simply meant that the nurse was deliberately attentive to clients during testing, including eye contact, relaxed and attentive body language, and verbal following of what clients said (Rosendahl and Ross, 1982). In the second study, nursing assistants indicated they preferred to care for elderly people who were more independent in self-care activities, cheerful and friendly, and appreciative of efforts made by nursing personnel. Nursing assistants were reluctant to care for clients who behaved in opposite ways (Elliott and Hybertson, 1982). Results of this study are consistent with studies done a number of years ago, one of which indicated that nurses valued clients less who made excessive demands through incontinence, littering the environment, failure to cooperate, disruptive behavior, and low self-care ability (Brown, 1969). In another study, nurses demonstrated fewer individualizing behaviors, such as screening for privacy during care, toward clients who scored lower in social participation and activities of daily living (White, 1974). These findings should alert nurses to identify clients with the fewest positive attributes as primary targets for rehabilitative–restorative nursing care.*

Both clients and nurses use the behavior of the other to reinforce or change their self-esteem and eventually their self-concept. Clients, for example, translate from nursing behaviors in a sequence that moves from "this is what the nurse does," through "this is what the nurse thinks of me," to "this is what I am." Similarly, nurses translate client behaviors toward them in a sequence that progresses from,

---

* Entire instruments should be administered to avoid the problem of items eliciting different responses when they are separated from the original whole instrument. The evaluative items can then be scored separately to represent the attitude measure.

---

* An exception may be the client who lacks potential for restoration due to a terminal illness or an illness with a very negative prognosis for self-help, such as amyotrophic lateral sclerosis. In these instances, measurable goals related to promotion of comfort in the broadest sense and maintenance of functional status should be identified to focus nurse actions in a positive direction.

This approach is consistent with nonemergency priorities and is the opposite of that employed in triage during civil and war-related crises.

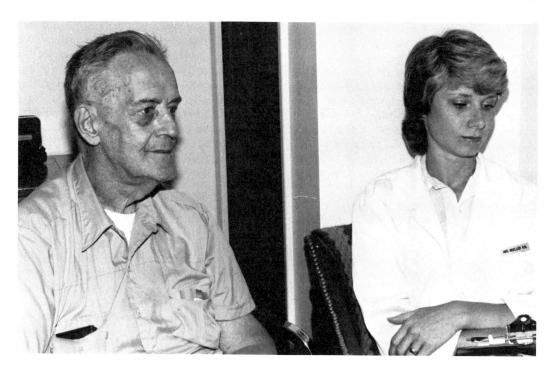

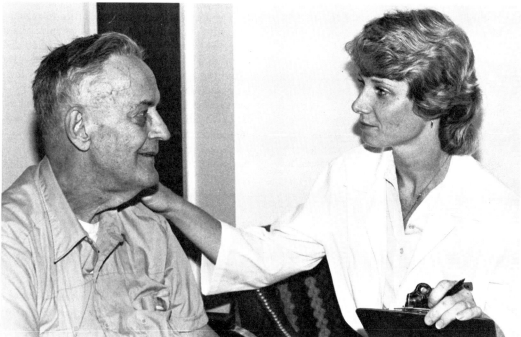

Figure 4.5. When nurses are attentive during client assessments, clients demonstrate higher levels of functioning.

"this is what the client does," through "this is what the client thinks of me," to "this is what I am."

Although the processes may seem identical, the outcomes tend not to be equal, with clients losing and nurses enhancing their self-esteem. This inequality occurs because the balance of power favors the nurse. In any setting (outpatient or inpatient), the nurse owns the information and skills clients require to alter their health status. In long-term care, inpatient settings the nurse's power is even greater because of losses clients sustain that result in their requiring such placements.

This section will consider attributes of elderly people and of nurses that prompt negative behavior in the environment of the elderly. Emphasis will be given to nurse–client encounters in long-term care settings. Institutions are simply settings in which events either happen or do not happen. Behavior is an ongoing, continuous activity that the environment maintains (supports), strengthens (increases), or weakens (decreases), depending on how it is structured (Hoyer et al., 1974, p. 151). Nurses are a large part of the institutional environment and, thus, bear a major share of responsibility for the nature of that environment.

Attributes of the Elderly that Elicit Negative Responses

Therapeutic goals in long-term care settings are frequently limited to maintaining intact skin using hygienic and nutritional measures, as well as frequent position changes (Elliott

and Hybertson, 1982; Robb, 1983). A number of practitioners and researchers have written about the general reluctance of nurses, physicians, and other health professionals to engage in practice involving the elderly (Gunter, 1971; Butler and Lewis, 1977; Ford and Sbordone, 1979; Brower, 1981). What characteristics of elderly people inspire these negative behavioral responses?

Physical Appearance

Physical age cues are so easy for others to perceive that they may influence interpersonal encounters as initial impressions are formed. Accurate assessment of the chronologic age of old people has been accomplished by both children (Britton and Britton, 1969) and adults (Kastenbaum et al., 1972). "Physical changes, including getting sick, slowing down, wearing out, and showing visible signs of age such as wrinkles and gray hair, are considered by the public as the principal causes of old age" (National Council on the Aging, 1974, p. 26). Figure 4.6 presents one cartoonist's view of the impact of physical age cues on perception.

Aging can be a genuine ordeal. Mentioning individuals' ages after 35 may remind them that they are nearer the end of life than the beginning. Changes in physical appearance are about the same for both men and women. However, a double standard of aging exists. Aging for men is an asset, since our society values men for what they do, not how they look. A handsome old man may be admired, since white hair and wrinkles do not conflict with his image as strong and intelligent (de Beauvoir, 1972,

Figure 4.6. An example of physical age cues influencing impressions. *(Berry, J. Berry's world. Pittsburgh Press, August 13, 1978. Copyright 1978 by Newspaper Enterprise Association, Inc. Reprinted by permission.)*

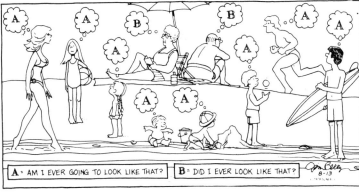

A = AM I EVER GOING TO LOOK LIKE THAT?   B = DID I EVER LOOK LIKE THAT?

p. 440). Fame, money, and power enhance male sexuality; each tends to increase with age. Men stay sexually interesting as long as they can make love. Women must meet stricter standards for appearance and age to remain sexually desirable. No one speaks of a beautiful old woman, in life or in literature. The terror of a woman's life is the moment represented in a statue by Rodin called "Old Age." A naked old woman, seated, pathetically contemplates her flat, pendulous, ruined body. Aging in women is a process of becoming sexually obscene—flabby bosom, wrinkled neck, thin white hair, waistless torso, and veined legs (Sontag, 1972, p. 37).

Both sexes care how they appear, and playing with body image can be fun. Beauty, fashion, and decoration are cultural imperatives—tattoos, scarification, and beards are examples. Past and present generations have been masochistic in pursuit of fashion, but women are more often the victims than men. Cultures tend to place a beauty compulsion on women and an achievement compulsion on men.

The double standard of physical aging has been the most significant force in making the marriage of an older woman to a younger man a deviant act, compared to marriage between older men and younger women. For a man, marriage to a young woman is good public relations. It emphasizes that he is still capable and desirable. An older woman who marries a man many years her junior has broken a strong taboo. She gets no credit for her courage. Instead of being admired for her vitality, she is often condemned as predatory, willful, selfish, exhibitionist, or pitiable. In cases of extreme age difference, her judgment may be questioned, especially if money is involved. Her spouse is labeled effeminate, neurotic, or opportunistic.

Older and old women may come to be accepted as desirable sex partners with the aging of the cohort that believed "anyone over thirty should not be trusted." This large group has continued to believe in itself (including its women) as it progresses through each decade beyond the 20s. The movement for women's rights has also helped to dispel some of the aversion to older women (Morrow, 1978).

Impact of physical age cues on behavior toward the elderly was investigated by Lawrence (1974). The results indicated that physical change cues were considered to a greater extent than dress, facial expression, body build, and stance when respondents formed impressions of older people than when impressions were formed about middle-aged or young people. Responses to photographs of young and old people interacting in various roles indicated that the young people were viewed as counselors, with the old people viewed as counselees. It was more appropriate, however, for a young man to give "professional" advice to an older man than to advise him about his business affairs. When an older man and younger woman were seen arriving at a cocktail party, most believed the couple had a relationship other than husband and wife. Very few said that the couple were dating.

The issue of contemptuous behavior expressed toward the aged was examined in a study of 95 societies randomly chosen from the 186 "distinctive world areas" in the Standard Cross-Cultural Sample (Murdock and White, 1969). Results indicated six reasons for contempt listed in order of declining importance: (1) lack or loss of children, (2) *deterioration of appearance,* (3) loss of physical strength and stamina, (4) gaining negative traits, (5) mental deterioration, and (6) lack or loss of skills, and/or obsolescence. The 18 kinds of contemptuous acts identified ranged from giving the elderly "scrap food" to killing them (Maxwell and Maxwell, 1979). At least 15 of these 18 contemptuous behaviors are commonplace in long-term care facilities. For example, excluding aged people from sexual relationships, deposing them from authority or influence, excluding them from work (Storlie, 1982), and subjecting them to poor medical care (Brown, Cornwell, and Weist, 1981; Steel et al., 1981; Buckeleu, 1982; Jahnigen et al., 1982).

Clothing is an important part of the image people present to the world. In institutional settings, this image is particularly important, as personnel turnover is often high and there is only limited opportunity for anything more than casual relationships. Dressing according to choice permits a person to express individuality of feeling and thought. Consider your own responses to the images of people in Figure 4.7.

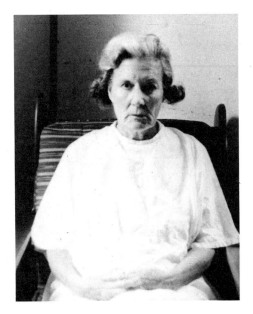
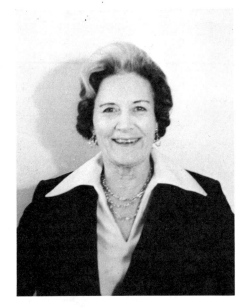
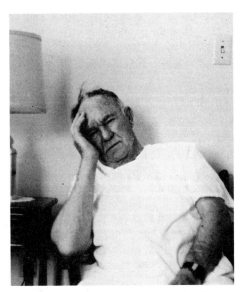
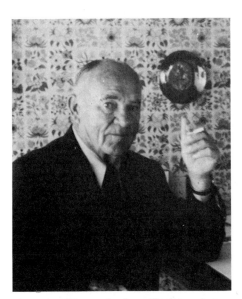

Figure 4.7. Appearance influences the way people respond to each other. *(Photographs by Nance Photo, Pittsburgh, PA.)*

Keeping institutionalized people in bed clothing even when they are fully ambulatory forces them to appear ill or tired, and inspires others to respond accordingly. Loss of personal clothing through theft or laundry procedures is often used to justify hospital attire for all but the most competent, affluent clients. If similar problems arose in the provision of syringes or enema canisters, they would be quickly resolved. Wearing of personal clothing is a psychosocial intervention and human right. Because it is not a medical therapy, the practice is not valued in institutional settings.

Death Potential
One factor that isolates the elderly from society and inspires negative attitudes may be their proximity to death. In the past, death was more evenly distributed across the lifespan because of unsafe work environments and uncontrolled disease processes. Today, more people in modern industrialized societies live to their 70s and 80s. It is primarily the old who die. Since death is a function of age, aging and the aged are symbols through which death is perceived and understood.

Aging and dying are usually two different processes. In a sense, it can be said that everyone is aging and dying from the time of conception. However, aging usually describes those changes in bodily capacities that make the individual increasingly likely to die from random accidental causes. Since no one dies of age-related changes in themselves, dying is described as the process leading from the incidence of the accidental cause of death to the state of being dead. This distinction makes it clear that the individual is *aging* from the time of conception, but he is *dying* after he acquires an "accidental" cause of death, such as an embolus, until he is dead from a cerebrovascular accident or myocardial infarction.

Several studies have compared death attitudes of the elderly with those of other age groups. Death seems to be less frightening for those who are older. This has been observed in a variety of situations, using a variety of measurement instruments (Kalish, 1976; Devins, 1979; Stevens, Cooper, and Thomas, 1980). However, some evidence indicates that the elderly think and talk more about death than people in other age groups (Cameron, Stewart, and Biber, 1973; Kalish and Reynolds, 1976).

The relationship between death anxiety and helping behavior is not simple—it depends on the kind of help, the kind of helper, and the kind of person being helped (Salter and Templer, 1979; Pinder and Hayslip, 1981). Elderly

people are increasingly dying in institutions (Kastenbaum, 1978; Katz, Zdeb, and Therriault, 1979). In these settings, Glaser and Strauss (1965) found a cloak of secrecy around dying clients that blocked all meaningful interactions and interventions involving the group. Patterns of disinterest and rejection of dying clients have been reported by others (Sudnow, 1967; Gottesman and Bourestrom, 1974; McMahon and Miller, 1980, Buckeleu, 1982). The number, length, and quality of contacts with nurses decrease, to the point where old people who are considered close to death may be unkempt and allowed to smell badly. One study of relationships among general anxiety, age, and measures of conscious and unconscious death anxiety suggested that with increased age, people tend to link death and aging unconsciously rather than consciously, so that the impact of death anxiety influences care provided to old people through denial (fears not admitted) and through displacement (fears expressed as negative behaviors toward old people) (Pinder and Hayslip, 1981). Salter and Templer (1979) asked how young people coped with fears of death triggered by the sight or thought of an old person. Results of their study suggested that young females tended to avoid the elderly and deny thoughts of aging and death in an effort to repress anxiety. Young males, however, tended to adjust their attitudes and behavior in a more realistic and adaptive way through actually helping elderly people by visiting them, taking them to religious and medical services, telephoning them, and running errands for them. These results are of particular interest since nursing remains a predominantly female profession.

Dependence
Very old people seem to be less involved with their physical and social environments. Some are very passive and dependent. Dependency in infants and children is expected to be temporary and to decrease. In the elderly, however, it is regarded as irreversible and increasing in nature. Since independence is an American ideal, "inappropriate" dependence is reason for rejection by most members of society—including those who are themselves de-

pendent. Nursing personnel have been shown to prefer caring for old people who are independent in grooming and ambulation and continent of bladder function (Elliott and Hybertson, 1982).

Unfortunately, instead of promoting independence on the part of the elderly, health professionals may create dependency (Mikulic, 1971; Baltes and Zerbe, 1967a; Lester and Baltes, 1978; Baltes and Barton, 1978). Twenty elderly women with hip fractures were studied to determine the factors associated with postoperative confusion (Phillips, Wolanin, and McFeaters, 1978). The study concluded that the behaviors and expectations of the nurses significantly influenced the appearance of withdrawing behaviors (apathy, hostility, unresponsiveness, and confusion) in certain clients. Those clients who were highly motivated to overcome large odds were held in very high esteem by nurses. Some of these clients who were, in fact, confused were not regarded as confused by the nurses. Passive clients tended to be held in low esteem. Sometimes they were labeled as confused when, in fact, they were not. The study suggests that confusion is but one of several coping behaviors an elderly client may adopt in time of crisis. Confusion may thus be predictable and preventable, especially if nurses are alert to those clients who are at the most risk—the passive, dependent old people. In a different arena, public policy-makers enforce dependency by denying old people work, money, and a place to live (Comfort, 1976, pp. 6–7).

Other Behaviors

To the casual observer, the actual behavior of the elderly does not appear to support a positive view of aging. The viewer who does not look closely may conclude that very old people are slow in thoughts, words, and actions. Ideas and requests are comprehended more slowly. Response time is extended. Older people appear to do less with their time. The range of their activities is likely to diminish. The lifespan of all organisms appears to be regulated by a biologic clock. Biologic evidence of loss and decline is substantial. Regardless of how positively disposed an individual is toward ag-

ing and the aged, that person would probably not elect to live within an old body (Manney, 1975, p. 4).

Physical deterioration, however, does not account for all the negative behavioral characteristics of old people. Some of these behaviors relate to psychosocial influences. These include perceptions of societal complexity, dangers, and reward systems, as well as social losses—losses of significant others, wealth, occupation. Not surprisingly, nursing personnel prefer clients, regardless of their ages, who are "appreciative, cooperative, friendly, affectionate, cheerful, satisfied, interested in the environment, and not manipulative or verbally abusive" (Glazer, 1981; Elliott and Hybertson, 1982). Findings like these inspire at least two questions for nurses to consider. Nurses should remember the message of the film, *Mrs. Reynolds Needs a Nurse* (Little, Pesznecher, and Baker, 1963)—reasons for "deviant" or "disruptive" behavior should be sought and care managed creatively so that clients' needs are met. If psychosocial factors give rise to negative behaviors in old people, cannot psychosocial interventions modify these behaviors in a positive direction? Deliberate use of "attending behavior" by nursing personnel can improve scores earned by elderly people on mental status tests (Rosendahl and Ross, 1982). Intimate contact with a loving companion-animal such as a dog or cat can stop an elderly client from swearing repeatedly and striking at people passing by his chair (Robb, Boyd, and Pristash, 1980). Participation in small group activities can set people free to be themselves and produce many positive changes in interpersonal functioning (Wolanin, 1977).

Myths

Myths and stereotypes about the elderly flourish* because this age group is relatively invisible. Few young people know any old people well, other than relatives. The elderly do not

* Experts in gerontology are not immune to myths. Erdman Palmore (1977; 1981), developed a quiz to test knowledge about aging and the aged. Even students of gerontology were unable to score 100 percent. Stereotypic patterns of thought and expectation are very pervasive.

appear in work, educational, or entertainment settings in proportion to the percentage of population they represent. They are expected to behave in certain ways merely because they have reached a certain age. Consider these phrases: "young for her age" to describe an older woman, "old for her age" to describe a girl, and "entering a second childhood" to describe a middle-aged man. Phrases such as "you can't teach an old dog new tricks" and "old biddy" reflect stereotypes. Fear associated with continuing sexuality inspires the phrase, "dirty old man." Euphemisms such as "golden ager" and "senior citizen" reveal hostility toward the status of being old. A vicious cycle is established, in which myths derived from minimal contact insure that minimal contact will continue.

Age stereotyping is destructive to the elderly because it mixes casual observations with factual knowledge. Since aging is seen primarily as a physical process, reversible psychosocial forces that have a detrimental impact are not recognized. Consider some popular stereotypes. Retirement is "necessary" because old people are no longer physically capable, not because economic considerations decree a reduction in the work force. Confusion and mental slowness are caused by "dementia," a physical condition, rather than by lack of appropriate stimuli and positive expectations for competence. Potential for growth and contribution goes unrecognized.

The belief that the situation of the elderly is caused by physical decline is widely accepted. As a result, the opposite possibility is rarely considered—that physical decline is precipitated by social rejection. The National Council on Aging survey (1974) indicated that negative images of the elderly are accepted by both young and old. However, old people have a more positive view of their individual situations than of the situations of old people in general. This suggests that Brubaker and Powers (1976, p. 445) may be correct in suggesting that the stereotype of "old" that an elderly individual will accept is closely related to previous positive or negative self-concept. Old people who do not regard themselves negatively base their self-concepts on such char-

acteristics as progressiveness, productivity, health, activity, attractiveness, flexibility, and organization (Catron, 1978).

The behavior and appearance of old people, coupled with a tendency to idolize youthful stereotypes, have led both young and old to dwell on the negative aspects of aging. In an effort to combat these negative views, many "gerontophiles" deny the real difficulties associated with aging. These orientations may be categorized as "there is nothing to be done" versus "anything is possible." Both coping strategies result in distorted behavior toward old people.

The following situations are fairly commonplace. Consider how individuals might respond based on their prevailing orientation toward old people.

SITUATION	PESSIMIST THINKS:	OPTIMIST THINKS:
An old man fails to cross the street before the traffic light changes	"Oh well, what do you expect of an old man?"	"If he exercised more, he could certainly do better."
An old lady starts to retell an account of the birth of her first child.	"I don't have time to waste hearing this story again."	"If I listen, she will feel better and become more able to deal with the present."
A senator, age 71, appears on the evening news as a result of a speech against mandatory retirement.	"That man is a remarkable exception to the way most old people are."	"More old people could be like that man if they tried."
An elderly lady arrives at the Social Security office only to find it closed for a federal holiday.	"Forgetting to call is typical of old people."	"With wider publicity she would not have made that mistake."

The pessimists in these cases tend to regard old people who function well as exceptions to the rule. If an elderly person has overcome a difficulty, the difficulty could not have been significant in the first place. The optimists tend to place the elderly person under a performance compulsion to try harder. If enough resources were mobilized, the difficulty could be alleviated.

Elderly people may be disadvantaged both by the very negative and very positive views. Evidence emerging from studies in gerontology suggests that controlled investigation can lead to clearly defined solutions for problems once believed to be irreversible in elderly people. On the other hand, premature adoption of unproven remedies can lead to disillusionment and waste of scarce resources.

Nursing Behaviors Toward the Elderly

Determination of nursing behavior toward any client group has been difficult. Barriers are imposed by clients' rights to privacy, and the need for unobtrusive measurement procedures. Direct observation of behavior has been used primarily by educators, supervisors, and researchers to evaluate effectiveness of nurse performance. However, the impact of the observer on the behavior of the subject being evaluated has been well documented.

Another obstacle to measurement of nursing behavior has been a lack of consensus as to what constitutes quality nursing care. The American Nurses Association (ANA) has defined standards of practice for a variety of settings (e.g., Standards of Gerontological Nursing Practice, ANA, 1976). Quality assurance programs have been established to insure compliance with these standards. However, in the real world the practicing nurse collaborates with several different groups—clients, physicians, head nurses, and peers. Each of these groups has a different idea of how a nurse should act. What is deemed good for the "organization" is often not good for the client.

Development of reliable and valid measurement instruments to assess the quality of care in long-term settings has lagged behind development of such instruments for acute care

settings. The issue of whether outcomes of health care should be determined by providers/ therapists or by clients has hardly been addressed. When reliable instruments are developed to measure the processes in which nurses engage while providing health care, and the outcomes clients achieve as a result, the nurses' behaviors can be more accurately evaluated and, perhaps, considered in relation to their attitudes.

Attempts to measure nurses' behaviors toward elderly clients have involved direct observation using trained observers (Mikulic, 1971; Hatton, 1977; Barton, Baltes, and Orzech, 1980; Simmons et al., 1981; Bossenmaier, 1982; Adelson et al., 1982). Methods, such as videotaping nurses' performances (Daubenmire et al., 1977), reviewing written records such as chart notes (Phaneuf, 1976; Steckel, 1976), and rating nurses' responses to simulations (McLaughlin et al., 1979; Holzemer et al., 1981), that have been used with clients in other age groups and settings have not been reported for elderly people receiving long-term care.

Observation categories used by Mikulic (1971) to categorize nurses' reinforcement behaviors (positive reinforcement, negative reinforcement, and absence of reinforcement) were the same as those used by Baltes and associates (Lester and Baltes, 1972; Barton, Baltes, and Orzech, 1980).

Hatton (1977) developed an elaborate observational coding scheme for behaviors considered responsive or not responsive to client needs. However, Hatton experienced difficulty in observing and categorizing nursing behaviors using this coding plan.

The Wandelt Quality Patient Care Scale (Wandelt and Ager, 1974) was modified for a study to determine the quality of nursing care provided in several long-term skilled nursing care facilities (Simmons et al., 1981). It examines quality of care from the client's perspective through observations of staff–client interactions. Modifications made in the scale consisted of deleting items observed infrequently in long-term care settings and reducing the number of categories in the rating scale to observed, not observed, and not applicable.

These changes may have affected the reliability and validity of the scale.

Nurse behaviors toward elderly clients in acute care hospitals were examined in an exploratory study by Bossenmaier (1982). Four areas of intervention were chosen because of their importance to nursing practice and to changes of normal aging: touch, verbal communication, control, and physical care. Operational definitions for these categories must be developed before they can be used in further studies. Results from this exploratory study suggested a number of deficiencies in the care nurses provided, as well as missed opportunities to provide care that was specifically planned for elderly people.

A "Health Professional–Geriatric Patient Interaction Behavior Rating Code" was developed to fill the instrument void in this area (Adelson et al., 1982). Results of initial developmental testing indicate this behavior rating code is a reliable and valid tool to grade health professionals' skills in relating to geriatric clients.

Caution must be used in saying that any of these observational plans measures "quality of nursing care." Studies involving several different quality of nursing care instruments in acute care (Ventura and Hageman, 1978; Ventura, Hageman, Slakter, and Fox, 1980) found small and insignificant associations between the various instruments. This suggests that the concept of "quality of care" has not been defined with adequate precision to permit valid measurement.

Suffice it to say that nurses' behavior toward the elderly leaves a great deal to be desired. The quality of nursing care in long-term care facilities has not been empirically determined, largely because of the developmental status of measuring instruments. Limited evidence, however, suggests that nurses who work in long-term care settings have not provided the quality of services required. The report of former HEW Secretary Elliot Richardson's Committee to Study Extended Roles for Nurses stated, "Nurses involved in long term care often function at less than the level for which they are prepared and less effectively than society has the right to expect" (Extending the Scope of Nursing Practice: A Report of the Secretary's Committee to Study Extended Roles for Nurses, 1971).

Frances Storlie, a nurse, wrote about nurses' behavior on the basis of in-depth study of life in six nursing homes.

> Through deprivation of a whole range of independent actions—the old person is told when to eat, when to wash, when to toilet himself, and when to sit, stand, or lie down—the adults lose touch with what they once were, and what they now are. Finally, they lose control over what matters most to them—their own bodies (Storlie, 1982, p. 555).

The anecdotes Storlie provides indicate some of the actions nurses take that contribute to this outcome. Nurses (1) do whatever is necessary to prevent visible physical damage to clients, especially damage from falls, infections, or failure to eat, (2) fail to allow meaningful decision-making by clients, and (3) employ any strategy that gets the work of keeping clients clean, covered and fed done within the first 3 to 4 hours of each tour of duty.

Elderly-directed behaviors by nurses in acute care have been studied even less than those of nurses in long-term care. One study, conducted in several different settings, examined the development of confusional states in elderly women undergoing surgery to repair hip fractures (Williams et al., 1979). Nurses were reported to use several comparatively easy-to-use interventions to reverse confusional states: verbal orientation, explanations and reassurance, and variation of sensory input.

In a second study, the researchers sought to learn whether nurses' behavior toward their clients approximated that of jailers toward their prisoners, and it was found that nurses did, in fact, behave very much like jailers. Basically, the imprisonment model describes the process by which the behaviors of a hospitalized elderly person are shaped through negative reinforcement into negative responses. As the person perceives him- or herself to be imprisoned, he or she emits negative behaviors that, in turn, stimulate the nursing personnel to punish that behavior. The net result is mutual withdrawal. An example of this sequence was provided.

> For the purpose of this example, the discriminating stimulus is that the patient must get out of bed. The patient, who is feeling the effects of imprisonment, may respond negatively with an angry or whining "No I don't want to get out of bed, what does it matter to you if I do?" or he may not respond verbally at all but may just look at the nurse (both are withdrawing type behaviors). To this, the nurse responds with an angry remark or may handle the patient more roughly than necessary (punishing behavior) or she may not give the patient any instruction or encouragement during the transfer procedure (punishing behavior). To this the patient emits more withdrawing behaviors such as crying, whining, or anger which punishes the nurse for her behavior. This behavior increases the likelihood that the nurse will attempt to avoid contact with this patient (positive reinforcement for the nurse). At the same time, the patient's withdrawing behaviors increase the likelihood that the nurse will seek justification for her behavior from her peers, for example by calling the patient unmotivated during report. As the nurse emits angry or distancing behaviors, she punishes the patient's behavior. Increased distance means that the patient not only does not receive the cues he needs to transfer comfortably and the social touching so important for the geriatric patient, but also the patient ends up sitting in the chair for a very long period of time because the nurse does not come back for a long period of time. Interestingly enough, in the long run, the patient's behaviors also turn out to be positively reinforced by the nurse's avoidance. Because the nurse stays out of the room longer, there is less opportunity for punishment both by angry words and rough handling, and also by having to get out of bed fewer times (Phillips, Wolanin, and McFeaters, 1978, pp. 7–8).

These two studies are as important in terms of what was not found as what was found. In neither study were nurses reported to treat the elderly as special people, particulary at risk of developing serious complications as a result of events occurring in the acute care setting. Elderly people received the same, potentially harmful venipunctures, medications, and schedules as anyone else. The ultimate solution for confusional states was to wait for the old people to move along, if not to their homes, then to long-term care facilities. Results of a third exploratory study, conducted to learn whether nurses recognized special age-related needs of elderly people receiving acute care, supported results from these two studies (Bossenmaier, 1982). Lacking special preparation in gerontologic nursing, acute care nurses are poorly equipped to advocate on behalf of the elderly and in opposition to decisions of physicians, a behavior that is required to prevent iatrogenical illnesses so often suffered by elderly clients during hospitalization (Steel et al., 1981; Gillick, Serrell, and Gillick, 1982; Jahnigen et al., 1982).

Accentuating the Positive

People who work with the institutionalized elderly usually have little contact with independent functioning old people of the type found in large numbers in Sun City, Arizona, or St. Petersburg, Florida. Having known a family member who aged "successfully" often does not overcome the negative perceptions of aging that tend to prevail in long-term care settings. In institutional settings, one group (the care-givers) is charged with responsibility for the safety and well-being of another group (the elderly clients). The "responsible" group tends to regard the other group as "irresponsible." Labels of irresponsibility commonly applied to elderly people institutionalized for health care are "in need," "invalid," and "incompetent." It has been found that nurses are more likely to give a diagnosis of organic brain syndrome to a client depicted as elderly rather than young. This tendency to misdiagnose elderly people increased when nurses had more extensive contact with institutionalized elderly people (Ciliberto, Levin, and Arluke, 1981).

Nurses may not accept the potential of an old person, even when made aware of it by others. An elderly man, newly admitted to a long-term care facility, was incontinent of urine on the first night. Without assessment to determine if this was a new or old problem, an external catheter was applied. When the man later said he needed to urinate, he was told to go ahead because he was wearing a catheter. No one considered the possibility that this man might be able to void continently, or that he might not understand the purpose of a catheter. He was labeled "confused" because he did not "realize" that he had a catheter in place. When they visited a week later, the family revealed that the man had not been incontinent prior to admission. The nurses, in fact, had taught him to be incontinent. This horror story illustrates that the potential of the elderly person too often goes unrecognized. Clients who are dependent for many of the activities of daily living are often labeled as "total cares." This term assumes a total lack of self-sufficiency. Few care-givers regard the elderly as self-sufficient until proven otherwise.

The biologic aspects of aging so pervade the perspective of nurses who work with the elderly that the spiritual, social, and cultural aspects of the process are acknowledged only at an intellectual level. Just as one process of aging cannot be understood in isolation from the others, old age itself cannot be understood apart from middle age, adulthood, youth, adolescence, childhood, and infancy. Each stage of life brings its gains and losses.

The idea that a client who demonstrates confused, disorganized behavior may be engaging in adaptive–protective behavior makes many nurses laugh. However, an evaluative study to determine effectiveness of a reality-orientation program found that as orientation improved, depression increased (Dennis, 1976). This suggests that disoriented behavior may sometimes be a protective response to the fear and uncertainty associated with facing losses and death. These findings do not imply that people should be maintained in a confused or disoriented state, or even helped to achieve that status. Rather, professionals must restore the client's control over his or her life. Quality nursing practice in long-term care settings will not be achieved until nurses address themselves to these issues.

Appreciation of Clients' Histories

Nurses often have difficulty in recognizing the relationship between what a person was and what he brings to the institution, such as hobbies, work history, or pattern of dealing with loss or stress. This information, however, is an important part of the nursing assessment. Without precise and detailed assessment and goals, accurate evaluation is impossible. A nursing assessment that omits the client's history of allergies is considered deficient, but if it omits a history of confusion, or the person's pattern of dealing with stress, no criticism is made. Indeed, the nurse who includes such information is apt to be accused of wordiness. Such information is essential, for example, to plan interventions to reduce or eliminate wandering behavior without resorting to physical or chemical restraints (Snyder et al., 1978; Hiatt, 1980; Monsour and Robb, 1982).

Detailed information about grooming and bedtime rituals is rarely obtained. A person with memory impairment can function quite well when cued to perform a familiar activity. If Ms. J is prompted by presentation of her denture cup, she will probably move on to clean dentures, remove hairpins, wash her face, use the toilet, and get into bed. However, the key word is *familiar*. The nurse must discover and share with others what is familiar for each client.

The scope and level of detailed information nurses need in order to implement and evaluate care for clients who have, or are likely to have, mental impairments can be understood by considering an analogous situation. If you expected to lose your ability to communicate, what information would you need to record ahead of time so that your life could go on exactly as when you were able to communicate?

Assessment Breadth and Depth

Assessment to screen a client's visual and auditory status is certainly within the nurse's capability. The techniques need not require special equipment. Such screening is rarely done for the elderly, despite publicity given to their problems of sensory impairment and deprivation. Snyder, Pyrek, and Smith (1976) screened 295 residents in a long-term care facility for both visual and mental status. Eighty-one percent of the residents had no record of previous eye care exams after coming to the facility. Only 3.7 percent of the residents screened had received vision care within the previous year;

12 percent had received vision care within the previous 4 years. After vision screening, 49.5 percent were recommended by the ophthalmologist for follow-up. The conclusion was that more can and should be done for the vision needs of the elderly in institutions, in terms of precise assessment and expanded interventive strategies (Snyder, Pyrek, and Smith, 1976, p. 493).

Some may argue that vision screening is the physician's responsibility, but the point is that it *wasn't done*. Why did the nurses not push for vision screening with the same enthusiasm they show in arranging supplementary nourishment for clients who lose weight? Was vision loss considered "normal," while weight loss was not? Were the clients' adaptive responses to impaired vision misinterpreted as characteristic of the aging process?

A clinical specialist in gerontologic nursing developed an assessment tool for a long-term care facility. Designed in checklist format, to increase complete data collection and reduce recording time, this tool was six pages long and took between 45 and 90 minutes to use. If specific problems, such as urinary incontinence, confusion, or skin breakdown were noted, special assessments, printed separately and requiring additional time to administer, were to be completed. A separate guide defined all of the terms used in the assessment form. The total package was about 1½ inches thick. During an orientation to the tool, one head nurse dropped the packet on the table saying, "Anything this heavy can't possibly be any good!" The head nurse group united (for the first time in years) to oppose using the assessment form. The form eventually adopted was a one-page form that did not call for objective or subjective data needed to arrive at conclusions. Instead, the form asked for conclusions such as ability to walk, eat, and bathe and provided no space to record supporting data. More than one head nurse commented that there was no need to know anything else about the residents because (1) there was nothing nursing could do about the problem (for example, confusion, urinary incontinence, or immobility) or (2) the problems belonged to some other discipline (for example, the psychiatrist, urologist, or physiatrist). These head nurses held to their position despite the specialist's plea that even 3 hours of initial assessment by nurses was not very much when clients often stayed for years!

Therapeutic Use of Self

An increasing amount of evidence is accumulating to indicate that many "aging" behaviors are reversible, and that environmental and biologic factors have an interactive effect upon decline and deterioration (Lester and Baltes, 1978, p. 23). Biologic or disease models of aging view behavioral deficiencies in the elderly as being generally irreversible. By tradition, the therapeutic tools of the physician are primarily medical or surgical. For the most part, nurses are restricted by law from prescribing medication and performing invasive procedures. The primary therapeutic tool of the nurse is the use of self to structure the environment.

Behavior management approaches provide an excellent opportunity for nurses to use themselves to help clients achieve goals. Behavior here refers to the entire range of overt behavior employed by nurses. Behavior management approaches are derived from the operant theoretical framework that explains the acquisition of undesirable behaviors with aging as a function of:

1. The presence of reinforcers following "undesirable" behaviors
2. The absence of punishers following "undesirable" behaviors
3. The presence of punishers or a lack of reinforcers following "desirable" behaviors

Any voluntary behavior can be modified by manipulation of its consequences.

Evidence of elderly clients' responsiveness to the behavior of nurses has been found, particularly in long-term settings. The observations indicate that nursing personnel more consistently provide positive reinforcement for dependent behaviors than for independent behaviors (Mikulic, 1971; Lester and Baltes, 1978).

Upon admission to a long-term care facility, one client participated actively in her bath. At the end of 11 days, she no longer helped herself. The nurse had not encouraged self-bathing behaviors through positive reinforcement (Mikulic, 1971). It is possible that clients may lack the strength or will to resist the patterning and expectations imposed by their environment. Thus, they conform. The opposite occurs when behavior therapy is used constructively. Clients are rewarded for behaviors regarded as conducive to their health and welfare, and behave accordingly.

A considerable body of evidence indicates that old people in institutions do not maintain their health status in the presence of "regular" or "routine" nursing care. Instead, their health status declines! Incontinence increases (Carpenter and Simon, 1960), disorientation and confusion increase (Robinson, 1974; Harris and Ivory, 1976; Citrin and Dixon, 1977), and self-care abilities decrease (Mikulic, 1971; Baltes and Zerbe, 1976b; Lester and Baltes, 1978; Baltes and Barton, 1978). Thus, the behavioral environments in long-term care facilities appear to reinforce dependent behavior by clients.

On a small scale, behavior management approaches have been successful in reversing dependent behaviors such as nontalking (Hoyer et al., 1974), noneating (Geiger and Johnson, 1974; Baltes and Zerbe, 1976b), nonexercising (Libb and Clements, 1969), non-self-care (Mishara, 1971), and nonwalking (MacDonald and Butler, 1974). Client behaviors often consid-ered annoying can be modified: "screaming" behavior (Baltes and Lascomb, 1975); self-injurious behavior (Mishara, Robertson, and Kastenbaum, 1973); and excessive use of the call light (Moore, 1977). Effort should be made to apply these approaches to large numbers of clients in a variety of settings, in order to reverse unnecessary dependency.

Paternalism

Paternalism is the right of people in authority "to interfere coercively or deceptively in the life of the ordinary citizen for his own good" (Halper, 1980, p. 472). Paternalistic practices remain central to health and social policy. Although nurses often say they value client participation, they practice differently. Greater client participation in decision-making involves extra work, and is often a challenge to nurses' authority. Arguments developed by Halper (1980) for and against paternalism are summarized in Table 4.1.

Any solution to the problem of paternalism needs to be developed with at least three considerations in mind. First, the elderly are not a homogeneous group. Given wide and numerous variations among the aged, social policy generalizations become dangerous. Second, diversity among the elderly does not eliminate the need for an overall political strategy. Such

TABLE 4.1 ARGUMENTS FOR AND AGAINST PATERNALISM

Arguments in Favor of Paternalism	Arguments in Opposition to Paternalism
1. Freedom is not the only route to happiness and may sometimes lead in the opposite direction.	1. Although an old person may not always discern and pursue his best interest, he will do so more often than will public officials or family members simply because he is the only one who really knows his wishes, needs, views, and so forth.
2. The rights of society must be balanced against those of the individual.	2. By reducing risks of existence a challenging life is denied to aged people.
3. In the modern world, a number of situations exist where an old person's ignorance or short-sightedness might have deleterious effects on the individual.	3. Paternalism provides a convenient rationalization for morally dubious self-interests of those who practice this behavior.
4. As long as paternalism is based on the urge to help others, this stance represents no real danger.	4. Paternalistic policies imply official intolerance of a citizen's shortcomings and a subordinate relationship that counter the presumption of equality.

a strategy is needed so that conflicting demands do not leave politicians and other officials uncertain as to how to respond, the net effect being that the elderly receive less than their fair share of goods and services. Third, a society that values freedom should be reluctant to part with that freedom. The burden of proof needs to rest with the paternalist and not the opponent (the old person) to justify the practice (Halper, 1980).

Career Choices

Only a tiny number of graduate nurses enter gerontologic nursing. Six to eight months after graduation 1.4 to 3.6 percent (depending on type of nursing program) work in nursing homes, whereas 91.1 to 95.8 percent work in hospitals (National League for Nursing, 1982, p. 130). Considering all registered nurses, only 8.0 percent (101,209) work in nursing homes compared to 65.6 percent (835,647) in hospital settings (U.S. Department of Health and Human Services, 1982). However, there are more nursing home beds (1,402,000)* (National Center for Health Statistics, 1979, p. 8) in the United States than short-stay hospital beds (1,096,322)† (National Center for Health Statistics, 1981, p. 183). This picture of a grossly insufficient number of registered nurses to care for the elderly in nursing homes is not altered appreciably by comparing the need for skilled (as opposed to personal or custodial) nursing care between nursing homes and hospitals. If 60 percent of the nursing home beds are designated as requiring skilled nursing care, and the occupancy rate is 89 percent, then 748,668 clients require skilled care in nursing homes daily.‡ If 100 percent of the hospital beds are designated as requiring skilled nursing care

and the occupancy rate is 74 percent (National Center for Health Statistics, 1981, p. 186), then 811,278 clients require skilled care in acute care settings daily. A difference of 4 percent more clients in hospitals does not require that approximately 66 percent of the registered nurses work in these settings and only 8 percent in nursing homes.

One reason for the small number of registered nurses in nursing homes is that present staffing standards are unrealistic or vague, leaving administrators free to cut costs by using fewer registered nurses. The Joint Commission on Accreditation of Hospitals sets no numerical standards, stating merely, "A facility shall maintain an organized nursing service with sufficient qualified nursing personnel to meet the needs of all patients/residents in the facility." If any clients require a skilled level of nursing care, "at least one registered nurse shall be on each shift 7 days a week" (Joint Commission on Accreditation of Hospitals, 1980, pp. 43–45). The present federal standard for skilled nursing facilities requires one registered nurse to cover the day shift only, 7 days per week, regardless of the size of the nursing home (42 C.F.R. 405.1120, 1976).

State requirements tend to be somewhat more exacting. However, wide variations are found from state to state. In Pennsylvania, any skilled nursing facility of between 60 and 150 clients must have one registered nurse on duty for each tour of duty. For skilled nursing facilities of 251 or more clients, two registered nurses are required per tour of duty (Pennsylvania Department of Health, 1982, p. 55). Connecticut requires at least one registered nurse on duty 24 hours per day, 7 days per week (regardless of facility size) plus, in chronic and convalescent nursing homes, one "licensed nurse" on duty per client-occupied floor at all times (Connecticut Department of Health Services, 1981, p. 14). A "licensed nurse" may be either a practical or registered nurse.

It is clear that something must be done to increase the number of health professionals, particularly registered nurses prepared in gerontologic nursing, who work with the elderly. The possibility occurs that if long-term care facilities stopped hiring those who simply want to work in "less demanding" settings and started

---

* Data from the National Nursing Home Survey, 1977.

† Data from the National Master Facility Inventory, 1978.

‡ Nursing home beds are distributed by certification status as follows: 21 percent skilled; 39 percent skilled and intermediate (dually certified); 28 percent intermediate; and 12 percent not certified. The annual occupancy rate for skilled nursing facilities is 92 percent; for dually certified facilities, 89 percent; for intermediate facilities, 87 percent; and for uncertified facilities, 89 percent; the rate for all facilities is 89 percent (National Center for Health Statistics, 1979, p. 8).

hiring professionals with expertise in gerontology or in caring for highly dependent clients, the prestige associated with caring for old people would rise. The orientation of health care for the elderly might shift from predominantly custodial to therapeutic.

Changing Clients' Behavior

A number of problems confront the nurse who seeks to promote changes in clients' behavior within natural (clinical) settings: (1) institutional constraints, (2) external pressure, (3) language, (4) the presence of two populations, (5) limited resources, (6) labeling, (7) perceived inflexibility, and (8) compromise (Reppucci and Saunders, 1974). This list is not exhaustive, nor are the problems mutually exclusive. The purpose of listing these barriers is not to imply that behavior change is impossible. The extensive body of literature reporting successful behavior management endeavors (refer to page 123) suggests that elderly people can be helped to change their behaviors. Nurses too are capable of changing their behaviors when they are rewarded for doing so. The barriers to change behavior, however, are formidable. Any effort is doomed to failure unless nurses carefully consider and resolve the obstacles. Strategies for dealing with barriers can be derived from the implications for nursing practice, research, education, and management presented in Chapter 6.

Institutional Constraints

Mr. F, age 86, screamed "all the time for no reason" according to the nurses. A review of records indicated that he had not had his vision or hearing tested for over a year. Before doing a detailed assessment of the screaming behavior and the antecedent and consequent conditions, the nurse submitted requisitions to have Mr. F's hearing and vision tested. (Sometimes "screaming out" serves as a source of sensory stimulation, especially when sensory capabilities are reduced.) Before the eye clinic call came for Mr. F, some 6 weeks later, his temperature rose to 101°F, he stopped screaming, and died. The reason was never discovered.

Even if the backlog of clients for the ophthalmology and audiology clinics had been less,

the average wait for corrective devices was 8–12 weeks in this institution. The nursing staff reasoned that despite the long wait to assess vision and hearing status, other assessment preliminary for other kinds of interventions would constitute poor use of nursing time.

External Pressure

In a natural environment, a number of forces exert pressure for change. These forces may be political, economic, or administrative in nature. The direction of behavior change seen as desirable by a nurse may not coincide with the direction of change caused by such external pressures.

Few people really know or expect that elderly people do not have to decline automatically after admission to an extended-care facility. Significant others tend to expect such a decline. To them, observable decrements in a client's self-care abilities provide justification for institutional placement. When nurses initiated a bladder continence program in a long-term care facility, the daughter of one of the program participants berated the nursing staff. "I know why you removed Daddy's catheter! You are getting ready to send him home. Well, you just put it back on because I can't afford to have him at home. Besides, I sold his bed."

Language

In order to begin a program of behavior management therapy, all personnel involved must speak a common language. Usually a period of orientation or training precedes the program, in which basic principles are taught and terms defined. The terminology is readily learned and voiced, but acceptance of the words and concepts may involve a clash with values held by the staff. When nursing personnel in one institution were oriented to a program for promoting urinary continence through positive reinforcements for staying dry, they immediately asked whether the clients were going to be "shocked or anything like that." Actually, punishment or aversive conditioning tends to be counterproductive in behavior management programs, especially those designed to promote independence in self-care activities. Once this particular program was underway, the nurse coordinator found that clients were being "reinforced" with cigarettes, candy, and the like, whether they were dry or not. The staff explained that they were accustomed to giving cigarettes to clients at certain times such as after meals or after bathing. To deny elderly people this "small pleasure" seemed cruel. The dilemma was resolved by relabeling "positive reinforcer" as "reward" and emphasizing that a reward is only given when the client accomplishes something deserving of a reward, like staying dry.

Two Populations

An investigator in a laboratory can work directly with one subject at a time and thus exert substantial control over elements of a behavior change program. In the clinical setting, the nurse who wishes to implement such a program must first change the behavior of nursing personnel and others who interact with the target client(s). Salaries, promotions, and employment security are obvious reinforcers to use in manipulating personnel behavior change. However, these powerful determinants of behavior are rarely subject to control by the individual nurse. Thus, less efficient techniques must be employed. Most of these can be categorized as persuasive communications: in-service training, modeling, and direct appeal.

In institutional settings serving the elderly, independent behavior is widely professed as a desired goal, but it is inadvertently extinguished in the day-to-day course of events, probably as a result of a number of factors. Educational programs focus mainly on the acute-care setting in which mechanical gadgetry, curative therapies, and a fast-paced schedule of diagnostic and remedial procedures predominate. Nurses in long-term care settings lack exposure to effective restorative and maintenance models for health care. Some elect to work in long-term care to fulfill their own dependency needs. These individuals are likely to promote dependent behavior by clients. Most nurses who must collaborate with others have said to themselves, "If I were the only one caring for Ms. M, she would do more for herself," or "When I am on duty, Mr. K puts on his own clothes, but when I'm off, he is dressed in pajamas." These comments point up the inherent problems of controlling a therapeutic approach that is implemented by many individuals.

Sometimes it is difficult to reach agreement on the desired behavior, especially when persons in authority expect decremental or minimal functional status on the part of the elderly. One physician assigned to a respiratory care unit refused to support a program of walking exercise for clients with chronic emphysema. His objection was that the men were old and tired, and that if he himself had chronic emphysema, he would not want to be made to walk. Without physician support to order screening tests and write exercise prescriptions, the program could not be implemented.

The nurse may or may not have control over formal reinforcers, such as privileges to leave a facility, and tangible reinforcers, such as candy and personal care items. Informal reinforcers established and maintained by the elderly client's peers usually cannot be controlled. Mr. G had been accustomed to making his bed before his transfer from a psychiatric long-term care facility to a nursing home. By the time the nurses in the nursing home learned this, Mr. G had made friends with a group of men who pointed out that "no one else around here makes his bed. Why should you?"

Limited Resources

Major emphasis in behavior management is placed on evaluating the behavior to be modified (frequency, pattern, intensity, duration) and identifying the reinforcers. In clinical settings serving the elderly, there are often too few staff members available for the task of recording behavior (actually a detailed assessment). Insufficient staff may make it difficult to deliver reinforcers at the appropriate time. Even with adequate staff, nursing personnel may view the recording of behavior as just another chore to be performed. Thus, they fail to record information, or record it inaccurately.

Labeling

In clinical (natural) settings that serve old people, a wide range of activities carry value-laden labels, such as education, recreation, therapy, etc. For example, a locked unit with a ramp leading outside to an enclosed courtyard may be viewed as a therapeutic environment for clients inclined to wander. In such an environment, mobility can be encouraged. Once the unit is viewed as beneficial and therapeutic, personnel tend to respond to its label rather than its function. No one is likely to listen to the behavior change agent who argues that placement on the unit is viewed as a "punishment" by confused clients who congregate at the locked door, saying, "let me out." Highly polished floors are viewed as a sign of a clean environment. Wheelchairs provide a safe and rapid means for transporting clients who are unsteady on their feet. Centralized physical and recreational services permit smaller numbers of therapists to serve larger numbers of clients. These elements add up to an environment in which nursing personnel, charged with safely escorting large numbers of clients in a limited amount of time, encourage residents to rely on wheelchairs. It is not easy to argue against the virtues of shiny floors and rapid, safe transportation!

Inflexibility
This area of difficulty might better be titled "responsible leadership." A variety of circumstances make behavior change in natural settings difficult. The nurse who wants to promote change must therefore work constantly to insure the basic integrity of the program without becoming unnecessarily rigid. Ability to be flexible within the theory of behavior change without arousing resentment from others who are cooperating in the effort requires a responsible and skillful leader.

Compromise
In applying behavior management approaches, compromises are inevitable. The nurse should be aware of the compromises that have occurred and should avoid those that could negate a specific behavior change program. One essential requirement in bladder training for the elderly is that the client have some urine in the bladder to succeed or to fail with. Thus, fluids must be forced at times when the client is to be rewarded for voiding continently. When this program was explained to nursing person-

nel, they replied that staffing was not adequate to permit them to force fluids at hourly intervals for more than four clients at a time. A compromise could be made to place only four clients in the program at one time (eight had been selected). A compromise could not be made to eliminate the forced fluid requirement.

Changing Nurses' Behavior
Nurses are expected to take independent action to insure:

1. Supervision of a total, comprehensive nursing care plan for the patient
2. Observation, interpretation, and evaluation of the client's symptoms and needs
3. Supervision of other personnel who provide client care
4. Implementation of nursing procedures and techniques
5. Provision of health guidance and education
6. Accurate recording and reporting of facts and evaluations of client care (Lesnik and Anderson, 1962; Creighton, 1975)

The only aspect of nursing practice in which nurses must depend on another profession for direction is in carrying out the orders of physicians for medications and treatments. When a nurse takes orders and direction or supervision from a physician, the physician must be licensed and the order must be legal. Furthermore, the nurse must understand the cause and effect of the order.

Despite a mandate to do more, nurses too often confine their practice to carrying out the physician's orders and attending to the physiologic and safety needs of clients. When and if time permits, psychosocial needs of clients are considered. "I don't have enough time" is the usual rationale for not changing nursing practices. This "no-time" mentality blinds nurses to alterations in practice that could be accomplished within constraints of limited time, limited access to reference materials, and lack of money to support systematic inquiry.

Evidence indicates that nurses do what is conspicuously demanded by the difficulty of their assignments. When assignment difficulty (defined in terms of tasks to be done for clients with various need levels) is low, they engage in activities unrelated to client care (Freund and Mauksch, 1975, p. 190). Many practicing nurses know that when the client population is low, the bedside stands get cleaned or the wheelchairs scrubbed. This pattern suggests deficits in knowledge on the part of the practitioner or deficits in leadership by administrative personnel. Nurses, like other human beings, tend to adopt practices that require the least amount of time and energy. Rewarded as doers rather than thinkers (Cross, 1977), they too often settle for quick or expedient answers, without grasping the advantage of taking the time, money, and effort required to develop alternative approaches.

Quick to blame physicians for excessive use of chemical and physical restraints for the elderly, nurses often overlook their own role in influencing physician practice. Persistent requests from the nurse to "restrain Mr. J for his own protection" or to "give Mr. N a tranquilizer because he yells all night and keeps everyone awake" are sure to result in physician compliance sooner or later. "After all," the physician may reason, "the nurse has to stay with the client, I don't." Rare is the nurse who says, "Give us a couple of weeks. I know of several instances where interpersonal approaches by nurses succeeded in reversing behavior like Mr. N's."

Nursing personnel must have the knowledge and skills requisite for creative problem-solving. They should be oriented toward independence and health rather than dependence and illness. It is important that nurses be supported by a system of primary assignments (to fix responsibility and accountability), analytic discussions (to focus on the basis for both the client's and nurse's responses), and group problem-solving sessions (to devise a consistent approach for all who encounter the client). In-service education should be designed to expand the nurse's ability to assess and intervene effectively. Such education must incorporate the newest assessment and interventive strategies identified through research. The likelihood of favorable actions by nurses is greater when:

1. Staff understand the dynamics of aging
2. Staff know what constitutes favorable actions

3. Staff actions are directed toward increasing the numbers of "valued" behaviors and traits displayed by patients
4. Favorable actions are reinforced by the organizational environment (White, 1977, p. 20)

Unfortunately, most efforts to change nursing behavior are directed toward the first two approaches (increasing knowledge) rather than the last two approaches (setting expectations and providing rewards consistent with expectations). Two exciting studies that involved nursing personnel contracting for rewards based on specific changes in their caring behaviors proved highly successful (Sand and Berni, 1974; Steckel, 1976). In the first study nursing assistants demanded information related to client inability and succeeded in getting five out of eight sedentary elderly clients to move significantly more in just 3 weeks. The total cost of the aides' rewards was only $122.00 (Sand and Berni, 1974). In the second study, nurses suddenly began to chart in such a way as to provide written evidence that they used the nursing process when they were permitted to choose nonmonetary rewards for achievement of charting goals (Steckel, 1976). When rewards became clearly available, nursing personnel apparently felt freer to demonstrate previously infrequent behaviors. In neither case was education used as the means to change behaviors. Clearly, nurses need to place greater reliance on reward systems, as opposed to educational programs, to change their behavior in desired directions.

The traditional orientation of nurses has been to accept or to flee from situations that do not permit them to practice in accordance with professional standards. Nursing is the health profession with the largest numbers and the greatest direct service commitment (24 hours per day, 7 days per week) in institutional settings. The time has now come to change this "accept or flee" orientation and fight for structural environments that support quality nursing practice. Practicing nurses tend to become deeply involved with immediate work situations and clients. They expend tremendous effort to do their best under the circumstances. Rarely do they look beyond their daily tasks to consider ways in which they might change the situation for the larger number of nurses and clients to come.

It has been suggested that some health professionals "overreact" to the process of aging and the aged by flatly denying the legitimate problems associated with growing old. Wershow (1977, p. 297) writes that

> for the present and foreseeable future there will remain a large number of persons suffering from organic brain syndrome (OBS), an irreversible disorder of learning and memory. Now that death and dying are more freely discussed, it is obvious that senile dementia, or chronic OBS, and the problems it presents remains a taboo topic. Only optimistic approaches to the problems are admitted into professional consideration.... Denial may be a functional defense mechanism in the face of impossible adversity in patients and their families. It is an indefensible reaction in a professional and scientific community.

Clearly, there is no easy answer to the problem of motivating nurses to use themselves to produce therapeutic changes in client behavior. Just as clearly, evidence indicates that nurses strongly influence the kinds of behavior they must deal with, even when the client is old. Old dogs *can* learn new tricks if they are dealt with patiently and with care. The elderly can learn new behavior if nurses choose to function as teachers. Nurses should place a priority on self-care classes for the elderly, and on environments that offer a consistent self-help focus. When nurses fail to take these steps, they force the clients into dependence and make them targets for negative attitudes and behavior.

CONCLUSION

In summary, attitudes—when we learn what they are and how to measure them—may prove to have no implications for the way elderly people are treated in this society. "A single number (or even a set of numbers within a multidimensional framework), ... cannot really begin to convey the richness and subtlety of a person's beliefs and attitudes about old people" (Kogan, 1979, p. 31). Too many factors, other than attitudes, may influence behavior to per-

mit behavior (1) to be predicted from attitudes and (2) to be changed by simply altering attitudes.

Nurses' behavior toward elderly clients is in serious need of modification. Members of the profession need to devote their efforts to (1) promoting self-care and control on the part of elderly people and (2) eliminating barriers imposed by other health professionals and by institutions that impede such actions by nurses.

One characteristic of all institutions is that decisions regarding what is best for residents rest formally in other people's hands (Goffman, 1961). Efforts to empower nursing home residents (Horn and Griesel, 1977; Devitt and Checkoway, 1982), professionalize other kinds of clients (Dewar, 1978), and encourage self-help activities (Levin, 1978; Gadow, 1979; Stein, Linn, and Stein, 1982) represent strategies to restore control to customers and diminish the power of health professionals and administrators. Although no one gives away power, nurses may find that by empowering their elderly clients, they increase their own power to act to change prevailing patterns of health-care delivery.

RECOMMENDED READINGS

Buckholdt, D.R., Gubrium, J.F. Therapeutic pretense in reality orientation. International Journal of Aging and Human Development 16(3):167–181, 1983. *Based on a 3-month period of intensive observations in a nursing home to identify aspects of staff work in the application of reality orientation with clients who were confused or disoriented. Presents the view that a clear separation between the work of care-givers and the problems of clients cannot be justified. That is, care-givers help to constitute the problems they endeavor to treat.*

Ernst, P., Beran, B., Safford, F., Kleinhauz, M. Isolation and the symptoms of chronic brain syndrome. The Gerontologist 18(5):468–474, 1978. *A literature review that supports the idea that isolation is a key contributing factor to mental disorders in the elderly regardless of underlying brain pathology. Effects of environment are stressed.*

Fishbein, M., Ajzen, I. Belief, Attitude, Intention, and Behavior: An Introduction to Theory and Research, Reading, MA, Addison-Wesley, 1975. *Presents Fishbein's model of behavior-attitude relations and ample supporting, research-based evidence.*

Essential reading for anyone seeking to measure and predict attitudes or behaviors.

McTavish, D.G. Perceptions of old people. In Mangen, D.J., Peterson, W.A. (eds.). Clinical and Social Psychology. Minneapolis, MN, University of Minnesota Press, 1982, vol 1. *Discusses and lists measures of attitudes toward and beliefs about old people. Many instruments are included in their entirety. Definition of the concept or variable, description of the instrument; method of administration; context of development and subsequent use; samples; scoring, scale norms, and distribution; formal tests of reliability/homogeneity; formal tests of validity, usability on older populations; sensitivity to age differences; scale development statistics; general comments and recommendations; and references are presented for each measure.*

Mikulic, M.A. Reinforcement of independent and dependent patient behaviors by nursing personnel: An exploratory study. Nursing Research 20(2): 162–165, 1971. *Presents an easy-to-replicate example of behavior observation in a clinical setting.*

Rosendahl, P.P., Ross, V. Does your behavior affect your patient's response? Journal of Gerontological Nursing 8(10):572–575, 1982. *Reports results of a study that provided support for the proposition that elderly people who receive attending behavior while answering a mental status questionnaire have higher performance ratings than elderly people who receive no attending behavior.*

Szasz, T.S. Illness and indignity. Journal of the American Medical Association 227(5):545, 1974. *Discusses the conflict between the pursuit of health and the pursuit of dignity. Points to ways health professionals emphasize health to the detriment of client dignity.*

Wolanin, M.O. The Cinderella effect: An administrative challenge. Concern 3(3):8–12, 1977. *Describes the importance of maintaining a setting in which the client can be himself as an administrative challenge. Identifies common features of various therapies commonly used with elderly people and explains why they all work.*

REFERENCES CITED

Adelson, R., Nasti, A., Sprafkin, J.N., Marinelli, R., Primavera, L.H., Gorman, B.S. Behavioral ratings of health professionals interactions with the geriatric patient. The Gerontologist 22(3):277–281, 1982

Ajzen, I., Fishbein, M. Attitudes and normative beliefs as factors influencing behavioral intentions. Journal of Personality and Social Psychology 21(1):1–9, 1972

Ajzen, I., Fishbein, M. Attitude–behavior relations: A theoretical analysis and review of empirical research. Psychological Bulletin 84(5):888–918, 1977

American Nurses Association. Standards of Gerontological Nursing Practice. Kansas City, MO, American Nurses Association, 1976

Axelrod, S., Eisdorfer, C. Attitudes toward old people: An empirical analysis of the stimulus-group validity of the Tuckman-Lorge questionnaire. Journal of Gerontology 16(1):75–80, 1961

Bader, J.E. Attitudes toward aging, old age, and old people. Aged Care and Services Review 2(2):1,3–15, 1980

Baltes, M.M., Barton, E.M. The Fate of Self-Skills in Nursing Home Residents. Paper presented at the 31st Annual Meeting of the Gerontological Society, Dallas, TX, 1978

Baltes, M.M., Lascomb, S.L. Creating a healthy institutional environment for the elderly via behavior management: The nurse as a change agent. International Journal of Nursing Studies 12(1):5–12, 1975

Baltes, M.M., Zerbe, M.B. Independence training in nursing home residents. The Gerontologist 16(5):428–432, 1976

Baltes, M.M., Zerbe, M.B. Reestablishing self-feeding in a nursing home resident. Nursing Research 25(1):24–26, 1976

Barton, E.M., Baltes, M.M., Orzech, M.J. Etiology of dependence in older nursing home residents during morning care: The role of staff behavior. Journal of Personality and Social Psychology 38(3):423–431, 1980

Berry, J. Berry's world. Pittsburgh Press, August 13, 1978

Bossenmaier, M. The hospitalized elderly. Geriatric Nursing 3(4):253–256, 1982

Britton, J.O., Britton, J.H. Discrimination of age by preschool children. Journal of Gerontology 24(4):457–460, 1969

Brower, H.T. Social organization and nurses' attitudes toward older persons. Journal of Gerontologic Nursing 7(5):293–298, 1981

Brower, H.T. A Study of Attitude Changes Toward the Aged by Registered Nurses Attending a Geriatric Nurse Practitioner Program. Unpublished report, 1977. (Available from Nova University, Center of Higher Education, 3301 College Avenue, Ft. Lauderdale, FL 33314)

Brown, M.I. Patient Variables Associated with Preferences Among Elderly Patients. Paper presented at ANA Nursing Research Conference, 1969

Brown, M.M., Cornwell, J., Weist, J.K. Reducing the risks to the institutionalized elderly. Journal of Gerontological Nursing 7(7):401–407, 1981

Brubaker, J.H., Powers, E.A. The stereotype of old: A review and alternative approach. Journal of Gerontology 31(4):441–447, 1976

Buckelew, B. Health care professionals vs. the elderly. Journal of Gerontological Nursing 8(10):560–564, 1982

Burge, J.M. A Descriptive Survey of Personality Traits, Social Characteristics, and Stereotype Attitudes Toward the Aged in Three Types of Nurses Giving Care to the Aged in Nursing Homes. Doctoral dissertation, University of Florida, 1976. Dissertation Abstracts International 37:4989-B, 1977, University Microfilms No. 77-8154, 125

Butler, R.N., Lewis, M.I. Aging and Mental Health, 2nd ed. St. Louis, MO, Mosby, 1977

Campbell, M.E. Study of the attitudes of nursing personnel toward the geriatric patient. Nursing Research 20(2):147–151, 1971

Cameron, P., Stewart, L., Biber, H. Consciousness of death across the life-span. Journal of Gerontology 28(1):92–95, 1973

Carpenter, H.A., Simon, R. The effect of several methods of training on long-term, incontinent, behaviorally regressed hospitalized psychiatric patients. Nursing Research 9(1):17–22, 1960

Catron, L. Personal Exemption from Aging. Paper presented at the 31st Annual Meeting of the Gerontological Society, Dallas, TX, 1978

Chamberland, G., Rawles, B., Powell, C., Roberts, M.J. Improving students' attitudes toward aging. Journal of Gerontological Nursing 4(1):44–45, 1978

Ciliberto, D.J., Levin, J., Arluke, A. Nurses' diagnostic stereotyping of the elderly. Research on Aging 3(3):299–310, 1981

Citrin, R.S., Dixon, D.N. Reality orientation: A milieu therapy used in an institution for the aged. The Gerontologist 17(1):39–43, 1977

Connecticut Department of Health Services. Regulation of Department of Health Services Concerning Deemed Status. Hartford, CT: State of Connecticut, Department of Health Services, 1981

Comfort, A. Age prejudice in America. Social Policy 7(6):3–8, 1976

Creighton, H. Law Every Nurse Should Know. Philadelphia, PA, Saunders, 1975

Cross, E.D. Nursing research in the Veterans Administration. Nursing Research 26(4):250–252, 1977

Cutler, N.E. Subjective age identification. In Mangen, D.J., Peterson, W.A. (eds.). Clinical and Social Psychology. Minneapolis, MN, University of Minnesota Press, 1982, vol. 1

Daubenmire, M.J., White, F.L., Heinzerling, K., Ashton, C.A., Searles, S.S. Synchronics: A Rotation System for the Quantitative and Qualitative Description of Presenting Behaviors. Columbus, OH, The Ohio State University Research Foundation, 1977

de Beauvoir, S. The Coming of Age. New York, Putnam, 1972

Dennis, H. Remotivation therapy for the elderly: A surprising outcome. Journal of Gerontological Nursing 2(6):28–30, 1976

Devine, B.A. Old age stereotyping: A comparison of nursing staff attitudes toward the elderly. Journal of Gerontological Nursing 6(1):25–32, 1980

Devins, G.M. Death anxiety and voluntary passive euthanasia: Influences of proximity to death and experiences with death in important other persons. Journal of Consulting and Clinical Psychology 47(2):301–309, 1979

Devitt, M., Checkoway, B. Participation in nursing home resident councils: Promise and practice. The Gerontologist 22(1):49–53, 1982

Dewar, T. The professionalization of the client. Social Policy 8(4):5–9, 1978

Dye, C.A. Attitude change among health professionals. Journal of Gerontological Nursing 5(5):31–35, 1979

Eisdorfer, C. (ed.). Annual Review of Gerontology and Geriatrics. New York, Springer, 1980, vol 1

Eisdorfer, C. Attitudes toward old people: A re-analysis of the item-validity of the stereotype scale. Journal of Gerontology 21(3):455–457, 1966

Eisdorfer, C., Altrocci, J. A comparison of attitudes toward old age and mental illness. Journal of Gerontology 16(4):340–343, 1961

Elliot, B., Hybertson, D. What is it about the elderly that elicits a negative response? Journal of Gerontological Nursing 8(10):568–571, 1982

Extending the Scope of Nursing Practice: A Report of the Secretary's Committee to Study Extended Roles for Nurses. (Department of Health, Education, and Welfare.) Washington, D.C., U.S. Government Printing Office, November, 1971

Fishbein, M., Ajzen, I. Belief, Attitude, Intention, and Behavior: An Introduction to Theory and Research. Reading, MA, Addison-Wesley, 1975

Ford, C.V., Sbordone, R.J. Psychiatrists' Attitudes Toward Older Patients. Paper presented at the 32nd Annual Scientific Meeting of the Gerontological Society, Washington, D.C., 1974

Futrell, M. Attitudes of Physicians, Nurses, and Social Workers Toward the Elderly and Toward Health Maintenance Service for the Aged: Implications for Health Manpower Policy. Doctoral dissertation, Brandeis University, 1976. Dissertation

Abstracts International 37(1B):149-B, 1976, University Microfilms No. 76-16, 253, 144.

Gadow, S. Advocacy nursing and new meaning of aging. Nursing Clinics of North America 14(1):81–91, 1979

Geiger, O.G., Johnson, L.A. Positive education for elderly persons: Correct eating through reinforcement. The Gerontologist 14(5):432–436, 1974

Gillick, M.R., Serrell, N.A., Gillick, L.S. Adverse consequences of hospitalization in the elderly. Social Science Medicine 16(10):1033–1038, 1982

Glaser, B.G., Strauss, A.L. Awareness of Dying. Chicago, IL, Aldine, 1965

Glazer, G. The "good" patient. Nursing and Health Care 2(3):144–164, 1981

Goffman, E. Asylums. Garden City, NY, Anchor, 1961

Golde, P., Kogan, N. A sentence completion procedure for assessing attitudes toward old people. Journal of Gerontology 14(3):355–363, 1959

Gottesman, L., Bourestrom, N. Why nursing homes do what they do. The Gerontologist 14(6):501–506, 1974

Green, S. Attitudes and perceptions about the elderly: Current and future perspectives. International Journal of Aging and Human Development 13(2):99–119, 1981

Greenshields, S., Roberts, P., Stewart, R.B. Attitudes Toward Old People: An Inquiry into Methodology. Paper presented at the 33rd Annual Scientific Meeting of the Gerontological Society, San Diego, CA, 1980

Gunter, L. Students' attitudes toward geriatric nursing. Nursing Outlook 19(7):466–469, 1971

Hagestad, G.O. Life-phase analysis. In Mangen, D.J., Peterson, W.A. (eds.), Clinical and Social Psychology. Minneapolis, MN, University of Minnesota Press, 1982, vol. 1

Halper, T. The double-edged sword: Paternalism as a policy in the problems of aging. Millbank Memorial Fund Quarterly/Health and Society, 58(3)472–499, 1980

Harrison, C.S., Ivory, P.B.C.B. An outcome evaluation of reality orientation therapy with geriatric patients in a state mental hospital. The Gerontologist 16(6):496–503, 1976

Hart, L.K., Freel, M.I., Crowell, C.M. Changing attitudes toward the aged and interest in caring for the aged. Journal of Gerontological Nursing 2(4):11–16, 1976

Hatton, J. Nurse's attitude toward the aged: Relationship to nursing care. Journal of Gerontological Nursing 3(3):21–26, 1977

Heller, B.R., Walsh, F.R. Changing nursing students' attitudes toward the aged: An experimental

study. Journal of Nursing Education 15(5):9–17, 1976

Hiatt, L.G. The happy wanderer. Nursing Homes 29(2):27–31, 1980

Hickey, T., Bragg, S.M., Rakowski, W., Hultsch, D.F. Attitude instrument analysis: An examination of factor consistency across two samples. International Journal of Aging and Human Development 9(4):359–375, 1978–79

Hicks, D.A., Rogers, C.J., Shemberg, K. "Attitudes" toward the elderly: A comparison of measures. Experimental Aging Research 2(2):119–124, 1976

Hinchliffe, E.B. An Experimental Study of the Effects of Classroom Instructions and Clinical Learning Experiences on the Attitudes of Students of Nursing Towards the Aged. Unpublished doctoral dissertation, The College of William and Mary in Virginia, 1979

Holtzman, J.M., Beck, J.D., Kerber, P.E. Dimensional Aspects of Attitudes Toward the Aged. Paper presented at the 32nd Annual Scientific Meeting of the Gerontological Society, Washington, D.C., 1979

Holzemer, W.L., Schleutermann, J.A., Farrand, L.L., Miller, A.G. Simulations as a measure of nurse practitioners' problem-solving skills. Nursing Research, 30(3):139–144, 1981

Horn, L., Griesel, E. Nursing Homes: A Citizens' Action Guide. Boston, MA, Beacon, 1977

Hoyer, W.J., Kafer, R.A., Simpson, S.C., Hoyer, F.W. Reinstatement of verbal behavior in elderly mental patients using operant procedures. The Gerontologist 14(2):149–152, 1974

Jahnigen, D., Hannon, C., Laxson, L., LaForce, F.M. Iatrogenic disease in hospitalized elderly veterans. Journal of the American Geriatrics Society 30(3):387–390, 1978

Joint Commission on Accreditation of Hospitals. Accreditation Manual for Long-Term Care Facilities, 1980 Edition. Chicago, IL, Joint Commission on Accreditation of Hospitals, 1979

Kafer, R.A., Rakowski, W., Lachman, M., Hickey, T. Aging opinion survey: A report on instrument development. International Journal of Aging and Human Development 11(4):319–333, 1980

Kalish, R.A. Death and dying in a social context, in Binstock, R.H., Shanas, E. (eds.), Handbook of Aging and the Social Sciences. New York, Van Nostrand Reinhold, 1976

Kalish, R.A., Reynolds, D.K. Death and Ethnicity: A Psychocultural Study. Los Angeles, CA, University of Southern California Press, 1976

Kastenbaum, R. Death, dying, and bereavement in old age: New developments and their possible implications for psychosocial care. Aged Care and Services Review 1(3):1–10, 1978

Kastenbaum, R., Derbin, V., Sabatini, P., Artt, S. "The ages of me": Toward personal and interpersonal definitions of functional aging. Aging and Human Development 3(2):197–211, 1972

Katz, B.P., Zdeb, M.S., Therriault, G.D. Where people die. Public Health Reports 94:522–527, 1979

Kayser, J.S., Minnigerode, F.A. Increasing nursing students' interest in working with aged patients. Nursing Research 24(1):23–26, 1975

Kilty, K.M., Feld, A. Attitudes toward aging and toward needs of older people. Journal of Gerontology 31(5):586–594, 1976

Kogan, N. Attitudes toward old people: The development of a scale and an examination of correlates. Journal of Abnormal Psychology 62(4):44–54, 1961

Kogan, N. Beliefs, attitudes, and stereotypes about old people: A new look at some old issues. Research on Aging 1(1):11–36, 1979

Kogan, N., Wallach, A. Age changes in values and attitude. Journal of Gerontology 16(3):272–280, 1961

Lawrence, J.H. The effect of perceived age on initial impressions and normative role expectations. International Journal of Aging and Human Development 5(4):369–391, 1974

Lesnik, M.J., Anderson, B.E. Nursing Practice and the Law. Philadelphia, PA, Lippincott, 1962

Lester, P.B., Baltes, M.M. Functional interdependence of the social environment and the behavior of the institutionalized aged. Journal of Gerontological Nursing 4(2):23–27, 1978

Levin, L.S. Patient education and self-care: How do they differ? Nursing Outlook 26(3):170–175, 1978

Libb, J.W., Clemets, C.B. Token reinforcement in an exercise program for hospitalized geriatric patients. Perceptual and Motor Skills 28(3):957–958, 1969

Little, D., Pesznecher, B., Baker, J. Mrs. Reynolds Needs a Nurse. Seattle, WA, University of Washington School of Nursing, 1963. (Film produced by Smith, Kline, and French Laboratories, Philadelphia.)

Lutsky, N.S. Attitudes toward old age and elderly persons, in Eisdorfer, C. (ed.), Annual Review of Gerontology and Geriatrics. New York, Springer, 1980, vol. 1

MacDonald, M.L., Butler, A.K. Reversal of helplessness: Producing walk-behavior in nursing home wheelchair residents using behavior modification procedures. Journal of Gerontology 29(1):97–101, 1974

Mangen, D.J., Peterson, W.A. (eds.): Research Instruments in Social Gerontology. Vol. 8, Clinical and Social Gerontology. Minneapolis, MN, University of Minnesota Press, 1982

Manney, J.D., Jr. Aging in American Society. Ann Arbor, MI, The University of Michigan-Wayne State University, The Institute of Gerontology, 1975

Maxwell, E.K., Maxwell, R.J. Explanations for Contempt Expressed Towards Old People. Paper presented at the 32nd Annual Meeting of the Gerontology Society, Washington, D.C., November 25–29, 1979

McLaughlin, F.E., Cesa, T., Johnson, H., Lemons, M., Anderson, S., Larson, P., Gibson, J., Delucchi, K. Nurse practitioners', public health nurses', and physicians' performances on clinical simulation tests: COPD. Western Journal of Nursing Research 1(4):273–295, 1979

McMahon, M., Miller, P. Behavioral cues in the dying process and nursing implications. Journal of Gerontological Nursing 6(1):16–20, 1980

McTavish, D.G. Perception of old people. In Mangen, D.J., Peterson, W.A. (eds.), Clinical and Social Psychology. Minneapolis, MN, University of Minnesota Press, 1982, vol. 1

Meyer, M.M., Hassameir, R.S., Bahr, R.T. A comparison of attitudes toward the aged held by professional nurses. Image 12(3):66, 1980

Mikulic, M.A. Reinforcement of independent and dependent patient behaviors by nursing personnel: An exploratory study. Nursing Research 20(2): 162–165, 1971

Mishara, B.L. Comparison of the Types of Milieu Programs for Rehabilitation of Chronic Geriatric "Mental" Patients. Paper presented at the 24th Annual Meeting of the Gerontological Society, Houston, TX, 1971

Mishara, B.L., Robertson, B., Kastenbaum, R. Self-injurious behavior in the elderly. The Gerontologist 13(3):311–314, 1973

Monsour, N., Robb, S.S. Wandering behavior in old age: A psychosocial study. Social Work 27(5): 411–416, 1982

Moore, E.M. Using contingency management to facilitate behavior changes in nursing home residents. Concern 3(3):13–15, 1977

Morrow, L. In praise of older women. Time 111(17):99–100, 1978

Murdock, G.P., White, D.R. Standard cross-cultural sample. Ethnology 8(4):329–369, 1969

National Center for Health Statistics. Health, United States, 1981. (DHHS Pub. No. (PHS) 82-1232.) Washington, D.C., U.S. Government Printing Office, 1981

National Center for Health Statistics. The National Nursing Home Survey: 1977 Summary for the United States. (DHHS Pub. No. (PHS) 79-1974. Series 13, No. 43.) Washington, D.C., U.S. Government Printing Office, 1979

National Council on the Aging. The Myth and Reality of Aging in America: A Study Conducted for the National Council on the Aging by Louis Harris and Associates. Washington, D.C., National Council on the Aging, 1974

National League for Nursing. NLN Nursing Date Book, 1981. New York, National League for Nursing, Publication Number 19-1882, 1982

Palmore, E.B. Attitudes toward the aged: What we know and need to know. Research on Aging 4(3):333–348, 1982

Palmore, E.B. The facts on aging quiz: Part two. The Gerontologist 21(4):431–437, 1981

Palmore, E. Facts on Aging: A short quiz. The Gerontologist 17(4):315–320, 1977

Pennsylvania Department of Health. Long Term Care Facilities Licensure Regulations. Harrisburg, PA, Pennsylvania Department of Health, Bureau of Quality Assurance, Division of Long Term Care, 1982

Phaneuf, M. The Nursing Audit: Self-Regulation in Nursing Practice, 2nd ed. New York, Appleton-Century-Crofts, 1976

Phillips, L.R., Wolanin, M.O., McFeaters, E.S. Confusion of the Hospitalized Elderly—The Imprisonment Theory. Paper presented at the 31st Annual Meeting of the Gerontological Society, Dallas, TX, November 1978

Pinder, M.M., Hayslip, B. Cognitive, attitudinal, and affective aspects of death and dying in adulthood: Implications for care providers. Educational Gerontology 6:107–123, 1981

Richardson, P.C., Cunningham, W.R. A Study of Factor Structure of Attitudes Toward Aging and the Aged. Paper presented at the American Psychological Association Meeting, Toronto, Ontario, 1978

Robb, S.S. Attitudes and intentions of baccalaureate nursing students toward the elderly. Nursing Research 28(1):43–50, 1979

Robb, S.S. The challenge of research. Journal of Gerontological Nursing 9(6):336–343, 1983

Robb, S.S., Boyd, M., Pristash, C.L. A wine bottle, plant, and puppy: Catalysts for social behavior. Journal of Gerontological Nursing, 6(12):721–728, 1980

Robinson, K.D. Therapeutic interaction: A means of crisis intervention with newly institutionalized elderly persons. Nursing Clinics of North America 9(1):89–96, 1974

Rosencranz, H.A., McNevin, T.E. A factor analysis of attitudes toward the aged. The Gerontologist 9(1):55–59, 1969

Rosendahl, P.P., Ross, V. Does your behavior affect your patient's response? Journal of Gerontological Nursing 8(10):572–575, 1982

Salter, C.A., Templer, D.I. Death anxiety as related to helping behavior and vocational interests. Essence 3(1):3–8, 1979

Sand, P., Berni, R. An incentive contract for nursing home aides. American Journal of Nursing 74(3):475–477, 1974

Schmidt, A. Predicting nurses' charting behavior based on Fishbein's model. Nursing Research 30(2):118–123, 1981

Simmons, V., Fittipaldi, L., Holovet, E., Mones, P., Geradi, R., Mech, A. Assessing the quality of care in skilled nursing homes. Journal of Long-Term Care Administration 9(2):1–17, 1981

Snyder, L.H., Pyrek, J., Smith, K.C. Vision and mental function of the elderly. The Gerontologist 16(6):491–495, 1976

Snyder, L.H., Rupprecht, P., Pyrek, J., Brekhus, S., Moss, T. Wandering. The Gerontologist 18(3):272–280, 1978

Sontag, S. The double standard of aging. Saturday Review 55(39):29–38, 1972

Steckel, S.B. Utilization of reinforcement contracts to increase written evidence of the nursing assessment. Nursing Research 25(1):58–61, 1976

Steel, K., Gertman, P.M., Crescenzi, C., Anderson, J. Iatrogenic illness on a general medical service at a university hospital. New England Journal of Medicine 304:638–642, 1981

Stein, S., Linn, M.W., Stein, E.M. The relationship of self-help networks to physical and psychosocial functioning. Journal of the American Geriatrics Society 30(12):764–768, 1982

Stevens, S.J., Cooper, P.E., Thomas, L.E. Age norms for Templer's Death Anxiety Scale. Psychological Reports 46:205–206, 1980

Storle, F.J. The reshaping of the old. Journal of Gerontological Nursing 8(10):555–559, 1982

Sudnow, D. Passing On: The Social Organization of Dying. Englewood Cliffs, NJ, Prentice-Hall, 1967

Taylor, K.H., Harned, T.L. Attitudes toward old people: A study of nurses who care for the elderly. Journal of Gerontological Nursing 4(5):43–47, 1978

Tollett, S.M., Adamson, C.M. The need for gerontological content within nursing curricula. Journal of Gerontological Nursing 8(10):576–580, 1982

U.S. Department of Health and Human Services. The Registered Nurse Population, an Overview from National Sample Survey of Registered Nurses, November, 1980. Washington, D.C., Bureau of

Health Professions, Health Resources Administration, Public Health Service, U.S. Department of Health and Human Services, Report No. 82-5, 1982

Ventura, M., Hageman, P. Testing the Reliability, Validity, and Sensitivity of Quality of Nursing Care Measures: Final Report. Washington, D.C.: Health Services Research and Development Service, Veterans Administration, 1978

Ventura, M.R., Hageman, P.T., Slakter, M.J., Fox, R.N. Interrater reliabilities for two measures of nursing care quality. Research in Nursing and Health 3(1):25–32, 1980

Wandelt, M., Ager, J. Quality Patient Care Scale. New York, Appleton-Century-Crofts, 1974

Wershow, H.J. Comment: Reality orientation for gerontologists. The Gerontologist 17(4):297–302, 1977

Whitbourne, S.K. Personal communication, January 7, 1983

Whitbourne, S.K., Wheeler, L., Sperbeck, D.J. The Relationships Between Information and Attitudes About the Aged. Paper presented at the Annual Scientific Meeting of the Gerontological Society, San Diego, CA, 1980

White, C.M. The nurse-patient encounter: Attitudes and behaviors in action. Journal of Gerontological Nursing 3(3):16–20, 1977

White, C.M. On the Association Between Selected Patient Characteristics and the Supportive Behavior of Nursing Personnel Toward Patients in Nursing Homes. Unpublished dissertation, Johns Hopkins University, 1974

Wilhite, M.J., Johnson, D.M. Changes in students' stereotypic attitudes toward old people. Nursing Research 25(6):431–432, 1976

Williams, M.A., Holloway, J.R., Winn, M.C., Wolanin, M.O., Lawler, M.L., Westwick, C.R., Chin, M.H. Nursing activities and acute confusional states. Nursing Research 28(1):25–35, 1979

Wingard, J.A. Measures of attitudes toward the elderly: A statistical re-evaluation of comparability. Experimental Aging Research 6(3):299–313, 1980

Wolanin, M.O. The Cinderella effect: An administrative challenge. Concern 3(3):8–12, 1977

5

Environmental Resources for Healthful Aging

Susanne S. Robb

Reading this chapter will enable the individual to:

1. Identify characteristics of the elderly, as a group, that influence their resource needs
2. List three commonly available resources that enable discovery of additional resources for the elderly
3. Recognize at least five issues in delivery of services to the elderly
4. Name the three largest sources of income for the elderly
5. Describe the advantages and disadvantages of income subsidies versus in-kind services
6. Indicate the advantages and disadvantages of age-segregated housing for the elderly
7. Define three methods of special financing for housing for the elderly
8. List two problems the elderly find with available food programs
9. Identify the primary source of transportation for the elderly
10. Discuss the wishes of elderly people regarding work opportunities
11. Name four leisure pursuits available to elderly people
12. List three factors that make criminal victimization more of a problem for the elderly than for other age groups
13. Identify three strategies for protecting the elderly from crime
14. Describe three factors that predispose elderly people to being victims of consumer fraud
15. List five approaches nurses might use to reduce or eliminate the problem of elder abuse
16. Discuss three needs that elderly people may meet through involvement in religion
17. Name five patterns of family relationships stemming from institutionalization
18. Identify three sources of significant others for elderly people without close family relationships

There are a variety of resources in the environment that enhance the old person's ability to participate in society. Personal characteristics, social institutions, objects, services, and people, because they are relevant to the choices or options of the elderly person, constitute resources. It is hard for most health professionals to maintain current and comprehensive knowledge about rapidly changing resources. Thus, the first sections of this chapter are designed to prepare the nurse to enter the resource system and locate appropriate resources *as the need arises.* The focus then moves to a discussion of enduring issues in service delivery. This information may help nurses to understand some of the barriers to a more adequate service delivery system. The last sections discuss resources of major importance to elderly people. Implications for nursing practice are presented as appropriate.

ENVIRONMENT, RESOURCES, AND SOCIAL SERVICES DEFINED

Environment can be categorized as *individual,* referring to what the person brings to the situation, or *social,* referring to what a society contributes to the situation. As people continually adapt to the environment, they alter and are altered by the environment. Many individuals tend to shift from an active to passive environmental orientation as they age (Neugarten, 1973, pp. 311–335; Lowenthal and Chiriboga, 1973, pp. 281–310). Residents in long-term care facilities, in particular, often accept

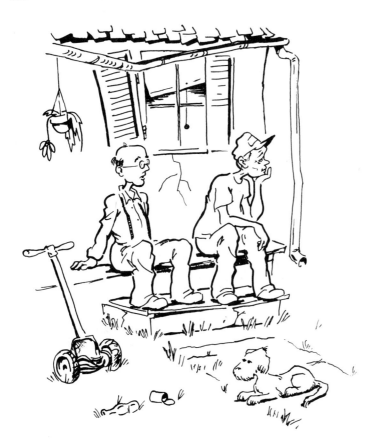

"No money, no energy to keep up the old place. Guess we'll have to go to the old folks home."

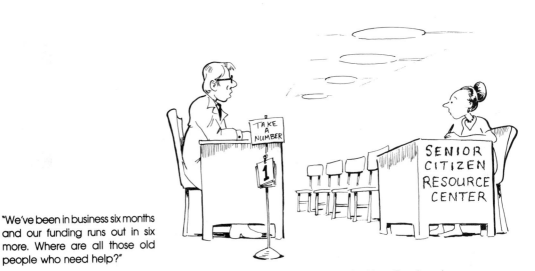

"We've been in business six months and our funding runs out in six more. Where are all those old people who need help?"

Figure 5.1 Needs and resources may not match. *(Drawings by Harry Trumbore.)*

whatever happens without question. When they identify a problem, these elderly people view the cause as being outside themselves, and respond fatalistically, as though they no longer have any control over the way life treats them.

Specific environmental experiences may strongly influence future responses to the environment. Today's elderly have lived through two world wars, a major economic depression, the rise of the technologic age, the expansion of the educational system, and the immigration era. These old people tend to be thrifty and insist on paying their way. Ethnic and religious origins are important considerations in making friends. To these people, employment and productivity are synonymous.

Individual resources that enhance the lifestyle of the elderly include good health, financial security, relationships with significant others, the ability to adapt to stress, and a sense of the purpose of life. *Societal resources* can be grouped according to the kind of human need. Money, health care, housing, home help, food, and transportation are usually considered the most essential supports. Other resources of nearly equal importance include law enforcement, activities, counseling/referral, and significant others. The five basic components of a home-delivered social–health support system are (1) health maintenance, (2) home help, (3) mobile meals, (4) transportation, and (5) crisis intervention, advocacy, and counseling (Bell, 1973, p. 395).

Social services are organized approaches to the relief or elimination of unacceptable conditions. Currently there are many resources/services available to the elderly, but they are not well articulated. Indeed, the social and health system in this country can best be described as a nonsystem. Providers of health and social care may agree on a common purpose, such as promoting optimum functioning, but they do not agree on the means of achieving this purpose. Elderly people who need help, however desperately, must be "of the correct age, sex, and race, with the right set of eligibility standards, living in the right location at the right time," or they will probably not receive the services they require (Krause, 1977,

p. 164). Figure 5.1 illustrates one instance of failure to match resources with client needs.

CHARACTERISTICS OF THE ELDERLY RELEVANT TO RESOURCE NEEDS

Understanding of the nature, purpose, and adequacy of resources available to the elderly needs to be based on at least six interrelated themes which seem to characterize old people.

1. The elderly are a heterogeneous group. There is no "typical" old person. Age alone is a poor predictor of abilities, behaviors, and needs. Wide variability exists in the social, psychologic, physical, and economic characteristics of old people, exceeding the range found in younger age groups. This diversity creates major challenges for planners of policies, programs, and services targeted for elderly people (U.S. Senate Special Committee on Aging, 1982; Final Report of the 1981 White House Conference on Aging, 1982a,b).
2. Elderly people in this country do not feel deprived and do not want to be treated in a patronizing manner. Today's elderly people want to be treated as individuals in a society where economic, social, and political institutions are being changed as a result of the changing age distribution. Experience and knowledge of the elderly should be considered a national asset and kept in the mainstream of American life (Final Report of the 1981 White House Conference, 1982).
3. Although most elderly people do not require special resources, some subgroups within this population experience a greater share of problems: blacks, Hispanics, the very old, women, and those without pensions.
4. Legitimate differences between old people and people in other age groups are often unrecognized when services are provided. Physical decrements do lead to losses of mobility or agility and perceptual capabilities. These losses create a widespread need for

affordable and readily available transportation.

5. There is sometimes a discrepancy between objective conditions and subjective perceptions. For example, the elderly tend to regard their homes as satisfactory housing. In reality, the home may be unsuited to the old person's physical abilities and located in a geographic area distant from needed services. The majority of America's elderly view themselves as healthy individuals, with between 56 and 68 percent rating their health as "excellent or good" (National Council on the Aging, 1981; U.S. Senate Special Committee, 1982a) despite the fact that a 1979 National Center for Health Statistics report indicated that over 80 percent of older people have at least one chronic condition (U.S. Senate Special Committee, 1982a).

6. American society, considered as a whole, continues to cling to negative myths about the elderly. Substantial majorities of younger adults (18 to 64 years of age) think that the high cost of energy, fear of crime, lack of money, and loneliness are very serious problems for most older people, while only minorities of the elderly cite these problems as being very serious (Aging in the Eighties, 1981). Health professionals, perhaps because of their disproportionate exposure to elderly people seeking medical and health services, tend to believe illness is the norm among old people (U.S. Special Committee, 1982a, p. 294). In contrast, a majority of old people regard themselves as healthy.

Considered together, these six themes mandate that nurses individualize their assessments to decide resource needs for each client encountered. Efforts to serve elderly clients and alleviate some of their hardships must be based on respect for who they are and what they have already accomplished.

The interplay between individual needs and environmental resources is illustrated by the situation of a veteran of World War I who was in his 80s when he retired from the job he took after he retired from his primary career em-ployment. Mr. C entered a VA long-term care facility because he considered himself too ill to live with his wife, who also experienced poor health. Subsequent assessment revealed that Mr. C was functionally able except for some unsteadiness on his feet. His wife had abused him psychologically for many years by accusing him of being unfaithful and then punishing him by demanding and receiving all of his money, forcing him to eat leftover food, and relegating him to a very small bedroom. Mrs. C really did not want Mr. C at home. By entering a long-term care VA facility, a benefit Mr. C believed he had earned, Mr. C was able to give his wife all but $50.00 worth of his social security check and all of the pension from his first work in industry, while relieving her of the burden of his care. Both parties seemed satisfied with this arrangement and Mr. C adjusted well in the VA facility.

However, because Mr. C was able to care for himself, his transfer to a state operated domiciliary facility was arranged. After an initial inspection visit, Mr. C was in full agreement with the transfer although the move would take him too far away for his former employer (and only visitor) to travel and force Mr. C to leave behind a dog who visited the VA regularly and spent most of each day in his company.

Three days after his transfer, Mr. C wrote the letter contained in Figure 5.2 to a physician at the VA facility.* This letter raises a number of questions concerning compromises between human and organizational needs. How often is pertinent information withheld from clients in order to influence their decisions in ways that benefit service providers? What will happen to Mr. and Mrs. C's health if the agreement they made is broken because his social security check is turned over to the state-operated facility? Is it reasonable for Mr. C to live on tax dollars (federal or state) when, in fact, his income through social security and private pension is adequate for both Mr. C and his wife if they live together? If Mr. C. stays

---

* Names have been changed or deleted to protect the identities of all concerned.

January 30, 1983

Dr. _____

Barbara Jones, the social worker at your place, told me that I would not have to pay anything here.

They told me I would have to pay so much per month.

The social worker called this morning and she said they are trying to get rid of the people that walk and that is why I had to come here.

That is not quite true because in the auditorium where they play bingo there are quite a few that walk, and also the cafeteria. So I do not know why I had to come up here.

I thought I was getting a private room like they showed me when I visited but they put me in with two other fellows which don't speak to one another and the people here are unfriendly. Most of them don't speak to one another.

I hope they fix it so I won't have to pay anything because my wife is sick and needs all of my money. I do not have any money to pay with.

I also can't get anything on my television. I am too far away in the country. I would have to get cable for $7 per mo.

I miss you and my dog. I want to come back.

M_____ C_____

Figure 5.2. Letter from a client illustrating the interplay between individual needs and resources available in the environment of the elderly.

at the state-operated facility without visits from his former employer, contact with "his" dog, and no television, will his health suffer?

ENTERING THE RESOURCE SYSTEM

Anyone who has ever had to deal with a bureaucratic agency or process, such as the refuse pickup center or a university registration office, knows the difficulties involved. Usually several calls are required, conflicting information is provided, and the contact people are less than empathetic. The majority of the elderly are reluctant to ask for assistance, for these and other reasons. Benefits and services earned through work, such as social security and Medicare, are quite acceptable. However, anything that has not been earned is suspect as a form of welfare. Considering both the difficulties in contacting resource agencies and the reluctance to ask for help, the probability of an elderly person obtaining needed services is slim at best. Therefore, nurses who recommend resource services to the elderly should do a preliminary screening to select the correct agency and to overcome such potential obstacles as travel arrangements, barriers to the handicapped, and lengthy waiting periods. Provided with a definite appointment, the name of a contact person, and adequate transportation arrangements, the elderly person is usually able to cope and much more likely to receive the needed service. When directing clients to services, the nurse should remind them to conserve their time, money, and energy by telephoning or writing before attempting a personal visit. After a reasonable length of time, the nurse should call to find out whether the referral was successful, and should intervene again if it was not.

The importance of identifying and using contact persons within the resource system cannot be emphasized too strongly. Nurses and clients alike should learn the name of the person with whom they are speaking so that they can deal with that individual on subsequent calls. Mrs. L, a wily 76-year-old, experienced

an unexpected and severe attack of arthritis. She wanted to see her physician but had no appointment. Without giving her name, she called the office to be sure she had names of the office staff correct. She asked for Miss G, the doctor's long-time receptionist, and learned that Miss G had left 6 months ago and been replaced by Mrs. K. Armed with this information, Mrs. L arrived for a 2:00 P.M. "appointment." When told she had no appointment, Mrs. L said, "Which one is Mrs. K? I made this appointment with you 5 weeks ago. Don't you remember, dearie?" Mrs. L was seen that day. People who work in agencies are far more likely to give correct information, send materials promptly, and honor promises when they know the requesting person has their name.

LOCATING THE APPROPRIATE RESOURCE

Both the client who is seeking a service and the nurse who wishes to make a referral are unlikely to be knowledgeable about specific resources available. A search should start with the most available sources of information: the "yellow" and "white" pages of the local telephone directory. The Yellow Pages index carries listings for "Aging Services and Facilities—see Senior Citizens Service Organizations" and "Agencies—see Social Service Organizations." Under "United States Government" in the White Pages, the Federal Information Center is listed. Under the State listings can be found resources such as "Health Department" and "Public Assistance and Welfare Offices."

Elected representatives to the federal and state legislatures are a second available source of information. These can be contacted through their local offices (to avoid a toll charge) or by letter at their capitol addresses. Governors may have toll-free lines to their information centers.

The card catalogue of the local library might yield "where to" information under topics such as "directories" or "services." "How to" information might appear under the topic of interest. To illustrate, books such as *How to Select*

A Nursing Home (U.S. Health Care Financing Administration, 1981) and *A Guide to Nursing Home Living* (Griffith and Strandberg, 1982) might be located under the heading "nursing homes."

As a rule, the smaller the community, the greater the possibility that workers in any service capacity are experts on available resources for the elderly. Such workers might include policemen or firemen, librarians, pharmacists, clergy, postmen, grocers, etc. If any of these people are elderly, they may even have used the service themselves. Some service centers may be resources in themselves, or may provide referral to the service desired. Examples include Social Security Offices, welfare/public assistance offices, and Area Agencies on Aging (AAA).

Larger cities often have special directories to a full range of service organizations: A typical example is *Where to Turn: Directory of Health, Welfare and Community Services in Allegheny County,* published by Information and Volunteer Services of Allegheny County, Pittsburgh, in 1974. This particular directory indexed services both by title of organization and by service type. Some directories provide listings for a particular service throughout the country. *The Discount Guide for Travelers over 55* (Weintz and Weintz, 1981) lists, by state, discounts for elderly people in hotels, motels, restaurants, transportation, sightseeing, and cultural attractions. The same information, but less detailed, is provided for Canada, Mexico, the Caribbean, and Europe. The *Directory of Adult Day Care Centers* (U.S. Department of Health and Human Services, 1980) provides a list of programs that provide adult day care throughout the country. This list is arranged alphabetically by state and identifies the address, telephone number, program director, sponsoring organization, funding source, and the nature of the service (social, maintenance, or restorative) for each program. The *National Directory of Retirement Facilities* (Huff, 1979) is a catalogue of nonprofit agencies and government-funded housing projects designed and developed for senior citizens. States are arranged alphabetically, as are locations within

the state. Each facility listing includes the name, address, and number of units. Levels of care are indicated for the private facilities. This directory was produced once, without specific plans for revision. Even after several years, however, the directory provides a good starting place for persons seeking information about retirement facilities.

Nurses should be able to gather information about the various services available in order to help the old person understand and explore available options. Maintenance of the elderly in the community with home-delivered or congregate organized services is easier to recommend then to do. The nurse must be able to accept the anxiety associated with encouraging an elderly person who may be angry, depressed, debilitated, and confused to live independently, rather than in a protective environment. Family members may be reluctant to assume responsibility for an elderly person, lest the responsibility increase. Specific skills the nurse will need to intervene include facilitation of communication, resolution of conflicts, identification of extrafamilial support resources, and selection of congregate noninstitutional housing with home delivered services when possible. Social workers are also prepared to intervene to link people with resources. The important point is that *someone makes the effort.*

ISSUES IN SERVICE DELIVERY

Availability

There are not enough services available to the elderly. For example, long-term, in-home care consists of services to the elderly who, because of chronic functional disabilities, need assistance with basic activities of daily living. The most common type of assistance needed by the elderly involves housecleaning or shopping. Many elderly also need assistance with personal care such as bathing and dressing. Between 10 and 22 percent of the elderly aged 65 years and over do not receive these kinds of services when they need them (U.S. General Accounting Office, 1981).

Traditionally, the service system in the United States has been oriented toward young people. In the past, dissatisfied youths threatened the social order while the elderly did not. The elderly were dealt with through income maintenance programs, such as social security and welfare assistance. Young people, on the other hand, received services such as job training, job placement, education, counseling and recreational programs. Nursing home entrepreneurs found that providing institutionally delivered services to the elderly was far more lucrative than providing home or community delivered services. The government itself regards the institutionally delivered services as more economical. The resulting bias has contributed to a concentration of services for comparatively healthy old people.

During the late 1960s, and 1970s, the elderly began to emerge as a political force. Services relevant to their needs and concerns began to change, at least to the extent that numbers of research and demonstration projects increased. However, these trends did not assure the availability of services. A serious imbalance in services presently exists between urban and rural settings. Many elderly people in rural areas have very small incomes, inadequate means of transportation, substandard housing, and poor health. In contrast with the urban elderly, however, these old people have a greater sense of happiness, greater family pride, and stronger family support. Rural neighborhoods are rated more favorably as places to live than are urban neighborhoods (Youmans, 1977; Schwartz, 1980; Grams and Fengler, 1981).

For the most part, rural communities lack resources to serve the elderly. One of the most widely available resources for the rural elderly are The Area Agencies on Aging (AAA), as outlined in the 1973 amendments to the Older Americans Act. AAAs were established to provide advocacy for the interests of the elderly, to plan and coordinate services (without actually providing them), and to locate untapped resources and information needed for comprehensive programs.

Minority group advocates claim that minority old people have been denied many existing services, and have been faced with programs insensitive to culturally related needs. Many believe that the ethnic and minority elderly require a different approach because of their language, life-style, socioeconomic status, and historic experiences in this country. For them, different services, or at least modified and feasible regulations and requirements to promote access, are needed. Facts to define the nature and extent of the problems experienced by old people in minority groups are also needed.

Services will expand for the elderly when mandated by political pressure. Political power wielded by the elderly has been a popular subject for study and speculation. The elderly tend to be more involved in political activities than younger people, but these activities need to be translated into political power. If the elderly can form coalitions with other interest groups, they may succeed in creating necessary political pressures. No public official cares to be the target of a demonstration by old people in wheelchairs!

Accessibility

Administrative coordination of human services in a cost-effective manner tends to favor physical centralization—that is, services grouped under one roof or in one central location. However, decentralization seems to be far more practical for the elderly, whose ability to travel may be limited to a block or two. Even if transportation to more distant locations were available (and it usually is not), psychologic and physiologic obstacles often interfere with utilization. Some old people, for example, cannot hold their urine long enough to ride 5 or 6 miles. Others fear criminal assaults on their property if they are away for any length of time. In addition, centralization of service suggests convenience for the provider, not the consumer. Since old people tend to be reluctant consumers of support services, they often use centralized services as a last resort, when problems have reached the point where they cannot otherwise be satisfactorily resolved.

The following case study illustrates some strategies that were useful in taking services to those in need. To reach out to the fiercely independent people living in a remote rural area of northwest Pennsylvania, workers from a social service outreach program set up centers in *each* town, however small. Residents simply would not travel 12 miles to the next town for socialization and recreation. Workers then went from door to door coaxing people to come to "Latestart," a 10-week program scheduled 3 days weekly from 9 A.M. to 3 P.M., for the purpose of discussing available resources. Those people who attended the first program spread word of services available to their acquaintances. When an information and referral center was eventually established, a manual telephone number "ASK US" was used, to avoid the complexity of a 10-digit toll-free number in an area where most residents were accustomed to dialing five (Jeselnick, 1978). These measures helped to reach people who would not have participated if the program had simply been located in a single town and publicized by conventional means such as newspaper, radio, or television.

Awareness

Significant others tend to minimize the needs of the elderly individual, in an attempt to prolong autonomous living. Old people often are unaware of what resources and services exist and do not perceive that they have serious needs. Very few of them spontaneously mention agencies or professionals as possible sources of help. In the Minneapolis Age and Opportunity Center, elderly clients respond to the center by using direct field services such as meals, home services, or transportation, but rarely counseling, which is crucial to establishing an effective client care plan (Krause, 1977, p. 167). Despite serious problems requiring immediate help, the elderly ask for very little. More than half the clients using the Well-Being service in Detroit were living on less than $3000 per year—yet only 15 percent asked for any sort of economic help (Barney, 1977, p. 312).

Getting elderly people into the system of helping services by direct appeal through addresses to clubs and church groups, mailings, leaflet distribution, and articles in local newspapers tends to be unsuccessful (Barney, 1977). Storefront operations seem to be more successful, especially when an effort is made to provide the help without attempting to exert control. The determination of the elderly to survive on their own is probably the strongest factor limiting even more widespread use of institutions. Thus, help should be provided in a way that augments self-reliance and maintains existing support systems. Information and problem-solving activities should be conveniently located wherever the elderly are. Suggestions and arrangements should be made for the least disruptive form of assistance available.

Intrusion, in the long run, should be minimal and mutually agreed upon (Barney, 1977). A telephone call from the referring nurse to determine whether the minimum assistance has permitted continuation of the client's preferred life-style may be quite sufficient. Helping in a nonintrusive way may seem at odds with nurses' knowledge about client needs and available resources. However, consideration of what the client *wants* and *will accept* should help to keep the nurse on target. Nurses who function in community settings may be more successful in their case finding efforts if they go door to door, rather than waiting in an office or clinic for a referral. This type of approach may seem highly intrusive, but the old person situated in his home is probably freer to make health-care decisions than the one who comes seeking care in a time of crisis.

Discontinuity

Services that do exist are fragmented, with a complex of public, non-profit, and profit-making private agencies providing the services needed by the elderly. Most are autonomous and focus on a single type of service or a single need area. As a result, the needs of old people are seldom assessed comprehensively, and no single agency is equipped to deal with all of them. This discontinuity in services has several consequences. First, the old person is forced to deal with several bureaucracies instead of one. Second, and perhaps more important, the agency fails to obtain a complete understanding of the client's problems. Case histories abound of people like the elderly widow who refused to leave her home, despite repeated robberies, lack of heat, and multiple health problems, because no one would care for her highly significant others—six cats and seven dogs. No agency was prepared to deal with her needs as she perceived them or in the manner in which she wanted them attended. Thus, she was declared incompetent and institutionalized. Within 6 months she died—clean, fed, and warm.

Further evidence of discontinuity in health-care services is found in the special health-care services provided for American Indians and Alaskan natives by the Indian Health Service (IHS) when the Indians live "on or near" reservations. Indians who reside in urban settings must seek medical services provided to urban groups in general (Williams, 1978, p. 13).

The record of ineffective government intervention in the social condition of elderly people has been accumulating at an appalling rate:

> Few if any contemporary Americans would argue with the assertions that: The Model Cities Program did not develop model cities; although Social Security provides retirement income to approximately 20 million persons each year, at least several million older Americans experience severe economic deprivations; Medicare does not make adequate medical care available to the aged; and the War on Poverty has not been won, it has been abandoned (Binstock and Levin, 1976, p. 511).

Inadequate government intervention is due partly to an absence of effective program models and partly to political considerations. Faced with an overload of competing demands for policies and programs, Congress has responded by quickly distributing funds to state and local governments, with only general rules governing their use. The effectiveness of policies and programs is therefore highly dependent on the implementing agencies. As the following situation and Figure 5.3 illustrate, results for the individual can be disastrous:

> This year's winter struck hard at Mary Northern, 72, who lived alone in a rundown, unheated house in Nashville. Alerted by neighbors, police took her against her will to a hospital. Miss Mary, as she is known, was found to have gangrene in both her frostbitten feet. Surgeons recommended amputation. Miss Mary refused.

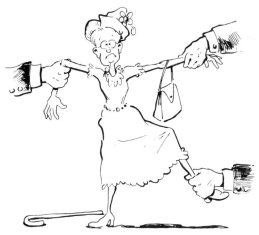

Figure 5.3. I don't believe your idea of help is in my best interest! *(Drawing by Harry Trumbore.)*

> Tennessee welfare workers petitioned for the operation over her protest. Her court-appointed lawyer resisted. The case went to the U. S. Supreme Court. Eventually, believing Miss Mary to be near death, the courts gave permission for the surgery. It was not needed. Miss Mary had developed pneumonia, and the antibiotics used to help her had also halted the gangrene.
>
> Under Tennessee's well-meaning law, Miss Mary is now liable for the costs of the suit brought, against her wishes, to have her feet cut off. Her only asset, beyond meager Social Security benefits, is her house, appraised by tax collectors at only $16,000 but located in a Nashville commercial district. A court hearing is scheduled for this week on whether to force her to sell the house to pay for having been protected. (Protecting Miss Mary, 1978, p. 24. Copyright 1978 by Time Inc. Reprinted by permission from *Time, The Weekly News Magazine.*)

Individualization

The issue of individualization is concerned with whether the elderly require services different from those needed by other groups. On the affirmative side of this question, aging processes increasingly differentiate people of the same chronologic age from each other. The young-old constantly bring new values, life-styles, and expectations to old age. Within the elderly population are groups with ethnic, cultural, national, and racial identities. The traditional approach in service delivery has been to fit the individual to the service. Since the elderly may have unique and changing needs, perhaps individualized services should be provided.

On the negative side of the question, an age-oriented focus to social policies and programs rather than a problem-oriented focus tends to reinforce negative stereotypes of the elderly as victims of social segregation, physical disabilities, and discriminatory attitudes. "The view of older persons as a status group with unique specialized needs tends to set up a dysfunctional tension between older Americans and the rest of society" (Etzioni, 1976, p. 21). According to this point of view, the elderly require special services only to the extent that they have special problems, not because of their age per se. It is doubtful, however, that any problem they experience is confined only to old persons. Thus, the service focus should be on the problem (poverty, poor health, inadequate transportation, and so on) and not the age group (old, young, middle-aged, and so on).

This same logic may be applied to the matter of special services for minority elderly groups. The plight of these groups has been described by many as one of "double jeopardy" (Jackson, 1970, 1971; National Council on the Aging, 1972). This refers to the additive negative effects of being both old and a member of a minority group. When an elderly person is a victim of double jeopardy, the experience of both age and social discrimination is supposed to leave the individual with relatively more problems than either racial or ethnic minorities considered separately. The rural elderly (who can also be regarded as a minority group) have been said to suffer from "triple jeopardy" in that they are old, poor, and isolated in communities lacking organizations to serve them (National Council on the Aging, 1972; Youmans, 1977).

An alternative to the double or triple jeopardy theory is that age exerts a leveling influence and tends to erase the differences found among those of a younger background, so that minority elderly are more like the majority (white, urban) elderly than their younger counterparts (Dowd and Bengtson, 1978).

Evidence suggests that both the jeopardy and leveling ideas may be correct. Information was collected for a study of ethnic variation between a large number of middle-aged and elderly blacks, Mexican-Americans, and Anglos living in Los Angeles County (Dowd and Bengtson, 1978). Elderly blacks and Mexican-Americans differed from Anglos with regard to self-assessed health and income, suggesting that these groups are indeed victims of double jeopardy. However, age appeared to exert a leveling influence on some ethnic variations over time. For example, frequency of interaction with relatives and, for blacks, life-satisfaction factors such as "tranquility" and "optimism," varied less from one ethnic group to another as the age of the groups increased.

In generalizing about the elderly in minority groups, at least three pitfalls must be avoided. The first is a tendency to overemphasize the presumed advantages of growing old in a culture or subculture considered to be traditional or family oriented, while failing to recognize legitimate hardships. The second is a tendency to focus on the problems and deprivations of the minority aged and to disregard the resources (shared culture, symbols, and rituals) these people bring to their aging experience. The third is a tendency to focus on the ethnic group rather than the problem. This can lead to depletion of resources in treating symptoms instead of causes.

Some differences between minority groups of elderly are indeed ethnic or racial in origin. However, many differences directly reflect poverty and poor education, rather than race, ethnicity, or culture in themselves. For example, a poor elderly black person may share more behavioral similarities with poor elderly white people than with wealthy black people. The influence of shared ethnicity may be restricted to a shared sense of peoplehood but not all behaviors (Adams, 1980).

The importance of the issue of individualized services to the nurse relates to the client's uniqueness and the nurse's objectivity. A general awareness of ethnic differences does not enable the nurse to understand the personal situation of the 81-year-old Mexican who is no longer able to work as a farm laborer and who indicates, when asked, that sometimes he does not eat because he has no money. Tremendous variation exists within ethnic categories. The wishes and desires of the client must shape the plan of nursing care, regardless of his or her ethnic origins.

Institutional Versus "Alternative" Services

Identification of the institution as a place of last resort for the elderly has contributed to emphasis on the need to develop "alternative" services to prevent institutionalization. Actually, the situation is not one of "either/or," as implied by the term "alternative." Institutions provide an essential service for those who need and wish to use them. Thus, the term *parallel services* is preferable to alternative services (Morris, 1974; Tobin and Lieberman,

1976). A continuum of flexible services packages should be available to provide elderly people and their significant others with an appropriate range of options. Approaches to service delivery can be categorized according to target and organization pattern: (1) individualized home delivered approach; (2) a congregate-organized approach; and (3) a congregate residence approach. Both the individualized home-delivered and congregate-organized approaches serve elderly people who live in an independent or quasi-independent situation, alone or with a few significant others. In congregate-delivered services, elderly people receive services in a group setting, such as a

TABLE 5.1 PARALLEL WAYS OF STRUCTURING THE DELIVERY OF SERVICES.

A Continuum of Service	Individually Delivered Home-Based	Congregate Delivered	
		Congregate Organized	Congregate Residence
From services for the comparatively well elderly	Outreach Information and referral Telephone reassurance Friendly visiting Work at home Senior Wheels to shopping, doctor, dentist, and social functions	Adult education Recreational senior center Nutrition sites (Wheels to Meals) Sheltered workshop	Senior housing (includes retirement hotels) Senior housing with recreation Senior housing with recreation and social services
Through services that provide alternatives for preventing premature institutionalization	Escort service Homemaker service (housekeeping, handyman, and so forth) Meals on Wheels	Multipurpose senior center (all of the above plus outreach, and health and social follow-up)	Sheltered care Halfway house
To services for those whose needs may demand institutional care or its equivalents	Home health care (visiting nurse, rehabilitation, speech therapy, dentist, and doctor) Foster home care Complete social and health care for bedridden person in a home	Outpatient day or hospital care	Mental hospital Institutional care (nursing home and home for the aged) Intermediate nursing care Skilled nursing care Short-term crisis care Vacation plan Terminal care

(Adapted from Tobin, S. S., Lieberman, M. A. Last Home for the Aged. San Francisco, Josey–Bass, 1976, p 226. Copyright 1976 by Josey–Bass Incorporated Publishers. Reprinted by permission.)

senior housing center or a long-term care institution. In the congregate residence the elderly live together for reasons including health, economy, and safety. The service continuum should extend from services for the comparatively well elderly through services for those who require institutionalization or its equivalent (Tobin and Lieberman, 1976, pp. 225–227). Such a service continuum, with approaches to service delivery, appears in Table 5.1.

Increasing consideration of parallel services to accompany institutional care has raised a number of questions concerning access, utilization, efficiency, and cost-effectiveness (Billings, 1982, p. 3):

1. Should only those at immediate risk of being placed in a nursing home be considered for noninstitutional care?
2. Does provision of home services weaken the support that families now provide their elderly?
3. What is the strength of family support?
4. Who should pay for needed care and how much?
5. At what point is it more cost-effective to provide care in an institution rather than in the home?
6. What percent of nursing home residents could be cared for in the community if care were available?

Although there has been some research into each of these questions, the findings have been difficult to validate and translate into public policy.

Cost-Effectiveness

Cost-effectiveness is often mentioned as the main factor governing the feasibility and desirability of providing parallel services for the elderly. The discussion usually proceeds as follows:

> Some older persons are hospitalized or are located in long-term care institutions unnecessarily and at very high cost. Alternatives to institutionalization surely can be found which probably provide more adequate care at lower cost. But commitment of more than a small fraction of our resources to these alternatives is not prudent because total system cost is already too high; new services will add to and not replace existing services, and thus there is no effective way to control utilization and related cost. Consequently, we must repeatedly convince ourselves that alternative types of care are cost-effective or, more specifically, that they are more economic than institutionalization (Maddox, 1977, p. 155).

Preoccupation with the cost factor diverts attention from the central issue: systematic coordination of services for elderly people. Without a comprehensive, integrated continuum of health and social services, community and home delivered/sponsored services probably do not reduce the total costs to society (Maddox, 1977, p. 157). Such programs may well require substantial financial investment by both private and governmental sectors, to provide for staff training as well as the time and materials needed for extensive assessment and creative implementation. However, experience in settings such as the Ebenezer Center for Aging and Human Development in Minneapolis, where sensitivity to the environment has been a major consideration in programming, suggests that costs may well be recovered through reduction of disruptive behavior and achievement of greater self-reliance on the part of elderly clients (Snyder, 1978).

Generally speaking, costs increase in the following order: home-care and day-care centers, after-care, nursing-home intermediate care, nursing-home skilled care, day hospital care, and hospital care. Exceptions occur when, for example, a terminally ill client is cared for at home with extensive support from the health team. Important considerations are overlooked when cost-effectiveness alone determines the choice of services available. In some instances, the client or his significant others may *prefer* home care. Apart from such wishes, there is ample evidence that a familiar environment has significant advantages—especially for the elderly. In a specific location, the client may have available a good home care program but poor skilled care facilities. Overemphasis on the "cost-effectiveness" and "either-or" aspects of institutional versus "alternative" services should not obscure the need to make resources/

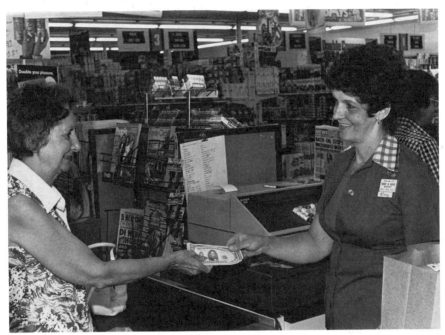

Figure 5.4. Inflation poses one of the biggest threats to aged income security. Finding that each basket of groceries costs more than the last causes worry, despair, and less adequate food intake. *(Photograph by Shawn Mertz, Pittsburgh, PA.)*

services readily available, accessible, and acceptable to the elderly.

INCOME

Adequacy

Nearly every older American is confronted by inadequate or at least insecure income. Many old people have adequate financial resources. However, a secure financial position does not insure an old age free of money worries. Inflation and a rising life expectancy raise unanswerable questions about how much should be spent and how much should be saved (Fig. 5.4). Elderly people with inadequate incomes are caught up in the crisis of poverty.

Satisfaction with monetary resources is directly influenced by relative and distributive justice whereas income itself only indirectly affects one's financial situation (Liang and Fairchild, 1979; Liang, Dvorhin, Kahana, and Mazian, 1980; Fengler and Jensen, 1981).

Elimination of poverty has been an announced goal of American domestic policy for a number of years. However, evaluation of progress toward this goal is hampered by the changing definitions of poverty, sometimes including cash income alone and sometimes including noncash income such as food stamps, rent subsidies, Medicare, and Medicaid.

Between 1959 and 1978, the percent of people aged 65 and over with incomes below the poverty level* declined from 35 percent to 14 percent (U.S. Bureau of the Census, 1980). By 1980, this percent increased to 16 percent because incomes failed to rise as fast as consumer prices during 1979 and 1980 (U. S. Bureau of the Census, 1982, p. 31). Older blacks and Hispanics continued to be far more likely to be living on incomes below the official pov-

* Poverty Level in 1980 was defined as $8,414 for a nonfarm family of four persons. In 1980, the farm–nonfarm distinction was removed (U. S. Bureau of the Census, 1982, p. 3).

erty level, with 38 percent of all older blacks and 31 percent of all older Hispanics so classified. Elderly people in nonmetropolitan areas were poorer (21 percent) than their metropolitan counterparts (12 percent) (U.S. Bureau of the Census, 1982, pp. 37–44).

Subjectively, the following percentages of groups aged 65 years and older regard lack of money as a very serious problem: white Americans (13 percent), blacks (42 percent), and Hispanics (52 percent). Considered as a group, 79 percent of individuals aged 65 years and over report they are unable to make ends meet or are just about getting by (National Council on the Aging, 1981).

Sources

Social Security

This program, started during the Great Depression in 1935, was intended to provide all workers and their families with a floor of income protection in the event that the worker was no longer able to earn income due to retirement and, later, due to premature death or disability. The remainder of the income required by a worker and his family was supposed to come through supplementary insurance, savings and investments, and other arrangements made voluntarily by the worker. Over the years, this program was modified to expand coverage, improve the quality of income protection for workers, and increase funding for the program. Social security retirement (Old Age Survivors Insurance/OASI), disability benefits (Disability Insurance/DI), and hospital benefits (Hospital Insurance/HI or Medicare) are paid for by contributions based on a percentage of a worker's earnings. During their working years, employees, employers, and self-employed people pay social security contributions into special trust funds. When earnings stop due to retirement, disability, or death of a wage earner, monthly cash benefits are paid to replace part of the earnings the individual or family has lost.

Retirement benefits under social security may be taken earlier than age 65 (at age 62). The person who elects to take benefits early receives permanently lower benefits than if retirement had been delayed until age 65.

Disability benefits are paid to the worker or his dependents if disability occurs before age 65. A person is considered disabled if unable to work and if the disability is expected to last (or has lasted) 12 months or is expected to result in death.

Survivors' benefits are available to families if a worker entitled to social security benefits dies before age 65. Monthly payments can be made to unmarried children up to age 18 if they are attending post-secondary school and to age 19 if they are attending elementary and secondary school; unmarried children aged 18 or older who were severely disabled before age 18 and who continue to be severely disabled; widows or dependent widows aged 60 or older; widows, widowers, or surviving divorced spouses if caring for the worker's child under 16 (or disabled regardless of age) who has been receiving a benefit based on the worker's earnings; widows or dependent widowers aged 50 or older who become disabled not later than 7 years after the worker's death, or in the case of a widow, within 7 years after she stops getting checks as a widow caring for the worker's children; dependent parents aged 62 or older; and a divorced wife at age 65 or older, or surviving divorced wife at age 65 or over, or surviving divorced wife at 60, or disabled surviving divorced wife at age 50 or older if the marriage lasted 10 years or more. In addition to monthly payments, a lump-sum payment may be made after the worker's death to either an eligible spouse or a child eligible to receive monthly survivors' benefits.

By the start of the 1980s, 95 percent of all jobs were covered by social security and the first generation of lifelong contributors was retiring and beginning to draw benefits. This program, that included the railroad retirement program, was the major source of income, accounting for 38 percent, of all income to aged units. An aged unit is either a married couple living together, one or both of whom is 65 or older, or an individual 65 or over who is not living with a spouse.

Concern about adequacy of the funding base for social security prompted the Omnibus Budget Reconciliation Act of 1981, which served to reduce benefits while maintaining the fundamental purpose of the program. In all of the rhetoric surrounding debates on how to finance social security, the question is frequently raised as to whether the present and future work force can support the retired, disabled, and/or ill aged populations. This question represents ageism on the part of those who ask it, since the same question is not asked with regard to the defense budget.

Retirement benefit adequacy for women has been a pressing concern because a high proportion of the elderly poor are widowed, divorced, or never-married women. This problem occurred, in part, because social security linked benefits to an individual's earnings and work history. Working women frequently interrupt their work histories to raise children. Women also have generally lower career earnings than men. Income paid to dependent spouses, widows with young children, and widows over age 60 years was paid as a percent of the earnings record of the principal earner. The net result has been inadequate benefits to divorced and widowed spouses and inequities in benefits for families with two earners.

Social security is a complex program that tends to change often as new legislation is enacted. The nurse who needs information about this program should contact any social security office. To locate the nearest office, consult the telephone directory under Social Security Administration or inquire at the post office.

Earnings

Earnings have decreased from the single largest source of income for the elderly (33 percent in 1963) to the second largest source of income (23 percent in 1978) (Epstein and Murray, 1967; Grad, 1981).

Assets

Personal assets (property) provide the next largest (19 percent) proportion of income to a large percentage of both elderly families and individuals. Income from property includes interest, dividends, net rent, estates, or trusts. A home is the most common asset possessed by the elderly. However, money invested in a home can be converted to cash only if the home is sold.

Pension Plans

Employer-sponsored pensions have increased in importance as a source of income to the elderly. Still, in 1978, these pensions remained the fourth largest source of income, providing only 16 percent of the dollars received by aged units. These pensions, with the exception of federal civil service and military retirement pensions, provide incomplete protection for inflation. Only 3 percent of private pensions provide small automatic annual adjustments (U.S. Senate Special Committee, 1982a). In many instances, coverage for a wife after the death of her husband is not included. In addition, private pension plans are not available to a large percentage of the work force.

Supplemental Security Income

Supplemental Security Income (SSI) is a federal program that replaced three state-administered public assistance programs to provide a national minimum income for the aged, blind, and disabled. Enacted as part of the 1972 amendments to the Social Security Act, SSI became available in 1974. The aim of the program is to provide monthly checks when they are needed so that anyone who is 65 or older, blind, or disabled can have a basic (minimum) cash income. This does not mean that all eligible people get the same amount. Some get less because they have income from other sources. Some get more because they live in a state that adds money to the federal SSI payment. In most cases, a person eligible for SSI is also eligible for Medicaid and other welfare services.

People who have little or no regular cash income and who do not own much property that could be converted into cash—such as stocks, bonds, jewelry, or other valuables—may get SSI. A home does *not* count as an asset. Previous public assistance programs required homeowners to sign a lien (a promise to repay money accepted from the state out of the proceeds from selling their homes in the future). Understandably, this practice deterred many people from using public assistance. With SSI, this requirement has been abolished. Personal effects (clothing) and household goods (furniture) also do not count. Insurance policies or a car may affect eligibility, depending on their value. People may earn a small amount while receiving SSI without any reduction in their checks. Information on the SSI program is available through local social security offices.

One measure of the success of SSI is the impact on users' health. One study found that SSI did aid people to recover good health, prevent a drop in the percentage in better health, and reduce age-specific mortality rates. The results supported a projection that, for example, in 1977 a white man living with his spouse would be at a 71 percent greater risk of death if his SSI benefits were cut by $3000 yearly. The obvious explanation for these findings is that people use some of their SSI money for preventive and curative health expenditures (Taubman and Sickles, 1983). Problems with the SSI program include underutilization, administrative difficulties, and inadequacy of the guaranteed minimum income level. This program provides only a very small share (2 percent) of income to the elderly.

Veteran's Benefits

Various benefits are available to veterans from the armed forces, ranging from disability benefits to GI home loans. Veteran's benefits include cash payments, compensation for service connected disability, pensions for nonservice-connected disability, and compensation and pensions for survivors. Other benefits and services include hospital and medical care, allowances for burial expenses, vocational rehabilitation, and educational assistance for wives and widows. Pensions are available to the war veteran at age 65, depending on the individual's income but not state of health. Nurses who wish to obtain more information or to refer clients should contact the local veterans' affairs office.

Other

Other sources of postretirement income include savings and cash support from significant others. Public assistance provides a source of economic relief for people with limited assets, who may be eligible for food stamps and reimbursement for travel to receive health care.

Special Needs

Several groups of elderly people have special economic needs. Elderly blacks, Hispanics, Asian-Americans, and American Indians tend to have a very poor financial status. Many of these minority-elderly are not eligible for social security benefits, since they have not accumulated the required quarters* of work to be eligible. Domestic and farm laborers have only recently been included in social security. Some workers spend lifetimes at jobs where employers are willing to risk nonpayment of social security benefits and split the difference with the worker. Although these workers make more money on the job, they lose when they are no longer able to work.

Elderly women have fewer income resources than elderly men. They seldom have pensions or opportunities for substantial income from work. Many never worked in covered employment, having worked as domestics. Women live longer than men, and live more of those years as widows than men do as widowers. Because men tend to marry women younger than themselves, more than 50 percent of women aged 65 and over are widowed, compared with about 14 percent of men who are widowers (U.S. Bureau of the Census, 1981).

Approaches to Adequate Income

There are two approaches to solving the money-related problems of the elderly: income subsidies and "in-kind" services. *Income subsidies* provide direct cash payments, such as Supplemental Security Income, Aid to Families with Dependent Children, and unemployment compensation. With income subsidies, the recipient is permitted to make his own choices about the acquisition of benefits.

"In-kind" services provide actual material goods and services rather than the cash with which to purchase them. In-kind services largely remove choice from the individual and place it

---

* Social security credit is measured in "quarters of coverage." Employees and self-employed people receive one quarter of coverage if a specified number of dollars is earned in a 3-month period. No more than four quarters of coverage may be earned in a year.

in the control of government agencies. Examples of in-kind services are food stamp programs, Medicare, sewage removal, and public education.

The issue of income subsidies versus in-kind services is one of the oldest in the history of social services. Factors to consider in this debate relate to (1) characteristics of the recipients, (2) economic factors, and (3) the government's role. How capable and willing are the elderly to acquire needed services in the marketplace if they have the cash to spend? If an old person is unable to go shopping for groceries because of physical incapacity or fear of personal harm, money is of little value. An elderly person who gives his money to his children, perhaps to convince all concerned that he "has plenty," is then unable to buy medication or rent a boat to go fishing.

Will the market be responsive to the needs of the elderly as consumers? Food, clothing, and shelter are available for the price. Many elderly people, however, need services such as home delivery of prepared meals, specialized housing, homemaking and household repair services, and convenient transportation. For enough money, virtually any service can be purchased. The problem for old people is that, even with cash assistance, money is a limited resource that must last for an indefinite period of time. The costs of many services needed by the elderly are too high when provided in the marketplace but are cheaper when provided as in-kind services.

The role of government in social welfare has been debated since this country was first settled. Is social welfare a normal function of modern society? Or should it be provided only when traditional institutions, such as the family and the market economy, no longer function adequately? Decision-makers at the national, state, and local levels, sampled from both the private and public sectors, tended to reject an income subsidy solution for most problems of the elderly. They did not view the elderly as too dependent or incompetent to use the cash resources, but they believed that the market was incapable of responding to many of the problems involved. Sadly, these decision-makers did not regard the government as able to

meet the special needs of old people any more effectively than the market (McConnell and Kasschau, 1977).

Unless the elderly as a group come to pose a major threat to the structure of capitalist–corporatist society, changes in the present structure of service programs and distribution of income are unlikely. Social service programs will affect only the most desperately needy parts of the population. Those services that require large numbers of people to run them will find funding increasingly difficult to secure, especially since they so rarely demonstrate the benefits their advocates initially promise (Zald, 1977, p. 121).

Implications for Nurses

When nurses care for financially deprived people, a value conflict often arises. Nurses and other health care providers prefer middle-class clients because of perceived similarities in characteristics and values (Mason, 1981). Thus, nurses need to clarify their values by answering relevant questions. What do I value? How do the client's values differ? Whose values are more important? Do I expect the client to conform to my values? What/whom is responsible for this client's poverty? Financial value conflicts may be increased when the poor client presents other sharp contrasts to characteristics of the nurse, such as age, race, or ethnic background.

Old people are often reluctant to admit to financial problems. The exact amount of income is probably less important than what the individual does with it. Assessment should therefore focus on income adequacy rather than precise dollar figures. An assessment sequence of "Have you noticed that the price of meat is rising?" followed by "Have you changed your meat-eating habits as a result?" will yield more useful information than "How much money do you spend on meat?" Negative response to several such questions often provide a clue that income may be a problem.

Of particular concern to nurses is how much the elderly person is able or willing to spend for health care. Here, a focus on relative values is more apt to be useful than a direct query related to dollar expenditures. "I'll bet you'd rather have _____ (some knitting yarn, a "shot and a beer,")" will provide more information than, "Are you going to get this prescription filled?" Too often health professionals "write off" the client who fails to act on their recommendations. "If Mr. K won't stop spending money on his children instead of his medication, then there is nothing more to be done" is a frequent stance taken by nurses, physicians, and others. For any regimen to be *successful* it must first be *acceptable* to the client. What should be asked of Mr. K is, "If you won't stop spending money on your children instead of your health, what will you do and how can I help you?" The client is responsible for his health, not the health professional. The health professional is only responsible for providing information so that the client can make an informed decision.

When the nurse believes that a money problem exists she does not necessarily have to determine its exact nature. Intervention should be primarily aimed at referring the client to someone with extensive knowledge of available financial resources. The knowledge and ability to make such referrals constitute the nurse's challenge in intervention.

HOUSING

The subject of housing as a resource for the elderly is complex. Ideally, such housing should promote physical, social, and psychologic well-being, while permitting privacy and continuity of life-style. Appropriate services should therefore include health and social services, an emergency communication system, recreational options, and an attractive environment. At a minimum, housing for the elderly should be convenient, comfortable, and physically safe. Unfortunately, many housing facilities in which the elderly live are operated for profit. Elderly residents often become victims of rent or tax increases, and may be subject to eviction when ability to live independently becomes questionable.

Matching the differing needs of the elderly with available housing resources is hampered by several problems. These include a lack of standard terminology to describe existing facilities, varied sponsorship (private for profit, private nonprofit, public), lack of certification for housing owners and managers, and diversity in location, support services available for residents, costs, and financing mechanisms.

Housing for old people was once considered to be no different from housing for other age groups. However, this orientation began to change in the mid-1960s to reflect special concerns with safety, reduction of maintenance, and minimization of cost. More recently, service considerations (meals, social services, health monitoring, recreational programs, and transportation) have further changed the concept of traditional housing.

Housing options for the elderly can be thought of in terms of a service continuum that ranges from no support (traditional owner-occupied or renter-occupied housing) through moderate service support (special housing, such as congregate or retirement) to extensive service support (institutions established primarily for health rather than residential needs). The latter are discussed under health-care resources.

A persistent issue in gerontology concerns segregation versus integration—that is, whether the elderly should be set apart as a group for education, leisure activities, housing, etc. Theorists tend to favor integration. On the other hand, services and programs for old people are usually provided on a segregated basis, and thus tend to promote age separation. A number of forces have encouraged the trend toward age-group isolation. The elderly were "left behind," first in the rural areas when many young people flocked to the city in search of work in business and industry, and later in the inner cities when young families moved to the suburbs. The rural to urban migration shift turned the focus from the extended to the nuclear family and, thus, smaller dwelling units. Federal housing policy has encouraged age-segregated housing by congregating large numbers of old people into single buildings, presumably for the sake of economy, efficiency, and safety.

Age-segregated housing may have unintended and undesirable social consequences.

The elderly may become more isolated, with no opportunity to dispel age-related stereotypes by casual daily encounters with people of various ages. Protection against crime is limited to events that occur within the building, and the elderly must still venture onto the streets and into commercial areas. Studies of elderly people in urban settings indicate that residents in age-segregated housing consider themselves more vulnerable to neighborhood problems than other community residents (Sherman, Newman, Nelson and Van Buren, 1975, Kahana et al., 1977). Alternatively, age-segregated housing has been found to enhance social interaction (Rosow, 1967) and well-being (Lawton, Nahemow, and Tsong-Min-Yeh, 1980).

Given the diversity of the elderly as individuals, the issue of age-segregated versus age-integrated housing does not require an "either–or" solution. Rather, both types of living options should be available to accommodate individual preferences.

Research concerning the environments that surround and influence the lives of elderly people is still in relative infancy (Howell, 1980). This situation is especially true in the area of housing. The following questions represent some of the specific research questions that remain to be studied (Howell, 1980; Newman, 1981):

1. What spatial experiences are in the mind rather than actually present in the daily behavior of older people?
2. How do environments, past and present, reflect self-concept?
3. What is the relationship between changes which people experience as they grow older and various housing adjustments?
4. Do different life events such as disability, widowhood, and retirement result in different housing adjustments?
5. What are the sequences and lags of life changes and housing changes?
6. How does provision of housing related services affect adjustment type and timing?

Types of Housing

This section describes the most frequently used types of housing for the elderly in the United States.

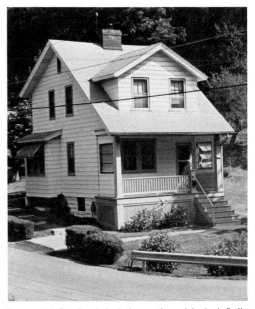

Figure 5.5 Real estate is less vulnerable to inflation until it is sold and converted to cash. *(Photograph by Shawn Mertz, Pittsburgh, PA.)*

Owner-Occupied

Most elderly people have paid off their mortgages and own their homes, will sacrifice to keep them, and derive benefits from home ownership that cannot be equaled by other housing arrangements as suggested by Figure 5.5. Special analyses of the 1976 Annual Housing Survey of the Department of Housing and Urban Development (Brotman, 1982, p. 16) indicated that approximately 70 percent of the elderly own their own homes, compared to 63 percent of younger people. The mortgage has been paid off in 84 percent of these elderly-owned homes. Older people tend to dwell in older housing, with generally less adequate service systems such as heating and cooling, single bathrooms, and higher maintenance costs. Estimates of flawed or inadequate housing vary from 10 to 30 percent (Brotman, 1982; Soldo; 1980). Black and Hispanic elderly families as well as divorced or never-married older men and women are substantially more likely to live in deficient housing. Home ownership among older households outside metropolitan areas exceeds the number of older renters by a margin of 4 to 1, compared to a margin of less than 3 to 1 among the general population (U.S. Senate Special Committee, 1982a).

Older households increasingly turned to mobile home living during the 1970s, so that by 1980 about 17 percent of all new mobile homes were occupied by the elderly compared to 0.9 percent of all new housing in general (U.S. Senate Special Committee, 1982a).

The traditional rule of thumb is that housing should not cost more than 25 percent of income. In 1976, 23 percent of elderly homeowners spent more than this proportion of their incomes on their housing, representing an excessive housing burden. Many homeowners keep their housing expenses low by neglecting needed repairs and maintenance.

Home ownership is important and beneficial to elderly people. Owning one's home is associated with older persons' wishes and needs to remain independent (Kummerow, 1980), maintain family tradition (Langford, 1962), derive status (Baer, 1976), and deny poor conditions as a positive adaptive mechanism (Lawton, 1980; O'Bryant, 1982).

Renter-Occupied
Approximately 30 percent of the residences occupied by the elderly are rental properties. In contrast to the owner-occupied households, which are usually made up of two or more persons, renters tend to be single people (Brotman, 1982).

Some elderly people choose to rent in facilities where they do not have to be responsible for housekeeping. Residence clubs and hotels or motels provide "hotel type" services at rates comparable to ordinary apartment rentals. Central dining facilities provide two to three meals daily, although individual units may have a hotplate and small refrigerator. Maid service, towels, linen, and other services, such as a nurse or physician on call, may be included in the monthly charge. Most of these facilities provide telephone and an intercommunication system. Sometimes residence clubs offer a program of social and cultural activities under the leadership of a program director.

Many of the elderly poor live in boarding homes or rooming houses that provide food, linens, and cleaning services but rarely provide health care. Since so many of the old people in these facilities have serious health problems and no other place to live, states are moving toward regulation of boarding homes, in an effort to prevent resident abuse and institute some supportive services.

A number of hazards may be associated with living in commercial residences. In some cases, physical facilities are not appropriate for the elderly. Elevators, doors, and hallways may be narrow. Lighting may be poor and fire protection measures inadequate. Some converted housing facilities are located in declining areas of central cities, where crime rates are high. As a result, the residents become virtual prisoners in their rooms, afraid to come out for food, clothing, or recreation. Low rates (occasionally as little as $10 per week) may be available only with double occupancy and use of a common bathroom. Ownership of these facilities tends to change frequently, disrupting continuity of operations and often leading to rate increases for occupants.

Two models, constant and accommodating, have been proposed to conceptualize person-environment change in situations where people do not own their homes (Lawton, 1977; Lawton, Greenbaum, and Liebowitz, 1980). In the constant model, housing managers plan admission and termination policies, as well as the physical environment and service programs, so as to maintain the relative level of independence of the original tenant group. Stringent health requirements are maintained. Tenants are asked to leave when they begin to require help to maintain their initial levels of independence. In the accommodating model, tenants may continue to reside in the setting as long as 24-hour nursing care is not required. As the tenants' level of independence declines, formal service programs are increased and physical-environmental changes instituted to protect the total milieu for marginal tenants. Results of a study to evaluate these two models indicated that neither model seemed appropriate. Instead, a balanced model involving intervention to strengthen informal networks was suggested (Ehrlich, Ehrlich, and Woehlke, 1982).

Too often, "life care" plans in commercial residences provide little more than shelter and food. Owners usually reserve the right to terminate the agreement if the resident becomes unable to live independently. Some facilities permit residents to work part time on the premises to supplement their incomes. However, the duties may be too much for the elderly person, and the wage paid is usually well below the federal minimum. In this way, the facility is able to operate with a small staff and payroll. Residents should be particularly wary of agreeing to a shared bank account with building owners "in case of illness and/or inability to handle one's affairs." Before beginning even a year of residency in commercial housing, the prospective resident should live at the facility for several weeks or months in order to verify acceptability of services. If such a trial period cannot be arranged, the prospective resident should look elsewhere for housing.

Special Housing

A variety of residential arrangements are currently being made available to the elderly (Weismehl, 1977). The concept of *congregate* or *group housing* is based upon the idea of a residential environment that assists the elderly in achieving independence, pleasure, security, and growth. The collective living arrangement of private places (individual rooms, apartments, or separate dwellings) and shared spaces (lounges, kitchen, dining areas, and laundries) is intended to foster mutual assistance among the residents. The program design calls for a service delivery system (meals, recreation, social service, transportation, and health monitoring) to permit elderly people to maintain or return to a semi-independent life-style.

The concept of congregate housing should not be confused with the specific program provided under the Housing and Urban Development Act of 1970 and the Community Development Act of 1974. This legislation served to identify congregate housing with meal service. The purpose of congregate or group housing is to provide "an assisted independent group living environment that offers the elderly who are functionally impaired or socially deprived

but otherwise in good health, the residential accommodation and supporting services they need to maintain or return to a semi-independent life style and prevent premature or unnecessary institutionalization as they grow older" (International Center of Social Gerontology, cited in Peace, 1981). Other names for this type of housing plan include "special housing," "purpose-built housing," "assisted residential housing," "collective housing," "pensioners' hotels," and so forth. All of these projects have in common grouped independent accommodation plus services. Communal meals, housekeeping assistance, and some personal care are almost always among the services provided. Group sizes range from 3 to 30 residents, with an average of 8 to 12 (Peace, 1981).

Sponsoring agencies usually require that prospective residents be ambulatory and reasonably fit, capable of most of the activities of daily living, and not in need of 24-hour supervision. Figure 5.6 depicts such a group. The degree of disability that can be tolerated in a given setting depends very much on the resources of the sponsoring agency. Seldom addressed is the issue of what to do when residents start to fail and become unable to continue in this form of independent or semi-independent living without a great deal of assistance. Forcing these people to move to an institution that provides more extensive care disrupts what may have become important relationships with significant others (Beaver, 1979).

Very few of the living arrangements for older people have been evaluated; fewer still have been studied using "before and after" designs to evaluate changes over time. The few studies that have been completed indicate that residents are satisfied with what they see as a safer, more supportive environment that offers them a degree of companionship (Peace, 1981b). However, then shared housing arrangements do not last long unless residents can reconcile desires for privacy and autonomy (Pritchard, 1983).

In the United States, as of 1981, the number of these group or shared homes was estimated to number 100, with most having come into existence since 1975. The Jewish Council

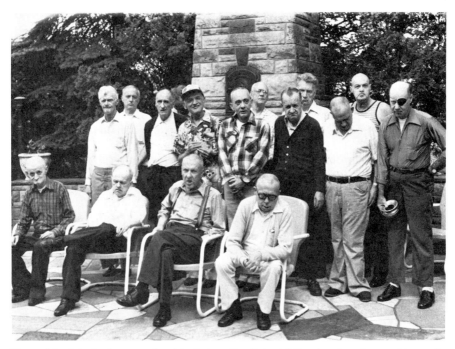

Figure 5.6. A typical group of residents from the Colonial Gardens "small group" home in Butler, Pennsylvania. *(Photograph by Shawn Mertz, Pittsburgh, PA.)*

for the Aging (JCA) in the Washington, D.C. area has operated a program of shared apartments for older people since 1974. The program provides eight three-bedroom apartments and four two-bedroom units. All units are rented. Each resident has his or her own bedroom and no more than two people share a bathroom. All residents share the living room, dining room, and kitchen.

These residents must be ambulatory, capable of self-care, and responsible for their own medication. They must also be able to use the stove and telephone and to share in light household tasks. Each resident group has a homemaker who works 20 hours per week, Monday to Friday. The homemaker does all of the grocery shopping for the apartment and cooks the main meal of the day. Residents prepare their own breakfasts and lunches. This homemaker also assists with changing bed linen

and washing laundry each week. Heavy cleaning is done every other week. A social worker visits weekly. JCA minibuses take residents on outings. The monthly cost to residents covers rent, utilities, telephone, food, and homemaker services (Peace, 1981, pp. 17–18).

Retirement communities are self-contained developments that admit only elderly people as residents. Entry age ranges from 55 to 65. Spouses can be of any age, and young people may visit for defined periods of time. Individual dwellings, apartments, and condominiums are usually available. Apartments may be designed for either housekeeping or nonhousekeeping. Some retirement communities offer multilevel housing facilities that provide a continuum of living arrangements, ranging from independent housekeeping through nonhousekeeping to nursing home, under one roof or within a defined campus-like area. These facilities are designed to serve residents as their needs change with advancing age or illness. Usually, residents can move freely from one level of housing to another. To promote a feeling of well-being, the units that serve the very dependent elderly tend to be set apart from those of the other residents.

Many retirement communities provide a country club atmosphere, with swimming pools, golf, tennis, and lakes. Recreation programs are usually extensive. A few communities provide health-care services through local clinics and hospitals. Since retirement communities may be located in convenient locations and may offer varying kinds of services, the prospective resident should plan to stay in the community for a month or more before making a commitment to buy or rent for an extended period.

Payment for Housing

Housing is the primary financial expenditure for the elderly. On the average, it accounts for more than one third of their budget. Because of their relatively fixed incomes, the elderly are particularly affected by shortages in affordable housing. As a rule of thumb, the elderly homeowner who devotes more than 30 percent of his income to housing is in need of assistance (U. S. Senate Special Committee, 1982a).

General Funding

Elderly homeowners receive sporadic relief from housing costs through measures such as tax relief, reduced interest rates, mortgage guarantees, and home repair or winterization programs. However, assistance to homeowners is difficult to arrange because of the effect of equity accumulation of government aid. Eventually a home will be sold, and the owner or his heirs will receive equity monies. The prevailing policy to date has been that equity should not be permitted to accumulate at taxpayer expense. Reverse mortgages have been proposed, which would provide the homeowner with income from the equity. Thus far, the elderly have displayed little interest in giving up their equity holdings (U.S. Senate Special Committee, 1982).

Elderly renters may be eligible for federally funded housing assistance payments, which allow lower-income families to occupy existing standard units while paying as little as 15 percent and no more than 30 percent of their gross incomes for rent. Others may be able to live in public low-rent housing. Public housing authorities in local communities certify eligibility of tenants for this type of housing, and the rents are based upon ability to pay. Waiting periods for admission tend to be long; a 2-year wait is typical. These facilities do not provide consistently available support services. As of 1975, only about one-fourth (270,000) of the total public housing units were specifically designed for the elderly. The major complaint about public housing involves victimization of tenants by criminals. Some of the units are located in declining neighborhoods with high crime rates.

Special Financing

Among the special types of financing for housing are *founders' fees, life lease contracts,* and *life care. Founders' fees* are used by nonprofit groups (usually church-related). The initial occupants, or "founders," of a housing facility pay sums ranging from $8000 to $35,000 or more. These fees permit the facility to be constructed. The resident, in turn, receives lifetime use of one dwelling unit and makes a contribution to the sponsoring religious group.

Life lease or life contracts involve payment of a specified sum based on life expectancy actuarial tables. Both founders' fees and life lease contracts guarantee lifetime occupancy of an apartment, but they do not provide for ongoing maintenance services, health-care plans, or other programs. Apartment ownership reverts to the facility owners after the resident's death. If a resident must move, some owners return a proportion of the original investment.

Life care financing plans are used infrequently by some retirement homes and residence clubs. Based upon actuarial tables of life expectancy and service costs, the elderly person pays an amount for total life care, which includes housing, meals, health, and personal care services. If the old person lacks sufficient cash, his assets, up to the equivalent of the total cost, may be turned over to the owner. The owner must provide care for the elderly person, regardless of cost, for as long as that person lives. Problems with this payment strategy relate to (1) failure of the facility, if owners are unable to live up to their part of the bargain, and (2) inadequate guarantees for quality of care.

Implications for Nurses

Nurses become involved in the issue of housing when they are part of teams that inspect residences, and when individual clients are found living in inadequate dwellings. The nurse's primary responsibility is to assess the situation and then make a referral to a social worker or agency representative who is more familiar with alternative housing arrangements and remedial strategies. Many elderly people live in old dwellings in need of repair and have difficulty paying rent or mortgages and taxes. The nurse should discuss living arrangements with each elderly client, helping them to plan for the future and the possibility of having to move to a more protective setting. This can be done by simply asking a few relevant questions. "How long do you expect to be able to live alone?" "Where will you live if _____ moves away/dies?" "Just supposing you had to move somewhere because your health was not good. Where would you go?"

Even though the client may be disturbed by discussion of a future in any setting other than his or her home, the fact of having brought the possibility out in the open may facilitate acceptance should a future move become necessary, as well as minimize the negative impact of such a relocation.

Loss of a home for an elderly person should be regarded as a crisis until careful assessment indicates no negative impact on the individual's health.

In addition to dealing with specific clients' housing problems, the task of nurses is to recognize the issues involved in housing for the elderly and to advocate necessary changes by speaking out from their perspectives as citizens as well as health professionals. Along with

income and health, housing is one of the "trinity" of factors that affect the quality of living for the elderly. One reason the concept of a spectrum of facilities has not materialized may be due to conflicts in the approaches of federal agencies responsible for housing and health, respectively. Approaching the problem of a spectrum of housing on the basis of medical assumptions results in a focus on institutional and acute medical care. An emphasis on housing needs alone tends to ignore needs of the frail elderly for special services. When a broad spectrum of housing options are made available to the elderly in conjunction with home health, personal care, and other support services, the possibility of keeping disabled or partially disabled people out of institutions is greatly enhanced.

FOOD

Food for the elderly in the community is often available through programs that deliver to the home or serve meals in a central location. Mobile meals programs for the home-bound elderly usually deliver one hot and one cold meal simultaneously, either 5 or 7 days a week. Delivery is usually made by volunteers, who also check on the recipient's general well-being and provide a few minutes of socialization. Problems with home-delivered meals involve the acceptability of the food in terms of individual tastes and the cost of the meals. Despite efforts to keep the charge low, some recipients believe they could feed themselves (if they were able) for less. Actually costs per meal vary from roughly 70 cents to 2 dollars. Delivery of meals to homes on a regular basis is one of the most essential support services to enable quasi-independent living.

Congregate-meal programs provide one meal a day, 5 days per week, in a location easily accessible to large numbers (50 to 150) of old people. Of course, the elderly must be sufficiently mobile to get from home to the center on a regular basis. Sometimes medication dispensing, health screening, counseling, referral, educational, and recreational services are provided in conjunction with congregate-meal programs.

A food-stamp program operated by state and local departments of public welfare, in conjunction with the Department of Agriculture, enables low-income households, regardless of age, to buy more food of greater variety. Participants receive at regular intervals an allotment of food stamps, which can be exchanged for a variety of foods at most area grocery stores. Food stamps may be used by people 60 years or older to buy home-delivered meals, if they meet eligibility requirements for both mobile meals and food stamp programs. Food stamps may also be used to buy food in approved restaurants that contract to sell meals to the aged at "concessional prices." To participate in a food-stamp program, the individual or head of the household must meet certain financial and nonfinancial criteria. The income test is based on poverty guidelines set by the Office of Management and Budget. Elderly people have been reluctant to take part in this program because of this test and because the program is part of the public assistance (welfare) program. Public assistance tends to be unacceptable to old people because they regard it as charity.

To overcome some of these barriers and encourage the elderly to improve their diets, a number of changes have been made in the food-stamp program. Elimination of the purchase requirement increased participation of eligible older people by 42 percent. This requirement obligated food-stamp users to pay cash for their stamps. The value of the stamps was higher than the amount paid. However, many people had difficulty accumulating the cash they needed to buy the stamps. The Supplemental Security Income (SSI) elderly cash-out demonstration project was tested in some states. Households consisting completely of persons 65 years of age or older, or persons receiving SSI benefits received a check equal to the value of what their food-stamp allotment would otherwise have been. The purpose of this project was to remove the following participation barriers: difficult application procedures, lack of transportation, and the "welfare stigma" associated with applying for and using food stamps

(U.S. Senate Special Committee on Aging, 1982b, p. 12).

TRANSPORTATION

Transportation is the least available of the essential services that permit independent or quasi-independent living for the elderly. Finding transportation is difficult in both urban and rural settings. The transportation situation for rural old people has been summarized in this way:

> You own your own car. For without it you are a prisoner in your own home. There is one four-lane stretch of highway—6 miles to be exact. One airport, no passenger rail service, though once that was plentiful and the area's lifeline. Throughout the 3200 square miles there are six taxicabs, and if you want to take a bus, you may have to travel 40 miles to get it (Jeselnick, 1978, p. 33).

The need to own a car can be just as great for the urban elderly, although perhaps for different reasons. Urban settings have more transportation systems: bus, cab, and rapid transit. Problems include costs, which are too high for elderly people's budgets, extended waits, which can involve exposure to bad weather and victimization by criminals, difficulty in boarding and exiting from vehicles, and long rides, which tax energy reserves. Old people in urban environments, therefore, are often as disadvantaged as the rural elderly who have no transportation systems available. Both must appeal to the generosity of significant others, or hope that a transportation program for the elderly is available. Older women are particularly disadvantaged in a society dominated by automobiles. Possession of automobiles and driver's licenses is substantially lower among women aged 65 and older than among older men.

Five basic types of transportation services have been identified as serving the elderly: conventional public transit, typically fixed route and schedule service; special systems, usually described as some form of dial-a-ride or demand-responsive system; coordinated systems encompassing both fixed route and dial-a-ride features, frequently "route deviation" systems; taxi systems typically operating with some form of reduced or subsidized rate; and a variety of volunteer-based programs (U.S. Senate Special Committee on Aging, 1982a). Specialized transportation systems comprise the major provider for elderly people. Most of these demand-responsive or dial-a-ride systems provide door-to-door service and require advance reservations (usually 24 hours). When these systems refuse to take reservations prior to 24 hours before transportation is required, elderly people experience planning difficulties. For the most part, these programs will only transport the elderly to destinations providing health or nutrition services or opportunities for personal shopping. Thus, travel for purposes of recreation or socialization is seldom possible.

For those who are able to use public transportation, many states and cities have programs that permit the elderly to ride free or at reduced fares by showing proof of age. People who participate in medical assistance programs (Medicaid) are eligible to travel free for the purpose of receiving health care. They are required to use the cheapest form of public transportation permitted by their functional abilities.

In 1979 the Department of Transportation developed regulations requiring accessibility (for example, wheelchair lifts) for all modes of transportation receiving public money within 30 years, with additional provisions for providing interim accessibility services during transition to complete accessibility. In 1981, however, the Department of Transportation pulled back these regulations after a court ruling by the U.S. Appellate Court of the District of Columbia determined that the regulations posed an excessive burden on local programs and exceeded the Department of Transportation's authority.

During the 1981 White House Conference on Aging, transportation was considered in context of conditions for continuing community participation of the elderly. Problems with both privately and publicly owned transportation concentrating on profitable/high use routes were acknowledged. For occasional and rural travel, reliance on friends and neighbors was considered as the best solution. Incentives for volunteer transportation were recommended by means of insurance rate reductions, expense reimbursement, and income tax reductions. Global recommendations were made, calling for adequate, accessible, transportation throughout the entire United States (Recommendations, 1982, pp. 137–139).

Given the transportation problems listed above, it is not surprising that the automobile is the primary source of transportation for the elderly (U.S. Senate Special Committee on Aging, 1982a, p. 434). As they age, many drivers notice problems such as visual or auditory impairments, slowed response rates, nervousness, crippling lack of confidence, and difficulty adjusting to new things.

Changes in driving conditions compound these problems. Old people seem to be bothered most by the speed of traffic, the number of cars on the road, and the difficulties of negotiating freeways and interchanges (National Council on the Aging, 1978, p. 220).

For nurses, the implications of the transportation needs of elderly people are fairly obvious. Vision, hearing, and other relevant physical abilities should be preserved and enhanced. Nurses can help elderly clients plan "best times" to drive and identify ways to minimize time spent on the road. Nurses can also support the elderly in their demands for more adequate public transportation.

LEISURE

Positive use of time in the later years includes volunteer work, political activism, and continued education, and any other pursuit that does not involve becoming a burden on anyone else. Productivity is not essential. Resources to support the old person who wishes to do "nothing" are widely available (Fig. 5.7). Even the most decrepit home provides a front step with a view of something to watch. Clinics, parks, and construction sites attract a fair share of elderly "people watchers." The important considera-

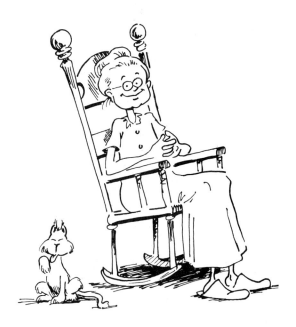

"Sometimes I sit and think and sometimes I just sit."

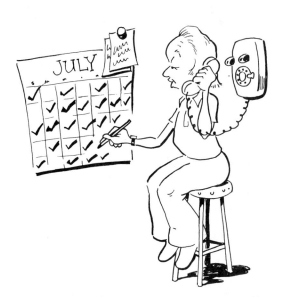

"Two weeks from Tuesday? I couldn't possibly. Next time please give me a little more notice."

Figure 5.7. Activity levels of older adults vary widely. *(Drawings by Harry Trumbore.)*

tion in evaluating use of leisure is whether the person is satisfied with his choice.

Work

The wishes of the elderly regarding work involvement are unclear. A Harris poll released on November 18, 1981 found:

1. Among all those working in the preretirement ages between 55 and 64 years, a majority of 79 percent were opposed to stopping work completely when they retired
2. Greater availability of part-time work was favored by 73 percent
3. Job-sharing opportunities were favored by 66 percent
4. Jobs involving a day or two per week to work at home were favored by 68 percent
5. Among people of all ages surveyed, 90 percent believed that nobody should be forced to retire because of age (U.S. Senate Special Committee on Aging, 1982a, p. 249).

The fifth highest priority recommendation selected by delegates to the 1981 White House Conference on Aging called for the elimination of mandatory retirement and other forms of discrimination against older workers. In addition, the recommendation called on employers to hire older workers on a part-time, temporary or shared basis, and emphasized flexible work schedules (U.S. Senate Special Committee on Aging, National Retired Teachers Association, and American Association of Retired Persons, 1982). Despite these expressed desires for more flexible work opportunities and the importance of earnings from employment to an adequate retirement income, a trend toward early retirement among older workers is a well-established fact. One-third of all social security beneficiaries retire at age 62 years. Since early retirement began, the number and percentage of persons of both sexes retiring early has steadily increased (U.S. Senate Special Committee on Aging, 1982a). Perhaps elderly people simply want the right to work, with freedom from the necessity to do so.

Employment opportunities for the elderly are limited, in comparison with those available for most other age groups. Extension of the mandatory retirement age from 65 to 70, and elimination of mandatory retirement in some instances, were important measures to improve work opportunities for the elderly. Creation of such opportunities has centered on provision of public service jobs by the federal government. For example, Title IX of the 1973 Comprehensive Services for Older Americans Amendments Act of 1965 established the Older Americans Community Service Employment program to promote part-time work in community service projects for low-income elderly.

Job redesign for older persons appears to be more advanced in England and Sweden than in this country. In job redesign, the older person's job is changed to fit that person's changing abilities. In other cases, the worker is relocated in a job better suited to his altered capabilities. Unfortunately, many companies in this country do modify jobs to meet the needs of elderly workers but do not want to publicize this information (U.S. Senate Special Committee on Aging, 1982a, p. 285).

Performance assessment is an important means for older workers who want to continue working. A standardized system of job requirements, goals, and performance standards helps both employers and employees make justifiable decisions about continued work. Performance rating systems that are comprehensive, communicative, rational, and fair have been upheld by the courts in age discrimination cases.

The U.S. Employment Service is probably the primary resource available to elderly job seekers. A network of approximately 2600 local employment security agencies facilitates the exchange of labor by coordinating information on job applications and job vacancies. Ideally, services that include testing, counseling, and referral to jobs and training are provided without a charge to all job applicants. Scarce agency resources, however, impose practical constraints on the services actually offered. More than 25 percent of older job seekers attempt to use the U.S. Employment Service. Only a small proportion of these receive services beyond the filing of a standard application (U.S. Senate Special Committee on Aging, 1982a).

Some employers retire employees and then rehire them as consultants or advisors on a part-time basis. Some retired workers are reemployed part time in adjunct roles or in seasonal periods. For example, a custodian might be rehired to work 2 hours a day during the evening or night. A secretary might be able to fill in during the summer for vacation relief.

Retirement

Few people venture into totally new activities in retirement (Fig. 5.8). Instead, preexisting interests tend to expand to fill the time left vacant by loss of the work role (Kasschau, 1976, p. 20). If individuals must assume new roles in retirement as substitutes for work activities, then formal socialization of elderly workers to the opportunities available is essential. Although most companies do not have preretirement planning, the numbers and percentage of those that do offer such planning has been increasing steadily. Among employers that do offer preretirement programs, about 30 percent cover a broad range of topics, 40 percent cover a more limited range of topics, and 30 percent cover only the narrowest range of topics—social security and company pension benefits (Kasschau, 1976; Robb, 1978; U.S. Senate Special Committee on Aging, 1982a, p. 283).

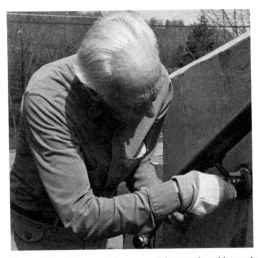

Figure 5.8. Retirement from one job may lead to work at another. *(Photograph by Shawn Mertz, Pittsburgh, PA.)*

Volunteering

Opportunities for volunteer work are widely available. A number of volunteer programs have operated exclusively or primarily with elderly volunteers, including the Foster Grandparent Program (FGP), Retired Senior Volunteer Program (RSVP), Senior Companion Program (SCP), and the Senior Corps of Retired Executives (SCORE)–Active Corps of Executives (ACE) organization. Some volunteer programs are available only to old people with low incomes. Participants are usually reimbursed for out-of-pocket expenses, such as travel to the volunteer activity. Some programs provide an hourly stipend, meals, an annual physical examination, and insurance benefits. Churches, hospitals, and long-term health care institutions have a long tradition of using volunteers to supplement regular staff. In 1974, a National Council on the Aging Study estimated that over 40,000 Americans aged 65 and over were serving as volunteers in educational institutions alone. More interesting was the fact that almost twice as many volunteers could have been recruited *if asked.*

Studies that compare elderly volunteers with nonvolunteers generally show that volunteers have much higher levels of life satisfaction, stronger will to live, and fewer symptoms of depression (Hunter and Linn, 1980–81). These differences are not explained by differences in health status or other background factors such as age, sex, income, or education. Although these differences create the impression that participation in volunteer activities causes improvement in psychosocial status, this impression needs to be tested. Such a test would require evaluating a group of elderly people who have symptoms of depression, anxiety or general dissatisfaction with life before and after their involvement in a program of volunteer activities. Information about the feasibility of involving nonvolunteers in volunteer programs is needed to guide nurses' practice.

The following example illustrates one instance where nurses acted to help elderly people help each other through volunteer efforts. The Department of Nursing of the State University of New York at Farmingdale collaborated with The Nassau County Department of

Senior Citizen Affairs and the Suffolk County Office for the Aging and, with partial funding from the New York State Office for the Aging, conducted a 5-year demonstration training project. The purpose of the project was to test the feasibility of developing older adult, non-professional volunteers as new personnel resources in home health care. A total of 250 older adults enrolled in the training programs. Most of the participants had no prior experience in working with older people and most were women. Six months after training, about 75 of those trained were actively engaged in providing home health support services on a voluntary basis to elderly relatives or home bound peers. A few were receiving a fee for their services. Those who were not active cited as reasons transportation problems, not wishing to be "tied down," and conflicting family responsibilities (Heller, Walsh, and Wilson, 1981).

Political Activism

Political activism is an emerging role for senior citizens. The question of whether or not the elderly are a growing force in American politics is controversial and the answer is unclear. Among the different views held are (1) the increasing proportion of old people within the population alone provides adequate evidence of "senior power" on a mass basis, (2) increasing proportions of old people *plus* the problems of age discrimination and economic hardships will prompt the elderly to develop as an organized political force, and (3) the elderly will not emerge as a viable political force in the foreseeable future because of their strong party identifications and ideologic conservatism (Miller, Gurin, and Gurin, 1980).

Analysis of voter participation in the 1976, 1978, and 1980 presidential and congressional elections revealed the following patterns despite a long-term trend toward lower voting turnouts. The highest percentage voting remained with the middle aged population, followed by the 65–74 group, the 75 plus group, and finally, the 18–44 group. In the 1980 election, whites voted in greater proportions than blacks, who voted in larger proportions than Hispanics. Overall, persons aged 65 and older

made up 15.4 percent of the voting age population but cast 16.8 percent of the votes (Brotman, 1981, p. 28).

Studies of political involvement on the part of elderly people do support the following conclusions:

1. People who are internally oriented, that is, who believe that their actions can change the outcome of situations and problems they confront in life, are more likely to be politically active than externally oriented people, who believe that the outcome of these situations and problems depends on factors beyond their control (Cox, 1980).
2. Identification with the age group of old people, plus a feeling that old people can increase their influence in society, promotes political participation and equalizes the extent of involvement despite social class differences (Trela, 1977–78; Miller, Gurin, and Gurin, 1980).

These findings suggest a couple of strategies for nurses to use in encouraging elderly clients to participate in political matters. One approach is to select clients with internal loci of control or take steps to increase clients' feelings of internal control. The second approach is to encourage clients to participate in organizations comprised largely of elderly people. Here, clients will be exposed to the views of others to whom they can relate and encouraged to express their own views.

Major senior-citizen organizations have been in existence only since the early 1960s. Political activities make up only a small part of the services and activities these organizations offer to members. Examples of national organizations for the elderly that engage in political activities are the Gray Panthers, The National Council on Aging (NCOA), and the combined American Association of Retired Persons–National Retired Teachers Association (AARP–NRTA).

The *AARP–NRTA* organization focuses on self-help through group health insurance, mail order pharmacy services, and money market opportunities. Lobbyists maintain liaisons with government officials and ensure that the organization presents testimony to congressional committees. The AARP–NRTA claims the largest voting block, with 13.3 million full-time members (Champlin, 1982b).

The *Gray Panthers,* founded by Maggie Kuhn as a coalition between young and old to protest the Vietnam war in the early 1970s, also lobby on Capitol Hill. However, this organization places an emphasis on vocal activism that takes the form of marches, protest signs, and press conferences. Gray Panthers rely on their numbers for political influence, rather than their money. Members are urged to write to their legislators. Coalitions are formed with other groups to increase the numbers; for example, the nursing home industry on long-term care issues and the insurance industry on health-care reimbursement. An estimated 60,000 people belong to the Gray Panthers (Champlin, 1982b).

The *National Council on Aging* is a nonprofit organization established to assist professionals who work with the elderly. The Council supports research on the problems of the elderly, provides training education and consultation for people who work with older people, and attempts to shape public policy regarding the elderly. Membership is open to both individuals and groups and in 1982 numbered between 3 and 4 million people (Champlin, 1982b).

Education
Free time in the later years might be spent in adult or continuing education. Local colleges and universities have a number of experimental educational and vocational programs for the elderly. However, the percentage of old people involved in classroom endeavors is quite small. Fewer than 2.5 percent of those people aged 65 years and over enroll for organized instruction, and those who do participate are largely from the higher socioeconomic groups (U.S. Senate Special Committee on Aging, 1982a, p. 447).

The 1970s produced a great deal of material on education and aging, most of which focused on education as self-enrichment. In the 1980s the trend has been toward programs geared to self-sufficiency for adults (including older adults) whose educational needs had been inadequately served.

Because educational levels have increased over time, older people are not as well educated as those in the following generations. In 1979, about half of all older Americans had less than a 10th grade education, about 9 percent were "functionally illiterate," having had no schooling or less than 5 years, and about 8 percent were college graduates (Brotman, 1982, p. 26). However, the increasing educational attainment of the older population was apparent in the increase of more than 1 year in the median number of school years completed that occurred between 1970 and 1980. Although these people may be too intimidated to return to a classroom situation, the elderly in the future may be more interested in returning to formal education because of prior exposure. Slightly more popular with old people are short-term educational programs, sponsored by their church, library, and secondary school, that teach crafts and skills or explore topics of interest, such as changes in tax laws that affect senior citizens.

Value orientation toward education must be considered in trying to attract elderly people to adult/continuing education programs. People aged 60 and over are usually socioculturally and improvement-learning oriented toward education. Among institutional characteristics that attract old people, the location and the nature of educational programs offered are the most important considerations (Daniel, Templin, and Shearon, 1977).

Although most elderly people are no longer concerned with converting their educational gains into wages, changes in the economy may reverse this situation. From a health service perspective, poorly educated older adults often have trouble finding out about services and, when they do, find the paperwork and bureaucratic hurdles built into such programs difficult to deal with. Nurses may be able to reduce some of these barriers by identifying education-related capabilities of elderly clients early in the assessment process.

Implications for Nurses
When trying to influence leisure patterns, the nurse must realize that the odds are against an elderly person's taking up new activities

unless an effort is made to socialize him to the activity. If asked, some old people will volunteer. Thus, the nurse must do more than simply suggest, "Mr. S, you ought to find something to do with yourself. How about the Gray Panthers?" If Mr. S has never been a joiner, is not familiar with the group, and receives no support, such as Gray Panther literature or an opportunity to discuss the impact of participation on his life-style, he will not act on the nurse's suggestion. If the goal is to change Mr. S's leisure habits, the nurse stands a better chance of success when she does the following:

1. Obtains a history of Mr. S's past use of leisure
2. Selects an activity that relates to his past interest and is appropriate for his current resources
3. Plans specifically with Mr. S for incorporation of the activity into his life-style

For example, if the history reveals an interest in bowling but Mr. S. is now confined to a wheelchair, the nurse might locate a bowling alley proprietor near Mr. S's home who would be willing to ask Mr. S to volunteer to work at the rental desk during "off hours" when help is difficult to hire. The proprietor might visit Mr. S to request his help in return for transportation to and from the bowling alley.

A fine line exists between respect for the client's right to choose and the health professional's responsibility to promote healthful behavior. Some nurses believe that if activity options are reasonably available to the elderly client they have no further role to play. However, dramatic improvements in morale have resulted when the nurse made a special effort to restructure the immediate environment to promote the old person's involvement in activities. The client who says he doesn't want a television may be saying he cannot see well, cannot hear well, and has no money. The sudden appearance of a wide-screen television with special volume control, provided by the television dealer as part of a "pilot project," might cause him to change his point of view. A "lost" kitten found on the doorstep with the morning paper may brighten the life of a lonely old person. The nurse who intervenes for the purpose

of changing leisure patterns in elderly people needs both creativity and the skills of a successful salesperson.

LEGAL RESOURCES

The Elderly as Victims

Criminologists and gerontologists agree that the American elderly are not a highly victimized group and that younger age groups are more likely to be criminally victimized (Cook and Cook, 1976; Antunes, Cook, Cook, and Skogan, 1977; Hochstedler, 1981). Victimization notes from the National Crime Survey conducted by the U.S. Department of Justice for the years 1973–80 indicated the elderly are victims of violent crimes such as rape, robbery, and assault at an annual rate of 8 per 1000 population while the rate for the under-65 population is 37 per 1000. For crimes of theft, which include personal larceny with or without contact, the rates are 24 per 1000 compared to 104 per 1000 for the under 65 population. Age is not the only factor that affects the likelihood of personal victimization. For example, victimization rates for personal crimes are relatively higher for males, younger persons, nonwhites, the poor, and for persons divorced, separated, or never married (Liang and Sengstock, 1981). Characteristics of the environment are also related to rates of personal victimization. These may include population density, inner-city location, proportion of one-person households, and age and affluence of the neighborhood (Liang and Sengstock, 1981; O'Brien, Shichor, and Decker, 1982–83).

However, significance of criminal victimization of the aged is not entirely a question of victimization rates. There are at least three factors that intensify criminal victimization as a problem for the aged. First, the aged are more fearful of criminal victimization than are younger age groups (Adams and Smith, 1976; Clemente and Kleiman, 1976; Ollenburger, 1981). In addition, women and residents of densely populated areas are more fearful than their counterparts (Clemente and Kleiman, 1976).

The second intensifying factor is found in

the differential impact of the criminal acts. The aged are generally a lower income group living on fixed incomes. Thus, even a small loss can have a large impact upon an elderly person (Cook, Skogan, Cook, and Antunes, 1978). The elderly are also more likely to be injured when attacked; they suffer wounds and broken bones less than others, but suffer more internal injuries and are more likely to lose consciousness or suffer cuts and bruises. They are not more likely to need medical care, but if they receive it, its costs will constitute a much larger proportion of their income than is the case for other age groups.

The third factor that magnifies the impact of victimization for the aged is the location of violent crimes. Compared to other age groups, the aged are more likely to be victimized in or near their homes (Antunes, Cook, Cook, and Skogan, 1977). This suggests that the elderly cannot avoid the places where they are most often victimized. To the extent that old people fear leaving their homes and avoid doing so, they become victims whether or not they are ever actually criminally victimized.

Two conclusions can be derived from studies completed in the area of victimization among the aged. First, wide variations that occur in victimization rates among different subgroups of the aged population (Liang and Sengstock, 1981) make it premature to dismiss criminal victimization as a social problem for the elderly simply because they have the lowest overall average victimization rate among all age groups. Second, attention needs to be focused on more than observed rates of victimization to include reduction of fear of crime and compensation for victims of crime.

The judicial system can be viewed as a means for making elderly people less desirable targets for criminals and others who set out to violate their rights when and if the punishments serve as deterrents to future perpetrators. However, among crimes reported by people of all ages, only 12 percent end up in arrest, 6 percent in conviction, and 1 percent in imprisonment (Powell, 1980, p. 30). Thus, the judicial system probably does not serve to make elderly people less vulnerable to crime.

Approaches to Protection

Approaches to prevent victimization by criminals can be categorized by whether they reduce the (1) availability, (2) vulnerability, or (3) desirability of the elderly person (Skogan and Kleca, 1976).

Availability

Many old people cope with fear of crime by staying home, often alone, in what amounts to a self-imposed prison sentence. Security-intensive retirement living centers have been suggested as a means to reduce the vulnerability of the elderly to crime. However, such segregation of the elderly may have undesirable consequences, leading to social isolation and feelings of false security. A better solution seems to be congregate living arrangements. Certainly old people who hope to deter burglars should follow the recommendations of local police departments: security locks, alarm systems, dog(s), possession engraving, and so on. Unfortunately, many of these deterrents are too expensive for the elderly.

Vulnerability

The elderly might be made less vulnerable by increasing their capabilities for self-help. Courses in self-defense are possible. However, crime victims of any age risk "backfire" injury if they try to resist a criminal assault. It is probably safer for old people to join in group activities and escort programs, which make attack by criminals more difficult. Increased police surveillance tends to be too costly for taxpayer pocketbooks.

Desirability

Desirability of the elderly as crime targets might be reduced if old people made it a habit to carry little or no cash. Deposit of welfare assistance and Social Security checks directly into the bank accounts of the elderly may also reduce target desirability. Increased penalties for those who commit crimes against the elderly are a possibility, but the merits of this approach must be balanced by drawbacks such as the social consequences of prolonged jail or prison sentences. Encouraging the elderly to report crimes and press charges against the criminal is not likely to be too successful, since many old people fear reprisal by the offender or others.

Role of the Law

The law has been both a friend and an enemy of the elderly. Recognition of the civil rights and legal needs of the elderly has led to the emergence of legal services as a component of social services. Court suits have compelled providers of social services to initiate or improve services to the elderly. The law has also been a tool for expansion of their rights and privileges.

Unfortunately, the law has also been used to hurt the elderly through incompetency and involuntary commitment proceedings, which share a number of similarities. Both tend to be directed at the elderly. Both are presumed to be benevolent legal actions to protect the person who is unable to manage his affairs wisely and who is not willing to admit his deficiency. Both lead to suspension of the individual's civil rights. Both are usually conducted as something less than genuine adversary proceedings. In both proceedings, psychiatric terminology with little legal precision is heavily relied upon.

One body of opinion believes that there is no such thing as a scientifically valid definition of mental illness (Szasz, 1961, 1970). Court rulings against involuntary commitment and legal attacks on incompetency proceedings reflect increasing doubt that treatment of "mentally infirm" persons can be successful. Involuntary treatment in a long-term care facility and appointment of a legal guardian to manage affairs may not be in the individual's best interests.

Incompetency actions place the elderly person's property under the control of the guardian. Those who bring incompetency proceedings are usually potential heirs to the old person's estate or hospitals seeking to recover the costs of treatment. Incompetence usually refers to memory loss. Most elderly people found to be incompetent are prohibited from making decisions about their financial affairs. They usually end up involuntarily committed to long-term care institutions. Their property is rarely protected against the day when they might be proven competent. Recommendations have been made to increase protection for these old people, who stand to lose their civil rights and also their liberty.

Affluent people have always been able to find a lawyer to act as their advocate. In recent years, the poor have also found reasonably adequate legal representation through community legal service groups. The middle class probably has the least access to legal representation; their incomes are too high to qualify them for free services but too low to afford the minimum fee schedules adopted by most bar associations. Like other agencies serving as resources for the elderly, legal service agencies are usually underfunded and inadequately distributed. Although most lawyers working in these agencies are burdened by excessive case loads, many people who could use the service are never reached.

Efforts have been made to tap unused legal training by utilizing law students under the supervision of retired or semiretired lawyers. In some situations, paralegal personnel have been trained to locate older people and screen them for legal needs. In other cases, an organization for the elderly that can afford the expense hires a lawyer, who then represents members of that group without charge. Thus, elderly people who belong to organizations should inquire about the availability of legal services.

A few cities and states have established small claims courts that prohibit either party from retaining an attorney. The plaintiff and defendant both tell their stories to a hearing examiner, who arbitrates a settlement. If the hearing examiner fails to arrive at a settlement, a judge decides the case. Small claims courts permit a consumer to sue a merchant without costly legal help and with a fair chance of winning.

The consumer movement has been helpful to the elderly in at least two ways. First, people who might have been too embarrassed or simply reluctant to seek help have begun to protest being defrauded, perhaps because they realize their problem is not unique. Second, the consumer movement has led to formation of groups that represent aggrieved consumers and publicize frauds.

Consumer Fraud

The elderly are also potential victims in the marketplace. They are usually less able to cope with problems familiar to most consumers: the average of 23 problems associated with each new car purchased; the computer billing errors that can only be corrected in person; or the rotten onions concealed on the bottom of the bag, to name a few.

Old people are particularly susceptible to frauds and confidence games, such as quack medicines, home improvement schemes, and real estate swindles. Despite a lack of reliable data to describe the scope of the financial, physical, or emotional impact of frauds against the elderly, testimony before the House and Senate Aging Committee has provided some clues. Such consequences range from small, but embarrassing, financial losses to actual loss of life from suicide, as a result of losing a life's hard-earned savings, and death caused by abandonment of traditional treatments in favor of "miracle cures" (U.S. Senate Special Committee on Aging, 1982a, p. 469). One investigation in California indicated that more than 90 percent of fraud victims are over 65, and most are women. Seven out of every 10 cases of medical fraud reported in California were against elderly people (Younger, 1976). Each of these problems relate to the purchase of goods and services and cost the consumer time, effort, and money—resources that are in short supply for many old people.

Factors that contribute to the vulnerability of the elderly to consumer frauds and deceptions include health concerns, limited incomes, home ownership, assumption of new roles, lowered awareness, limited mobility, isolation, sensory impairment, and limited education (U.S. Senate Special Committee on Aging, 1982a, pp. 469–471). Illness or fear of illness prompts use of phony or unproven "cures." Limited incomes encourage investment in bogus investment schemes. A majority of old people own homes built before 1940. These homeowners, especially those who live in poverty or near poverty, are victimized by a common and lucrative fraud—phony home repair. A large segment of the elderly population are widows who lack experience making economic decisions, although they may be very proficient in some consumer areas. Consequently, in their widowhood, they become more susceptible to home repair and investment fraud. As a group, elderly people tend to be less aware of unfair business practices (Perloff and McCaskey, 1978). Limited mobility renders them liable to fraudulent practices that appear to provide easy accessibility, such as work-at-home and door-to-door schemes. Living and feeling lonely increases the vulnerability of some elderly people to con artists who appear friendly and offer their companionship as a means of gaining access to the home. Vision and learning impairments reduce elderly peoples' ability to receive consumer information and conduct transactions with confidence. These reduced abilities are further decreased when elderly people lack reading and writing skills.

Measures to protect elderly people from fraud and deception have been slow in developing. In 1982 the Senate Special Committee on Aging was holding hearings on the problem and introducing legislation to strengthen the U.S. Postal Service's ability to combat frauds involving the mail. By evaluating each elderly client's risk-for-fraud profile in terms of the factors listed above, nurses may be able to initiate teaching and arrange for resources to meet specific needs (such as chore or home-repair services) that will enhance the client's ability to resist fraudulent schemes.

Guardianship

When people are not capable of making decisions that affect their lives, the legal system may be asked to empower another person to make decisions for that individual through the process of guardianship. Judicial criteria for determining functional impairment require clarification. However, several tests of competence, often overlapping, have been used (Kapp, 1981, p. 366):

- Can the person make choices concerning his life?
- Are the outcomes of these choices "reasonable"?
- Are these choices based on "rational" reasons?
- Is the person able to understand the implications of the choices made?
- Does the person actually understand the implications of the choices?

A judicial finding of incompetence signifies that a person, because he is not able to make rational decisions, cannot care adequately for himself or his property. A court-appointed guardian (a person, an association, or a corporation) assumes total control over the individual's personal and business decisions. For the most part, guardianships are created without adequate administrative or statutory mechanisms to ensure that guardianship proceedings are conducted in accordance with due process and result in the least restrictive alternative for the elderly (Morrissey, 1982, p. 301). At a typical hearing, the party requesting the incompetency decision (petitioner), that party's attorney, and the judge are the only ones present, who take active roles in the decision-making process. Medical evidence is weighed heavily in determining incompetency without any clear indication as to how a given diagnosis actually affects the person's ability to manage his affairs. The individual whose competency is being decided is seldom present or represented by counsel. In just a few minutes, in an informal setting, the individual may lose such basic rights as the right to vote, initiate litigation, execute a contract, or engage in business or professional activities. The decision is rarely reversed; even when it is, the individual is stigmatized with the label of "incompetent" for the remainder of his life.

The following situation represents a typical instance of guardianship assignment.

Mary Eustace, a frail widow in her early eighties, informally entrusted most of her personal and business affairs to her son-in-law. Her daughter, an only child, had died many years earlier. As it became more and more difficult for Ms. Eus-

tace even to write checks or sign papers because of her increasing frailty, her son-in-law suggested she grant him a power of attorney. She did this, still in full possession of her faculties.

Eventually, and of her own volition, she entered a nursing home. After several months there, she told her son-in-law that an aide had suggested that if Ms. Eustace would deed her house and estate to her, she (the aide) would take Ms. Eustace back to her home and care for her there the rest of her life. Ms. Eustace—by now confused about her age, condition, and everything else—had decided to agree to this arrangement.

Inasmuch as her son-in-law still held the power of attorney, he discussed the matter with Ms. Eustace's physician, who declared her to be now mentally incompetent. Her son-in-law (who was not her heir) petitioned the court to appoint him her guardian. This was granted and he managed her affairs until she died six months later (Kapp, 1981, p. 366).

Resources the elderly might use to protect their rights in guardianship proceedings are almost nonexistent (Kapp, 1981; Morrissey, 1982). One possibility is the *guardian ad litem* or counsel or both, who almost every state requires be appointed to represent the allegedly incompetent or incapacitated person. The guardian ad litem is not a representative of the court; his purpose is to protect the individual's liberty from being taken away via a guardianship. The Commonwealth of Virginia developed a manual to help educate guardians ad litem about the elderly and ways to make the proceedings more formal and adversarial in nature (Morrissey, 1982).

Nurses might want to address the problem of inadequate protection of the rights of elderly more actively than they have in the past. As a beginning, nurses might visit courts where such proceedings are held and review the book, *A Piano for Mrs. Cimino* (Oliphant, 1980). A next step might be to inform attorneys, judges, and others about myths concerning "senility" and normal aging. Research could be conducted to answer questions such as, How often are people declared incompetent resistant to the guardianship? To what extent do attorneys assume an advocacy and adversarial role in guardianship proceedings? What proportion of guardianships are established solely because the individuals cannot care for health-related needs? Nurses could introduce a model statute on public guardianship.

Elder Abuse

Elder abuse is another crime that victimizes elderly people and that has received increasing attention in the 1980s. One survey of 1000 health professionals in Massachusetts revealed that almost every profession considered had come into contact with or suspected elder abuse by family members. One hundred eighty-three respondents reported citing elder abuse during the previous 18 months and indicated incidents tended to happen repeatedly to the same person (Crime, 1980). Twenty interviews with 77 victims of elder abuse revealed five types of abuse: direct physical abuse (20 percent), physical neglect (23 percent), financial abuse (55 percent), psychologic neglect (23 percent), and psychologic abuse (58 percent). Many cases, as evident from the overlapping percentages, suffered multiple types of abuse. Children were the abusers in over half of the cases, while the remaining half were spouses, grandchildren, siblings, roomers, and landlords (Elder abuse study, 1982).

Abuse of the elderly represents a problem in which resources to help victims are almost nonexistent. Legal, medical, and social restraints make prevention of the problem more difficult than its detection. Financial assistance for state prevention, identification, and treatment programs has not been available. A few demonstration projects have been established on a temporary basis. An example is the Elder Abuse Project operated by the Elder Home Care Services of the Worchester, Massachusetts area (Champlin, 1982a). This program worked with 60 abuse victims in the first year, sending a homemaker or personal care-giver into the home on a regular basis. The victims were thus provided with adequate care while the home environment was monitored to discourage further neglect or abuse.

Elder abuse is a problem where concerned nurses play an important part in developing service and support options. At least two nurses have published detailed assessment guides and suggested actions nurses can take to intervene in specific cases and to prevent the problem of elder abuse (Johnson, 1981; Falcioni, 1982). Nurses need to join other concerned people in demanding the resources required to prevent elder abuse. Resources commonly identified in the literature (Phillips, 1980a,b; Hickey and Douglass, 1981; Hooyman and Tomita, 1981; Johnson, 1981; Champlin, 1982a; Elder abuse study, 1982; Falcioni, 1982; Sengstock, Barrett, and Graham, 1982) include:

1. Programs of public education to increase awareness of professional and lay members
2. Relief services for care-givers
3. Mandatory reporting legislation similar to child abuse legislation in every state
4. Protective services similar to those available for child abuse victims, such as a system of foster care, court-appointed guardians, and shelters
5. Research to discover how definitions of abuse are translated into identification of abusers, determination of characteristics that predispose individuals and their care-givers to a pattern of abuse, and so forth
6. Counseling for *both* abuser and abused

RELIGION

Role of Religion

Religion may be a resource to help the elderly resolve questions of the meaning of life and of adversity or good fortune. Involvement in religion may also provide a source of leisure activity. Evidence suggests that religion is not likely to be initially adopted in old age. Thus, people who have been religious during their earlier years may be able to benefit from their involvement. However, essentially nonreligious people are unlikely to turn to religion for support simply because they have grown old (Fig. 5.9).

There is little consensus about whether religious behavior, sometimes called religiosity, in old age results from the aging process itself or from generational differences reflecting changes in the emphasis that society places upon religion (Riley and Foner, 1968). Win-

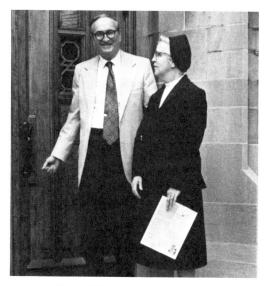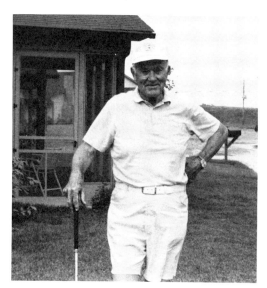

Figure 5.9. Sunday morning reveals formalized religion to be relevant for some elderly people and not for others. *(Photograph by Nance Photo, Pittsburgh, PA.)*

grove and Alston (1971) studied church attendance of five cohorts (groups) of white people by viewing their rates of attendance at six points in time between 1939 and 1969. They concluded that although variation in attendance was related to age, each group demonstrated a unique attendance profile. Nearly all groups experienced their peaks in church attendance between 1950 and 1960, a period of limited religious revival in the United States. Thus, factors other than age influence church attendance patterns: sex, specific cohort membership, and the prevailing social view of religion. Ethnicity may also be an important influence on church attendance. Both blacks and Mexican-Americans have been found to be more active in attending church than whites (Antunes and Gaitz, 1975).

Various definitions of religiosity from one study to another make results difficult to interpret. For example, in one review of 14 studies (Moberg, 1965b) that defined religious behavior by church attendance, the reviewer found four that indicated an increase in religious practices with age, eight that found a decrease starting at age 60 years, and two studies that found religious practices to be consistent throughout the life cycle, except for a decline in very old age.

Religion may provide meaning and identity (Moberg, 1965a,b; Moberg and Taves, 1965; Edwards and Klemmack, 1973; Cutler, 1976; Blazer and Palmore, 1976; Guy, 1982; Heisel and Faulkner, 1982). However, religion, "can also promote ethnocentricity and even infantilism" (Tellis-Nayak, 1982, p. 360). Attitudes toward religion have been found unrelated to personal adjustment (Havighurst and Albrecht, 1953; Barron, 1961). Religiosity does not protect people from loneliness or fear of death, nor do lonely people necessarily tend to turn to religion (O'Reilly, 1958). Strong beliefs, either in terms of religion or atheism, have been equally associated with reducing death fears (Kalish, 1976).

Religious Cults

In recent years, religious cults have begun active programs to recruit older members. Defining a cult is problematic in that it is difficult to discern "healthy" from "harmful" and "religious choice" from "brainwashed belief." One definition characterizes cult as a belief system/group in which coercion and deception are used to solicit members. Heavy emphasis is placed upon donation of material possessions or large amounts of physical labor for the good of the group. Members generally swear allegiance to a leader with absolute authority, who forbids questioning of decisions (Rudin and Rudin, 1980). Examples of cult groups include the Unification Church founded by the Reverend Sun Myung Moon, the Church Universal and Triumphant (CUT), the International Society for Krishna Consciousness (Hare Krishna), The Way International, The Divine Light Mission, Church of God, Church of Scientology, Church of Armageddon (Love Family), The Tony and Tusun Alamo Christian Foundation, and The Body of Christ (Rudin and Rudin, 1980).

The responsibility of health professionals is to enable older persons to protect themselves from coercion. What cults offer older people, rather than what they take from them, is perhaps more important. Cult membership may provide opportunities for elderly people to (1) give and feel essential, (2) separate themselves from discredited major institutions such as the scientific community, the military, big business, academia, and the family, (3) pursue a total and perfect solution to an unsatisfying and imperfect world, or (4) enjoy structure and direction in a society that is seen as confusing and rapidly changing. The most important cause of cult appeal, however, is probably the need to be a part of a caring community—a way to connect with others to dispel loneliness and alienation that people may experience at any age.

It appears that the most vulnerable target group for cult recruitment is the person, young or old, who has made no meaningful connection with an established religion, who is in search of spiritual values and transcendent meaning, who is willing, even yearning for strict discipline and authority, and who may be burdened with guilt about affluence, sex, or drugs. Such a person may enthusiastically make the sacrifices necessary to maintain the love of the cult leader and of his peers within the group. In an age of dislocation, when everything and everyone seems rootless and in flux, when one's own family is seen as superficial and vapid, one's own religion

as irrelevant and relativistic; and society as chaotic and uncaring, the absolute claims, guarantees, and promises of cult life are appealing (Rudin and Rudin, 1980, pp. 116–117).

Implications for Nurses

The phenomenon of religious commitment has been defined as consisting of five dimensions: experiential, ideologic, ritualistic, intellectual, and consequential (Glock, 1962; Glock and Stark, 1965). High religiosity in one dimension does not necessarily mean that the person will be religious in another dimension.

Nurses need to examine various dimensions of religiosity during assessment in order to understand clients' religious commitments. Depending on the importance of religion to the individual, the nurse can aid the elderly person to achieve optimum support from religion by providing transportation to religious group gatherings or alternative methods of religious fulfillment when failing health precludes travel. When religion proves to be irrelevant to individual clients, the nurse needs to draw upon other sources of support when the individual needs to cope with various life crises. When nurses want to intervene to discourage client involvement in cults, a strategy based on substituting benefits the older person receives from cult membership needs to be considered.

SIGNIFICANT OTHERS

A number of societal forces have influenced the family's role in caring for aging members. Demographic trends have reduced the number of relatives to whom an old person may turn for assistance. At the same time, parents are more likely to live out the full number of years theoretically available to them. Some of the extremely old live long enough to pose a threat to their children, who themselves wish to retire free from financial obligations and demands on their time. The changes in women's roles, particularly the change from homemaker to wage earner, have created obligations that compete with responsibilities to elderly parents.

Economic forces have decreased the power

of the elderly to demand support from their children. When our economy was agriculturally based, the parent could retain title to the property in exchange for support until time of death. Our present post-industrial society, with its growing welfare system, has freed adult children and their parents from economic dependence on each other. The elderly no longer have financial power over their children, nor are they totally dependent upon them for financial support. Substitution of emotional for economic bonds appears to be an acceptable trend. Indeed, parents now seem to expect more from their offspring in terms of social and affective support than in instrumental and economic assistance. Parents' expectations of responsibilities to be assumed by adult offspring are inversely associated with morale, at least in modern, urban settings (Seelback and Sauer, 1977). This suggests that elderly people with "extended" expectations are out of tune with the expectations of their children. When children neglect them, or fail to live up to parental expectations, the parents' morale suffers more than if their expectations had been consistent with norms characteristic of small (nuclear) families.

Regardless of parental expectations, however, family resources often become overextended in the day-to-day supervision of elderly relatives. There are simply too few adult children to share the responsibilities. Relatives with the best of intentions often find that custodial care of an elderly parent is too much to assume in the face of competing responsibilities. When relationships with the old person have been unsatisfactory in earlier years, relatives are not likely even to attempt such care.

Often overlooked is the possibility that significant others may not act in the best interests of the elderly person. Mr. and Mrs. N had been married over 50 years when he began to show signs of memory loss and to change his sleeping habits so that he was frequently up at night. Mrs. N, who viewed her own health as "not good," gradually changed her patterns to fit Mr. N's. She began to sleep only when Mr. N slept, and had food delivered so she could "keep an eye on Mr. N lest he injure himself

or wander away." Exhausted after several months, Mrs. N called her daughter-in-law, a social worker, to ask if "some kind of tranquilizer might help or if Mr. N should be put in a nursing home." The daughter-in-law visited and found that with the exercise of getting out of the house daily for an extended period of time and a glass of sherry at bedtime, Mr. N was able to sleep through the night. Believing that the situation had improved, the daughter-in-law returned home. Two weeks later, Mr. N was placed in a nursing home, where he developed pneumonia and died within 3 weeks. The exact reason for this decision was never revealed to the daughter-in-law who, because of living far away from the situation, was reluctant to ask too many questions. One possible explanation is that the mother-in-law found the exercise regimen more burdensome than the less effective interventions with which she was more familiar. A second explanation is that the mother-in-law had already made up her mind to place Mr. N in a nursing home before she asked for help from her daughter-in-law. Unconscious commitment to this intention may have led the mother-in-law to sabotage the exercise and sherry interventions. Perhaps too, the interventions that were effective initially (while the daughter-in-law was present) were not effective after several days. Sometimes a person who enters a nursing home or dies leaves behind years of neglect, intentional or unintentional. Perhaps if interventions had been started at the first signs of memory loss or if Mrs. N had been able to share the burden of care with someone, Mr. N might have been able to stay at home longer. Sometimes a person who enters a nursing home or dies leaves behind years of neglect.

The case of Mr. and Mrs. N raises a number of questions. How many impaired elderly people are maintained at home without the benefits of memory development techniques, a bladder continence program, or contact with people outside the home? Is failure to seek services for such elderly people sometimes deliberate on the part of significant others?

Despite these considerations, the family remains the major caretaker for the ill old person. In the United States, from two to three times as many people are cared for at home as are cared for in institutions of all kinds* (Brotman, 1981, p. 12). Families have been estimated to provide 70 to 80 percent of the long-term care services in this country (Shanas, 1979; U.S. Special Committee on Aging, 1982a). This fact is often overlooked, perhaps because of the trend toward separate households. However, separation of generations into separate households is probably due more to adequate income than to weakening of family ties. People move apart when housing is available and affordable, and because the telephone and readily available transportation make maintenance of family ties feasible even at a distance.

Support for the family in providing care for its elderly members has recently been considered as a policy alternative in the United States. The idea of awarding cash payments and tax credits to families who assume responsibilities for the elderly is a reaction against the long-term care institution, with its negative connotations and high costs. This policy direction, however, may conflict with the wishes of some families.

The view of the family as an alternative resource to government-provided programs differs among whites, blacks, and Mexican-Americans (Bengtson, 1976). Whites, who tend to have fewer children, speak generally about the importance of "family or individual" responsibility, as opposed to "government" responsibility. However, they strongly oppose living with or being financially supported by children. In contrast, Mexican-Americans have the highest number of children, interact with them more frequently, and expect them to help out as needed. Blacks mention the importance of family or individual responsibility for meeting the needs of the elderly slightly less often than Mexican-Americans. However, like whites, both groups attributed much greater responsibility to "government" in providing for needs.

---

* Based on 5 percent of the elderly population residing in institutions in 1977 and 10 percent confined to bed at home or needing help in the house or neighborhood to 19 percent confined to bed, needing help in the house or neighborhood, or needing help outside the neighborhood.

The government was viewed by all three groups as most responsible for health care, and slightly less responsible for providing transportation (Bengtson, 1976).

For elderly Native Americans, the family structure appears to facilitate service utilization. In a study of 160 Native Americans (Murdock and Schwartz, 1978), more than half were found to live with their children. Perception of service needs, awareness of service agencies, and use of agency services were highest for those who lived with children. Thus, children may help their elderly parents to learn about services and to take advantage of them. Apparently, while Native Americans are less reluctant to live with children than some of the other ethnic elderly, they are willing to use public services when made aware of them.

Despite fragmentation of the family with regard to material and child-rearing roles, the parent-caring role may remain intact. A pattern seems to be emerging in which social institutions take over the financial support and health care of the elderly, while middle-aged children provide social and emotional support. That is, caring *about* is not necessarily the same as caring *for* the elderly person.

Working with Significant Others

Given the presence of significant others, nurses have a responsibility to educate those interested individuals about the changes of aging and appropriate functions for the elderly. Particularly when an old person resides in a long-term care facility, visitors often are not helped to understand that this is an acceptable setting for the elderly person, or to identify ways to show that they care about the individual. Many institutions for the poor elderly do not even provide individual telephones so that residents can keep in touch with significant others. Change is needed in this and other practices that deter contact between clients and significant others.

In some instances, families do not enjoy their visits to elderly relatives in long-term care facilities. Families of old people who were disheveled or confused seemed to have less enjoyable visits (York and Calsyn, 1977, p. 503). Families may need help in learning how to make such visits more satisfying. Instead of staying away when family members are visiting, nurses can intervene to assess what happens during the visit and determine family and client response to the experience. This might yield rewards in the form of more frequent family visits or more definitive involvement by the family in the actual care of the client.

Nurses often fail to utilize the expertise gained by the family in caring for the elderly person before he came to the nursing home. Despite chronic understaffing, nurses tend to feel that they are not doing their job if visitors make the client's bed, bathe him or, even "worse," take his temperature. To correct this situation, classes on aging might be held at times when the number of visitors is high—usually evenings and weekends—with both clients and family in attendance. This approach, even more than one-to-one teaching, could yield real gains for nurses, in return for a minimal investment of time and effort. Since families experience the greatest difficulty in coping with mental deterioration and mood disturbances, one of the topics for a class should be brain failure and associated behavior changes. A second focus should be on how to make visits productive and enjoyable. Too many families complain that they just sit and stare at their elderly relative for the duration of the visit. Surely an hour or more of one-to-one contact with an old person can be made to serve a more constructive purpose.

Unfortunately, both institutionalization *and* independent living may be interpreted by the elderly as abandonment by significant others. The fairness and truth of this judgment are debatable. Society offers few direct supports for those who elect to care for aging relatives. Problems in delivery of the few services available to support independent or quasi-independent living for old people make institutionalization the alternative with the least risk. Elderly people with support from significant others tend to be institutionalized as a "last resort" when social and financial resources are depleted and need to help with activities of daily living becomes great (Barney, 1977).

Most elderly people enter nursing homes directly from hospitals (York and Calsyn, 1977,

p. 502). Thus, physicians and social workers are important in influencing the decision for institutionalization. When this alternative is advised by the physician and seconded by the social worker, few families are likely to elect any other course of action. Families aware of other services are often reluctant to utilize them (York and Calsyn, 1977, p. 502). Nurses are in a position to encourage such utilization, but should be wary of taking this action. Waiting lists for good alternative services tend to be long. When funding is uncertain, as is often the case, services are apt to be terminated or cut back abruptly.

When families do elect to use alternative services, or to continue participation in the day-to-day care of aging relatives, the nurse is in a position to provide maximum support. Translated into action, this means teaching, supplying names and telephone numbers of community-based resource people, and follow-up calls to verify the acceptability of the decision or supply additional information or referral service. For example, the family might need to become familiar with principles and techniques of memory development to cope with the old person's mental deterioration. Physical devices, such as a lock to prevent use of the stove when no one is available to supervise, may have to be found and purchased.

Long waiting lists for admission to nursing homes often discourage families from searching for exactly the right setting for their elderly relative. Many do not even visit the facility before the old person is placed. Availability of a bed and location are the two principal factors influencing choice of a home (York and Calsyn, 1977, p. 502).

Families who decide to institutionalize elderly relatives ought not be made to feel guilty about their decision. Indeed, nurses can provide family members with a chance to discuss feelings about their decision by providing openings such as "Deciding to bring your (father, uncle) here probably wasn't easy for you."

Evidence indicates that families do not abandon the elderly person who is institutionalized. Rather, they continue contact through visiting and telephoning. York and Calsyn (1977, p. 503) found the mean number of visits to be 12 per month, with only two families visiting less than twice monthly. The number of visits were correlated with the amount of telephone contact, and the amount of preplacement family involvement was related to the amount of postplacement contact.

Families may become closer and more united as a result of placing an elderly person in an institution. Smith and Bengtson (1978) interviewed 100 parent–child pairs and identified six general patterns that reflected consequences for family relationships stemming from institutionalization:

1. Renewed closeness and strengthening of family ties (30 percent)
2. Discovery of love and affection (15 percent)
3. Continuation of closeness (25 percent)
4. Continuation of separateness (20 percent)
5. Quantity without quality interactions (10 percent)
6. Abdication—institutions as a dumping group (0 percent)

Improved parent–child relationships after the elderly parent is placed in an institution may relate to:

1. Alleviation of preadmission trauma
2. Improved physical and/or mental status of the parent
3. An opportunity to spend time together in recreational and interpersonal activities rather than caretaking ones
4. The parent's involvement with other residents in the institution

Finding Significant Others

Some elderly people have such negative relationships with their relatives that they might as well not have relatives at all. Others lack families and even acquaintances. This phenomenon increases as the person moves from old to very old age. Study results suggest that the greater the age difference (younger or older) between people, the greater the social distance they feel. Furthermore, people feel more socially distant from the elderly, regardless of their own age (Kidwell and Booth, 1977). That is, the elderly tend to feel distant from each other.

A confidant relationship may be more important to the quality of life than the quantity of interactions with family or friends (Strain and Chappell, 1982). A confidant is someone an individual confides in or talks to about himself or his problems (Powers and Bultena, 1976). A confidant relationship implies the following elements of quality: intimacy, dependency, regularity of interaction, and freedom of choice (Cantor, 1979). These qualities differentiate a confidant relationship from more casual, less demanding relationships with others. In searching for sources of social resources for elderly people, nurses need to consider peer and intergenerational relatives as possible confidants for clients. When clients need to choose between quantity and quality in relationships with others, the nurse may find counseling in the direction of quality relationships to be more effective.

Finding significant others for these solitary elderly people is not easy. One possibility is to organize the elderly to help each other. For example, small groups (about four to eight people) of elderly people might share the rent or mortgage on a home with enough room for both private spaces and shared living areas. The chances are good that someone will be home at all times to deter robbers. Not everyone will experience the same illness or incapacity at the same time, so one will be able to help another cope with poor health. Shopping and household chores can be shared.

The nurse is in a position to help overcome social distance barriers and bring the elderly together in self-help groups. Once the group is operational, the nurse can withdraw support. The nurse should not attempt to include mentally impaired persons in such groups. Observations of institutionalized elderly suggest that physically handicapped and physically able individuals will tend to help each other. However, mentally impaired and mentally able individuals avoid each other.

The idea of the elderly helping each other also has value for institutional settings. The nurse must again be prepared to facilitate formation of the group. The purpose of the group might be to take a stand on some issue such as client rights or the quality of food, to assist fellow residents in activities of daily living, or to engage in a recreational pursuit. Establishment of self-help groups for the elderly in institutional settings is particularly worthwhile because the nurse can invest a few hours initially to promote an activity that will eventually save her time (doing what the elderly can do for themselves) and frustration (wishing she could attend to more of the needs of the elderly than working conditions permit).

Occasionally, significant others can be found through "friendly visitor" programs. This type of program is probably one of the oldest social welfare services. Voluntary organizations, especially church-related groups, often sponsor this service, which provides visitors trained to listen and to identify problems or situations requiring referral. Elderly people may also be encouraged to use available telephone services. "Hot lines" exist for people who are depressed, lonely, or suicidal. Health information is available by telephone in some areas. Miss J, age 93 and living alone, was the only survivor of her family, except for a distant cousin. She began to talk to herself and to imagine that terrible things were happening. A telephone call interrupted her thoughts. A pleasant voice inquired as to how she was and what she was doing. The conversation lasted less than 5 minutes. However, Miss J began to look forward to the daily call and the weekly visit by her friendly visitor. Knowing that someone cared and would check on her was enough to support Miss J's independent spirit. She managed to live several more years before she died in her sleep at home.

Another possibility for providing the elderly with significant others rest in the area of companion animals (Fig. 5.10). The pet could be any small animal (to control cost of food and management of waste). A small dog tends to be the most effective and embodies the overwhelming argument for this type of therapy. Who else is totally dependent and capable of providing unconditional love to an elderly person? The elderly need to be needed and loved. Evidence indicates that people who have not moved or spoken in years respond to dogs (Corson et al., 1975; Robb, Boyd, and Pristash, 1980).

Several research and program reports in-

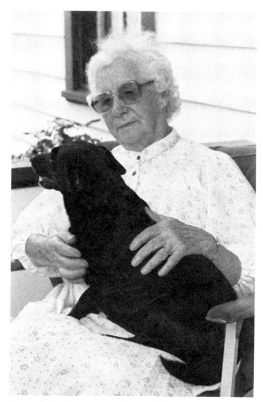

Figure 5.10. Dogs can help an old person feel needed and wanted; they provide unconditional love. (Photograph by Shawn Mertz, Pittsburgh, PA.)

dicate that companion animals, particularly dogs, are feasible in long-term care facilities (Arkow, 1982; Robb and Miller, 1982; Stauffer, 1982). Nurses can help in these projects simply by supporting the approach. Those with allergies to animals should transfer off the units where pets are located. Some nurses have found it difficult to conceptualize the long-range impact of pet therapy in the face of short-term anticipated problems. This myopic view has been responsible for blocking several pet therapy projects.

Other transitional objects, such as plants and even wine bottles (Talbott et al., 1976), have been found to increase socialization behavior among the elderly. A *transitional object* is some physical item that is especially significant to the individual. Contact with transitional objects decreases anxiety, reinforces sense of self, and links the person to the past. The impact of transitional objects appears to be less dramatic than that reported with small dogs (Mugford and M'Comisky, 1975; Robb, Boyd, and Pristash, 1980). Evidence suggests that the ability of transitional objects to provoke responses from the elderly is related to the animation or responsiveness of the object. On a continuum, animals are more responsive than plants, which are, in turn, more responsive than inanimate objects such as fake plants or stuffed animals.

Children are potential significant others. Old people and children can sometimes establish more satisfactory relationships than either group can establish with adults in their middle years. The reasons for this may involve congruence between needs and potentials. Children enjoy listening, and the elderly enjoy talking. Old people need encouragement to be active and take risks; children need encouragement to pause and rest, and to consider safety during play. These two age groups can be brought together by establishing nursery schools close to places where elderly people live in large numbers, such as high-rise apartments and nursing homes.

CONCLUSION

The fundamental assumption of deinstitutionalization programs and community-based services is that problems of the aged are caused by a lack of services. However, shifting programs and funding does nothing to remedy the underlying value system that disenfranchises the elderly and gives rise to stresses of low income and loss of employment and social supports. What shifting programs and funding does do is to maintain the present approach that treats individuals with services and thereby supports an expending service economy. Services are provided not so much to produce results as to provide a substitute for adequate income maintenance policies (Estes and Harrington, 1981). When nurses support institutional or community-based services, or both, they need to realize that none of these "alter-

natives" will solve the losses of income and social support that foster dependency on the part of old people.

Disconcerting though the thought may be, future development of social resources relevant to the elderly will be characterized by change. Specific services and delivery systems will vary in number and focus as the result of a number of forces; the needs of the elderly, knowledge about the aging process, the economy, and the political power of the elderly comprise a few of the factors that will shape the future of resources for the elderly. Regardless of changes in the society-provided resource structure, the task of the nurse will remain the same. As suggested in Figure 5.11, the nurse needs to assess the elderly individual's need for and readiness to accept help. The nurse needs to know the client well to accomplish this task. Knowledge of specific resources available is of secondary importance. Once the client's need is clearly identified, the nurse needs to know the process to follow to locate the right

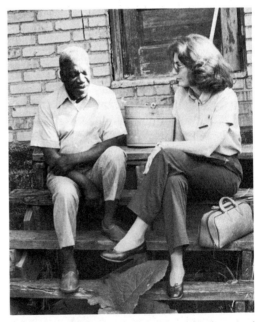

Figure 5.11. "With some help you could get more of the things others enjoy," said the nurse. "Who says we want 'em?" replied the offended elderly person. *(Photograph by Shawn Mertz, Pittsburgh, PA.)*

resource. This process starts by accessing the resource system through common, familiar entry points such as the telephone directory and/or a social worker. Once the right resource is located, the elderly person and the resource need to come together. The nurse's responsibility at this point is a follow-up contact to discover the amount of help received by the client and, if necessary, to start the process over again.

RECOMMENDED READINGS

Aging 331–332:2–28, 1982. *This issue focuses on companion animal–human interactions, with five articles titled as follows:*
1. Katcher, A.H. Are companion animals good for your health? A review of the evidence, pp 2–8
2. Stauffer, S.B. Pet programs for the elderly: Rewards and responsibilities, pp 9–14
3. Nussman, J., Burt, M. No room for pets, pp 15–17
4. Lago, D., Knight, B., Connell, C. Pact: A pet placement organization for the elderly living at home, pp 19–25
5. Jessee, E.M. Pet therapy for the elderly, pp 26–28

Holder, A. Involuntary commitment incompetency, and consent. IRB 5(2):6–8, 1983. *Distinguishes between the status of involuntarily committed and incompetent people and discusses The National Commission's Report on Research Involving Those Institutionalized as Mentally Infirm.*

Human Values and Aging Newsletter. Available from Institute on the Humanities, Arts, and Aging, Brookdale Center on Aging of Hunter College, 425 East 25th Street, New York, NY 10010. *Content is defined by the title. Each issue contains several short articles that address value dilemmas such as:*
Can rights be wrong? 5(1):1–2, 1982
Whose money is it anyway? Ethical issues in the transfer of assets, 4(2):2–5, 1981
Perspectives on older women, 3(4):2–4, 1981

Informal support systems. The Gerontologist 23(1):51–70, 1983. *A series of three articles, on the topic indicated in the title, that serve to describe the extent of social support available to noninstitutionalized elderly people.*

Johnson, D. Abuse of the elderly. Nurse Practitioner 6(1):29–30, 32, 34, 1981. *Provides an overview of the elder abuse problem but is more valuable for the detailed screening protocol for identification of abuse and neglect of the elderly, intervention suggestions, and a list of preventive measures.*

Lusk, P., Maule, H.L. Life care: No longer a viable concept? Journal of Gerontological Nursing 8(9):526–528, 1982. *Provides a comprehensive review of the problems inherent in life care homes. Useful for nurses advising clients about pros and cons of entering into life care arrangements.*

Matthews, S.H. Participation of the elderly in a transportation system. The Gerontologist 22(1): 26–31, 1982. *A case study that serves to illustrate several matters related to resources for elderly people: (1) operation of a successful transportation system, (2) "death" of the system precipitated by changes in government-sponsored funding for transportation, and (3) benefits of providing services to elderly people without regard for need.*

Phillips, L.R. Elder abuse—What is it? Who says so? Geriatric Nursing 4(3):167–170, 1983. *Presents ethical questions that arise when nurses try to use standard definitions of abuse in classifying frail home-bound elderly people.*

Reports by the Special Committee on Aging, U.S. Senate or the Select Committee on Aging, U.S. House of Representatives on aging that are issued annually. *Useful as reference material, these reports are available by writing to one's senator or congressman. The volume is typically 300 or more pages of facts and figures about the elderly and their needs in terms of income, employment, health, social services, crime, education, and other topics. Federally sponsored programs that address these needs are usually described and evaluated.*

Symposium: Aging and the family. The Gerontologist 23(1):24–50, 1983. *Five articles on this topic that deal with the role of the family in the economic well-being of the elderly, autonomy and independence, family ties in cross-cultural perspective, and other topics.*

REFERENCES CITED

Adams, J.P. Service arrangements preferred by minority elderly: A cross-cultural survey. Journal of Gerontological Social Work 3(2):39–57, 1980

Adams, R., Smith, T. Fear of Neighborhood. National Opinion Research Center Report 127C on the Social Change Project. Chicago, IL, National Opinion Research Center, 1976

Antunes, G.E., Cook, F.L., Cook, T.D., Skogan, W.G. Patterns of personal crime against the elderly. The Gerontologist 17(4):321–327, 1977

Antunes, G., Gaitz, C.M. Ethnicity and participation: A study of Mexican-Americans, Blacks, and Whites. American Journal of Sociology 80:1192–1211, 1975

Arkow, P. "Pet therapy": A Study of the Use of Companion Animals in Selected Therapics, 3rd ed. Colorado Springs, CO: The Humane Society of the Pikes Peak Region, 1982

Baer, W.C. Federal housing programs for the elderly. In Lawton, M.P., Newcomer, R.J., Byerts, T.O. (eds), Community Planning for an Aging Society. Stroudsburg, PA: Dowden, Hutchinson, and Ross, 1976

Barney, J.L. The prerogative of choice in long-term care. The Gerontologist 17(4):309–314, 1977

Barron, M.L. The Aging American. New York, Crowell, 1961

Beaver, M.L. The decision-making process and its relationship to relocation adjustment in old people. The Gerontologist 19:567–574, 1979

Bell, W.G. Community care for the elderly: An alternative to institutionalization. The Gerontologist 13(3):349–354, 1973

Bengtson, V.L. Families, Support Systems, Ethnic Groups: Patterns of Contrast and Congruence. Paper presented at the 29th Annual Meeting of the Gerontological Society.

Billings, G. Alternatives to nursing home care: An update. Aging 325–326:2–11, 1982

Binstock, R.H., Levin, M.A. The political dilemmas of intervention policies. In Binstock, R.H., Shanas, E. (eds), Handbook of Aging and the Social Sciences. New York, Van Nostrand Reinhold, 1976

Blazer, D., Palmore, E. Religion and aging in a longitudinal panel. The Gerontologist 16(1):82–85, 1976

Brotman, H.B. Every Ninth American. In Developments in Aging: 1979, A Report of the Special Committee on Aging, United States Senate. Washington, D.C., U.S. Government Printing Office, 1980

Brotman, H.B. Every Ninth American. An unpublished report prepared for the Special Committee on Aging, United States Senate, Washington, D.C., 1981

Brotman, H.B. Every Ninth American, 1982 edition: An Analysis for the Chairman of the U.S. House of Representatives Select Committee on Aging. Washington, D.C., U.S. Government Printing Office, 1982

Cantor, M.H. Neighbors and friends: An overlooked resource in the informal support system. Research on Aging 1:434–463, 1979

Champlin, L. The battered elderly. Geriatrics 37(7):115–121, 1982a

Champlin, L. Militant elderly: The wave of the present. Geriatrics 37(9):125–130, 1982b

Clark, M., Anderson, B. Culture and Aging. Springfield, IL, Charles C. Thomas, 1967

Clemente, F., Kleiman, M. Fear of crime among the aged. The Gerontologist 16(3):207–210, 1976

Cook, F.L., Cook, T.D. Evaluating the rhetoric of crisis: A case study of criminal victimization of the elderly. Social Service Review 50:632–646, 1976

Cook, F.L., Skogan, W.G., Cook, T.D., Antunes, G.E. Criminal victimization of the elderly: The physical and economic consequences. The Gerontologist 18(4):338–349, 1978

Corson, S.A., O'Leary Corson, E., Gwynne, P.H., Arnold, L.E. Pet-facilitated psychotherapy in a hospital setting. In Masserman, J.H. (ed), Current Psychiatric Therapies. New York, Grune and Stratton, 1975

Cox, H. The motivation and political alienation of older Americans. International Journal of Aging and Human Development 11(1):1–12, 1980

Crime. Aging International 7(3):2–3, 1980

Cutler, S.J. Membership in different types of voluntary associations and psychological well-being. The Gerontologist 16(4):335–339, 1976

Daniel, D.D., Templin, R.G., Shearon, R.W. The value orientations of older adults toward education. Educational Gerontology: An International Quarterly 2:33–42, 1977

Dowd, J.J., Bengtson, V.L. Aging in minority populations: An examination of the double jeopardy hypothesis. The Gerontologist 33:427–436, 1978

Edwards, J.N., Klemmack, D.L. Correlates of life satisfaction: A reexamination. Journal of Gerontology 28(4):497–502, 1973

Ehrlich, P., Ehrlich, I., Woehlke, P. Congregate housing for the elderly: Thirteen years later. The Gerontologist 22(4):399–403, 1982

Elder abuse study. Information on Aging 25:13–14, 1982

Epstein, L.A., Murray, J.H. Aged Population of the United States: 1963 Social Security Survey of the Aged, Staff Paper No. 19. Washington, D.C., Social Security Administration, Office of Research and Statistics, 1967

Estes, C.L., Harrington, C.A. Fiscal crisis, deinstitutionalization, and the elderly. American Behavioral Scientist 24(6):811–826, 1981

Etzioni, A. Old people and public policy. Social Policy 7(3):21–29, 1976

Falcioni, D. Assessing the abused elderly. Journal of Gerontological Nursing 8(4):208–212, 1982

Fengler, A.P., Jensen, L. Perceived the objective conditions as predictors of the life satisfaction of urban and non urban elderly. Journal of Gerontology 36(6):750–752, 1981

Final Report of the 1981 White House Conference on Aging, Volume 2. Washington, D.C., U.S. Government Printing Office, 1981

Glock, C.Y. On the study of religious commitment. Religious Education 57:s98–s110, 1962

Glock, C.Y., Stark, R. Religion and Society in Tension. Chicago, IL, Rand McNally and Company, 1965

Grad, S. Income of the Population 55 and Over, 1978. Washington, D.C., Social Security Administration, Office of Research and Statistics, 1981

Grams, A., Fengler, A.P. Vermont elders no sense of deprivation. Perspective on Aging 10(1):12–15, 1981

Griffith, J., Strandberg, T. A Guide to Nursing Home Living. Charleston, IL, Generation, 1982

Guy, R.F. Religion, physical disabilities, and life satisfaction in older age cohorts. International Journal of Aging and Human Development, 15(3): 225–232, 1982

Havighurst, R.J., Albrecht, R. Older People. New York, Longmans, Green, 1953

Heisel, M.A., Faulkner, A.O. Religiosity in an older black population. The Gerontologist 22(4):254–358, 1982

Heller, B.R., Walsh, F.J., Wilson, K.M. Seniors helping seniors: Training older adults as new personnel resources in home health care. Journal of Gerontological Nursing 7(9):552–555, 1981

Hickey, T., Douglass, R.L. Mistreatment of the elderly in the domestic setting: An exploratory study. American Journal of Public Health 71(5):500–507, 1981

Hochstedler, E. Crime Against the Elderly in 26 Cities. Washington, D.C., U.S. Department of Justice, Bureau of Justice Statistics, 1981

Hooyman, N.R., Tomita, S. A Model for the Prevention, Detection, and Treatment of Elderly Abuse and Neglect. A paper presented at the 34th Annual Meeting of the Gerontological Society of America, Toronto, Canada, November, 1981

Howell, S.C. Environments and aging. In Eisdorfer, C. (ed), Annual Review of Gerontology and Geriatrics. New York, Springer, 1980, vol 1

Huff, R.L. National Directory of Retirement Facilities. Washington, D.C., Housing, Program Department, NRTA-AARP, 1979

Hunter, K.I., Linn, M.W. Psychosocial differences between elderly volunteers and nonvolunteers. International Journal of Aging and Human Development 12(3):205–213, 1980–81

Information and Volunteer Services of Allegheny County. Where to Turn: Directory of Health, Welfare and Community Services in Allegheny County. Pittsburgh, Information and Volunteer Services of Allegheny County, 1974

Jackson, J.J. Aged Negroes: Their cultural departures from statistical stereotypes and rural-urban differences. The Gerontologist 10:140–145, 1970

Jackson, J.J. Compensatory care for the black aged. In Minority Aged in America. Occasional Paper No. 10. Ann Arbor, MI, Institute of Gerontology, University of Michigan–Wayne State University, 1971

Jeselnick, Y. Fierce independence hampers aid. Perspective on Aging 7(1):33–34, 1978

Johnson, D. Abuse of the elderly. Nurse Practitioner 6(1):29–30, 32, 34, 1981

Kahana, E., Liang, J., Felton, B., Fairchild, T., Harel, Z. Perspective of aged on victimization, "ageism," and their problems in urban society. The Gerontologist 17(2):121–129, 1977

Kalish, R.A. Death and dying in a social context. In Binstock, R.H., Shanas, E. (eds), Handbook of Aging and the Social Sciences. New York, Van Nostrand Reinhold, 1976

Kapp, M.B. Common concern: Legal guardianship. Geriatric Nursing 2(5):366–369, 1981

Kasschau, P.L. The elderly as their planners see them. Social Policy 7(3):13–18, 1976

Kidwell, I.J., Booth, A. Social distance and intergenerational relations. The Gerontologist 17: 412–420, 1977

Krause, D.H. Integration of components of health and social services, in Exton-Smith, A.N., Evans, J.G. (eds), Care of the Elderly: Meeting the Challenge of Dependency. New York, Grune and Stratton, 1977

Kummerow, M. Marketing. In Scholen, K., Chen, Y.P. (eds), Unlocking Home Equity for the Elderly. Cambridge, MA, Ballinger, 1980

Langford, M. Community Aspects of Housing for the Aged. Ithaca, NY, Cornell University Center for Housing and Environmental Studies, 1962

Lawton, M.P. An exological theory of aging applied to elderly housing. Journal of Architectural Education 31:8–10, 1977

Lawton, M.P. Environmental change: The older person as initiator and responder. In Datan, N., Lohman, N. (eds), Transitions of Aging. New York, Academic, 1980

Lawton, M.P., Greenbaum, M., Liebowitz, B. The lifespan of housing environments for the aging. The Gerontologist 20(1):56–64, 1980

Lawton, M.P., Nahemow, L., Tson-Min-Yeh. Neighborhood environment and the well-being of older tenants in planned housing. International Journal of Aging and Human Development 11(3):211–227, 1980

Liang, J., Dvorhin, L., Kahana, E., Mazian, F. Financial well-being among the aged: A further elaboration. Journal of Gerontology 35:409–420, 1980

Liang, J., Fairchild, T. Relative deprivation and perception of financial adequacy among the aged. Journal of Gerontology 34:746–759, 1979

Liang, J., Sengstock, M.C. The risk of personal victimization among the aged. Journal of Gerontology 36(4):463–471, 1981

Lowenthal, M.F., Chiriboga, D. Social stress and adaptation: Toward a life-course perspective, in Eisdorfer, C., Lawton, M.P. (eds), The Psychology of Adult Development and Aging. Washington, D.C., American Psychological Association, 1973

Maddox, G.L. The unrealized potential of an old idea, in Exton-Smith, A.N., Grimley Evans, J. (eds), Care of the Elderly: Meeting the Challenge of Dependency. New York, Grune and Stratton, 1977

Mason, D.J. Perspectives on poverty. Image 13(3):82–85, 1981

McConnell, S.R., Kasschau, P.L. Income versus in-kind services for the elderly: Decision makers' preferences. Social Service Review 51(2):337–356, 1977

Miller, A.H., Gurin, P., Gurin, G. Age consciousness and political mobilization of older Americans. The Gerontologist 20(6):691–700, 1980

Moberg, D.O. Religion in old age. Geriatrics 20:977–982, 1965a

Moberg, D.O. Religiosity in old age. The Gerontologist 5:78–87, 1965b

Moberg, D.O., Taves, M.J. Church participation and adjustment in old age, in Rose, A.M., Peterson, W.J. (eds), Older People and Their Social World. Philadelphia, Davis, 1965

Morris, R. The development of parallel services for the elderly and disabled. The Gerontologist 14(1):14–19, 1974

Morrissey, M. Guardians adlitem: An educational program in Virginia. The Gerontologist 22(3):301–304, 1982

Mugford, R.A., McComisky, J.G. Some recent work on the psychotherapeutic value of cage birds with old people, in Anderson, R.S. (ed), Pet Animals in Society. New York, Macmillan, 1975

Murdock, S.H., Schwartz, D.F. Family structure and the use of agency services: An examination of patterns among elderly Native Americans. The Gerontologist 18:475–481, 1978

National Council on the Aging. Triple Jeopardy: Myth or Reality? Washington, D.C., National Council on the Aging, 1972

National Council on the Aging. Fact Book on Aging: A Profile of America's Older Population. Washington, D.C., The National Council on the Aging, 1978

National Council on the Aging. Aging in Eighties: America in Transition. Washington, D.C., National Council on the Aging, 1981

Neugarten, B.L. Personality change in late life: A developmental perspective, in Eisdorfer, C., Lawton, M.P. (eds), The Psychology of Adult Development and Aging. Washington, D.C., American Psychological Association, 1973

Newman, S.J. Exploring housing adjustments of older people. Research on Aging 3(4):417–427, 1981

O'Brien, R.M., Shichor, D., Decker, D.L. Urban structure and household victimization of the elderly. International Journal of Aging and Human Development 15(1):41–49, 1982–83

O'Bryant, S.L. The value of home to older persons: Relationship to housing satisfaction. Research on Aging 4(3):349–363, 1982

Oliphant R. A Piano for Mrs. Cimino. Englewood Cliffs, NJ, Prentice-Hall, 1980

Ollenburger, J.C. Criminal victimization and fear of crime. Research on Aging 3(1):101–118, 1981

O'Reilly, C.T. Religious practices and personal adjustment. Sociology and Social Research 42:119–121, 1958

Peace, S. "Small group" housing in the community, Part II: Variations on sheltered housing. Ageing International 8(2):16–20, 1981

Perloff, R., McCaskey, P.H. Nonmonetary Costs Associated with Consumer Fraud and Dissatisfaction of the Elderly. Paper presented at the 1978 American Council of Consumer Interests Conference, Chicago, 1978

Phillips, L.R. The Relationship of Social Supports and Physical Status to Maltreatment of Frail Elderly Adults. Paper presented at the 8th Annual Nursing Research Conference, University of Arizona, Tucson, AZ, September, 1980a

Phillips, L.R. Abuse/Neglect Versus Good Relationships Among Frail Elderly Home Bound Individuals. Paper presented at the 33rd Annual Meeting of the Gerontological Society, San Diego, CA, November, 1980b

Powell, D. The crimes against the elderly. Journal of Gerontological Social Work 3(1):27–39, 1980

Powers, E.A., Bultena, G.L. Sex differences in intimate friendships of old age. Journal of Marriage and the Family 38:739–747, 1976

Pritchard, D.C. The art of matchmaking: A case study in shared housing. The Gerontologist 23(2):174–179, 1983

Protecting Miss Mary. Time 111(16):24, 1978

Recommendations, post-conference survey of delegates. Final Report of the 1981 White House Conference on Aging, Vol 3. Washington, D.C., Superintendent of Documents, 1982

Riley, M.W., Foner, A. Aging and Society, Vol 1: An inventory of Research Findings. New York, Russell Sage Foundation, 1968

Robb, S.S. The nurse's role in retirement preparation. Journal of Gerontological Nursing 4(1):25–28, 1978

Robb, S.S., Boyd, M., Pristash, C.L. A wine bottle, plant, and puppy: Catalysts for social behavior. Journal of Gerontological Nursing 6(12):721–728, 1980

Robb, S.S., Boyd, M., Pristash, C.L. Study of the Effect of Objects on an Animation Continuum on Social Behavior of the Elderly. An unpublished report. VA Medical Center, Pittsburgh, 1980

Robb, S.S., Miller, R.F. Pilot Study of Pet-Dog Therapy for Elderly People in Long Term Care. A final report submitted to Health Research and Development Service, VA Central Office, Washington, D.C., March, 1982

Rosow, I. Social Integration of the Aged. New York, The Free Press, 1967

Rudin, A.J., Rudin, M.R. Prison or Paradise: The New Religious Cults. Philadelphia, Fortress, 1980

Schwartz, D. Hamlet dweller–city dweller. Geriatric Nursing 1(2):128–132, 1980

Seelbach, W.C., Sauer, W.J. Filial responsibility expectations and morale among aged parents. The Gerontologist 17:492–499, 1977

Sengstock, M.C., Barrett, S., Graham, R. Abused Elders: Victims of Villains or of Circumstances. Paper presented at the 35th Annual Meeting of the Gerontological Society of America, Boston, MA, November, 1982

Shanas, E. The family as a social system in old age. The Gerontologist 19:169–174, 1979

Sherman, E., Newman, E.S., Nelson, A., Van Buren, D. Crimes Against the Elderly in Public Housing: Policy Alternatives. Albany, NY, School of Social Welfare, State University of New York at Albany, 1975

Skogan, W.G., Kleca, W.R. The Fear of Crime. Washington, D.C., American Political Science Association, 1976

Smith, K.F., Bengtson, V.L. Positive Consequences of Institutionalization: Solidarity Between Elderly Parents and Their Middle-Aged Children. Paper presented at the meeting of the Gerontological Society, Dallas, November, 1978

Snyder, L.H. Environmental changes for socialization. Journal of Nursing Administration 8:44–49, 1978

Soldo, B.J. America's elderly in the 1980's. Population Bulletin 35(4):1–48, 1980

Stauffer, S.B. Pet programs for the elderly: Rewards and responsibilities. Aging 331–332:9–14, 1982

Strain, L.A., Chappell, N.L. Confidants: Do they make a difference in quality of life. Research on Aging 4(4):479–502, 1982

Szasz, T.S. The Myth of Mental Illness: Foundations of a Theory of Personal Conduct. New York, Hoeber-Harper, 1961

Szasz, T. The Manufacture of Madness. New York: Harper and Row, 1970

Talbott, J.A., Stern, D., Ross, J., Gillen, C. Flowering plants as a therapeutic/environmental agent in a psychiatric hospital. Horticultural Science 11(4): 365–366, 1976

Taubman, P., Sickles, R.C. Supplemental social insurance and the health of the poor. Center for the Study of Aging Newsletter 5(3):10–11, 1983

Tellis-Nayak, V. The transcendent standard: The religious ethos of the rural elderly. The Gerontologist 22(4):359–363, 1982

Tobin, S.S., Lieberman, M.A. Last Home for the Aged: Critical Implications for Institutionalization. San Francisco: Josey–Bass, 1976

Trela, J.E. Social class and political involvement in age graded and non-age graded associations. International Journal of Aging and Human Development 8(4):301–310, 1977–78

U.S. Bureau of the Census. Characteristics of the population below the poverty level: 1978. Current Population Reports, Series P-60, No. 124. Washington, D.C., U.S. Government Printing Office, 1980

U.S. Bureau of the Census. Marital status and living arrangements: March, 1980. Current Population Reports, Series P-20, No. 365. Washington, D.C., U.S. Government Printing Office, 1981

U.S. Bureau of the Census. Characteristics of the population below the poverty level, 1980. Current Population Reports, Series P-60, No. 133. Washington, D.C., U.S. Government Printing Office, 1982

U.S. Department of Health and Human Services. Directory of adult day care centers. Washington, D.C., U.S. Government Printing Office, 1980

U.S. General Accounting Office. Improved Knowledge Base Would Be Helpful in Reaching Policy Decisions on Providing Long-Term, In-Home Services for the Elderly. Washington, D.C., Superintendent of Documents, 1981

U.S. Health Care Financing Administration. How to Select a Nursing Home. Washington, D.C., U.S. Government Printing Office, 1981

U.S. Senate Special Committee on Aging. Developments in Aging, 1981, Vol 1. Washington, D.C., U.S. Government Printing Office, 1982a

U.S. Senate Special Committee on Aging. Developments in Aging: 1981, Vol 2. Washington, D.C., U.S. Government Printing Office, 1982b

U.S. Senate Special Committee on Aging, National Retired Teachers Association, and American Association of Retired Persons. Survey of Delegates to the 1981 White House Conference on Aging: A Preliminary Report. Washington, D.C., Superintendent of Documents, 1982

Weintz, C., Weintz, W. The Discount Guide for Travelers Over 55. New York, Dutton, 1981

Weismehl, R. Congregate living: A further extension of the service continuum. Concern 3(5):17–20, 1977

Williams, B. Social, Economic and Health Characteristics of Older American Indians, Part 2 of 2

(Department of Health, Education, and Welfare Publication No. (OHDS) 78-20289). Washington, D.C., U.S. Government Printing Office, 1978

Wingrove, C.R., Alston, J.P. Age, aging, and church attendance. The Gerontologist 11:356–358, 1971

York, J.L., Calsyn, R.J. Family involvement in nursing homes. The Gerontologist 17(6):500–505, 1977

Youmans, E.G. The rural aged. Annals, AAPSS. 429:81–90, 1977

Younger, E.J. The California experience: Prevention of criminal victimization of the elderly. Police Chief 43(2):28–30, 32, 1976

Zald, M.N. Demographics, politics, and the future of the welfare state. Social Service Review 51(1):110–124, 1977

6

Environmental Resources for Health Care of the Aged

Susanne S. Robb

Reading this chapter will enable the individual to:

1. Describe characteristics of an ideal health care delivery system
2. Distinguish between the terms "level" and "locus" of care
3. Explain the concept of channeling
4. Compare and contrast at least five programs or services that may be included in a community-based health care system
5. Describe four models of adult day care
6. Identify at least two sources of funding fo homemaker/chore service programs
7. Compare and contrast at least three programs or services that may be included in an institution-based health-care system
8. List the three main sources of payment for health care in order of priority
9. Name the top three health programs or services that receive money from elderly people
10. Identify one measure nurses can take to decrease health care costs for elderly people
11. Distinguish between structure, processes, and outcomes in relation to measuring quality of care

12. Describe the impact of at least five structural factors on quality of long-term care
13. List at least four actions that nurses can take to deliver improved service to long-term care clients
14. Indicate similarities and differences between nursing, education, quality assurance, clinical research, and management processes
15. Describe two risks to nurses who try to enforce adherence to patients' rights
16. Discuss differences and similarities between acute and long-term models of health care delivery

This chapter considers resources in the environment of the aged that, compared to those resources discussed in the preceding chapter, are more specifically related to health care after illness and/or disability have become realities. Health-care programs that provide various levels of care are discussed in reference to their usual location in either community- or institution-based settings. Sources of payment for health care are identified, along with their implications for nursing practice. Finally, implications derived from the numbers and kinds of health-care resources that are presently available, or needed for the future, are presented in terms of actions required by nurses (Fig. 6.1).

TOWARD THE IDEAL

An ideal long-term care system "would provide care of the right level, at the right time, in the right setting, at the maximum quality achievable within the state of the art, and would do it most cost effectively" (Weissert, 1979, p. 564). Thus, the long-term care system would be continuous, comprehensive, appropriate, and accessible. A balance would exist between provider-perceived "needs" and consumer preferences. An incentive system of reimbursement would reward achievement of the above

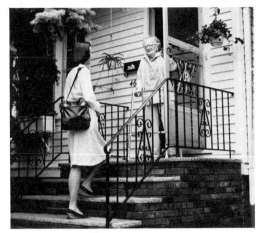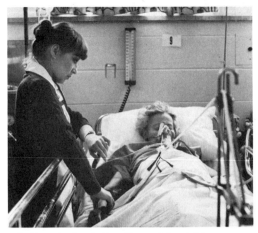

Figure 6.1. Health care of the right level, at the right time, in the right setting, at the right price, and of the right quality is difficult to find. *(Copyright 1983 by Robert Goldstein, New Milford, NJ. Reproduced by permission.)*

objectives within limits imposed by societal preferences concerning the appropriate division between public and private responsibilities. The system would provide some or all of the following services: needs assessment; preventive care; restoration of physical and social functioning to maximum achievable limits or maximum reduction in the rate of deterioration of physical and social function; provision of supportive services to people whose physical, psychologic, and social disabilities make them dependent; and maintenance at the maximum state of well-being or the maximum achievable quality of life for all (Weissert, 1979, p. 564).

Our present "system" of health-care delivery is a nonsystem that falls far short of achieving these desired attributes. Of all the difficult health-care issues facing this nation, none is more complex or urgent than the formulation of a viable policy of long-term health and medical care for the elderly and the chronically ill and disabled. Traditionally, health-care resources have been organized to deal with acute illnesses. Illnesses of the elderly, however, tend to be degenerative and chronic. Increases in the number and proportion of elderly people as well as the costs, fraud, and abuse associated with acute and long-term institutional care prompted a search for other services in other kinds of settings. For a time, services such as home health care, domiciliary, respite, hospice,

and adult day care were expected to provide a "quick fix" for these high costs (Billings, 1982). However, hopes that what is called "alternative care" would result in overall cost savings had to be modified. Under the present financing system, alternative services are "add-ons," not previously available, that do not substitute for more expensive nursing home care and may not delay entry into a nursing home. However, the quality of life for elderly people who receive care in the community appears consistently better than for those people who enter long-term care facilities (Chappell and Penning, 1979; Weissert, 1979; Hicks et al., 1981).

A distinction exists between *level* of care and *locus* of care. Level of care—for example, skilled, intermediate, or unskilled care—is based upon the nursing and medical needs of clients. The term unskilled simply refers to care provided by people who lack formal training and experience. Locus of care—institution or community—is decided by the social, economic, and environmental resources of clients, as well as the client's own choices and needs. The distinction between a community- and institution-based locus of care is based upon whether the client spends 24 hours per day in the setting (institutional) and ownership/control of the setting. Institutional settings are not usually owned by those they serve, and client participation in managerial decisions is negligible. This section organizes health-care resources/programs first by their locations and then by levels of care within each location. This organization is depicted in Table 6.1. Neither respite nor hospice care fit neatly within the scheme because both may be given in either location and both involve widely varying levels of care.

No degree of need, whether physical, psychologic, social, or economic, automatically dictates the setting in which care must be provided. Almost all levels of care, in fact, can be given at home. Our present policy of care of the aged was shaped by the Medicare and Medicaid legislation and has a strong institutional bias. Our present policy rhetoric strongly favors shifting the balance toward community-based programs.

A continuum of care refers to a coordinated and comprehensive range of health services at the local level for everyone 65 years of age and older. To become a continuum of care, any system of services must resolve problems of (1) access to services, (2) integration among services, and (3) accountability by service providers to the funding agency, to each other, and to their clients (Ishizaki, Gottesman, and MacBride, 1979, p. 385). These goals are achieved through a standardized assessment of clients' functioning needs, a written service plan, linkage services, regular case review, and plan revision. The channeling experiments represented an effort to evaluate such a system of care. For example, the ACCESS program in Monroe County, New York, and TRIAGE program in Connecticut sought to take direct responsibility for entire populations within their jurisdiction to ensure that all persons received what care and assistance they needed.

Channeling refers to the coordination and management of long-term care. Key elements

TABLE 6.1 A CONTINUUM OF CARE ORGANIZED BY BOTH LEVEL AND LOCATION OF CARE

Level of Care	Location of Care	
	Community Based	Institution Based

Skilled	Home care
	Hospital based
	Community agency based
	Day hospital (Model 1)
	Adult day care (Restorative;
	  Model II and III)
	After-care
	Clinic care
	Emergency care
		Acute care hospitals
		Rehabilitation centers
		Nursing homes (skilled
		  nursing facilities)
		Hospice*
		Respite*

Intermediate	Personal care
	Homemaker/chore care
	Adult day care (social;
	  Model IV)
		Nursing homes
		  (intermediate care
		  facilities)

Unskilled	Apartments (with some
	  supportive care)
	Senior-citizen centers
	Small group housing
	  (small capacity)
	Foster home care
	Boarding homes
	  (small capacity)
	Halfway houses
		Domiciliaries
		Personal care homes
		Boarding homes
		  (large capacity)
		Small group housing
		  (large capacity)

*Care/service is not consistently provided in an inpatient setting and substantial portions of the care may be provided by lay people without special education and experience.

of channeling are (1) emphasis on client-focused services and (2) an altered set of relationships among health, mental health, and social service agencies within the target community. A case management approach starts with comprehensively assessing an individual's needs, planning for his care, arranging for services, and periodically monitoring and reassessing his health.

Channeling was initially used on a wide scale in 1974 by the Wisconsin community care project. In 1976, the Georgia alternative health services project was started to test the cost-effectiveness of a coordinated system of community-based care. In 1980, the Department of Health and Human Services began the planning phase of a multiyear national channeling demonstration project. Each of 10 sites performed four care functions: outreach and case finding, screening, comprehensive assessment of needs, and case management. The goal was to help clients gain access to a wider array of services than was previously available to them. Within these demonstrations, the effects of an alternative reimbursement mechanism on service utilization and the impact of the channeling project on service development were of major interest.

The question of whether channeling is a solution to the problem of fragmented care has not been clearly answered. Even though channeling improves coordination of long-term care services, the procedure may uncover needs for more services and the channeling intervention itself may increase overall costs.

The usefulness of a continuum of services probably depends on the presence of a high-quality, institutionally based service capable of diagnostic and rehabilitative functions, temporary admissions for respite care (relief for care-givers), and high quality of service for that group of people whose social and health needs might be better met in institutions (Kane and Kane, 1980, p. 252).

COMMUNITY-BASED CARE

Community-based care produces a kind of enthusiasm that is less prevalent in institutional settings. It emphasizes differences among individuals and offers stimulation to both the provider and the consumer of health care.

Home Health Care

With adequate support from significant others, home health care can be viewed as the ideal form of "alternative" care. A spectrum of services—psychologic, social, personal, and medical—are provided in a single setting, the home, to people with moderate to severe incapacity. Significant involvement of family or friends occurs. These programs are sponsored by free-standing visiting nurse organizations or by hospitals.

In the first half of the 1900s, public health nurses played a key role in home care, with support from public funds and private insurance plans. Then the trend turned toward institutionalization, especially with the advent of Medicare and Medicaid. Medicare payment for home care has been directed toward medically oriented services for acute episodes: skilled nursing care; physical, occupational, and speech therapies; social services; home health aide assistance; and medical supplies and appliances. Under Medicaid, home health services vary by state, but all states must cover nursing, home health aide services, medical supplies, equipment, and appliances. Unlike Medicare users, Medicaid recipients do not have to be home bound or require skilled care to qualify.

Problems related to home health care include cost, adequacy, availability, comprehensiveness, and eligibility requirements. Sometimes third-party reimbursement of the cost is linked to the clients' need for *skilled* as opposed to *custodial* care. Skilled nursing care usually involves some technical procedure or professional judgment, coupled with the client's ability to progress toward a therapeutic goal. Goals and procedures aimed at maintenance, usually the most appropriate for the elderly, are not considered to require skilled services. In any event, third-party reimbursement does not continue indefinitely. Payment stops after a certain number of visits or days. The client must then assume the cost or lose the service. Publicly funded health services are available without charge to the consumer. However, these services tend to concentrate on health promotion (infection control and maternal–child health) rather than chronic illness. One requirement for these services is the presence of a caretaker in the home. However, many elderly people live alone, and therefore cannot use the program. The shortage of physicians has left home visiting teams without a representative from the medical profession. The use of nurse practitioners may be a solution to this problem.

Day Care

Unlike many European countries, where day care is often supported under national health programs, major day-care initiatives in the United States have come from the community rather than federal or state funding programs. In 1980 there were about 600 adult day-care programs in 46 states with an average daily census of about 13,500. These figures represent a tripling of such programs since 1977 (Billings, 1982, pp. 7–8).

Coincident with growth of the adult daycare movement has been development of an organization to promote these programs. The National Council on the Aging created a National Institute on Adult Day Care in 1979. This institute serves as a focal point for adult day care at the national level, with six purposes that may be summarized as promotion of adult day care as a component of long-term care, and information generation, collection, and dissemination to facilitate development of day-care programs and formulation of program standards.

> Adult daycare is a generic term that applies to a variety of programs offering services that range from active rehabilitation to social and health related care. Various terminology is applied: day care, day treatment, day health care, psychiatric day treatment, partial hospitalization, and day hospital care. Adult daycare is coordinated with, and relates to, other agencies and services such as senior centers, in-home services and institutional and hospital care (National Institute on Adult Daycare, 1980, p. 1).

A number of models have been proposed for day-care services. These models are useful conceptually, but they should not prevent flexibility in evaluating participants' needs or adaptability in addressing local community needs. One such categorization plan that offers four types of programs is summarized in Table 6.2 (O'Brien, 1981, p. 284). A second categorization plan identifies three types of models: restorative, maintenance, and social or psychosocial (Trager, 1979, pp. 7–8).

A restorative center/model is described as one that is oriented to patients who are "in need of extensive rehabilitation—who would be in a skilled nursing facility if the center services were not available; who can be returned to self-care or shifted to lower-level services within an established time period" (Trager, 1979, p. 7). The program focus is goal-oriented and time-limited (3 to 4 months).

Centers that emphasize rehabilitation or restoration follow established patterns: in initial assessment in order to determine the participant's potential for achieving treatment goals; in provision of established treatment regimes; and in review of plans and progress at established intervals. These centers tend to accept a higher proportion of wheelchair patients who are in the younger age range and maintain a relatively high staff-to-patient ratio, with greater emphasis on the services of health professionals and on health-care services. The TransCentury Report indicated that these centers served a relatively large group of stroke patients with multiple chronic conditions (TransCentury Report, 1975).

An example of the maintenance model is described as "not as staff-intensive" as the restorative model. All participants have an initial assessment. Reassessment of those in maintenance care is based on the expectation that service will be extended over longer periods of time than those in the restorative level. Maintenance services emphasize socialization, reality orientation, recreation and podiatry. The center uses the services of volunteers, drawing from its own clientele for volunteer services.

The social (or psychosocial) model is a center located in a retirement area. Some of these programs were originally established as multipurpose senior centers intended to provide relief for families in which there is an elderly family member. Within 2 years, these programs evolved into free-standing Adult Day Health-Care Centers. The client population is largely very elderly (84–98 years old) and con-

TABLE 6.2. FOUR MODELS OF ADULT DAY CARE

	Model I	Model II	Model III	Model IV
	Day Hospital	**Long-Term Care Facility**	**Long-Term Care Facility**	**Community Based**
Clients	Severely disabled, acute posthospital	Seriously disabled (mental or physical) posthospital, postnursing home	"At risk population"	Socially isolated "frail elderly," slightly disabled
Services offered	Intensive restorative medical and health services; physical, occupational, speech therapies; physician services provided directly by program	Intensive restorative medical and health services; physical, occupational, speech therapies; physician services not provided directly by program; activities, nutrition	Long-term health maintenance services, including nursing, activities, nutrition	Psychosocial activities in a protected environment, nutrition
Days per week offered	5 days	5 days	5 days	5 days
Estimated cost	$70–90/day	$20–30/day	$10–25/day	$5–15/day
Time limit	Yes	None	None	None
Expected outcome	Higher level of physical functioning	Higher level of functioning—both mental and physical	Prevention of premature institutionalization, relief to families, promotion of health	Prevention of mental deterioration and physical breakdown, promotion of health
Family responsibility	Family gives care on weekends and at night	Family gives care on weekends and at night	Family care provides health supervision in home during days not at program	Family provides supervision at home if necessary
Community supports	Usually necessary	Usually necessary	Offered when necessary	Not usually necessary

(Adapted from the four modules of adult day care defined by Edith Robins in "Operational Research in Geriatric Day Care in the United States," a paper presented at the 105th International Gerontological Congress, Jerusalem, Israel, June 1975, with the permission of the author. Appears in: Adult Day Care: A Practical Guide by Carole Lium O'Brien. Monterey, CA, Wadsworth Health Sciences, 1982.)

sists primarily of people who live alone in hotels or small apartments. The major emphasis is on socialization. The program objective is to keep people in the community as long as possible. No direct health services are provided, although a registered nurse directs the program and makes an initial home visit for assessment purposes. The group process is used extensively and effectively at the center and participants play a large part in determining what the center program will be.

A national study (Weissert, 1975) of 10 prototypical day-care programs found the following common structural features, summarized in the book *Adult Day Care* by Weiler and Rathbone-McCuan (1978).

Common criteria for admission to day-care programs exclude participants who are:

- bedridden
- totally disoriented
- potentially harmful or disruptive
- alcoholics or addicts
- devoid of medical need
- residents of mental institutions
- residents beyond the program's geographically defined service area, unless the residents provide their own transportation
- younger than 55 years old

Exceptions made by some programs are:

- participants of all ages accepted
- a personal physician is not required
- persons who live in mental institutions, nursing homes, or personal care homes accepted
- participants must be oriented to person, but not necessarily to place and time
- participants can be disruptive, as long as they are not harmful to themselves or others

Additional restrictions imposed by some programs require that participants must:

- be over 60 years old
- have a family member or significant other to provide supervision and care during program hours
- be eligible for one of three levels of institutional care
- be eligible for Medicaid or able to pay own bills

- not be frequently/habitually incontinent
- not require constant supervision due to disorientation
- be able to use a walker in an emergency, if he or she is wheelchair-bound
- not be subject to cardiac arrest
- not require a special diet

Basic services offered by all programs of adult day care include:

- general nursing devices
- referral to community services, including emergency services in a hospital or physician's office, ambulance transportation, hospital inpatient care, rehabilitation center, mental health facility, senior citizens center, nursing home, community health center, visiting nurse/homemaker service, health specialists/consultants
- social work services
- recreation activities
- assistance with activities of daily living
- supervision of personal hygiene
- lunch

One common feature of adult day care in this country is that characteristics vary widely from one program to another. No statement can be made about client characteristics, services, staffing, or costs without at least one exception (Weiler and Rathbone-McCuan, 1978). Standards and regulations for adult day care are not uniform from one state to another. Funding, or rather the lack of funding, is a primary issue in the adult day-care program movement. Most centers must rely on a combination of two or more sources of funding and exert considerable effort to assure continuation of those sources (O'Brien, 1981, pp. 284–285). For a variety of reasons that include uncertain funding, restrictive eligibility requirements, and limited ranges of services (including transportation), sufficient numbers of clients for day-care programs are sometimes difficult to locate (U.S. House of Representatives Select Committee on Aging, 1980, p. 19). Perhaps people do not trust that the programs or their eligibility to use them will last long enough to make enrollment worthwhile.

Major areas requiring further study have not changed since 1979, when they were outlined in the report of two national adult day-care conferences (Trager, 1979, p. 74):

1. Estimate of the population requiring adult day-care services
2. Personnel requirements for the provision of adult day care of good quality
3. Studies of space requirements for participant groups of different size in programs with different service emphases
4. Studies of optimum requirements in program setting
5. Methodology for integration of uniform long-term care data systems and adult day-care program records
6. Effective, uniform methods for funding reimbursement and determining costs of adult day care.

Multipurpose Senior Citizen Centers

Multipurpose Senior Citizen Centers are one of three major service programs sponsored by the Administration on Aging (AoA) under Title III of the Older American Act (OAA). The other two programs are nutrition services and social services. A multipurpose center in the OAA is "a community facility for the organization and provision of a broad spectrum of services, including provision of health, social, and educational services, and facilities for recreational activities for older persons" (Pfeiffer, 1977, p. 85). Funds appropriated for this program have been shared by many programs authorized under Section 308 of the OAA. Thus, typical multipurpose centers established, using federal monies, under this program have been started as model or demonstration projects, with additonal funds contributed from state and local sources. After the first year or two, federal support has been markedly reduced or discontinued and survival of the centers has been dependent upon other funding arrangements. Typical services offered within these centers are nutrition (via a substantial noon meal), recreation, and socialization. The program emphasis is social rather than health-related. These centers provide adult day care in a pattern most accurately described by the "Social Model" discussed in the preceding section on "Adult Day Care."

Day Hospitals

The term, day hospital, is used more widely in Great Britain than in the United States and covers more functions. The Department of Health and Social Security requires two day hospitals per 1000 people aged 65 years and older (Brocklehurst, 1977). A day hospital may mean a "medical out-patient clinic with access to meals, or occupational and physiotherapy departments for in-patient and out-patients, or purely out-patient rehabilitation, or diversional day care of patients for the relief of family stress at home, or all of these activities may be combined in the same unit" (Martin and Millard, 1975, p. 119). The distinction between a "day hospital" and a "day center" is that the former provides most of the services of an in-patient hospital without care at night or over the weekend. The day center provides a place for socialization but does not include nurses, physicians, or other therapists on the staff (Brocklehurst, 1977, Dall, 1978).

In the United States, "after-care" programs and outpatient surgical programs qualify as day hospitals. After-care programs provide services to clients who visit the hospital for 3- to 4-hour sessions three to five times each week to achieve specific therapeutic goals. These programs are transitional and are designed to facilitate discharge from hospital to home. Outpatient surgery was not begun as a service to the elderly, but rather as a way to avoid costly inpatient care for people of all ages. However, the elderly may have the most to gain from outpatient surgery because they benefit from maintaining continuity in their residences and care-givers. Efficient use of hospital personnel permits the cost-reduction associated with after-care and outpatient surgical programs. Like most ambulatory care programs, however, these programs assume clients have transportation whenever necessary to go from home to the hospital. In dealing with elderly clients, this assumption is often unwarranted.

Clinics, Physicians' Offices, and Emergency Rooms

Elderly people require more medical help than the general public. In 1980, noninstitutionalized elderly people, age 65 and over, reported an average of 4.2 office visits to physicians per year, compared to 2.7 visits for the population of all ages (McLemore and Koch, 1982). Results from the first National Health and Nutrition Examination Survey (National Center for Health Statistics, 1980, pp. 8–9) indicate that a total of 69 percent of the people aged 65–74 years had talked with a doctor in a private office, compared to 63.2 percent of the general population. In contrast, the elderly group was less likely than the general population (5 percent versus 8 percent) to have talked with a doctor at a clinic or a hospital emergency room. Regardless of setting, the 65- to 74-year-old group saw physicians most often for reasons of sickness or illness (40 percent), regular check-ups (33 percent), follow-ups (13 percent), injury (4 percent), injections and prescriptions (2 percent), and other reasons (8 percent of the visits). This pattern was the same as that for people of all ages.

Elderly people aged 65 years receive less dental care than people of all ages, with an average of 1.5 dental visits per person per year, compared to 1.7 visits for people of all ages, and a longer interval between visits to the dentist, with 42.4 percent waiting 5 years or more, compared to 13.7 percent for people of all ages (National Center for Health Statistics, 1982, p. 26). Reasons for this pattern are not clear since their reasons for visiting dentists, reasons for not seeing dentists, and their levels of satisfaction with the care and the waiting period are similar to those for people of all ages (National Center for Health Statistics, 1980).

Unlike other community-based services discussed in this section, clinics, physicians' offices, and emergency rooms were not developed specifically for the elderly. Each is fairly available in all but very remote rural areas and may be used by people of all ages.

Foster Care

Foster care is usually given in a private home occupied by an individual or family who provides rooms, meals, housekeeping, minimal surveillance, and personal care to a nonrelated elderly person for a monthly fee. Often the placement agency tries to match the characteristics of client and host. The host participates on the basis of both altruism and need

for additional income. Other names for foster care include "adult foster care," "personal care homes," "residential care homes," "board and care homes," and "community placement." These labels serve to distinguish adult foster care from foster placement for children, emphasize the community placement feature of the care, suggest the personal attention directed to individuals rather than groups, and indicate an absence of a consensus on an operational definition of the concept (Steinhauer, 1982).

Foster care is not a new concept. It has been in practice in Europe for hundreds of years, with the earliest known use recorded in 1250 in Gheel, Belgium. Families in the town accepted clients with mental problems into their homes for care. "Boarding out" these same kinds of clients was introduced into the United States in 1857 by Dorothea Dix. In 1885 Massachusetts became the first state to establish a program for people with geropsychiatric problems. The Binghamton State Hospital in New York instituted a program for elderly people in 1935 in response to sharply increasing numbers of old people (Steinhauer, 1982). The Veterans Administration (VA) has one of the oldest programs of foster home placement for veterans who, because of health conditions, are not able to resume independent living and have no suitable family resources to provide the needed care. This VA program began in 1951 as the Personal Care Home Program and is now titled The Residential Care Program. Care is provided in private homes selected by the VA, at the veteran's own expense. Social workers and other health professionals provide periodic follow-up visits and the veterans are outpatients of local VA facilities. In 1981, the approximate average daily census of this program was 12,500 (U.S. Senate Special Committee on Aging, 1982b; Steinhauer, 1982).

Foster care represents a natural way of responding to human needs for shelter and care. Thus, many informal structures have evolved without a formal plan. The incidence and prevalence of foster care is difficult to document. Regulation of adult foster care programs through inspection and licensure has not been uniformly addressed by the states (Steinhauer, 1982, pp. 294–295).

Funding arrangements for foster home care are variable. The VA, for example, expects veterans to use their own money whereas government support is a primary source of payment in other foster home programs. Usually state support is provided when other sources of payment, such as Social Security Benefits, Supplemental Security Income, and private pensions prove inadequate.

The issue of whether families or individuals who serve as hosts in foster home arrangements can avail themselves of respite care and emergency placements to secure relief from day-to-day burdens of caring for a nonfamily member has not been settled. This question, along with the questions of program definition, structure, regulation, and financing, requires attention from persons involved in long-term care planning.

Foster care tends to be underutilized partly because clients are not aware that this type of program is available. A second reason is that many potential care-providers are reluctant to open their homes to elderly people when they regard these people as destructive to their own family life. In addition, the care-giving relationship may end with the elderly person's death (Dunkle, 1982).

For adult foster care to become a more available option for the elderly, nurses need to view this type of care as a positive option for certain elderly people and assist in matching care recipients' needs and personalities to home environments. The foster family needs to be approached by professionals in the same way as natural families. Sometimes, two families will be involved with the client and his/her care decisions: the client's natural family and the foster family.

Homemaker/Chore Services and Personal Care Services

Homemaker/chore services focus on the client's home management needs. Homemaker services include performing routine light housecleaning, such as dusting, mopping, vacuuming, doing laundry, changing bed linens, washing dishes, and preparing meals. Chore services include running errands and shopping for groceries and medications. Persons who provide homemaker/chore services are usually the same individuals who provide personal care services to clients (U.S. General Accounting Office, 1981, p. 8).

Many elderly people have unmet needs for these types of services. Studies by the General Accounting Office in 1976 and 1978 indicated that between 16 and 22 percent of the sampled elderly population did not receive needed homemaker/chore services (U.S. General Accounting Office, 1981, p. 9).

Personal care services focus on the client's need for assistance with basic daily living activities such as bathing, oral hygiene, grooming, dressing, skin and foot care, and feeding and toileting. Home health aides who provide these services also remind clients to take prescribed medications.

General Accounting Office studies done in 1976 and 1978 found that the unmet need for person care services ranged from 10 to 22 percent of the populations sampled.

Both personal care and homemaker/chore programs are usually implemented by paraprofessionals under the guidance of professional supervisors. A typical team includes a nurse, a social worker, and a home health aide. A smaller team may consist of the home health aide plus either the nurse or the social worker as supervisor. Nutritionists and physical therapists may also serve as team members. Physicians are rarely involved.

Usually the aide visits on a part-time basis, two to three times each week for 1 to 4 hours. Support to the elderly client between visits may be provided by a volunteer staffed telephone checkup service. Supervisors visit on an as-needed basis.

Problems with homemaker/chore and personal care services are related to the great demand for service, which often forces clients to wait weeks or months to enter the program. Inadequate funding for these programs leads to recruitment of people willing to work for minimum wages, abbreviated training programs, and curtailment of aide supervision. Clients complain of aides who fail to come as scheduled and/or do little or nothing to help. When agency funding is reduced or stopped, clients must fend for themselves and/or go on a waiting list for entry to a long-term care facility.

Four federal programs—Medicare, Medicaid, and Title Twenty, under the Social Security Act and Title Three under the Older Americans Act—offer personal care and homemaker/chore services in the home, although these services are not their primary mandate. Each program has restrictions that limit the numbers of people who qualify for the services. Table 6.3 provides a comparison of essential characteristics of these four programs.

The most significant issue facing planners concerned with meeting the long-term, in-home needs of the elderly is how to contain cost without unreasonably restricting the availability of such services. "Various studies generally agree that in-home services prolong life and

maintain or increase the elderly's independence. They disagree, however, on whether providing long-term, in-home assistance has any impact on the number of elderly who are or would be receiving long-term care in nursing homes" (U.S. General Accounting Office, 1981, p. 24).

INSTITUTION-BASED CARE

In the United States, the proportion of elderly people admitted to short-stay hospitals has increased steadily since the advent of Medicare. Admission rates for long-stay hospitals and nursing homes, which rose immediately after the passage of Medicare, have declined in re-

TABLE 6.3 COMPARISON OF ESSENTIAL CHARACTERISTICS OF FOUR FEDERAL PROGRAMS FUNDING IN-HOME HOMEMAKER/CHORE AND PERSONAL CARE SERVICES

Characteristics	Social Security Act			Older Americans Act
	Title XVIII	Title XIX	Title XX	Title III
Services authorized:				
Nursing	Yes	Yes	No	Yes
Therapy	Yes	Yes	No	Yes
Home health aide	Yes	Yes	Yes	Yes
Homemaker	No	No	Yes	Yes
Chore	No	No	Yes	Yes
Medical supplies and appliances	Yes	Yes	No	No
Program eligibility requirements:				
Client must meet age requirement	Yes	No	No	Yes
Client must meet income requirement	No	Yes	Yes	No
Client must need part-time or intermittent skilled nursing care	Yes	No	No	No
Client must be homebound	Yes	No	No	No
Services to client must be authorized by a physician in accordance with a plan of care	Yes	Yes	No	No
Services must be included in state plan	*	Yes	Yes	Yes
Administration	Federal	State	State	State
Funding	Open ended	Open ended	Capped	Capped

*Federally administered program—no state plan required.
(U. S. General Accounting Office. Improved Knowledge Base Would Be Helpful in Reaching Policy Decisions on Providing Long-Term, In-Home Services for the Elderly. Washington, D.C., Superintendent of Documents, 1981, p 26)

cent years. This decline reflects strict standards for certification of the client's eligibility for Medicare payments, as well as the withdrawal of some nursing homes from the Medicare program in protest over the level of reimbursement. Admissions to boarding homes have increased as the admissions to nursing homes have declined. As support services to elderly people in all types of residential settings increase, there is a lessening of distinction between the congregate residence for the well elderly which offers some health services, and the health care facility in which old people in comparatively poor health reside for extended periods of time.

Hospital Care

Although the elderly comprised only 11 percent of the population in 1980, they used 30 percent of all short-stay hospital days used and stayed an average of 14 days per episode of hospitalization compared to 9 days for people of all ages. Nevertheless, a substantial amount of the elderly—82 percent, compared to 90 percent of people of all ages—reported having had no hospital episodes (National Center for Health Statistics, 1982, pp. 26–27).

The *swing-bed concept* refers to a practice of using the same hospital beds to provide both acute and long-term care as needed. This concept was developed in an effort to fill excess hospital beds left empty as a result of shortened hospital stays mandated by utilization review and third-party payers concerned about escalating acute-care costs.

There are several variations of the swing-bed concept in acute-care hospitals: (1) any bed in any location and at any time may be used for long-term clients, (2) a hospital with a designated long-term care section may also use acute beds for long-term care when needed, (3) part of the hospital may be converted for long-term care clients, and (4) an entire facility may be converted to a long-term facility (Miller, 1980, p. 97).

Problems associated with the use of swing-beds concern failure to plan for the differences inherent in long-term as opposed to acute care. Staff orientation and training are required to enable personnel to facilitate therapeutic goals of long-term clients. Meal trays served at the bedside are not appropriate in long-term care where socialization is a common client need and dining is an important means of encouraging socialization. The architecture and general atmosphere of long-term care units need to promote independence and meetings between residents. Access to outdoors plus alarm systems to alert staff to the fact that residents who may be confused are entering unprotected areas are both required.

The success of swing-bed policies has been mixed. On the positive side, swing beds do meet a need for services, as more elderly people require long-term care and hospital beds sit idle in the absence of clients needing acute care. However, the quality of care provided in swing-bed hospitals in at least three states was inferior to the care provided in nursing homes. Among the categories in which nursing homes scored higher were emotional, restorative, and social services, as well as numbers of care and client problem levels. The costs of providing an acceptable quality of long-term care to swing-bed occupants make swing-bed hospital care more costly in the long run than providing care in an existing skilled nursing facility (Rosenthal, 1980).

Long-Term Care Facilities (LTCFs)

These facilities are institutions in which people live for an extended time while they receive medical and social services. By this definition, both intermediate and skilled nursing facilities are long-term care facilities.

An *intermediate care facility* (ICF) is an institution (or distinct part of an institution) licensed under state law. It provides, on a regular basis, health-related care and services to clients who do not need the kind of treatment that a hospital or skilled nursing facility is designed to provide but who because of their mental or physical condition require care and services above the level of room and board (Congressional Budget Office 1977, p. 52). A *skilled nursing facility* (SNF) is an institution (or a distinct part of an institution) that is primarily engaged in providing post-hospital, convalescent, rehabilitation care, usually on a short-term basis (Congressional Budget Office, 1977, p. 52).

Nursing homes and *homes for the aged* are less clearly defined. They can be viewed as places where personal care services are provided in a protective environment. Both intermediate and skilled nursing facilities are casually referred to by the general public as "nursing homes," as are domiciliary facilities, boarding homes, personal care homes, and even rooming houses. Actually, nursing homes are designed to provide skilled nursing and medical care, while homes for the aged place less emphasis on such care. Homes for the aged usually admit clients who are healthy and independent, and then provide for some health-care services in response to changing needs.

Domiciliary care is a term covering a variety of living arrangements that include varying numbers and kinds of basic services to residents. At a minimum, services include shelter, food, and some supervision. Additional optional services consist of recreation, sheltered work, personal care, and grooming. Domiciliary care usually excludes nursing care or medical supervision even though residents may be physically or mentally disabled. Domiciliaries are most commonly licensed by state departments of social services. They are not eligible for reimbursement through either Medicare or Medicaid. The Veterans Administration provides domiciliaries as part of its continuum of services. Other names for domiciliary care facilities include "board and care" homes, "adult foster care," "personal care homes," "family care," and "homes for the aged." These facilities provide an appropriate alternative for people who do not need skilled nursing care, at one end of the scale, as well as for those who are not able to function in their own homes, at the other end of the scale.

These facilities have been increasing in size because of (1) the rapid increase in the population over 75 years of age, (2) the availability of federally supported income maintenance programs for the elderly, blind, and disabled, and (3) the release of many elderly and mental clients from state institutions. Domiciliary care facility residents tend to be younger

and are more likely to be male than the nursing home population (Billings, 1982).

In recent years, these types of facilities have received considerable attention as a result of congressional hearings and investigative media reporting that has documented the unsafe and unsanitary conditions, as well as resident abuse and neglect, occurring in some of these facilities. Thus, demands for more comprehensive higher-quality standards and enforcement of standards in the regulation of domiciliaries have escalated. An analysis of state regulations reported in 1983 (Reichstein and Bergofsky, 1983) indicated that a number of important requirements affecting the health, safety, and well-being of domiciliary care residents were not met. The only area where a majority of the regulations were met concerned the physical plant. However, even in this area, regulations tended to omit fire safety precautions and needs of the handicapped. A model code was recommended as a means of providing more comprehensive and uniform regulations from state to state instead of the present diversity. A second objective a model code could achieve is simplification of the standards in order to eliminate unnecessarily restrictive provisions that create difficulties for providers and place obstacles in the way of potential providers. However, standards are only one part of regulation and regulation alone does not guarantee quality of care.

Personal care homes, compared to domiciliary care homes, usually provide more assistance with activities of daily living. At any one time, approximately 5 percent of the elderly in the United States live in skilled and intermediate care facilities. However, the proportion of the elderly who are likely to spend some time in an institution has been estimated to be close to 25 percent (Kastenbaum and Candy, 1973; Wershow, 1976; Palmore, 1976).

Under what circumstances do and should people be institutionalized for long-term care? Four influencing factors are (1) the need for assistance, (2) the availability of financial resources, (3) the presence of social supports, and (4) the expression of personal preference. Institutionalized people who have both social support and financial support tend to be clearly in need of help with activities of daily living. They enter the institution only when resources are exhausted or death appears imminent. People lacking in social and financial supports tend to be more capable of independence in these activities. They enter the nursing home prematurely as "protection" for the future. Thus, a socioeconomic need is met with a health-care solution (Barney, 1977, pp. 309–310).

Respite Care

Respite care is usually defined as a service that provides temporary institutional care on an intermittent basis for chronically ill or disabled elderly people being cared for at home. This concept, however, needs to be extended to include homemaker/chore, personal care, and adult-sitter services provided in the home to enable regular care-givers to have a break or leave the setting for a time.

Kinds of situations where this type of care seems required include those in which (1) significant others wish to take a vacation or break from the continuing responsibility inherent in providing support, (2) a temporary crisis or medical emergency removes the care-giver from the home, or (3) care-givers are unable to leave the home unless someone else is present.

With institutionally centered respite care, the elderly person is admitted to a 24-hour care center (usually a nursing home) for a few days per week, weekends, vacations, or emergencies. Relief from the work and responsibilities involved in care of an old person with health impairments is as necessary for the care-giver as it is for the parent with preschool children. The outcome of a planned, convenient break through a respite care program may be improvement in a relationship that is very important to the elderly person. Such programs may also reduce the necessity for institutionalization as a permanent arrangement.

The potential demand for respite care is not known. The New York State Health Planning Commission informally estimated that two-thirds of a bed per 1000 people over age 65 might be a reasonable indicator (Howells, 1980, p. 2).

Problems with respite care include finding facilities that offer this care and then paying for it. Third-party payment for respite care is available primarily in connection with special demonstration projects.

Hospice Care

A hospice is not a place, but rather, a flexible concept of service. This type of care can be given in a variety of settings: a free-standing hospice facility, an area within a hospital or long-term care facility; or at home as part of a program sponsored by a hospital, nursing home, or community-based agency.

Impetus for hospice programs came from deficiencies in conventional care of the terminally ill: (1) inadequate control of pain, (2) continuation of expensive and often painful medical procedures unwanted by the client, and (3) provision of care in an institution when clients preferred to be at home.

In hospice programs, emphasis is placed on palliative and supportive care to meet the special needs of dying clients and their families during the final stages of illness. A range of health services is available from a multidisciplinary team 24 hours a day, 7 days a week. A high priority is placed on adhering to clients' wishes. Volunteers often assist with client care and administrative tasks.

Although the hospice concept originated in 1842 in France, the first U.S. hospice facility was not opened until 1974. The number of these facilities increased rapidly to an estimated 700 by 1982 (Billings, 1982, p. 8). Some private insurers provide coverage for this type of care. The Joint Commission on Accreditation of Hospitals announced an accreditation program for hospices starting in 1983.

The growth of hospice programs has prompted an important question. Why could not existing medical practices have been changed to permit care to be determined by the wishes of dying people rather than the wishes of the medical profession (Billings, 1982; Greer, 1983)? The "hospice concept" may be considered as synonymous with "good" nursing care. In time, clients other than those who are dying can be expected to notice the differences between the hospice and their own health care settings. When this awareness dawns, the following demand may well be heard: "Do I have to be dying to have some say about my care?" Meanwhile, some elderly people expected to die within a short, defined period of time (usually within 6 months) may find themselves in hospice settings.

Small Group Housing

As an alternative to institutional forms of care, almost every developed country has "congregate" or "sheltered" housing schemes to provide for assisted group living. Actually, such housing can occur within institutional settings (Peace, 1981) as well as in the community. Small group housing in community settings was discussed earlier in this chapter under "Special Housing."

In order to combat the institutional malaise that occurs in homes for the aged, homes are constructed or remodeled to permit "small group living" to occur. Most of this change is occurring in Great Britain (Peace, 1981). "Home Close," which opened in 1969 in Cambridgeshire, England provided five self-contained flats (apartments) for groups of eight (mixed sex). Each flat contained six single bedrooms, one double bedroom, a dining/sitting room, a kitchen, bathroom, two toilets, and a utility room with appliances required to wash and disinfect soiled linen, bedpans and commodes. Residents were encouraged to bring their own furniture. A centralized main kitchen, medical room, Chief Residential Care Officer's office, and laundry were provided. *Considerations of convenience from the staff's point of view were regarded as secondary* in avoiding features common to institutions. Residents prepare most of their own meals, make their own beds, maintain a tidy environment, and make decisions about assigning tasks (Peace, 1981). Evaluation of this program revealed that residents, despite greater physical disabilities, were more physically active and mobile, made greater use of the kitchen, did more housework, conversed more among themselves, and were less likely to be seen "doing nothing" than residents in two traditional homes (Peace and Harding, 1980). Problems with this living arrangement

centered on slow adjustment on the part of residents to the new life-style, including some resentment at not being "looked after" (Peace and Harding, 1980).

Probably those homes that are designed for "small group housing" operate more effectively, but the concept has been adopted successfully in traditional homes. The issue of what will happen as the resident population becomes more disabled remains to be solved.

PAYMENT FOR HEALTH CARE*

Sources

The trend toward public financing for health care has had dramatic consequences for the elderly. Less than half of the total personal health care expenditures for elderly people are covered by Medicare. The Medicare share has increased slightly from 35 percent in 1970 to 45 percent in 1980. Despite Medicare's increasing share of costs, however, the elderly person's individual responsibility for his or her total health care bill is growing, from $503 in 1970 to $1436 in 1980. These figures represent an increase from 17 to 19 percent of total income and are approaching the same share of personal income that health care costs consumed in 1965, before Medicare (20 percent). Figure 6.2 depicts types of expenditures and sources of funds for personal health care for the elderly.

Although approximately 90 percent of the population is covered by some form of health insurance, benefits vary widely and leave substantial areas uncovered. In 1965, Congress expanded the Social Security program begun in 1935 by adding two significant amendments on health care and services. The first, Title 18, established Medicare—a federal program of hospital and medical insurance to serve as the basic protection against the high costs of health

---

* Unless otherwise stated, statistics reported in this section are from the Health Care Financing Administration (HCFA), unpublished data for 1982, and were reported in an information paper prepared by the staff of the Special Committee on Aging, United States Senate (U.S. Senate Special Committee on Aging, 1982b).

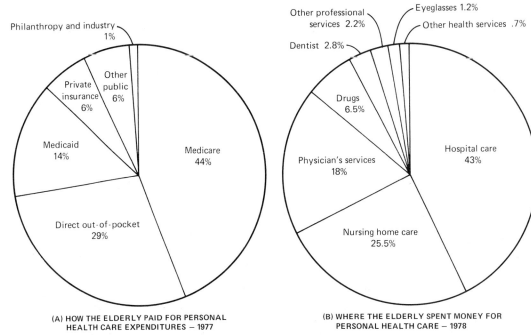

(A) HOW THE ELDERLY PAID FOR PERSONAL
HEALTH CARE EXPENDITURES — 1977

(B) WHERE THE ELDERLY SPENT MONEY FOR
PERSONAL HEALTH CARE — 1978

Figure 6.2. Types of expenditures and sources of funds for personal health care for the population aged 65 years and over. *(Adapted from Brotman, HB. Every Ninth American (1982 edition): An Analysis for the Chairman of the U.S. House of Representatives Select Committee on Aging, 1982, pp 9–10. United States Senate Special Committee on Aging. Health Care Expenditures for the Elderly: How Much Protection does Medicare provide? Washington D.C., U.S. Government Printing Office, 1982b, p 6.)*

care for elderly Americans. However, increasing numbers of elderly, inflation of health-care costs, increased scope and depth of services, and uncontrolled increases in charges by physicians and other providers threatened stability of the trust fund established to pay Medicare hospitalization benefits. Between 1965 and 1970, physicians' fees rose 39 percent and hospital charges rose 110 percent (Butler, 1975, pp. 174–224). These increases suggest that Medicare only insured that providers would be paid and not that clients would have a means to pay for the care they needed! The second amendment to the Social Security program, Title 19, established Medicaid—a federal–state program to help provide medical services for the medically indigent needy.

Medicare coverage is available in two parts. Part A (hospital insurance) is free to eligible people aged 65 and over and covers hospital

care, post-hospital extended care, and home health benefits. Part B (medical insurance) requires eligible elderly people to pay a portion of the cost in the form of monthly premiums. It covers physician care, hospital outpatient services, physical therapy, diagnostic tests, ambulance service, and the like. There are four major sources of health-care costs for the elderly not paid by Medicare: (1) uncovered premiums, (2) shared costs, (3) charges in excess of Medicare payments for covered services, and (4) premiums.

1. *Uncovered Services.* Since Medicare's focus is primarily on covering acute care, many services remain outside the scope of benefits. These services range from basic preventive services to long-term care. As an example, pneumococcal vaccine was recently included as a covered service. However, other preventive measures, from flu injections to physical ex-

aminations, remained uncovered. The nursing home benefit is restricted to 100 days, leaving longer-term skilled care and lower levels of chronic care uncovered. The acute care hospital benefit is limited to 150 days. Drugs, basic dental service, eyeglass, hearing aid, and special diet costs are not covered by Medicare.

2. *Shared Costs.* Medicare requires that users share costs in a number of situations, including a deductible for hospital services ($260 in 1982), copayments on hospital and nursing home services, and a $75 per year initial deductible and 20 percent coinsurance on physician and outpatient services. Copayments for hospital services are imposed starting with the 61st day of care and equal one-fourth of the hospital deductible for the 61st through the 90th day. This sum amounted to $65 per day in 1982. From the 91st through the 150th day, the copayment is one-half of the deductible—in 1982, $130 per day. For nursing home care, the copayment starts on the 21st day of care and is equal to one-eighth of the hospital deductible. This sum was $32.50 in 1982.

3. *Charges in Excess of Medicare Payments for Covered Services.* When physicians bill a Medicare client directly for services ("unassigned claims"), the beneficiary must then pay not only the 20 percent coinsurance, but any amount beyond what Medicare considers "reasonable" (as determined by law and regulation) for that claim. Approximately 50 percent of all physicians bill clients directly.

4. *Premiums.* Although not included in total personal health care expenditures, beneficiaries also pay a monthly premium for Medicare coverage for physician services. This premium rises automatically each year and in 1982 was $11.00 per month.

Medicaid is a grant-in-aid program, in which federal, state, and sometimes local government share the costs of medical care for people of all ages with low incomes. Within certain federally imposed limits, each state determines benefits and eligibility. Thus, benefits and eligibility vary from one state to another. Medicaid complements the hospital insurance (Part A) provision of Medicare by paying all or part of the deductible and coinsurance amounts for low-income aged people

who are insured. It also complements the voluntary medical insurance (Part B) provisions of Medicare by paying the monthly premiums for Medicaid recipients. Medicaid may also supplement the Medicare insurance program by providing additional benefits for people who are eligible. These benefits include such things as days of skilled nursing home care, home health services, physicians' services, inpatient hospital services, outpatient hospital services, and other laboratory and x-ray services. The exact nature of these supplementary benefits varies from state to state. Supplementary benefits are not available until benefits from Medicare has been exhausted.

Eligibility for Medicaid is determined by a means test, which is a deterrent to many potential elderly users. When old people in institutional settings have exhausted other financial resources, they are faced with the choice of discharge or application for Medicaid benefits. Long-term care facilities are reluctant to take clients on Medicaid, because reimbursement rates are lower than those of Medicare and private insurance companies.

The entire gap between personal health-care expenditures and coverage is not necessarily absorbed by the beneficiary, however. Over 70 percent of the elderly have some sort of supplementary coverage, including both private insurance and Medicaid. The Veterans Administration, the Hill–Burton Act, and state-funded mental hospitals also help elderly people receive health services.

Private insurance's share of total personal health expenditures for the elderly was 6.6 percent in 1977 (Fisher, 1980). Most of this coverage is designed to pay for Medicare deductibles and coinsurance amounts. A number of policies pay for hospital stays beyond the 150-day lifetime limit allowed by Medicare. However, few supplemental policies pay for outpatient drugs or long-term care, interventions that create large expenses for elderly people.

Premium rates for private insurance have increased steadily over the years. A typical annual rate for someone aged 65 and older prior to Medicare in 1965 was $180 to $240. In 1982, the rate ranged from $300 to $400 for only a supplement to Medicare. As might be expected, coverage is directly related to income, with the more affluent elderly more likely to have private insurance.

Although Medicaid covers over 13 percent of the health costs to the elderly, most of the expenditures are for the small proportion of elderly people using the long-term care benefit. Most elderly people (80 to 85 percent of Medicare beneficiaries) do not participate in Medicaid because they cannot pass the means test for low-income.

The major source of payment for health expenditures not paid by Medicare is direct out-of-pocket payment by the beneficiary. The elderly were responsible for 29 percent of their total personal health care expenditures in 1977, which came to about $768 per person in 1980. These direct out-of-pocket costs include neither the Part B Medicare premium costs that reached $146.40 in July, 1982, nor the cost of supplemental medical insurance premiums, which ranged between $300 and $400 per year in 1982 (U.S. Senate Special Committee on Aging, 1982b, p. 6).

The best known resources that the elderly use for health care are (1) Medicare, (2) private insurance, (3) personal out-of-pocket money, and (4) Medicaid when the first three resources have been used to their fullest, or, in the case of personal funds, nearly depleted. A less publicized source of payment for health care is the Hill–Burton Act. This federal law has given hospitals millions of dollars for construction since 1946. To insure that hospitals built with public money offer benefits to the public, the act requires that hospitals receiving this money provide certain amounts of "free and below cost" care to people who cannot afford to pay. In 1978 the Hill–Burton Act was replaced by Title 16 of the National Health Planning Resources and Development Act, which also contains the free care and community service requirements. Hospitals have traditionally been reluctant to honor their obligation to provide "free and below-cost" care. Nurses and clients who wish to learn which hospitals must provide such care should contact their State Health Department, the agency responsible for ensuring compliance with the Hill–Burton law.

Implications for Nurses

Nurses should be aware that health care is an expensive and unpopular commodity. Very few people can afford health care without the help of "third-party payment" (insurance). Even fewer people enjoy spending money for health care. Clients should be asked whether they expect that their health insurance will cover the costs of whatever health care they are receiving. Any client who appears to be at risk of exceeding limits of coverage should be told about alternative resources. The nurse can provide this information directly or through referral to a social worker.

When clients object to using Medicaid because of the means test, the nurse is free to try to convince them to do otherwise. However, chances of success are small. The nurse who believes that old people should receive health care as a matter of right (for simply having lived 65 or more years) might make an effort to influence legislators to abolish eligibility requirements for the elderly.

Since the cost of health-care services are high and the elderly, despite Medicare and private insurance, pay a substantial proportion of their expenses themselves, nurses must make every effort to keep costs to a minimum. Physicians should be reminded to prescribe generically. Nursing therapies should be evaluated in terms of their costs to the client and preventive measures should be stressed. Clients who wish to establish or act upon living wills for purposes of cost containment should be supported by the nurse.

IMPLICATIONS OF HEALTH CARE RESOURCES FOR LONG-TERM CARE NURSING

Special consideration of nursing practice in long-term care settings is warranted first because nurses are the most constant health care providers in these settings (Fig. 6.3). Nurses perform the work of other disciplines when members of those disciplines are off duty or otherwise occupied. Second, in long-term care settings, the care provided by the nurse is more neces-

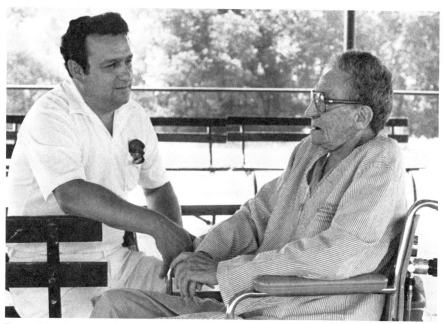

Figure 6.3. Nurses are the most necessary health discipline in long-term care. *(Photograph by Shawn Mertz, Pittsburgh, P.A.)*

sary than the treatments provided by the physician. Care can frequently refer to complete and lasting eradication of all manifestations of a disease, but it also means to relieve, support, and rehabilitate to make life rich and useful, even in the presence of continuing disease or disability (Lambertson, cited in Spanier, 1979, p. 739). In long-term care facilities, it is this latter definition of care that is so crucial.

In recent years, nursing has become disenchanted with traditional approaches to health and illness care. This disenchantment has led nurses to re-examine the concept of health and their role in providing health care to clients. In general, nurses are aligning themselves with health and wellness. However, as physicians refocus their efforts toward disease control and long-term survival, their practice may become more like the caring practice of nurses.

The vital part that nurses play in caring for the elderly can be described by considering a hypothetical example of a 7-day strike in a long-term care facility by all personnel except nurses. Nurses are prepared either through life experiences or formal training to cook, serve trays, wash dishes, mop floors, empty trash, assist clients to exercise and engage in therapeutic activities, make referrals to other agencies, and interact with clients and their families to obtain social histories. Medications and treatments ordered by physicians would continue to be given. New physical illness crises would be managed by transferring clients and/ or by applying nursing interactions. With fewer new medications and invasive therapies, clients might even fare better! Now consider a hypothetical, 7-day strike by only nursing personnel. Which *one* profession could step in to administer the large volume of medications as well as to bathe, dress, toilet, and feed clients? It is extremely doubtful that all of the professions combined (physicians, social workers, physical therapists, dietitians and occupational therapists) could handle the work involved. Unless the striking nursing personnel were brought back or replacement nursing personnel were found within the week, chaos would result and clients would soon show visible signs of the absence of nursing care.

A second example of invaluable service that nurses can offer elderly people can be found in a home assessment of urinary incontinence project. A nurse practitioner visits the client's home to conduct a comprehensive assessment that includes a detailed history, focused physical examination, quantification of the incontinence in terms of amount and frequency, and, if the problem remains after assessment, referral for invasive diagnostic studies by a physician, or teaching for reversal or improved containment of urine leakage (Robb, 1983). What other health profession is prepared to conduct a 95-page, computer-ready, assessment in clients' homes by applying communication skills to convince clients to tolerate the tedious and potentially embarrassing assessment and teaching skills to enable clients to keep complex and detailed records of urination and fluid intake? Until this project began in this country, most of these clients had been abandoned as hopelessly incontinent due to "age" and left to cope as best they could with pads, mops, and catheters.

If they would seize the opportunity to emphasize and publicize the results of their efforts, nurses might be able to control their practice in long-term care. With such a change, the term *nursing* home might come to mean a place where nurses eagerly seek employment to practice without undue constraint and clients deliberately seek the services of nurses. At present, the term *nursing* home represents an embarrassment to the profession. The term exists because physicians often decline to become involved in addressing day-to-day needs of clients. Physicians tend to operate "behind the scene" and make brief appearances on stage to justify billing clients or third-party payers for visits and treatments. Nurses are left to absorb the blame for inadequate services. Nurses are hampered in their efforts to provide proper care because they do not control the resources (supplies, equipment, physical environment) needed

for the task (DeSantis, 1982). Given this situation, the main implications for nursing practice in providing long-term health care concern the discovery and promotion of factors that affect outcomes achieved by clients. These factors can be categorized in terms of their relationship to either the structure (quality and quantity of resources) or the process (uses of resources) applied to achieve care outcomes (an end result of care defined as a behavior change in the client) (Donabedian, 1978).

Measuring Quality of Care

The focus of quality of care determination changes constantly to include one or more of the components listed in Linn and Linn's (1980) research model for the evaluation of quality of care, presented in Figure 6.4. The focus of medical care is on the prevention, detection, and arrest of pathologic processes (Schlotfeldt, 1975, p. 22). Health care goes further to include "care directed toward high-level wellness through processes that encourage alteration of personal habits or the environment in which people live. It occurs after health stability is present and assumes disease prevention and health maintenance as prerequisites or by-products" (Brubaker, 1983, p. 12). Examples of personal habits that may require alteration include smoking, using mind-altering substances, eating, and exercising.

A second term that requires definition is "quality." There is much ambiguity and confusion, even among professionals in the field, about what really constitutes quality care. This ambiguity is more apparent among the general public, who make demands on regulatory agencies and legislators to improve quality, without completely knowing what it is they expect. Some expect newer buildings, absolute safety, and environmental sterility. Others want more diagnostic thoroughness, more vigorous medical treatment, and life support machines and techniques that are available and used. At the same time, all recognize the lack of quality inherent in the restriction or denial of human rights, personal choice, comfort, and ordinary human relationships. All of these expectations are good and desirable, but sometimes they are mutually exclusive, at least in practice.

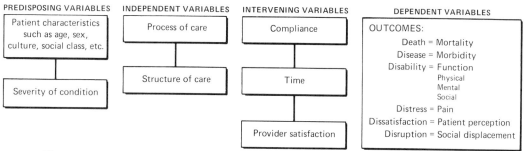

Figure 6.4. A research model for the evaluation of quality of care. (Linn, M.W., Linn, B.S. *Qualities of institutional care that affect outcome. Aged Care and Services Review 2(3):17, 1980. Copyright 1980 by the Haworth Press, Inc. All rights reserved. Reprinted by permission.)*

The trend is to define "quality" as the effect of care on the health of the individual and the population (Kane et al., 1983; Linn and Linn, 1980). Although outcome can be defined many ways, the classification of Elison described by White (1967) and supplemented by Sanazaro and Williamson (1968) contains most of the outcomes commonly considered in studies: death (mortality), disease (morbidity), disability (physical, social, and mental function), distress (pain), dissatisfaction (client's perception), and disruption (social displacement).

The refusal to consider as acceptable any outcome other than cure, even when the expectation is only implicit, makes it difficult to see how chronicity, deterioration, and death can ever be dealt with in a positive manner. An added complication to our expectations of quality is the possibility that much of our discomfort and outrage about the quality of long-term care has to do with our collective guilt and rage that any of us has to become disabled, deteriorate, or die.

Structural Factors Associated with Quality Care

In Donabedian's (1978) framework, structure refers to the quality and quantity of resources and the input of personnel, equipment, and facilities. Factors named in response to the following question tend to be structural variables: "What do nurses and others have to work with?" Bricks and mortar, ownership, and supply and equipment factors may seem to be beyond the control of nurses. However, persistent and vigorous efforts can change even a gloomy

structural picture for the better. An example exists in the work done by the Committee to Improve Kane Hospital, a small group comprised of disgruntled health professionals that included nurses. Publication of the report in 1975 detailing structure, process, and outcome problems, *Kane Hospital: A Place to Die*, led to U.S. Senate hearings and an audit by the General Accounting Office. Extensive process-related changes followed soon after the inquiries during 1976–78. By 1979, a variety of external pressures, generated by the report, forced county officials to proceed with plans to replace what was, before the public scandal, a 2000-bed facility with four "mini-Kane Hospitals" of approximately 300–400 beds each. Thus, nurses working with other people did influence change in the size and location of a nursing home (Robb, Peterson, and Nagy, 1979).

Admittedly, even though common sense tells us that structural factors of an institution ought to affect the quality of care, studies in this area have not been very definitive. Part of the failure to identify expected relationships is due to the way quality of care has been measured. Too often, structure and process factors have been studied in relation to each other, without any attempt to evaluate them against client outcomes. Considered as a group, however, these studies do provide useful information to guide people involved in long-term care planning and regulation.

Size

Size is one of the structural variables often studied in relation to institutional care. Overall results fail to indicate whether small or large facilities are superior. Very small facility size (under 50 beds) was found to be conducive to direct staff–client contact and, in turn, to very high quality rehabilitative programs (Ullman, 1981). With more clients, staff have been observed to exercise more control over client behavior (Cohen and Streuning, 1965; Moos, 1972; 1974). In larger facilities, clients experience lower discharge rates and fewer days back in the community (Linn, 1970). As nursing home size increases, client activity and communication decline (Greenwald and Linn, 1971), as does client satisfaction, friends within the home, and monthly contacts with these friends (Curry and Ratcliff, 1973). Kart and Manard (1976) found that increasing size in old age homes increased commitment of resources to clerical, administrative, and other impersonal activities that had an adverse effect on personal services to residents.

On the other hand, Moos and Ingra (1980) found that resident cohesion, independence, and self-exploraton increased as facility size increased. Winn and McCaffree (1976) reported that more beds, more staff, certification for more levels of care, and higher occupancy rates were all associated with homes perceived to be effective and efficient. Size was positively associated with quality of care defined as more registered nurse hours and higher expenditures for nursing care, dietary services, and other direct client care expenditures (Greene and Monahan, 1981).

In short, it is unclear what position nurses should take regarding the optimum size of long-term care facilities. It has not yet been resolved whether large homes can provide good care without being dehumanizing and whether small homes can give good care if they have fewer available resources.

Profit-Making Status

All else being equal, for-profit facilities provide lower levels of care than do nonprofit facilities. Distantly headquartered chains provide lower levels of care than locally owned facilities (Greene and Monahan, 1981). The strong and negative association between quality of care

and for-profit operation that was found in a study of 24 skilled nursing facilities in a metropolitan area in Arizona suggests the issue of profit-making requires further study and that vigorous public involvement in proprietary home operation is extremely important (Greene and Monahan, 1981). The quality of care measure in this study was comprised of the following items: registered nurse nursing hours, registered nurse expenditures, client dietary expenditures, and other client direct care expenditures all standardized on a per client-day basis. Results of this study are supported by those from a number of previous studies that found better care in nonprofit old age facilities. Townsend (1962) studied quality of care in 173 British long-term care institutions and found that voluntary nonprofit homes provided what was considered better care; proprietary homes provided average levels of care; and public homes gave the poorest care. A study of 80 facilities in St. Louis also reported that nonprofit old age homes were superior in terms of social milieu, staff attitudes, and other favorable characteristics than for-profit homes (Beattie and Bullock, 1964). Holmberg and Anderson (1968) found that clients in nonprofit homes were older but less impaired mentally than clients in for-profit homes. Yet another study found more physician hours per client in nonprofit than for-profit homes (Anderson, Holmberg, Schneider, and Stone, 1969).

In the past, the impact of profit-seeking on the quality of care provided in long-term care facilities has attracted considerable interest. For proprietary homes in particular, the opportunity and need exist to seek profits through reducing direct care costs (that is, by reducing the quantity or quality of services, or both) for a population that is essentially a captive one. A study done a number of years ago (Levey et al., 1973) found no relationship between for-profit operation and the quality of care. These findings have been used by nursing home owners to discourage regulation of their facilities as unnecessary. Thus, the newer study by Greene and Monahan (1981) is an important one that supports the personal experiences of surveyors and others who visit large numbers of long-term care facilities that are owned and operated for a variety of purposes.

Cost

A survey of 126 Minnesota nursing homes found that the quality of care was inversely related to the percentage of welfare clients in facilities and directly related to daily per capita facility expenditures (Anderson, Holmberg, Schneider, and Stone, 1969). A subsequent study of Massachusetts facilities supported results of the Minnesota study (Levey et al., 1973). Kosberg (1973), in studying 214 Chicago area nursing homes, found that nonaffluent and minority elderly were most often institutionalized in old age facilities that were lacking in treatment resources. More affluent elderly people tended to reside in facilities with more treatment resources (personnel and equipment). In evaluating the quality of care in 24 nursing homes in the Phoenix area, Greene and Monahan (1981) found that facilities that spent more money for administrative costs tended to provide higher levels of direct client care. Considered as a group, these studies provide some evidence that spending more money for care translates into the provision of better care.

Professionalism

To think that long-term care should cost comparatively little, based on the notion that anyone can care for old people, especially if they "just" need personal assistance and custodial care, is naive. Efforts to train the large numbers of nurses' aides now in long-term care institutions is based on this notion. It is as if this kind of nursing can be taught in a few weeks to any well-meaning person. Nursing, in addressing both the quality and cost of care, defends the need for more professional nurse involvement as being both quality and cost accountable. The more skilled the care-giver, the less time is wasted, the fewer costly mistakes are made, and the greater is the possibility of the client being restored to health. Although there is no clear answer to the question of how many registered nurses are "enough," the studies summarized below indicate that more registered nurses mean higher quality care.

STUDY #1

Purpose: "To examine variations in the quality of care given to individuals who are residents of skilled nursing facilities in Maryland, even though the residents are classified as requiring the same level of care. Factors were identified which had good relation to the construct 'quality of care' and were examined to determine their influence on the quality of care in the study population. These factors were location of facility, type of ownership, patient/staff ratios, numbers of licensed personnel, education of nursing administrator, ratios of skilled/intermediate patients, and number of support services" (Bingham, Fittipaldi, Holvoet, Mech, Mones, and Simmons, 1977, p. 58).

Conclusions: "Lower patient/staff ratio on a nursing unit increased the quality of care on that unit. The quality of care increased when the ratio of patients classified as requiring skilled care was lowered in respect to intermediate or residential level patients within the nursing home" (Bingham, et al, 1977, p. 59).

Quality Measure: Wandelt Quality Patient Care Scale

Source: Bingham, R., Fittipaldi, L., Holvoet, E., Mech, A., Mones, P., Simmons, V. Assessment of Quality Care in Skilled Nursing Facilities. Baltimore, University of Maryland, Master of Science in Nursing Thesis, 1977.

STUDY #2

Purpose: To consider the quality of care in several nursing homes over time, based on client's conditions both before and after admission to the home.

Conclusions: "Homes with more RN hours per patient were associated with patients being alive, improved and discharged from the home. Better ratings on meal services were related to being alive and improved. A higher professional staff-to-patient ratio, better medical records and more services were related to being discharged from the nursing home" (Linn, Gurel, and Linn, 1977, p. 337)

"RN hours specifically were related to outcome whereas hours per patient of other service providers or the total staff patient ratio were not so related. Nursing hours (including RNs, LPNs, and aides) were 2.47, 2.26, 2.40 and 2.27 for improved, the same, deteriorated and dead respectively. It has been reported that 3.2 hours per each patient is deemed to be borderline for severely ill patients who require almost total nursing care in nursing homes."

"Although staffing hours appear to be quite high in the homes where more of the patients deteriorated, these homes also had more severely ill patients with cancer. Therefore when means were adjusted for differences in severity of the patient's condition, the staffing favored the improved patient groups. The actual differences in amount of RN nursing time per patient for each of the outcome groups appears similar. However, the difference between .25 in the improved patient group and .22 in the group where patients died represents one more RN in terms of total staffing. In fact, a difference of about 10 percent more or less RN nursing staff exists between all of the outcome groups" (Linn, Gurel, and Linn, 1977, p. 341)

Quality Measures: Subjects were classified on follow-up as improved, the same, deteriorated, or dead. They were also classified as discharged from the nursing home, still in the home or readmitted to the hospital.

Source: Linn, M.W., Gurel, L., Linn, B.S. Patient outcome as a measure of quality of nursing home care. American Journal of Public Health 67(4): 337–344, 1977.

STUDY #3

Purpose: To analyze organizational variables related to the quality of nursing care in *hospitals.*

Research Question: Does the number of RN hours influence the quality of nursing care?

Conclusions: "The study of correlates identified a series of variables, and interrelationships among them, that significantly influenced quality of nursing care. Most important among these were a number of variables characterizing the organizational structure of the patient care unit. RN hours per patient day, continuity of care as reflected in the primary nursing organization, and coordination of the parts of the patient care system all related positively to quality, while the size and patient census of the unit as well as non-professional staffing related negatively to quality of care. Beyond these influences, leadership and unit staff satisfaction contributed to high quality. These variables, and hence their effect on quality, are all subject to administra-

tive influence. Variables external to the nursing service, such as hospital size and complexity, appear to influence quality mainly through their relation to the organizational structure of patient care units, to both unit and supervisory staff attitudes, and to leadership style" (Haussmann, Hegyvary, and Newman, 1976, p. 64).

Provision for Privacy

The large volume of literature on the topics of territory or space needs of the elderly clearly supports the need for privacy for residents in long-term care facilities [see, for example, Lawton and Bader (1970); Gioiella (1978); Johnson (1979); Firestone, Lichtman, and Evans (1980); Nelson and Paluck (1980); Rawnsley (1980); Louis (1981); and Rowles (1981)]. The arguments for private rooms and bathrooms in long-term care facilities are compelling. The psychologic and social functions of residents may be impaired to the point of confusion and depression when they are forced to share intimate living spaces (bedrooms and bathrooms) with strangers. There is a "sector-related trend in the quality of the psychosocial environment, with residents in voluntary or non-profit homes faring better than their counterparts in proprietary homes and much better than residents who live in facilities that offer services primarily to Medicaid beneficiaries. Specifically, residents in voluntary homes are able to bring personal possessions into the facility to continue to maintain previously held ties and associations; Medicaid beneficiaries live in environments that are lowest in the psychosocial dimensions of care. The latter residents experience the greatest degree of discontinuity and isolation, have the least privacy, their needs are provided for minimally, and they have limited opportunities for activity and social involvement" (Harel and Noelker, 1978, pp. 204–205).

A study of confusional states in elderly clients with hip fractures showed that clients "in private rooms tended to do better on memory testing than those in rooms shared with others" (Williams, Holloway, Winn, Wolanin, Lawler, Westwick, and Chin, 1979, p. 25). Without private rooms, loss of personal possessions is next to impossible to control. Whether from confusion or malice, people take each others' possessions in institutions. Private rooms with closed, if not locked, doors greatly reduce this behavior.

Residents themselves prefer private rooms. Lawton and Bader (1970, p. 52) found that almost no institutional resident who has a single room wishes to share one. On the other hand, among all who have roommates, 47 percent wish a single room. Gratification of sexual needs is virtually impossible without a private room. Failure to provide private rooms for each resident is to give architectural support to the myth that the elderly have no sexual needs. Without private rooms, dependence on staff is fostered to a greater extent than is necessary. The undue influence of staff can be minimized most effectively by limiting the range and scope of staff contacts with residents by maximizing resident choices. Resident options are most effectively increased if they have personal toilets, showers, and bedrooms (Lipman and Slater, 1977, p. 150).

The idea that clients should share bedrooms in order to help each other only holds true for the physically disabled. The mentally disabled cannot help each other and the rational residents refuse to interact with the confused residents (Lipman and Slater, 1977, p. 150). Separation of mentally alert clients from nonalert and confused clients has been associated with higher quality nursing home environments (Kane and Kane, 1976).

Resident Mix

The answer to the question, "Should clients with psychiatric diagnoses and cognitive impairment problems be mixed with physically impaired residents in nursing homes?" has no clear answer (Bergman, 1983). What criteria are used to decide whether or not people have "schizophrenia" or "Alzheimer's disease"? What happens when a resident fails mentally, that is, becomes disoriented, wanders, and is generally unable to perform activities of daily living? How is the mentally alert, nonconfused resident affected by these behaviors? What is the care-giver's responsibility toward meeting the psychosocial needs of both groups? If the two groups are segregated, who becomes the role model for the mentally impaired group? If the groups are mixed, is it fair to expect that the physically impaired but alert residents will help the psychosocially impaired residents? Clearly research is required to develop answers to these important questions.

At present, mentally and physically impaired residents are mixed together in some long-term care facilities and segregated in others. Evidence in support of either position can be found. However, the integration position tends to be supported by what people believe should happen whereas the segregation position is supported by a few research-based studies of what actually happens when the groups are mixed.

Hochschild (1973) found that older people living in group situations gained a sense of meaningfulness from developing their own activities. However, the congregate residence approach does not appear to benefit the more impaired elderly. Segregating the impaired forces them to identify with others who are also frail and dependent. This identification reduces the individual's ability to overcome physical and mental incapacities (Tobin and Lieberman, 1976, pp. 225, 227).

Mrs. S, who was nearing her 74th birthday, had occasional lapses of memory (as do most adults). She feared that she would become hopelessly confused and unable to live independently in her apartment. After a hip fracture, Mrs. S was sent to an extended-care facility to receive physical therapy. Here she encountered many women her age who were quite confused, and others who were wheelchair dependent. Mrs. S came to believe that she would be less likely to fall again if she transported herself by wheelchair. She stopped attending physical therapy. She began to focus on "losing her mind" by counting memory lapses. When friends from her apartment building visited, Mrs. S talked about how she was "not like them" anymore and that they were "exceptions" to the fate of most old people.

Mr. M, who was 84 years of age, quite alert, and fully capable of self-care, was placed in a six-bed room with Mr. T who was confused. Mr.

T had his days and nights reversed. Every night at 2:00 A.M. Mr. T wakened his five roommates by calling out, "Everybody up; time to get up" and turning on his radio. Over a 4-month period, the outcome of this arrangement was that the five roommates, including Mr. M spent most of the day sleeping and a small part of each day complaining to the nurses about Mr. T. After 4 months, Mr. T died. No one who shared his room expressed any regret.

Homes that attempt to mix residents, regardless of type of disability, have reported that the rejection of active "confused" elderly is a major problem. When "confused" residents enter rooms of other residents or take their possessions, the behaviors are regarded as crimes and not as symptoms of illness (Peace, 1981a). When "confused" wanderers and nonconfused residents were placed on a locked unit during a period of transition within a VA long-term care facility, Cornbleth (1977) found that the wanderers became more physically active (the desired outcome), while the other residents became less active as they stayed closer to their beds.

Given that segregation of severely impaired old people exists in institutions and that this practice has some positive benefits for both staff and residents, Maxwell (1979) proposed that there is a natural impulse that is part of a phylogenetic residue to avoid the mentally impaired elderly. Many animals demonstrate avoidance reactions in the presence of strange objects or people, and the more advanced the animal, the more disturbed the animal seems to be.

A study was made of the effects on mental and emotional status, sensory perception, and capability for needs of daily living when a mentally incompetent resident was placed as a roommate with a competent resident (Wiltzius, Gambert, and Duthie, 1981). A significant change occurred in mental and emotional statuses, but not in sensory or daily living task performance abilities, and the result was that the competent resident deteriorated!

Public Scrutiny

With increasing interest in nursing homes by licensing and regulating agencies, written standards have been developed and applied.

The effect of these standards of quality of care is not clear. A study of Massachusetts nursing homes reported a great increase between 1965 and 1969 in the proportion of facilities in compliance with regulatory standards for eight out of nine quality-of-care measures (Levey et al., 1973). However, the measure on which compliance declined during this time related to the personal care of clients (for example, client is clean, has clean clothes, is well groomed, has clean bedside unit). The facility-oriented items, such as personnel records, diet orders, and medical records, were the characteristics that improved dramatically.

Personal connections between the nursing home industry and its regulators and bureaucratic weariness have been effective deterrents to adequate regulation (Mendelson and Hapgood, 1974). *Lack of continued effective public pressure is the most basic reason for the failure of nursing home regulation.* Ombudsmen and other advocacy-oriented programs tend to be funded by tax monies. Thus, when these programs prove too successful in upholding resident rights, representatives of the nursing home owners are usually able to lobby successfully to abolish or weaken the programs. The effort mounted by social workers, owners, and others to correct major deficiencies in care at Kane Hospital in Pittsburgh (Kane Hospital: A Place to Die, 1975) was successful initially but eventually waned. These advocates became exhausted and discouraged from the combined work of raising money to support their work, accumulating evidence of the problems, informing the general public, and meeting with public officials who proved unreliable in taking corrective action. Added to the demands of full-time jobs and managing personal lives, this work simply proved overwhelming. The Committee to Improve Kane Hospital (supported by private contributions from senior citizens and religious organizations) became Citizens for Nursing Home Reform (supported jointly by private contributions and state tax monies), and then became Advocates for Better Care (supported entirely by state tax dollars). After about 2 years of operation, Advocates for Better Care was abolished in favor of an ombudsman program situated within the state department of health. This program is situated in the state capitol and thus is remote from the local scene where nursing homes operate. Limited travel funds restrict travel and force more of a telephone "hot-line" operation. Many nursing home residents do not have access to personal telephones or require help to use the telephone.

In summary, researchers have been successful in identifying characteristics of good long-term care facilities, but researchers, practitioners, and regulators operate in a vacuum when they confront the task of creating such a facility.

Process Factors Associated with Quality Care

Process involves an assessment of how resources are used and can be equated with client management or practice as seen in records, reports, and direct observation (Donabedian, 1978). Separation of process variables from structural variables is sometimes difficult. For example, staff behaviors are usually considered as a process variable because they indicate how care is given. Yet staff behaviors may also represent the training and competence these health providers received, a structural variable. Process factors tend to be those variables named in response to the following question, "What do nurses and others do with and for clients?" This section will present some processes used by nurses that have been shown to affect client outcomes.

Promoting Client Control

One area that seems to have a great deal to do with client outcomes is the freedom of choice or the amount of control clients experience in their daily activities. There is a large body of literature concerning the philosophy and theory of freedom (see, for example, Hillery, Dudley, and Morrow, 1977) and reporting positive effects of giving residents freedom and control even of "small" aspects of their environment in institutions (Schulz, 1976; Mercer and Kane, 1979; Sperbeck and Whitbourne, 1981; Perlmutter and Langer, 1982; Solomon, 1982). Indeed, the evidence supporting enhancement of resident control is quite convincing. An example is found in the results of the study by Mercer and Kane (1979). One group of nursing

home residents was exposed to an intervention that was designed to increase choice and control while a second group of residents received care as usual. The interventions included a request from the administrator for residents to assume more responsibility, an opportunity to choose a plant to care for, and an invitation to participate in a newly established resident council. The experimental group improved significantly over the control group on all three measures: activity levels, social behaviors, and hopelessness.

Resident councils are becoming increasingly popular as a means of giving clients a voice in operation of long-term care facilities. However, a study of resident council activities in central Illinois found that, although councils can facilitate communication and discussion of some resident problems, they generally do not alter facility policy or transfer power to residents (Devitt and Checkoway, 1982). Councils can be a vehicle to permit resident participation, but, in themselves, they do not ensure such participation.

Another strategy for nurses to use to increase client control is to promote aggressiveness. Nurses can and should prepare old people for institutional living by providing information and exposure to the future situation. This type of preparation is helpful in reducing psychologic symptoms, such as anxiety. However, it has little effect on the rate or degree of more severe problems, such as diminished self-care abilities and approaching death. To minimize these severe problems associated with institutionalization, the nurse should reduce or minimize the client's passivity, and support or stimulate aggressive/assertive behavior (Tobin and Lieberman, 1976, p. 232). Possible ways to increase aggressiveness include (1) providing assertiveness training sessions for people newly admitted to a long-term care facility and (2) increasing the individual's sense of mastery (planned opportunities for client decision-making, adherence to client's wishes, bargaining with the client, refusal to do for the client what the client is capable of doing, and the like.)

The nurse should identify the best mechanism for the elderly person to use in coping with the crisis of relocation to a long-term care facility, and should support its use. For example, Mrs. G responded with thinly disguised rage, saying that the decision was "hers alone" and was "for the good of the children," despite the fact that she had kept her own mother in her (Mrs. G's) home and "loved her to the end." Blaming others or rationalizing that the decision is entirely one's own are appropriate means of containing rage and mobilizing psychologic resources helpful for dealing with the demands of a new environment.

In working with families, health professionals may err on the side of oversupport for either the elderly person or his or her significant others, so that the other party feels guilty. In general, significant others who are likely to be younger or in better health should be helped to tolerate abuse or to withdraw from the situation gracefully when the interaction with the elderly person is dysfunctional for both parties (Tobin and Lieberman, 1976, p. 231). Nurses can explain that as an elderly person adapts to institutional living, significant others, especially children, become important in different ways. For example, parents talk about their children's successes to fellow residents, and thus achieve status among their peers. Children who carry on traditions and values help the elderly person to regard life as meaningful and to accept the inevitability and appropriateness of death (Tobin and Lieberman, 1976, p. 231).

Using Nursing, Education, Clinical Research, Quality Assurance, and Management Processes*

Five of the processes that nurses use frequently to influence client outcomes are derived from the fundamental problem-solving process. Table 6.4 presents a summary of these processes and permits easy comparison of similarities and differences between them. Detail about the nursing process was presented in Chapter 1 and is therefore not presented in this section.

Education. The education or teaching-learning process is comprised of the following major

phases: (1) determination of learning needs, (2) delineation of the learner's goals and capacities to learn, (3) provision of content, and (4) evaluation of the degree of goal attainment. This process is applied by nurses in long-term care to change the behavior of clients and their significant others, staff and students in both nursing and other health disciplines, and beyond these usual targets to those empowered to allocate health resources such as legislators, health planners, and administrators.

The educational needs of each of these groups are different. Clients and their significant others need to learn about their specific health impairments and disabilities. People who require long-term care are less entitled to health information than presumably well or healthy people. People with chronic disease or disability are entitled to as much information as they want, presented in a way that will enable them to assume responsibility for their own care. Staff and students need to keep informed of emerging concepts of long-term care. Those people who allocate resources required in long-term care need to know what nurses, apart from the other health professionals, do that makes a difference in client outcomes.

The purpose of any educational effort, regardless of the target, is behavior change. Nursing should not lose sight of this fact. The common pitfall of equating the providing of information with the act of learning must be avoided. Learning does not take place unless behavior is changed. The importance of reinforcement in producing behavior change cannot be overemphasized. People—nurses, clients, and others—do what they are rewarded for doing. The impact of positive reinforcement on nurses' use of the nursing process has been studied (Steckel, 1976). The charting of 23 nurses was observed and measured for a 3-week period. Each nurse was informed as to her performance, asked to set a goal for charting, and permitted to choose a reward contingent on achieving that goal. During the next 3 weeks, charting was again observed and measured. These two periods were again repeated. Results demonstrated a marked increase in charting during each reinforcement period and a decline during the second baseline period that was lower than the first baseline.

---

* This section (pp. 216–232) was coauthored by Mary Ann Mikulic, RN, MN, Clinical Specialist in Rehabilitation Nursing, at VA Medical Center, Seattle, WA.

TABLE 6.4 PROCESSES USED FOR PROBLEM SOLVING, NURSING, EDUCATION, QUALITY ASSURANCE, CLINICAL RESEARCH, AND MANAGEMENT

Basic Questions for Problem Solving	Nursing Process	Education	Quality Assurance	Clinical Research	Management
What is the problem question?	Assess client status	Define what client knows	Evaluate preliminary data (complaints, records, reports)	Evaluate preliminary data (pilot study, audit of outcome criteria, clinical experience)	Evaluate preliminary data (complaints, records, reports)
	Define problem establish goals	Define what client wants to know; establish goals	Define common problems or questions concerned with organization process, or outcomes of care	Define problem and population	Define problem or questions as experienced by manager(s)
What and how are solutions/answers sought?	Plan intervention	Select methods of teaching	Determine significant criteria/standards	Review literature	Select possible solution
			Develop a reliable, valid efficient data collection tool	Select framework	
				State hypothesis(es)	
			Develop a reliable data collection plan	Operationally define variables	
			Collect evidence to decide if criteria are met	Test manipulations and tools	
				Select design	
			Analyze audit findings	Define sample	
			Identify deficiencies	Define data collection procedure	
			Select corrective intervention		
	Implement intervention	Provide content	Implement corrective intervention	Implement study and collect data	Apply solution

(continued)

TABLE 6.4. (Continued)

Basic Questions for Problem Solving	Nursing Process	Education	Quality Assurance	Clinical Research	Management
Do the answers resolve the problem/question	Evaluate client's attainment of goals	Evaluate client's attainment of goals	Evaluate corrective intervention	Analyze or evaluate data in terms of hypothesis(es)	Evaluate resolution of problem
	Repeat process if goal(s) not attained; communication of results to persons involved	Repeat process if goal(s) not attained; communication of results to persons involved	Revise significant criteria	Interpret and communicate results widely	Repeat process if problem(s) not resolved; communication of results optional
Other differentiating elements:				Link to theory(ies)	
Primary aim	Obtain results for the client on hand	Obtain results for the client(s) on hand	Determine the efficiency and quality of nursing care delivered to the public	Generalize results to a larger population than the sample studied	Obtain results for the client(s) or employee(s) on hand
Plan	Written in sufficient detail so continuity of care is insured	Written in sufficient detail so continuity of teaching is insured	A plan for the overall agency quality assurance program is required. Plan for specific studies to be conducted under that overall plan may be written before they are done or indicated as part of the report of findings	Written in sufficient detail so study could be duplicated	May or may not be written; variable levels of detail

Setting	Clinical	Clinical or classroom	Clinical or offices of a service setting	Laboratory or clinical (usually not the same one as where problem/question occurred)	Clinical (usually the same as one where problem occurred)
Number of target people	One client	One client or groups of clients	Groups of employees, clients, physical plant, policies or procedures	Usually groups of clients; occasionally one client	Employees or clients alone or in groups
Control	Control of factor other than those of interest difficult to achieve or absent	Control of factor other than those of interest difficult to achieve or absent	Variable effort to control for factors other than the variables under study	Elaborate effort required to control for factors other than the variables under study	Control of factors other than those of interest difficult to achieve or absent
Analysis	Descriptive statistics (frequencies) if any	Descriptive statistics, if any	Descriptive statistics unless representative sampling is used	Descriptive and inferential statistics	Descriptive statistics, if any

Thus, reinforcement increased nurses' use of the nursing process (Steckel, 1976). Possibly the rewards removed some of the punishers operant in the environment that served to extinguish writing the nursing process. Positive reinforcement has been used to change a number of undersirable behaviors, ranging from incontinence in clients who are severely retarded (Azrin and Foxx, 1971) to screaming in an 80-year-old resident in a nursing home (Baltes and Lascomb, 1975).

In evaluating effectiveness of educational endeavors, the method should measure behavior change in the target/learner rather than retention of facts or changes in beliefs or attitudes that give no indication of whether health behavior has changed or not. Educational efforts directed toward clients are more likely to succeed when the various factors that influence clients' health behaviors are considered. The decision of people to use preventive services is based upon a number of factors, which may be categorized as (1) personal (e.g., perceptions of the importance of health, estimate of vulnerability, value of early detection), (2) interpersonal (e.g., concern of significant others, family patterns of utilizaiton, expectations of peers), and (3) situational (e.g., cultural acceptance of health behaviors; social group norms and pressures) determinants.

The distinction between "client education" and "self-care education" will become increasingly important as clients become more like consumers and less like patients (Levin, 1978). In client education the focus is on what the professional thinks the client should know. New knowledge and skills are provided to remedy client deficiencies. Activities under the control of the individual such as diet, dental prophylaxis, and sleep habits are behaviors to be changed. Content relates to insultive diseases and disabilities caused by biologic, psychologic, and environmental factors. The desired result is that the client's behavior is modified to improve health status.

Self-care education is more consistent with a holistic approach and rehabilitation concepts of self-help and independence. The focus in self-education is on what the client perceives as his needs and goals. The content capitalizes on knowledge and skills the person already has. Personal health status is considered more in relation to environmental factors and the problem of assaultive diseases (those caused by health-care providers) than factors embodied within the individual. Thus clients are not made to feel so guilty about their health behaviors. Instead they are encouraged to use their skills to bring about social change as well as to reduce personal risk.

Modeling high-quality, comprehensive care is a powerful approach for promoting learning on the part of both clients and nursing staff. When people actually see the nurse refusing to do for a client that which he can do for himself, they are more likely to follow suit in their practice. Significant others can learn a great deal about transferring the client from bed to chair by simply observing the nurse. By demonstrating a positive approach to long-term care, the nurse can do much to dispel negative connotations in the minds of other nurses and health professionals.

It is not enough to transfer skills and concepts. The educational method itself must include the experience of gaining fundamental control over one's destiny as a practicing nurse. Decision-making, knowledge-transfer, and change strategies must be practiced with the same intensity as transfer techniques and the detection of breath sounds.

The old adage that people learn by doing is not without foundation. Thus simulations such as those used to demonstrate the consequences of sensory impairment, gaming, and practice of skills under authentic conditions are powerful teaching strategies a nurse in long-term care may wish to use to stimulate maximum learning on the part of clients and nursing staff.

Educating the public about nursing's contribution to long-term care is a challenging task and one that nurses have not done well in the past. To counteract the assumptions, myths, and untruths that prevail, a deliberate marketing strategy is required. Fundamental to marketing a product is the need to have an identifiable and preferably a quality product. Nursing has a mission of its own that is unlike the missions of the other health disciplines.

This fact needs to be better understood by nurses as well as by the public. At the turn of the century, when nurses were making hospitals safe for clients and were preventing illness and lowering mortality rates in public health, nurses were better known for their contributions than they are today. Nurses in long-term care must be clear in their own minds as to their purpose and program and provide care of acceptable quality. Then the education of the public can proceed.

An important strategy is to publicize what nurses know and do. Summaries of research that support nursing's contributions, such as the studies that show nurse practitioner–social worker teams to be more cost-effective than physicians in providing primary care to the chronically ill (Kane, Jorgenson, and Pepper, 1974; Kane, 1976) need to be prepared in nontechnical language and given to legislators and others who allocate money for health-care services. Face-to-face contact with health planners and legislators to tell them clearly about what nursing has to offer long-term care clients can also be an effective means for influencing public opinion of nurses.

Quality Assurance. Concern with the cost of medical and health care has given rise to an era of evaluation to encourage provision of quality care. "Quality review" refers to collection of facts that attest to the present quality of care provided whereas "quality assurance" refers to a larger program that includes actions and review of actions taken to ensure that quality of care is provided. Professional standards review organizations, health systems agencies, and utilization review are all programs associated with the cost-containment quality of care promotion effort.

Instruments have been developed to measure the quality of nursing care. They include approaches for evaluating the quality of care delivered to people who are treated on a long-term basis. Many of these instruments require further development and testing to establish reliability and validity. It is also necessary to measure both the processes nurses use in giving care and the outcomes clients achieve. Evaluation of nursing process without docu-

mentation of the effects of nursing actions in client outcomes leaves the evaluator without a clear rationale for administrative action. Evaluation of outcomes with determination of process leaves nurses vulnerable to the charge that some other process contributed to the result.

Appraisal methods include direct observation and interview. Sources of data may be the setting, clients, staff, and records. From the client's perspective, the most desirable approach to evaluating quality of care is one that benefits him the most while bothering him the least (Plant, 1977). The Patient Appraisal and Care Evaluation (PACE), developed by the Department of Health, Education, and Welfare's Division of Long-Term Care and incorporated in the Patient Care Management System, is directed toward evaluating attainment of time-limited client outcomes (Abdellah, Foerst, and Chow, 1979). The basic features include a client history and assessment, need or problem list, plan of care, and goal achievement analysis. The multidisciplinary assessment form includes client behavior, activity preferences, activities of daily living, medical history, and discharge plans.

The terms quality assurance and quality research are used in overlapping ways. Although they have much in common, the situations in which they are carried out, the conditions under which they are performed, and the rigor in the methodology used are often different. The nursing quality assurance study is a systematic approach for evaluating nursing care by determining whether selected criteria related to nursing care process, client outcomes, or structural influences are met. This is accomplished through retrospective evaluations of client records or through concurrent observations of nursing care process, outcomes or structure. The nursing quality assurance study is more similar to research than either the nursing process or education since it consistently focuses on groups of clients and on multiple problems. Audit prepares nurses for involvement in research, since evaluation of outcomes of care is the first step in the research process (Padilla, 1979, p. 46).

In comparison, the nursing research process is more intimately related to theory development and testing and involves a representative sample and a more consistently systematic collection of information so that results are replicable and generalizable beyond the group initially studied. Clinical research is differentiated from nonclinical (basic) research on the basis of its purpose: whether it is knowledge for the sake of knowledge or knowledge for a specific purpose, namely, knowledge to direct nursing practice (Newman, 1982, p. 88).

Research. The full potential of nursing's contribution to those in need of long-term care is contingent upon a scientific basis for nursing practice. Increasing attention is being focused on developing new knowledge through research and on mechanisms to ensure its use in clinical practice.

Research responsibilities of the nurse in long-term care practice, as in acute care, may include communicating and implementing research findings within the practice setting, participating in studies, critiquing research reports, and assisting student and employed researchers to identify problems requiring investigation. Knowledge of the research process and the use of research tools and techniques are appropriate and essential aspects of the nursing role because evaluation of practice requires systematic data collection, analysis, and interpretation.

This section broadly defines what nurses need to study that is relevant to long-term care and presents a model for utilization of research results in practice settings. The importance of communicating research results to persons who formulate health policy is emphasized.

Virtually nothing has been studied in its entirety. In many instances, results of studies that relate to clinical practice are derived from research with serious methodologic flaws or simply from single studies. Replication is required before such results can serve as a basis for nursing practice. Thus, the list of problems requiring research and related to nursing care needs of people in long-term care could be quite long. It is important to realize the transactional nature of research. It is dependent on interactions involving gaps in basic knowledge, the adequacy of current methodologies, advancing technology, evolution of programs, and the sociopolitical climate. Broadly speaking, research is needed to study the process, structure, and client outcomes related to the provision of long-term care. Contributions to long-term care from research require that researchers, clinicians, and consumers be realistic in their expectations. Researchers need to become more sophisticated in translating research evidence that may be useful in directing policies and practices. Clinicians and consumers, on the other hand, must develop a sense of patience. Research requires time and support.

Probably the most important conclusion to be drawn from a review of the research done to date is that careful evaluation of professional nurses' activities directed toward clients in long-term care is required. Too many activities are undertaken without solid evidence that they are of benefit to the recipient. Thus, evaluative research designs need to be an integral part of each new program and service nursing provides to the long-term care population. Evaluative research in long-term care nursing is required at two levels. On the one hand, evaluation of specific nursing interventions is required. This microtype evaluation would examine the effectiveness of actions such as injection techniques, memory development programs, and continence training. The second level of evaluative research that is required is a macrotype that concerns the study of larger nursing programs such as nurse-administered units and nurse practitioner programs.

Nursing must prove through systematic study that the more skilled the care-giver, the less the waste of time, the fewer the costly mistakes in care, and the greater the possibility of restoration of the client (Schwab, 1976). Nursing cannot continue just to say these things are true, but must prove them.

The need for systematic initial assessment of people requiring long-term care, subsequent in-depth assessment in identified need areas, and periodic reassessment to measure progress toward goals is evident. Increased use of objective, quantified tools to facilitate assessment is appropriate for a number of reasons: (1) to provide adequate data for care planning, (2) to ensure a strategy for measuring outcomes in a field where outcomes are difficult to identify, and (3) to provide a data base for research purposes. Caution must be exercised, however, in using data that have been collected in the absence of proper controls.

Many of these tools have been developed in the field of rehabilitation, which, like nursing, is concerned with the effects of chronic illness or disability on the individual's functioning. Examples presented range from the simpler screening tools like the Barthel Index (Mahoney, 1965) and the PULSES (Adapted version) (Granger, 1979) to the more comprehensive, as well as more objective, Klein–Bell ADL Scale (Klein and Bell, 1982). Although lengthy, this scale gives an in-depth realistic appraisal of what the client can and cannot do for himself and which functions must be performed or taught by nursing personnel or others. Hence, it not only provides significant information about client needs, it can also be used to speak accurately to the use of adequate staff. Further it sequences the behavior of the various activities in a manner that can be utilized in developing teaching strategies to address the concept of successive approximations to the desired or target behavior. Further, when employed in settings that have interdisciplinary teams or even where both nursing and occupational therapy are available, use of the tool serves to improve communication between the disciplines on the client's behalf. Thus, this type of assessment can contribute to a nurse's fulfillment of the practice, managerial, educative, and research roles simultaneously.

Other scales such as the Ward Function Inventory (Norton, Romano, and Sandifer, 1977) address the deficits and needs of specific client groups. The Social Dysfunction Rating Scale (Linn et al., 1969) attempts to quantify the more complex area of social functioning.

Given the multidisciplinary nature of long-term care, collaboration among the various health disciplines in the conduct of research is expected and encouraged. Such cooperative efforts are particularly needed in research related to quality assurance in long-term care

where the contributions of the various professions to client outcomes are difficult to distinguish.

Although research can contribute to empirically derived information necessary to make decisions, information alone is not sufficient to impact upon the problems and issues in the field of long-term care. For example, knowledge about sensory impairment in elderly people with proven intervention strategies related to the use of color, lighting, and food is not utilized very often. Models for research utilization in clinical practice have been developed from at least two large projects: The Western Interstate Commission for Higher Education Regional Program for Nursing Research Development (Krueger, 1978; 1979) and the Conduct and Utilization of Research in Nursing Project (CURN) (Horsley, Crane, and Bingle, 1978). The latter project identified six phases to the research utilization process:

> The first phase involves two interrelated activities: identifying nursing practice problems which need solution and assessing valid research bases to utilize in practice. Generally speaking, people tend to identify problems and then seek solutions. However, the reverse can also occur. For example, new knowledge can alter one's perception of an event so that a specific practice, previously judged as satisfactory, now becomes questionable or problematic. Thus, nursing service departments must structure mechanisms which 1) identify and evaluate current nursing practice problems existing within the department and, 2) provide access to persons, organizations, and written material as sources of valid research bases. Note that we are not suggesting that the nursing service department is or should be responsible for evaluating the validity of the research base. At this point in time, that function should rest with academe, research consultants and organizations, or professional associations.

> The second phase of the research utilization process is directed toward evaluating the relevance of the research based knowledge as it pertains to the identified clinical practice problem, the organization's values and current policies, and the potential costs and benefits to accrue from its use. A set of probabilities should be established concerning the potential for organizational adoption of a practice innovation which

will be derived from the research base under consideration. The second phase ends when the probability for organizational adoption has been determined.

The major activity during the third phase is to design a nursing practice innovation which meets the needs of the clinical problem and does not exceed the scientific limitations of the research base. The innovation describes the intervention as it is to be carried out and prescribes the clinical limitations to be imposed. The design also contains a plan for implementation. The plan should include the following: a time frame; identification of a single unit on which a trial of the innovation will be implemented; identification of all key personnel related to the actual implementation; means for identifying and acquiring adequate resources (personnel, equipment, time, money); provision for staff training if necessary; and finally provision for adequate evaluation of the effects of the innovation. The fourth phase comprises an actual clinical trial evaluation of the innovation on an individual nursing unit. The trial should include baseline measures of the predicted outcomes. Adequate monitoring must be provided to ascertain the occurrence of unanticipated events. The evaluation should include as many dependent variables from the research base as are clinically reasonable. Divergence between the research base and the innovation trial data concerning these variables should be treated as a serious problem which needs resolution before the meaning of the evaluation can be fully ascertained.

The fifth phase, occurring after completion of the trial and evaluation, is directed toward making a decision to adopt, alter, or reject the innovation under consideration. The quality of the decision is totally dependent upon the adequacy and accuracy of the evaluation measures carried out during the clinical trial. A decision to reject the innovation completes the cycle of the process and it begins again at phase one with a new research base. A decision to alter the innovation returns the process to phase two, three or four depending on what the evaluation data indicate as the cause for the faulty trial. A decision to adopt the innovation leads to phase six—the development of means to extend the innovation to other appropriate nursing units within the hospital. This requires additional consideration of the issues involved in phases two, three, and four. The total process may recycle, to begin review of another research base before, during or

after the initial innovation is fully implemented on the appropriate nursing units. (Horsley, Crane, and Bingle, 1978; copyright 1978 by Concept Development, Inc. Reprinted by permission.)

The process is somewhat costly. It requires that nursing administrators establish enduring mechanisms, such as standing committees, policies, and procedures, to support the practice of evaluating research findings and raise the substantial resources, defined as personnel, equipment, and funds, needed to conduct evaluations. Benefits that may be expected to result from these investments include improved client care and outcomes, validation of current research findings, and direction for future nursing research investigations.

Research may be communicated for practice as indicated above. Research may also be communicated for scientific purposes from one scientist to another, for the purpose of gaining greater insight into the empirical world from the competent response of an expert and critical audience.

A third purpose of communicating research, one that is perhaps of greater importance to nurses in long-term care, is to influence public opinion and public policy. Much nursing research addresses social problems that relate to long-term care (e.g., loneliness and isolation, incontinence, confusion, status, and other impediments to the quality of life). Nurses cannot continue to ignore or complain passively about health policies formulated by people who know little or nothing about knowledge derived from nurses' research. Medical scientists have been very successful in using the media to communicate results of research supported by tax dollars. Nurses need to follow suit. As citizens, nurses in long-term care are not powerless when they communicate their empirically demonstrated accomplishments to legislators and others who formulate health policy.

Management. Nurses working in any facet of health or medical care need managerial skills. However, these skills are perhaps more essential to the nurse who provides long-term as opposed to acute care simply because so much requires changing. This section will define management, identify factors that impede nurses' functioning as effective managers in long-term care, and present selected strategies for the improved exercise of managerial responsibilities.

Management is defined broadly to include the acts of taking control of resources dominating or influencing people by tact, artifice, or confrontation, and directing, governing, or wielding power or influence. The primary purpose of management processes in long-term care is to succeed in accomplishing the numerous changes required (1) to promote the use of services that parallel institutional care, (2) to influence the allocation of resources within the medical and health-care delivery systems, (3) to effect control and direction of nursing care activities, and (4) to permit nurses freedom to act in support of nurses' and client's rights. Approaches that comprise management processes usually follow the general paradigm of problematic inquiry that was presented by Dewey in his famous analysis of reflective thinking, *How We Think* (Dewey, 1933, pp. 106–108). Steps involve identification of the problem or question, determination and testing of solutions or answers, and decisions as to whether the answers resolve the problem or question.

The management dilemma of nurses in long-term care cannot be separated from that of nurses engaged in other aspects of care delivery. The nursing profession suffers from a critical shortage of nurses prepared to be effective change agents. Too often, student nurses are socialized to use their power cooperatively and collaboratively to keep the system operative. They need to be taught to use their power to change a system that requires changing. As employees, nurses frequently function to perpetuate the status quo. Reasons for this state of affairs relate to the kinds of people who select nursing as a career and to the early socialization provided in nursing education programs. Too often, nurses emerge from basic preparation programs better prepared to serve the "system" than themselves or their clients. They frequently are unprepared to take risks and use the power, derived from money or numbers, necessary to develop their roles. In the past, nursing had power.

At the turn of the century, the social and professional power of nursing was becoming increasingly visible. Nurses were making hospitals safe for patients, and it was their skills, more than any other factor, that influenced physicians and patients to see these institutions as appropriate places for care. In public health too, nurses were again a primary force, preventing illness and lowering mortality rates as they applied the principles of their scientific knowledge. The "trained nurses" of that day were highly valued for their expertise; communities as well as physicians increasingly came to feel they could not do without this most useful professional and humanistically oriented group (Ashley, 1973, p. 638).

Prior to the advent of antibiotics, skilled nursing care was essential if clients were to recover from infections. Many nurses functioned independently in community settings. It is unfortunate that there are societal forces that have impinged upon the freedom of nurses to function as leaders defined as change agents. However, the nursing profession has latent power by virtue of its numbers. Nurses represent a majority in the health field. The challenge confronting nurses in long-term and other care areas is to use their power to compel changes necessary to reshape the values of our society so that health care is properly provided. Indeed interaction among nurses, consumers of health services, and other concerned groups is crucial to ensure acceptable, accessible, economical, and holistic health-care delivery.

Nurses can increase their numbers and thus their power base by aligning themselves with consumers of nursing services. However, numbers alone mean nothing in terms of power unless those numbers are organized. Much has been written about theories of change, knowledge dissemination and knowledge utilization. For the most part, however, such theories require further testing and development before they can serve as a blueprint for actually producing change.

One promising model for organizing people to build strength and power is being developed by the Industrial Area Foundation (IAF), an organization founded by the late Saul D. Alinsky (Alinsky, 1969, 1971). This model is based upon the following assumptions.

1. A leader is someone who controls and can deliver organized money or organized numbers of people or both
2. Some people are leaders, the rest are followers
3. Leaders can be organized to build a power base: followers cannot
4. Economic, cultural, and community pressures originate in money institutions that shape our daily lives
5. Money controlled by these institutions comes from people, including nurses and consumers of health and medical care
6. As long as nurses and other people exhaust themselves in struggles with middle level people like politicians, bureaucrats, and advisory personnel, the alignment of power will remain the same

The following elements comprise the IAF organizing model. *Religious* institutions form the center of the organization. These institutions have the people, the values, and the money. Without the values embodied in such institutions, organizations tend to be controlled by activists and become involved in movements or relationships that may create the impression of action while going nowhere. *Money,* derived from a solid dues base that builds from year to year, is another requisite element. Without dues money, organizations spend most of their time raising money. *Trained,* skilled organizers who are systematically trained over a period of 3 to 5 years are essential to find and develop a strong collective leadership. The bulk of the money goes to attract these expert ("lead") organizers and not to rental of operating quarters, production of brochures, or the hiring of extraneous personnel such as lawyers, public relations consultants or clerical staff. *Collective leaderships* of about 50–200 leaders, each of whom represents institutions, comprise the core of the organization. These leaders are people who can deliver either people or dollars to the organization and are committed to an internal training process for the purpose of preparing primary leaders to find and train other leaders. Expansion of leaders serves the interests of collective power. *Leadership training* is conducted to develop specific skills, such as how to distinguish between leaders and followers, how to analyze institutions, and how to negotiate with other decision-makers. *Multi-issue programs* are required to attract the requisite numbers of supporters to compel change. *Research,* defined as careful fact-finding to discover who makes decisions and who controls money, is a necessary element for planning effective interventions to bring about change. *Action* refers to the focusing of organizational energy to effect certain results and to enable the organization to grow in ability to deal with increasingly complex issues and to win more substantial victories. *Reflection,* or ongoing evaluation, are essential to enable leaders to correct errors and to execute focused actions over a period of time (Chambers, 1978, pp. 17–23).

Despite the developing nature of this model, its use has permitted a number of people who once felt as powerless as nurses in long-term care to achieve substantial changes. For example, in Pittsburgh 200 parish leaders made their way through a blizzard to meet with area bankers. The residents did not carry picket signs. Instead they carried institutional and family pledges to invest $5 million in a bank to be built in their community. When the bankers came to understand the numbers of people and their dollars, they saw that their self-interest lay in opening a branch bank in a community the people represented. In a similar effort, the Spanish-American community in East Los Angeles obtained an agreement from a major grocery chain to build a store in the area.

Nurses in long-term care, as well as other areas of nursing, would do well to consider ways in which they might become a part of existing organizations or develop new organizations based upon successful organizational models. If today's nurses want more for themselves and their clients, they need to act to satisfy their own demands instead of waiting to have them recognized and gratified by others.

Although not likely to produce the magnitude of change possible with use of the IAF model, a number of other strategies may be useful in bringing about changes on a smaller scale in long-term care. Already, substantial nursing initiatives in this area have been made, such as ambulatory nursing clinics and nurse-administered rehabilitation units. Highly competent, specialist nurses are the ones to establish admission standards and care regimens and make decisions about who is to be admitted to these units. Nurses assume responsibility for obtaining the services of other professionals when they are required. Independent nurse practitioners or practice groups may be expected to follow their own case loads of clients when third-party reimbursement for such services becomes a reality. Such innovations in the delivery of nursing care may be instrumental in helping to reconceptualize the potential contributions of the profession in improving the delivery of health services to people with long-term health problems or to groups at risk.

Nurses tend to define their role in encounters with other disciplines as seeking and relaying information when requested or volunteering impressions related to "difficult" clients. The multidisciplinary meeting where all concerned sit down and plan is a rare event. Sometimes when professional nurses attend team meetings, they participate more as "information providers" than "planners." They give a brief report when their turn comes and then sit silently through discussions and debates that involve the rest of the team. The status difference between nurses and the rest of the long-term care professionals is intensified by the fact that other professionals often criticize nurses for not doing their job correctly. A quotation from 1967 can still be heard all too often:

> Nurses are too authoritarian; they are too concerned with petty routines rather than the important needs of the patients; they maintain rigid ward schedules which interfere with other parts of the rehab program; they are lazy and do not want to do their work. Therapists sometimes talk as if their efforts to retrain patients were being deliberately sabotaged by the ward staff (Roth and Eddy, 1967, p. 45).

Although nurses profess to have little control over more formally developed plans made in relation to clients, they experience considerable control of the informal planning process. This mode of operating is illustrated in the case of Mr. R, age 89, a patient who yelled, usually at the top of his voice and frequently for long periods. This behavior took place at night and kept other residents awake. Mr. R explained his own behavior by saying that he "wanted attention." The nursing staff requested that the physician order a tranquilizer. The "proper" dose to quiet Mr. R left him extremely lethargic. The nursing staff was pleased with the success of their intervention. A number of alternative interventions were not feasible due to constraining factors. Minimal staffing precluded nurses spending time with Mr. R. Volunteers were not available consistently at the times Mr. R needed companionship. Pets were not permitted in the facility. There was no soundproofed room where Mr. R might be permitted to scream freely. Significant others were not available. Clearly the intervention selected was not in Mr. R's best interests. What is equally disturbing is that the nurses never considered applying their managerial talents to illustrate the need for better staffing or modification of the physical plant.

A second example illustrates more adequate management of clients' care. The problem in a long-term care facility was audiology and ophthalmology departments that were unresponsive to requests to test acuities on elderly clients with brain failure or disruptive behavior. Vision and hearing tests were not included in annual physical examinations. The nurse believed that sensory deprivation might be a contributing factor in the disruptive behavior. Previous efforts to obtain such screening had been unsuccessful in that the screening was often delayed for months due to "too many requests" and residents failed to cooperate with the screening when transported away from familiar surrounding to a facility 7 miles away for testing. Because of these problems, the head nurse had been reluctant to request vision and hearing testing. She considered trying to do some testing herself. When other disciplines fail to do their part, nurses tend to fill in the gap by doing the task themselves, or they give up. Neither solution is appropriate for the client's well-being in the long run. In this situation, the nurse decided to use numbers of clients to make the system responsive.

Requests for testing were prepared for each of the residents, signed by the physician, and submitted with a cover memo requesting that the testing be performed in the facility where the residents lived and with a member of the staff present to promote client cooperation. Research results suggesting the value of such testing were also cited in the memo. The department heads for both audiology and vision screening were able to use the requests and cover memo to obtain additional staff to do the testing as requested by the nurse. The nurse had made the system work for her . . . and for her clients.

Work has become a cultural pressure that is used to shape the values of nurses. Pressure derives from beliefs that overcrowded schedules, actions, and visible results are more important than their opposites. Nurses become so involved in these imperatives that they tend to address pervasive problems like incontinence on a case-by-case basis by citing individual reasons for the problem and trying individual interventions instead of assessing the institution-wide rate, summarizing the contributing factors, and intervening according to the greatest need and likelihood of success. Reacting to crises becomes the rule rather than planned action to alleviate the problems that give rise to crises. Thus nurses become masters at hiding linen, reheating cold trays, and nagging physicians. They are far less adept at negotiating with supply, dietary, or medical personnel to compel corrective action.

Special efforts are required to counteract the tendency of nurses to function as producers rather than managers. One promising strategy is for nurses to distance themselves from their work. "Working vacations" provide an opportunity to work in another setting for a period of time (e.g., 1 to 2 weeks) in order to experience alternative approaches to providing care and to gain perspective on the nurses' own work situation.

To convey the message that they are powerful people who make decisions, nurses might adopt some of the strategies discussed in books like *Things Mother Never Told You: Corporate Gamesmanship for Women* (Harrigan, 1977) or presented in assertiveness training programs.

Convene meetings whenever possible rather than waiting for them to be called. Sit at the head of the meeting table. Do not take good minutes or make good coffee if delegated these "housekeeping" chores. Stop service as a mediator between the client and the "system." When clients complain that the window sills are dirty, the appropriate response is to supply them with the name and telephone number of the department head responsible for housekeeping and not to personally dust the window sills. By providing a host of services that other disciplines should provide but do not, nurses may help a client but they do a great disservice to themselves (and ultimately their patients), in that they are left with little opportunity to practice *nursing*.

Potentially, nursing has more than the other health disciplines to offer those for whom cure is not a realistic goal, by virtue of the close relationship between the needs of the long-term care client and the nature of nursing. Is nursing destined to play a significant role in any efforts to deliver health services to people with long-term illness or disability? The answer depends on the ability of nurses, individually and collectively, to organize the resources of numbers and money, their own and others, into an active power base.

Serving as Client Advocates

Periodically, nurses should reconsider whom they serve. A number of long-term care facilities supply excellent care to the elderly, but many are deficient and some are seriously so. "Three major themes run through the many criticisms of long-term care facilities. First, the level of care is generally low and at best only keeps the person alive. Second, the environment is dehumanizing and frequently downright dangerous. Third, personnel—from administrators to aides—are poorly trained" (Manney, 1975, p. 154). Each of these criticisms is illustrated at intervals by major scandals. Homes burn down, clients are poisoned by spoiled food, home administrators are found to be embezzlers, and clients die in bed and remain undiscovered for several days.

The danger in reasoning that "the old are old and there is nothing to be done" is illustrated by the experience of a social worker who questioned the status quo in a nursing home that supplied seriously deficient care. This social worker was told by her supervisor that she (the social worker) was "afraid of growing old" and "ridden with guilt" because she was still young and vital. She was told to examine her attitudes carefully if she really believed that many of the residents did not belong in an institution and could be rehabilitated in any way. Doubting the truth of the supervisor's remarks, this social worker, along with two nurses, thoroughly and accurately documented problems identified within the facility for a year. This evidence was then presented anonymously to a concerned advocacy group in the community. Ultimately, the home was extensively investigated. Pressured by a series of temporary licenses, the administrators managed to upgrade the quality of care by a considerable margin. If these health professionals had accepted the supervisor's reasoning, serious health care delivery problems might have persisted for many years.

Nurses, as potential advocates for patients, need to know

1. What the clients' rights are
2. The mechanisms for enforcement of regulations
3. The risks involved in advocacy on their client's behalf

The nursing home patients' bill of rights incorporated in Federal Medicare and Medicaid regulations (42 C.F.R. 405.1121k and 42 C.F.R. 449.12) reflects a public concern that the personal liberties of institutionalized elderly people are frequently denied. These rights, and the "Interpretive Guidelines" issued by the Department of Health, Education, and Welfare (HEW),* are all concerned with the individual liberties and dignities of nursing home residents. They have nothing to do with the quality of health and personal care provided, which is covered elsewhere in the regulations. The rights

from the Medicare and Medicaid regulations are listed in Figure 6.5. The patients' bill of rights from the American Hospital Association (Fig. 6.6) is included for the purpose of comparison and reference for nurses in non-Medicare/Medicaid settings.

Federal regulations pertaining to nursing home clients are endorsed at three primary levels. The first level is the administrator of the home, whose enforcement effort has three components:

1. Establishment and use of a procedure to protect rights
2. Provision of clear notice to clients about their rights and related procedures
3. Education of the staff about patients' rights

Thus, copies of the patients' rights regulations should be readily available to the nurse. Vagueness of the complaint-handling procedure in the HEW guidelines and frequent insertion of the exception, "when medically contraindicated," are the major factors permitting administrators to do what they wish about clients' rights. The second level of enforcement is the inspectors who survey nursing homes as a condition of Medicare/Medicaid participation. This enforcement effort is hampered by the limited nature of the inspection process and the inappropriate penalty of decertification. The third enforcement level is made up of individual clients who bring private lawsuits in state or federal courts. Although private litigation is becoming recognized as legally viable, this mechanism is practically unavailable to the typical elderly nursing home resident. This resident faces a variety of obstacles: isolation from the community, including lawyers; lack of physical and psychologic energy; problems of proof when staff unite to depict the old person as mentally incompetent; a probable lack of funds to pay legal fees; and the law of damages which places small value on injury to someone with a low life expectancy.

Given these enforcement problems, nurses who advocate adherence to patients' rights may experience difficulties. Administrators may consider it cheaper to replace a nurse who asks too many questions than to provide patients'

* Since the time these guidelines were written, the name of the Department of Health, Education, and Welfare (HEW) has been changed to the Department of Health and Human Services (HHS).

A PATIENT'S BILL OF RIGHTS

(k) *Standard: Patients' rights.* The governing body of the facility establishes written policies regarding the rights and responsibilities of patients and, through the administrator, is responsible for development of, and adherence to, procedures implementing such policies. These policies and procedures are made available to patients, to any guardians, next of kin, sponsoring agency(ies), or representative payees selected pursuant to section 205 (j) of the Social Security Act, and Subpart Q of Part 404 of this chapter, and to the public. The staff of the facility is trained and involved in the implementation of these policies and procedures. These patients' rights policies and procedures ensure that, at least, each patient admitted to the facility:

(1) Is fully informed, as evidenced by the patient's written acknowledgment, prior to or at the time of admission and during stay, of these rights and of all rules and regulations governing patient conduct and responsibilities;

(2) Is fully informed, prior to or at the time of admission and during stay, of services available in the facility, and of related charges including any charges for services not covered under titles XVIII or XIX of the Social Security Act, or not covered by the facility's basic per diem rate;

(3) Is fully informed, by a physician, of his medical condition unless medically contraindicated (as documented, by a physician, in his medical record), and is afforded the opportunity to participate in the planning of his medical treatment and to refuse to participate in experimental research;

(4) Is transferred or discharged only for medical reasons, or for his welfare or that of other patients, or for nonpayment for his stay (except as prohibited by titles XVIII or XIX of the Social Security Act), and is given reasonable advance notice to ensure orderly transfer or discharge, and such actions are documented in his medical record;

(5) Is encouraged and assisted, throughout his period of stay, to exercise his rights as a patient and as a citizen, and to this end may voice grievances and recommend changes in policies and services to facility staff and/or to outside representatives of his choice, free from restraint, interference, coercion, discrimination, or reprisal;

(6) May manage his personal financial affairs, or is given at least a quarterly accounting of financial transactions made on his behalf should the facility accept his written delegation of this responsibility to the facility for any period of time in conformance with State law;

(7) Is free from mental and physical abuse, and free from chemical and (except in emergencies) physical restraints except as authorized in writing by a physician for a specified and limited period of time, or when necessary to protect the patient from injury to himself or to others;

(8) Is assured confidential treatment of his personal and medical records, and may approve or refuse their release to any individual outside the facility, except, in case of his transfer to another health care institution, or as required by law or third-party payment contract;

(9) Is treated with consideration, respect, and full recognition of his dignity and individuality, including privacy in treatment and in care for his personal needs;

(10) Is not required to perform services for the facility, that are not included for therapeutic purposes in his plan of care;

(11) May associate and communicate privately with persons of his choice, and send and receive his personal mail unopened, unless medically contraindicated (as documented by his physician in his medical record);

(12) May meet with, and participate in activities of, social, religious, and community groups at his discretion, unless medically contraindicated (as documented by his physician in his medical record);

(13) May retain and use his personal clothing and possessions as space permits, unless to do so would infringe upon rights of other patients, and unless medically, contraindicated (as documented by his physician in his medical record); and

(14) If married, is assured privacy for visits by his/her spouse; if both are inpatients in the facility, they are permitted to share a room, unless medically contraindicated (as documented by the attending physician in the medical record).

All rights and responsibilities specified in paragraphs (k) (1) through (4) of this section—as they pertain to (a) a patient adjudicated incompetent in accordance with State law, (b) a patient found by his physician to be medically incapable of understanding these rights, or (c) a patient who exhibits a communication barrier—devolve to such patient's guardian, next of kin, sponsoring agency(ies), or representative payee (except when the facility itself is representative payee) selected pursuant to section 205(j) of the Social Security Act and Subpart Q of Part 404 of this chapter.

Figure 6.5. Regulations for skilled nursing facilities with Medicare or Medicaid programs. *(Source: From 42 C.F.R. 405.1121(k). Prepared by the Department of Health, Education, and Welfare, 1974. A roughly parallel set of rights for intermediate care facilities is found in 42 C.F.R. 449.12 (1976).)*

A PATIENT'S BILL OF RIGHTS

The American Hospital Association Board of Trustees' Committee on Health Care for the Disadvantaged, which has been a consistent advocate on behalf of consumers of health care services, developed the Statement on a Patient's Bill of Rights, *which was approved by the AHA House of Delegates February 6, 1973. The statement was published in several forms, one of which was the S74 leaflet in the Association's S series. The S74 leaflet is now superseded by this reprinting of the statement.*

The American Hospital Association presents a Patient's Bill of Rights with the expectation that observance of these rights will contribute to more effective patient care and greater satisfaction for the patient, his physician, and the hospital organization. Further, the Association presents these rights in the expectation that they will be supported by the hospital on behalf of its patients, as an integral part of the healing process. It is recognized that a personal relationship between the physician and the patient is essential for the provision of proper medical care. The traditional physician-patient relationship takes on a new dimension when care is rendered within an organizational structure. Legal precedent has established that the institution itself also has a responsibility to the patient. It is in recognition of these factors that these rights are affirmed.

1. The patient has the right to considerate and respectful care.

2. The patient has the right to obtain from his physician complete current information concerning his diagnosis, treatment, and prognosis in terms the patient can be reasonably expected to understand. When it is not medically advisable to give such information to the patient, the information should be made available to an appropriate person in his behalf. He has the right to know, by name, the physician responsible for coordinating his care.

3. The patient has the right to receive from his physician information necessary to give informed consent prior to the start of any procedure and/or treatment. Except in emergencies, such information for informed consent should include but not necessarily be limited to the specific procedure and/or treatment, the medically significant risks involved, and the probable duration of incapacitation. Where medically significant alternatives for care or treatment exist, or when the patient requests information concerning medical alternatives, the patient has the right to such information. The patient also has the right to know the name of the person responsible for the procedures and/or treatment.

4. The patient has the right to refuse treatment to the extent permitted by law and to be informed of the medical consequences of his action.

5. The patient has the right to every consideration of his privacy concerning his own medical care program. Case discussion, consultation, examination, and treatment are confidential and should be conducted discreetly. Those not directly involved in his care must have the permission of the patient to be present.

6. The patient has the right to expect that all communications and records pertaining to his care should be treated as confidential.

7. The patient has the right to expect that within its capacity a hospital must make reasonable response to the request of a patient for services. The hospital must provide evaluation, service, and/or referral as indicated by the urgency of the case. When medically permissible, a patient may be transferred to another facility only after he has received complete information and explanation .concerning the needs for and alternatives to such a transfer. The institution to which the patient is to be transferred must first have accepted the patient for transfer.

8. The patient has the right to obtain information as to any relationship of his hospital to other health care and educational institutions insofar as his care is concerned. The patient has the right to obtain information as to the existence of any professional relationships among individuals, by name, who are treating him.

9. The patient has the right to be advised if the hospital proposes to engage in or perform human experimentation affecting his care or treatment. The patient has the right to refuse to participate in such research projects.

10. The patient has the right to expect reasonable continuity of care. He has the right to know in advance what appointment times and physicians are available and where. The patient has the right to expect that the hospital will provide a mechanism whereby he is informed by his physician or a delegate of the physician of the patient's continuing health care requirements following discharge.

(continued)

Figure 6.6. The Patient's Bill of Rights as revised by the American Hospital Association in 1975. *(Source: A Patient's Bill of Rights. Copyright 1975, by the American Hospital Association. Reprinted by permission.)*

11. The patient has the right to examine and receive an explanation of his bill regardless of source of payment.

12. The patient has the right to know what hospital rules and regulations apply to his conduct as a patient.

No catalog of rights can guarantee for the patient the kind of treatment he has a right to expect. A

hospital has many functions to perform, including the prevention and treatment of disease, the education of both health professionals, and patients, and the conduct of clinical research. All these activities must be conducted with an overriding concern for the patient, and, above all, the recognition of his dignity as a human being. Success in achieving this recognition assures success in the defense of the rights of the patient.

Figure 6.6. (Continued)

rights regulations translated into braille for the blind. Certainly, mechanisms operating within the home should be fully utilized. If the nurse finds these procedures ineffective, complaints can be anonymously registered with the regional office of Health and Human Services (HHS). Such complaints must be very specific, including client's name, date, time, and problem. At the same time, the nurse should be very careful to protect his or her identity, since information leaks from inspectors to facility administrators are commonplace. A strong community-based advocacy organization may provide nurses with an alternative channel for complaints. Sometimes, clients or their significant others are freer to complain than the nurse. Support from the nurse in the form of information about enforcement mechanisms can be the factor that makes these individuals take action.

Changing the Model of Service Delivery

One of the more frequently proposed strategies to enable nurses to function more effectively in long-term care is a change in the model of health-care delivery. The chance to give empathic care and apply rehabilitation measures to enhance the quality rather than the quantity of life has been hampered by reliance on the medical model instead of the long-term care model.

Table 6.5 provides a comparison of some frequently identified differences between the traditional and proposed models of care. The traditional model has been labeled "Acute Care/Medical" and the proposed model, "Long-Term/Holistic." The term "medical model" refers to basing clients' treatment primarily on medical

diagnoses and treatment plans that include medications or surgery. The new care model regards social and related needs as primary and medical needs as secondary. Medical needs are not disregarded in this model, however. Rather, they no longer provide the organizing focus governing allocation of resources, scope of service, nature of policies, and so forth. "Success" is determined on the basis of the client's level of functioning in relation to multiple parameters. Effects of intervention are evaluated on the basis of the client's previous activity levels. Thus, the whole person becomes focus of care. Each person's needs and problems are judged in relation to his or her situation, rather than against absolutes (such as the number cured or rehabilitated). Psychosocial services are regarded as being equally as important as nursing and medical services. Nurses and aides are part of a home and should dress accordingly. Not many home dwellers wear white clothes every day. Confusion on the part of who is who (staff versus residents) is considered good because the dilemma contributes to residents being treated like people first and clients second. Residents are permitted visitors at convenient and varied times—including children and companion animals. The environment is considered to be free of traditional boundaries so that design, policies, and programs are shaped by the residents' wants and needs rather than the convenience of care providers.

Although the distinction between the medical and social/functional models is clear, it is not clear which outcomes are to be maximized in programs at the cost of what other outcomes (Kane and Kane, 1980, p. 253). For example, what are the relative benefits of recreational activities versus primary medical

TABLE 6.5 COMPARISON OF ACUTE CARE/MEDICAL AND LONG-TERM/HOLISTIC MODELS

Characteristic	Setting	
	Acute/Medical	Long-Term/Holistic
View of behavioral deviation*	Deviation attributed to pathophysiologic changes	Deviation attributed to factors within both the individual and the environment
Aim/goal of intervention	Eradication of all manifestations of a disease	Relief, support, and rehabilitation to enhance functional abilities even in the presence of continuing disease or disability
Medical/physical needs	Primary	Secondary
Psychosocial needs	Secondary	Primary
Settings for delivery	Hospitals/medical centers	Home, day centers, long-term care facilities including nursing homes, domiciliaries, and personal care homes
Controlling therapist	Physician	Team (comprised of health professional staff and clients)
Activity of therapist	Provide medications and surgical procedures to correct behavioral deviations	Use self to facilitate clients' potential for self-care and self-growth
Role of client	Subordinate to the physician, powerless *patient,* and acted upon by the "wiser" intervener. Client values are not important in therapeutic consideration. A dependent, regressive relationship is the rule	Partner to the nurse with equal status as a human being and decision-maker for matters related to health and illness care. Client values are a major therapeutic consideration. Independence and progression in self-care are encouraged
Success	Number cured or rehabilitated	Number with actual level of functioning consistent with potential level
Decision-making	Physician makes decisions for staff and clients	Team, comprised of staff and clients, makes decisions by consensus
Accountability	To tasks and procedures	To residents

*Behavioral refers to both easily observable and difficult-to-observe actions of individuals. Walking, maintaining an intact skin, and recalling information are examples of easily observable behaviors. More difficult-to-observe behaviors include hematocrit, blood urea nitrogen, and glucose levels.

care? To choose between these alternatives, a basis for deciding their relative effectiveness is required but is not presently available.

Predicting future functional status for clients and/or health and medical service utilization has proved to be an exceedingly difficult task. Robert Kane and associates have been extensively involved in research to enable a shift in the nursing home reimbursement system from retrospective payment, based upon services provided to eligible clients, to one of prospective payment, based upon outcomes clients are expected to achieve (better, the same, or worse than expected). A great deal more research is required before such a shift is likely to occur (Kane et al., 1983). At present, however we define illness or impairment, the definition does not necessarily translate into disability or demand for health services. Two people with what appear to be similar degrees of impairment may show markedly different degrees of disability and achieve different outcomes in different settings and levels of care.

Concerns that have inspired various health care models have helped to create an adversary atmosphere in which nurses and physicians, supporting humanism and science, respectively, may be in opposition. Frequently, health professionals are divided into a "superior" group comprised of physicians, who control the industry through manipulation of monetary resources and treatment of diseases, and an "inferior" group, comprised of the other health professions, including nurses, who desire greater input by manipulating their numbers to provide care for the sick as well as promote health for all people. The client is the obvious loser in this adversary environment. The commonly proposed solution is "collaboration, communication, and complementarity among all branches of the health profession" (Engel, 1978, p. 175).

The main problem with this proposed solution is that people who hold power (some physicians) seldom elect to share that power via collaboration for mutually agreeable decision-making. A second problem is that collaboration and complementarity obscure the contributions of any one discipline to client outcomes. When contributions of no one discipline are identifiable, then the fee for service usually is paid to the agency/administrators and used to support salaries for staff. However, the physicians retain the right to bill clients or third-party payers directly, not because of client outcomes clearly attributable to physician services, but, rather, because they control the decision-making process.

Despite the often-expressed criticism of the medical model and wishes for a replacement (Melin and Hymans, 1977; Kane and Kane, 1981; Somers, 1982), this model continues to dominate long-term care facilities. The training and experience of many registered nurses contribute to the durability of this medical model. These nurses were trained in acute care settings where they received their impetus to practice largely from the physician's orders. Dependence upon this model blinds nurses to realities of the institutional long-term care environment. Medical necessity is given as the reason for clients entering these facilities, but for the most part, clients' acute illnesses have been stabilized and medical diagnoses have been made some time previously. Clients really enter long-term care facilities because of functional disabilities, familial disunity, physical and social losses, changing status of the family, and financial considerations. The medical orders that accompany the clients often have little to do with their requirements for nursing care. However, nurses spend most of their time with medications, other medical treatments, and care directed to basic physiologic needs. Very little time is devoted to making the comprehensive and detailed assessments that are required to capitalize on the clients' resources and minimize the effects of clients' deficits.

In short, the traditional medical model can hamper nurses' efforts to care for the elderly. Unfortunately, because of the prevailing power structure that supports health and medical care delivery in this country, any departure from this model of care delivery will be slow in coming.

CONCLUSION

The terms health care and health services have been used throughout this chapter more out of hope for the future than as a reflection of past or current practices. Serious issues related to long-term health care face the country and the nursing profession. As a result of historic attitudes toward some diseases requiring extended care, a model of care has developed based upon sickness, degeneration, and abandonment. Health services for most elderly clients include treatment for existing diseases (secondary prevention) or rehabilitation to limit the impact of disease processes (tertiary prevention). A greater emphasis is needed on the prevention of illness and maintenance of health (primary prevention). Professional nurses are prepared to assume responsibility for primary/ preventive health care. However, society has been reluctant to fund this type of care. Thus, elderly people who want to maintain or improve their health status before an acute or serious episode of illness occurs must be very aggressive in identifying resources available to them.

As it is presently delivered, the elderly might be better off without too much "illness care." Too many of the physicians and nurses who treat old people do not have the special background of knowledge needed to care for the elderly. Medical and nursing publications frequently report studies in which findings reveal excessive or inappropriate use of medications or inadequate screening—particularly in the institutionalized elderly, an essentially captive population. Interpersonal therapies that might help the elderly cope with the physical, social, and personal processes of advanced age are rarely provided: psychoanalysis, education, counseling, advocacy, and so on.

In its general usage, long-term care refers to care provided in institutions for extended periods of time. Parallel services provided outside of institutions have been slow to develop. For the profession to meet long-term and other health care needs of the elderly, nurses must organize themselves to achieve power, defined as the ability to act. The fragmented and imperfect resources that presently exist for health and medical care require improvement. The work that nurses do as educators, clinicians, researchers, and managers will not lead to improvement in resources unless nurses are able to act against many forces that maintain the status quo.

RECOMMENDED READINGS

American Nurses Association. Professionalism and the Empowerment of Nursing. Kansas City, MO, American Nurses Association, 1982. *A collection of seven papers presented at the 1982 ANA Convention, examining the need to empower the nursing profession, the means to achieve it, and its potential for increasing the quality of health care.*

Billings, G. Alternatives to nursing home care: An update. Aging 325–326:2–11, 1982. *A comprehensive review of many types of parallel care arrangements that include family support, a housing spectrum, domiciliary care, and many others. Pros and cons of each arrangement are discussed.*

Forum. The Gerontologist 23(3):229–242, 1983. *Two articles, listed below, present issues, accumulated facts, and directions for future research regarding relocation:*
  1. Horowitz, M.J., Schulz, R. The relocation controversy: Criticism and commentary on five recent studies, pp 229–234
  2. Borup, J.H. Relocation mortality research: Assessment, reply, and the need to refocus on the issues, pp 235–242

Kane, R.L., Bell, R., Riegler, S., Wilson, A., Kane, R.A. Assessing the outcomes of nursing home patients. Journal of Gerontology 38(4):385–393, 1983. *Describes the development of measures of nursing-home clients' functional status in the following areas: physiologic, activities of daily living, affective, cognitive, social, and satisfaction. Information was obtained directly from the clients using demonstrated ability in place of self-report wherever possible. Such measures are required for reimbursement and evaluative progress in long-term care.*

Kane, R.L., Kane, R.A. Alternatives to institutional care of the elderly: Beyond the dichotomy. The Gerontologist 20(3):249–259, 1980. *Presents one way to advance beyond the dichotomy of institutional versus community based care. This approach is based upon a system of reimbursement in which the client's own progress, compared to preestimated prognostic guidelines, is used as a basis for calculating nursing home payments.*

Kane, R.L., Kane, R.A. Values and Long-Term Care. Lexington, MA, D.C. Heath, 1982. *Methods for measuring and reconciling sometimes conflicting preferences of clients, families, health-care professionals, and others concerning long-term care of the frail elderly. What services should be provided? Who will provide them, where, when, and for how long? How do we weigh increased physical activity if it carries the expense of pain and discomfort? How do we evaluate the preferences of the cogni-*

tively impaired? Models and equations of economists and psychometricians are applied to experiences of the practitioner. Incorporates information about Kane and Kane's efforts to predict outcomes of nursing home clients.

Mongeau, S. (ed.). Directory of Nursing Homes. Phoenix, AZ, Oryx, 1982. *Useful as a reference rather than cover-to-cover reading, this directory gives the name, address, telephone, level of care provided, number of beds, ownership, and other facts about more than 15,000 state-licensed long-term facilities.*

Ralston, P.A. Learning needs and efforts of the black elderly. International Journal of Aging and Human Development 17(1):75–88, 1983. *Results of a study that investigated the self-perceived educational needs and activities of adults age 65 and older and compared black elderly with white elderly respondents. The number of significant race differences suggested the cultural orientation of blacks may have an effect on their interest and participation in educational endeavors.*

Storlie, F.J. The reshaping of the old. Journal of Gerontological Nursing 8(10):555–559, 1982. *A realistic portrayal of the constraints and limitations of life in a nursing home. Alternatives for the future are discussed.*

Tesfa, A. What does it take to let them go home? Journal of Gerontological Nursing 8(12):692–695, 718, 1982. *A review of six major barriers to the development of home health services and strategies for eliminating them.*

Vladeck, B.C. Unloving Care: The Nursing Home Tragedy. New York, Basic, 1980. *An example of the muckraking literature that has captured the attention of the American public.*

REFERENCES CITED

Abdellah, F.G., Foerst, H.V., Chow, R.K. PACE: An approach to improving the care of the elderly. American Journal of Nursing 79(6):1109–1110, 1979

Alinsky, S.D. Rules for radicals: A practical primer for realistic radicals. New York, Vintage, 1971

Alinsky, S.D. Reville for Radicals. New York, Vintage, 1979

Anderson, N.N., Holmberg, R.H., Schneider, R.E., Stone, L.B. Policy Issues Regarding Nursing Homes. Institute for Interdisciplinary Studies, Minneapolis, MN, American Foundation, 1969

Ashley, J.A. This I believe about power in nursing. Nursing Outlook 21(10):637–641, 1973

Azrin, N.H., Foxx, R.M. A rapid method of toilet training the institutionalized retarded. Journal of Applied Behavior Analysis 4(2):89–99, 1971

Baltes, M.M., Lascomb, S.L. Creating a health environment for the elderly via behavior management: The nurse as a change agent. International Journal of Nursing Studies 12(7):5–12, 1975

Barney, J.L. The prerogative of choice in long-term care. The Gerontologist 17(4):309–314, 1977

Beattie, W.M., Bulloch, J. Evaluating services and personnel in facilities for the aged, in Leed, M., Shore, H. (eds.), Geriatric Institutional Management. New York, Putnam, 1964

Bergman, J. Mentally ill in nursing homes? Yes if. . . . Geriatric Nursing 4(2):98–110, 1983

Billings, G. Alternatives to nursing home care: An update. Aging 325–326:2–11, 1982

Bingham, R., Fittipaldi, L., Holvoet, E., Mech, A., Mones, P., Simmons, V. Assessment of Quality Care in Skilled Nursing Facilities. Baltimore, MD, University of Maryland, Master of Science in Nursing thesis, 1977

Brocklehurst, J.L. The British experience with the day hospital, in Pfeiffer, E. (ed.). Daycare for Older Adults. Durham, NC, Center for the study of Aging and Human Development, Duke University, 1977

Brotman, H.B. Every Ninth American, 1982 Edition: An Analysis for the Chairman of the U.S. House of Representatives Select Committee on Aging. Washington, D.C., U.S. Government Printing Office, 1982

Brubaker, B.H. Health promotion: A linguistic analysis. Advances in Nursing Science 5(3):1–14, 1983

Butler, R.N. Why survive? Being Old in America. New York, Harper and Row, 1975

Chambers, E. Organizing for Family and Congregation. Huntington, NY, Industrial Areas Foundation, 1978

Chappell, N.L., Penning, M.J. The trend away from institutionalization: Humanism or economic efficiency. Research on Aging 1(3):362–387, 1979

Cohen, J., Streuning, E.L. Simple minded questions and twirling stools. Journal of Consulting Psychology 29(3):278–280, 1965

Congressional Budget Office. Long-Term Care for the Elderly and Disabled. Washington, D.C., U.S. Government Printing Office, February, 1977

Cornbleth, T. Effects of a protected hospital ward area on wandering and nonwandering geriatric patients. Journal of Gerontology 32(5):573–577, 1977

Curry, T.J., Ratliff, B.W. The effect of nursing home size on resident isolation and life satisfaction. The Gerontologist 13(3):295–298, 1973

Dall, J.L. Helping old people to continue being at home: The contribution of the day hospital. Royal Society of Health Journal 98:10–11, 1978

Department of Health, Education, and Welfare. Title 42 C.F.R. 405.112k, January 17, 1974 (amended October 3, 1974 and June 5, 1975).

Department of Health, Education, and Welfare. Title 42 C.F.R. 449.12, March 29, 1976

DeSantis, G. Power, tactics, and the professionalization process. Nursing and Health Care 3(1): 14–17, 24, 1982

Devitt, M., Checkoway, B. Participation in nursing home resident councils: Promise and practice. The Gerontologist 22(1):48–53, 1982

Dewey, J. How We Think. Lexington, MA, D.C. Heath, 1933

Donabedian, A. Needed Research in the Assessment and Monitoring of Quality of Medical Care. Washington, D.C., National Center for Health Services Research, DHEW, NO. (PHS) 78-3219, 1978

Dunkle, R.E. Problems in utilizing adult foster care homes. Clinical Gerontologist 1(2):74–75, 1982

Engel, G.L. The biopsychosocial model and the education of health professionals. Annals of the New York Academy of Sciences 21(310):169–187, 1978

Firestone, I.J., Lichtman, C.M., Evans, J.R. Privacy and solidarity: Effects of nursing home accommodation on environmental perception and sociability preferences. International Journal of Aging and Human Development 11(3):229–241, 1980

Fisher, C.R. Differences by age groups in health care spending. Health Care Financing Review 1(4):65–90, 1980

Gioiella, E.C. The relationships between slowness of response, state anxiety, social isolation and self esteem and preferred personal space in the elderly. Journal of Gerontological Nursing 4(1):40–43, 1978

Granger, C.W., Albrecht, G.L., Hamilton, B.B. Outcome of comprehensive medical rehabilitation: Measurement by PULSES Profile and the Barthel Index. Archives of Physical Medicine and Rehabilitation 60(4):145–154, 1979

Greene, V.L., Monahan, D.J. Structural and operational factors affecting quality of patient care in nursing homes. Public Policy 29(4):400–415, 1981

Greenwald, S., Linn, M.L. Intercorrelation of data on nursing homes. The Gerontologist 11:337–340, 1971

Greer, D.S. Hospice: Lessons for geriatricians. Journal of the American Geriatrics Society 31(2):67–70, 1983

Harel, Z., Noelker, L. Sector related variation on psychosocial dimensions in long term care for the aged. Social Work in Health Care 4(2):199–203, 1978

Harragan, B.L. Games Mother Never Taught You: Corporate Gamesmanship for Women. New York, Warner, 1977

Haussman, R.K.D., Hegevary, S.T., Newman, J.F. Monitoring the Quality of Nursing Care: Part II, Assessment and Study of Correlates. Bethesda, MD, U.S. Department of Health, Education, and Welfare, Health Resources Administration, 1976

Hicks, B., Raisz, H., Segal, J., Doherty, N. The triage experiment in coordinated care for the elderly. American Journal of Public Health 71(9):991–1003, 1981

Hillery, G.A., Dudley, C.J., Morrow, P.C. Toward a sociology of freedom. Social Forces 55(3):685–700, 1977

Hochschild, A.R. Unexpected Community. Englewood Cliffs, NJ, Prentice-Hall, 1973

Holmberg, R.H., Anderson, N.N. Implications of ownership for nursing home care. Medical Care 7(4):300–307, 1968

Horsley, J.A., Crane, J., Bingle, J.D. Research utilization as an organizational process. Journal of Nursing Administration 8(7):4–6, 1978

Howells, D. Reallocating Institutional Resources: Respite Care as a Supplement to Family Care of the Elderly. Paper presented at the 33rd Annual Meeting of the Gerontological Society, San Diego, CA, November, 1980

Ishisaki, B., Gottesman, L.E., MacBride, S.M. Determinants of model choice for service management systems. The Gerontologist 19(4):385–388, 1979

Johnson, F.L.P. Responses to territorial intrusion by nursing home residents. Advances in Nursing Sciences 1(4):21–34, 1979

Kane Hospital: A Place to Die. Pittsburgh, PA, The Action Coalition of Elders, 1975

Kane, R.L. Is good nursing home care feasible? Journal of the American Medical Association 235(6):516–519, 1976

Kane, R.L., Jorgenson, L.A.B., Pepper, G.A. Can nursing home care be cost effective? Journal of the American Geriatric Society 22(7):265–272, 1974

Kane, R.L., Kane, R.A. Long-Term Care in Six Countries: Implications for the United States. Washington, D.C., U.S. Government Printing Office, 1976

Kane, R.L., Kane, R.A. Alternatives to institutional care of the elderly: Beyond the dichotomy. The Gerontologist 20(3):249–259, 1980

Kart, C.S., Manard, B.B. Quality of care in old age institutions. Gerontologist 16(3):250–256, 1976

Kastenbaum, R.S., Candy, S. The four percent fallacy: A methodological and empirical critique of extended care facility program statistics. Aging and Human Development 4(6):15–21, 1973

Klein, R.M., Bell, B. Self care skills: Behavioral measurement with Klein-Bell ADL Scale. Archives of Physical Medicine and Rehabilitation 63(7): 335–338, 1982

Kosberg, J.I. Differences in proprietary institutions' care for affluent and nonaffluent elderly. The Gerontologist 13(4):299–304, 1973

Krueger, J.C. Utilization of nursing research? The planning process. Journal of Nursing Administration 8(1):6–9, 1978

Krueger, J.C. Research utilization: What is it? Western Journal of Nursing Research 1(1):72–75, 1979

Lawton, M.P., Bader, J.E. Wish for privacy by young and old. Journal of Gerontology 25(1):48–54, 1970

Levey, S., Ruchlin, H.S., Stotsky, B.A., Kinloch, D.R., Oppenheim, W. An approach of nursing home care. Journal of Gerontology 28(3):222–228, 1973

Levin, L.S. Patient education and self-care: How do they differ? Nursing Outlook 26(3):170–175, 1978

Linn, B.S. State hospital environment and rates of patient discharge. Archives of General Psychiatry 23(4):346–351, 1970

Linn, M.W., Gurel, L., Linn, B.S. Patient outcome as a measure of quality of nursing home care. American Journal of Public Health 67(4):337–344, 1977

Linn, M.W., Linn, B.S. Qualities of institutional care that affect outcome. Aged Care and Services Review 2(30):1–14, 1980

Linn, M.W., Sculthorpe, W.B., Evje, M., Slater, P.H., Goodman, S.P. A social dysfunction rating scale. Journal of Psychiatric Research 6(3):299–306, 1969

Lipman, A., Slater, R. Homes for old people: Toward a positive environment. The Gerontologist 17(2): 146–156, 1977

Louis, M. Personal space boundary needs of elderly persons: An empirical study. Journal of Gerontological Nursing 7(7):395–400, 1981

Mahoney, F.I., Barthel, D.W. Functional evaluation of the Barthel Index. Maryland State Medical Journal 14(2):61–65, 1965

Manney, J.D., Jr. Aging in American Society: An Examination of Concepts and Issues. Ann Arbor, MI, The Institute of Gerontology, The University of Michigan–Wayne State University, 1975

Martin, A., Millard, P.H. The new patient index—A method of measuring the activity of day hospitals. Age and Ageing 4(5):119–122, 1975

Maxwell, R.J. Doomed status: Observations on the segregation of impaired old people. Psychiatric Quarterly 59(1):3–14, 1979

McLemore, T., Koch, H. 1980 summary: National Ambulatory Medical Care Survey. Advance Data from Vital and Health Statistics of the National Center for Health Statistics 77:1–7, 1982

Melin, R.C., Hymans, D.J. Developing a health-care model for long-term care facilities. Journal of Nursing Administration 7(9):12–14, 32, 1977

Mendelson, M.A., Hapgood, D. The political economy of nursing homes. Annals of the American Academy of Political and Social Science 415(9):95–105, 1974

Mercer, S., Kane, R.A. Helplessness and hopelessness among the institutionalized aged: An experiment. Health and Social Work 4(1):90–116, 1979

Miller, D.B. Swing beds can work—with good planning. Hospitals 54(10):97–103, 1980

Moos, R. Evaluating treatment environments: A social ecological approach. New York, Wiley, 1974

Moos, R., Ingra, A. Determinants of sheltered care settings. Journal of Health and Social Behavior 21(1):88–98, 1980

National Center for Health Statistics. Basic Data on Health Care Needs of Adults Ages 25–74 Years, United States, 1971–1975. Hyattsville, MD, DDHS Publication No. (PHS) 81-1668, 1980

National Center for Health Statistics: Current Estimates from the National Health Interview Survey: United States, 1981. Hyattsville, MD, DHHS Publication No. (PHS) 82-1569, 1982

National Institute on Adult Daycare. 1980 Rules of Operation of the National Institute on Adult Daycare: A Program of the National Council on the Aging. An unpublished report by the National Council on the Aging, 1980

Nelson, M.N., Paluck, R.J. Territorial markings, self-concept, and mental status of the institutionalized elderly. The Gerontologist 20(1):96–98, 1980

Newman, M.A. What differentiates clinical research? Image 14(3):86–88, 1982

Norton, J.C., Romano, P.O., Sandifer, M.G. The ward function inventory (WFI): A scale for use with geriatric and demented inpatients. Diseases of the Nervous System 38(2):20–23, 1977

O'Brien, C. Adult day health care and the bottom line. Geriatric Nursing 2(4):283–286, 1981

Padilla, G.V. Incorporating research in a service setting. Journal of Nursing Administration 9(1):44–49, 1979

Palmore, E. Total chance of institutionalization among the aged. The Gerontologist 16(6):504–507, 1976

Peace, S. Small group living in institutional settings: Alternative living arrangements for the elderly—Part I. Ageing International 8(1):13–16, 1981

Peace, S.M., Harding, S.D. The Haringey group-living evaluation project. Research Report No. 1. North London, England: Survey Research Unit, Department of Applied Social Studies, Polytechnic of North London, 1980

Perlmuter, L.C., Langer, E.J. The effects of behavioral monitoring on the perception of control. Clinical Gerontologist 1(2):37–43, 1982

Pfeiffer, E. (ed.). Daycare for Older Adults. Durham, NC, Center for the Study of Ageing and Human Development, Duke University, 1977

Plant, J. Various approaches proposed to assess quality in long term care. Hospitals 51(17):93–98, 1977

Rawnsley, M.M. The concept of privacy. Advances in Nursing Science 2(2):25–31, 1980

Reichstein, K.J., Bergofsky, L. Domiciliary care facilities for adults: An analysis of state regulations. Research on Aging 5(1):25–43, 1983

Robb, S.S. Home Assessment of Urinary Incontinence in the Elderly. An unpublished study protocol for research funded by the Health Services Research and Development Service, Veterans Administration, HSR&D project number 82-054, 1983

Robb, S.S., Peterson, M.D., Nagy, J.W. Advocacy for the aged. American Journal of Nursing 17(6): 1736–1738, 1979

Rosenthal, J.M. Early returns on the federal and state swing-bed experiments. Hospitals 54(10): 98,100,102–103, 1980

Roth, J.A., Eddy, E.M. Rehabilitation for the Unwanted. New York, Atherton, 1967

Rowles, G.D. The surveillance zone as meaningful space for the aged. The Gerontologist 21(3):304–311, 1981

Sanazaro, P., Williamson, J. End result of patient care: A provisional classification based on reports by internists. Medical Care 6(3):123–130, 1968

Schlotfeldt, R.M. Long-term care in perspective: Shared control of the system among health professionals. In American Academy of Nursing. Long-Term Care: Some Issues for Nursing, Kansas City, MO, American Nurses Association, 1975

Schulz, R. Effects of control and predictability on the physical and psychological well-being of the institutionalized aged. Journal of Personality and Social Psychology 33(5):563–573, 1976

Schwab, M. Issues on long term care and implications for the nursing profession. In United States Department of Health, Education, and Welfare. Assessing health care needs in skilled nursing facilities: Health professional perspectives. Long Term Care Facility Improvement Monograph No. 1. Rockville, MD, U.S. Department of Health, Education, and Welfare, Office of Nursing Home Affairs, 1976

Solomon, K. Social antecedents of learned helplessness in the health care setting. The Gerontologist 22(3):282–286, 1982

Somers, A.R. Long-term care for the elderly and disabled: A new health priority. New England Journal of Medicine 307(4):221–226, 1982

Spanier, R. Nurses and physicians-goals complimentary, not exclusive. Forum on Medicine 2(8): 739–741, 1979

Sperbeck, D.J., Whitbourne, S.K. Dependency in the institutional setting: A behavioral training program for geriatric staff. The Gerontologist 21(3):268–275, 1981

Steckel, S.B. Utilization of reinforcement contracts to increase written evidence of the nursing assessment. Nursing Research 25(1):58–61, 1976

Steinhauer, M.B. Geriatric foster care: A prototype design and implementation issues. The Gerontologist 22(3):293–300, 1982

Tobin, S.S., Lieberman, M.A. Last Home for the Aged: Critical Implications for Institutionalization. San Francisco, CA, Josey–Bass, 1976

Townsend, P. The Last Refuge. London, Routledge and Kegan Paul, 1962

Trager, B. Adult Day Health Care—A Conference Report. (Report of a project supported by Grant #1 R13 HS 02580-01 from the National Center for Health Services Research.) Hyattsville, MD, National Center for Health Services Research, 1979

Ullman, S.G. Assessment of facility quality and its relationship to facility size in the long-term health care industry. The Gerontologist 21(1):91–97, 1981

U.S. General Accounting Office. Improved Knowledge Base Would Be Helpful in Reaching Policy Decisions on Providing Long-Term, In-Home Services for the Elderly. Washington, D.C., Superintendent of Documents, 1981

U.S. House of Representatives Select Committee on Aging. Adult Day Care Programs. Hearing before the subcommittee on health and long-term care of the Select Committee on Aging, House of Representatives. Washington, D.C., U.S. Government Printing Office, April 23, 1980

U.S. Senate Special Committee on Aging. Development in Aging, 1981. Washington, D.C., U.S. Government Printing Office, 1982a, vol 1

U.S. Senate Special Committee on Aging. Health Care Expenditures for the Elderly: How Much Protection Does Medicare Provide? Washington, D.C., U.S. Government Printing Office, 1982b

Weiler, P.G., Rathbone-McCuan, E. Adult Day Care: Community Work with the Elderly. New York, Springer, 1978

Weissert, W. Adult Day Care in the U.S.: A Comparative Study: A final report funded by contract #HRA-B6-74-148. Rockville, MD, National Center for Health Services Research, Health Resources Administrations, Public Health Service,

Department of Health, Education, and Welfare, 1975

Weissert, W.G. Rationales for public health insurance coverage of geriatric day care: Issues, options, and impacts. Journal of Health Politics, Policy and Law 3(4):555–567, 1979

Wershow, H.J. The four percent fallacy: Some further evidence and policy implications. The Gerontologist 16(1),Pt 7:52–55, 1976

White, K.L. Improved medical care statistics and health services system. Public Health Reports 82(9):847–854, 1967

Williams, M.A., Holloway, J.R., Winn, M.C., Wolanin, M.O., Lawler, M.L., Westwick, C.R., Chin, M.H. Nursing activities and acute confusional states. Nursing Research 28(1):25–35, 1979

Wiltzius, F., Gambert, S.R., Duthie, E.H. Importance of resident placement within a skilled nursing facility. Journal of the American Geriatric Society 29(9):418–421, 1981

Winn, S., McCaffree, K.M. Characteristics of the nursing home perceived to be effective and efficient. The Gerontologist 16(5):415–419, 1976

7

Life Changes Experienced by the Aged

Barbara Elliott Spier

Reading this chapter will enable the individual to

1. Discuss common life changes the aged experience related to productivity, relocation, relationships with others, and death
2. Identify stressors frequently encountered by the aged person experiencing a particular life change
3. Identify factors which influence adaptation to life changes

Throughout life individuals are confronted by a series of physiologic, psychologic, and sociologic changes. As discussed in Chapter 3, there are many specific theories related to these areas that describe the process of aging. Developmental theories encompass aspects from the physiologic, psychologic, and sociologic dimensions of man. Life experiences common to the aged can be studied from a developmental perspective or in relation to life changes.

Because developmental theories tend to be progressional, with limited flexibility, this chapter presents life changes of the aged rather than developmental tasks. Although many theorists have written about the developmental progression of the aged only the views of Neugarten, Erikson, and Peck are discussed in relation to life changes (Fig. 7.1).

Life changes commonly experienced by the aged include those related to productivity, relocation, relationships with others, health, and death. The mentioned changes with the exception of health are discussed in detail in this chapter. Changes related to health are identified throughout the book. The role of the nurse in relation to life changes of the aged is described in Chapter 8.

DEVELOPMENT THEORIES RELATED TO LIFE CHANGES OF THE AGED PERSON

The focus of the development theories of Erickson, Peck, and Neugarten differ. Erikson describes the later years, or the last stage of the life cycle as a time when the aged face "integrity versus despair" in relation to life experiences. Peck identifies three specific stages that the aged experience. According to Neugarten, age is not relevant to the major life events of the adult. Further discussion of each of these views follows.

Erikson's Theory
Erikson's theory describes development of the healthy personality over the entire lifespan. In the normal development of the healthy personality Erikson has identified eight stages. At each of these stages there is an issue or a psychologic conflict that is of particular importance:

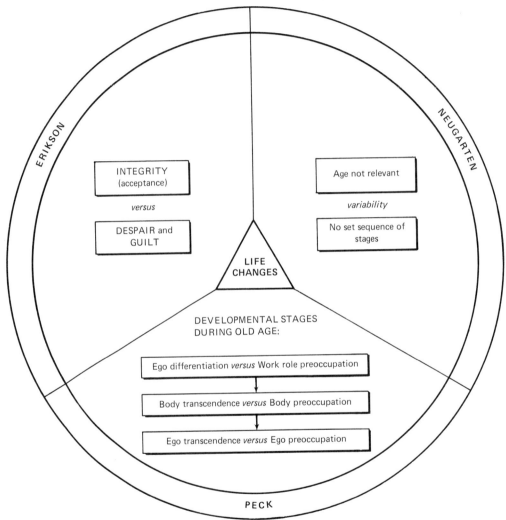

Figure 7.1. Life changes as related to Erikson's, Peck's, and Neugarten's developmental theories.

- Developmental stages of childhood
    Basic trust versus mistrust
    Autonomy versus shame and doubt
    Initiative versus guilt
    Industry versus inferiority
    Identity versus identity diffusion
- Developmental stages of adulthood
    Intimacy and distantiation versus self-absorption
    Generativity versus stagnation
    Integrity versus despair and disgust

Each of these issues or psychologic conflicts is of primary importance during one stage of development, with lesser importance during other stages. For example, during adolescence the primary issue is that of identity. However, identity is also important during the stages that precede and follow adolescence. As life changes are experienced by aged persons they risk loss of some of their identity. Maintenance of identity is necessary for the achievement of self-esteem. It may be necessary for the nurse to intervene to promote the maintenance of identity of the aged person.

Erickson originally indicated that success in resolving conflicts of a particular stage was not possible unless the conflicts of the preceding stages had been successfully resolved (Erikson, 1959). Recently it has been recognized that there may be regression, stagnation, and a continuing conflict between the extremes within each stage (Fiske, 1980).

Erikson's stage of integrity versus despair and disgust has the greatest significance for the older adult. *Integrity* is defined as "the acceptance of one's own and only life cycle and of the people who have become significant to it as something that had to be and that, by necessity, permitted no substitutions" (Erikson, 1959). The person who successfully achieves integrity accepts the experiences that have occurred during his or her lifetime and takes full responsibility for his or her own life.

With achievement of integrity, there occurs acceptance of life changes related to productivity, relocation, relationships with others, and health. The changes would be perceived positively and the person would make the most of them. For example, a retired person who achieves integrity would seek other means of productivity to satisfy his needs. Negative views of retirement are likely to be held by persons who demonstrate despair and disgust. They would probably blame others for difficulties such as inadequate income and would be unlikely to derive satisfaction from alternative roles. These persons were probably not satisfied prior to retirement. Erikson would relate this to lack of resolution of previous development stages.

According to Erikson's theory, persons achieving integrity accept significant events in the course of life experience without any wish that they might have been different. When the individual does not achieve integrity, despair follows, often accompanied by dismay that there is not enough time remaining to start all over. In some cases, disgust is substituted for despair. The disgust may be manifested as displeasure with particular institutions or individuals. Persons who succeed in achieving integrity should be able to assume the roles of both leader and follower (Erikson, 1950).

Peck's Theory
Peck divides the second half of life into several different stages of psychological learning and adjustment:

- Development during middle age
    Valuing wisdom versus valuing physical powers
    Socializing versus sexualizing in human relationships
    Cathectic flexibility versus cathectic impoverishment (emotional flexibility)
- Development during old age
    Ego differentiation versus work-role preoccupation
    Body transcendence versus body preoccupation
    Ego transcendence versus ego preoccupation

Peck has identified several stages that occur during "Old Age." During the stage of ego differentiation versus work-role preoccupation, the person about to retire is expected to redefine and reexamine self-worth, in hopes of achieving satisfaction from a broad range of activities rather than only from the specific work-role. To make a successful adaptation to old age, each individual is expected to establish "a varied set of valued activities and valued self-attributes" (Peck, 1968). This, in turn, should enable the person to gain satisfaction and a sense of self-worth from the pursuit of any one of several alternatives.

The issue of body transcendence versus body preoccupation relates to the individual's view of his physical discomforts and incapacities. Does the person dwell on them, does the person continue to enjoy life in spite of them? Some people become increasingly concerned with their physical state while others, with the same physical problems, minimize their discomforts and focus instead on the satisfaction they receive from their psychosocial activities and interactions.

According to Peck, the last adjustment to old age is that of ego transcendence versus ego preoccupation. As a person grows old there is enhanced awareness that life is finite. Those who adjust successfully to this awareness do not dwell on the prospect of death. Instead, they continue to make contributions that will improve the lives of those who live after them (Peck, 1968).

Neugarten's Theory

According to Neugarten, development of the adult is not limited by stages or age.

Because of the great variability that occurs among adults in relation to major life events, Neugarten (1979) indicates that "age is becoming less relevant and age norms less limiting." The timing of marriage, child-rearing, and grandparenthood varies tremendously. Other social changes related to life experiences include increases in the number of career changes, women in the working force, divorces, remarriages, and single-parent families. Neugarten questions the value of "describing adulthood as an invariant sequence of stages, each occurring at a given chronologic age." With aging, life becomes more complex and more enriched. Neugarten states, "Identity is made and remade: issues of intimacy and freedom and commitment to significant others, the pressures of time, the reformulation of life goals, stocktaking and reconciliation and acceptance of one's successes and failures—all

of these preoccupy the young as well as the old" (Neugarten, 1979, p. 891).

FACTORS AFFECTING REACTION TO LIFE CHANGES

What factors affect adaptation to life changes? One very significant factor is the extent to which the person's life focused on the change that has occurred. If previous activities and life-style have been closely related to the phase of life that is undergoing change then the change will have greater significance. In some instances a change may even affect the individual's self-image. The number of changes required, the degree to which changes must be made, the timing of the changes, and the amount of control the person has in relation to the changes all have an effect on the person's adaptation to the changes.

Most aged persons adapt well to the life changes that are encountered. Those who have adapted well to life changes in the earlier stages of development usually continue to adapt well as they grow older. People tend to utilize the same or similar coping mechanisms throughout their lives. The effectiveness of these mechanisms during the earlier years is a factor in the individual's ability to cope with the life changes of the later years. Many people are able to make a quick and complete adaptation to change. Others need an extended period of time to adapt and their ultimate adaptation may be incomplete. The availability of a person's usual coping mechanism is also an important factor. Changes in the person's health, support systems, or environment may interfere with the effectiveness of usual coping mechanisms or with the individual's ability to utilize them.

The health status of the person encountering the change as well as the health status of the person's significant others greatly influences the need for and adaptation to change. Since the nurse frequently encounters persons experiencing health-related problems it is important that the nurse assess the adequacy of the usual coping mechanisms to determine the extent of nursing intervention required. Health-related stressors may necessitate changes in relation to productivity, environment, and relationships with significant others. Vice versa, changes in any of these areas may be detrimental to the person's health.

Reactions to life changes are influenced by whether events are perceived as being positive or negative. Most life changes have both positive and negative aspects. To a certain extent, the individual's ability to adapt successfully is influenced by his focus on either the negative or the positive aspects of the change. Those who focus on the positive aspects and who play down the negative will adapt more readily, as long as they can be realistic in their planning. Persons who dwell on the negative aspects, on the other hand, may regard a particular developmental change as an overwhelming loss. A life change that is perceived as a loss of something valued precipitates grief. Engel (1964), Kübler-Ross (1969), and others have described stages of the grieving process. Although these stages are often associated with dying, they are also applicable to persons mourning any significant loss. (For a description of the stages refer to page 265.)

The timing of life changes is significant in determining reaction to change. Many life changes experienced by the aged person have been anticipated and planned for. As long as events occur when they are expected, most elderly persons adapt to related life changes and function to their fullest despite them to achieve integrity.

Peck's stages of development during old age are related to productivity, physical health, and an emotional awareness that one is aged. The aspect of Peck's theory that deals with productivity is focused on learning and adjustment in conjunction with changes associated with their work role. For many aged persons changes in the work role may have either a positive or negative impact on several areas of life. These include self-worth, leisure, income, and relationships with others. The second stage described by Peck is related to physical health. The third stage deals with the realization that the end of life is approaching. Either or both of these issues may create changes in relationship with others and may or may not necessitate relocation. Those who do not adapt successfully to the third stage dwell on

the prospects of death. Many factors influence adaptation to the stages described by Peck. One of the primary factors is the degree of successful adaptation to the changes that have occurred previously in the life of the person.

The number of events, as well as the kind of planning made to deal with them, may affect adaptation to developmental changes. For one person, a particular developmental task may be interrelated with several others. For another person, the same task may be the only source of change. An example might be the loss of a spouse. Compare the situations of Mrs. A and Mrs. B, both of whom have recently become widows.

Mrs. A (age 70)	Mrs. B (age 70)
Significant Others	
No children.	Two children within 60 miles.
Not involved in group activities.	Active in several organizations.
One sister lives 700 miles away.	Two brothers within 30 miles.
Few close friends.	Many close friends.
No pets.	Dog.
Income	
Social security.	Social security.
Husband's pension benefits ceased with his death.	To receive widow's pension benefits.
$5000 total savings.	Receives regular stock dividends and interest from large investment and savings.
Productivity	
Cared for invalid mother who died one year ago.	Officer in two groups. Member of many committees in church and community.
Perceived productivity activities primarily as those to meet husband's needs.	Frequently baby sits with grandchildren and performs tasks to assist children.

Mrs. A is more likely than Mrs. B to have difficulty in adjusting to the loss of her spouse. Mrs. A's problems are multiple and of a greater magnitude. Not only has she lost her spouse, but her financial resources are very limited; she has lost what she perceives to be her major role; and she has few support systems to assist her during this time of crisis. Mrs. B's situation is very different. Even though she has lost her husband, she will continue to have adequate financial resources, she has several roles that will encourage her to be productive, and she has multiple sources of support during her crisis period.

Similar losses may thus vary greatly in their impact on each person. When working with the aged, the nurse must view each client as an individual in identifying problems and their impact, as well as choosing methods of helping the client to cope with problems.

PRODUCTIVITY

Many aged persons experience changes related to productivity. A combination of factors, including employment, relationship with significant others, social activities, and health will determine whether productivity increases or decreases. Most older members of our society have been strongly influenced throughout their lives by the work ethic. Self-worth and self-esteem have largely been determined by the individual's ability to occupy his time with useful endeavors. Whether or not changes in role, changes in society, or changes in capabilities become a problem for the aged person depends upon the availability of opportunities for productivity, the value that the individual places on productivity, and whether a productive role enables the person to meet other needs such as socialization. Role change, reactions to retirement, planning for retirement, leisure activities, and maintaining income are issues that are related to productivity and are discussed below. The emphasis is on retirement, however, as this area has been researched the most.

Role Change
Opportunities for productivity may diminish suddenly, gradually, or may not seem to diminish at all. For some people, opportunities for productivity actually increase. Sudden losses

may be attributed to retirement, changes in health, automation, or relocation. As opportunities for productivity decrease in one realm, they may increase in another. Consider a woman who perceives her primary role to be managing the household. As her children become independent, she may become involved increasingly in activities outside of the home that would enable her to continue to be useful. Some individuals who have been highly motivated and under tremendous pressures from multiple roles welcome a release from their responsibilities and enjoy being able to pursue their interests at a leisurely pace.

Changes in our society have resulted in changes in productivity. During the life-span of our present senior citizens, many technical developments have eased the job of performing household tasks. For example, electric appliances and convenience foods have lightened the task of meal preparation. Automatic washers and dryers and permanent-press fabrics permit clothes and linens to be cared for in a few hours, when formerly this task often took more than a day. Changes in society have also led to many changes in employment. Industrialization has resulted in a decrease in the number of persons in the work force, and in the number of years and hours they work. People now spend less time in a formal productive capacity, and they have increased opportunities to take part in leisure activities.

Work and adaptation to leisure have been studied by many. A study by Daum, Freedman, and Canter (1977) indicated that, for older persons, work is more than just a source of income. According to their study, the elderly are also motivated to work because of benefits to their self-concept.

Uhlenberg (1979) indicates that engaging women over the age of 65 in constructive roles is probably the most effective means of reducing premature dependency and senility.

When identifying conditions under which role change is perceived as being stressful, George (1980) suggests that changes in roles that are personally significant are more stressful than changes in roles in which there is not a substantial identity involvement. Although retirement may be traumatic initially, George and Maddox (1977) found that the subjects they studied were able to adapt over time.

Reactions to Retirement

Retirement has tremendous significance for many aged persons. Often it is associated with the onset of old age, the final phase of life. Although some persons plan for retirement, and even eagerly anticipate it, others view retirement as a sudden shock that is damaging to both self-image and self-esteem (Fig. 7.2). A person who retains a self-concept of youthfulness may associate retirement with being old. Faced with retirement, such a person may realize for the first time that life is not infinite.

For many people, retirement is much more than the simple loss of a work role. It is often accompanied by changes in productivity, income, and relationships with significant others. Although most persons adjust well to retirement, this event often leads to significant changes in the life-style of the retiree and the retiree's spouse.

Health problems affect the aged person's ability to continue working and to experience satisfaction with retirement. Quinn (1981) found that health limitations dramatically increased the probability of both complete and partial retirement. A study of satisfaction with retirement by Barfield and Morgan (1978) demonstrated that retired persons who are less healthy experience decreased life satisfaction.

In our society, reactions to retirement are influenced by importance that has been attached to the work ethic. There has been a tendency to disapprove of those who have not worked steadily and those who have had employment difficulties throughout their lives. At the opposite end of the spectrum is the "workaholic," whose life usually focuses upon his job. Many workaholics have never known true leisure. Because their time and energy are constantly channeled to their work role, these persons often keep family relationships and social interactions to a minimum. In some cases, the person's dedication to the job interferes with the development of other normal roles. There are even workaholics who have never experienced a vacation for the sole purposes of rest and relaxation. These people often identify

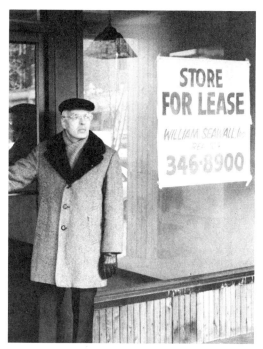

Figure 7.2. A man who has recently retired stands outside the storefront where his small business was formerly located. Although he has planned ahead for his retirement and is looking forward to it, such major changes are never easy. *(Photograph by Ed Spier, Murrysville, PA.)*

themselves so closely with their jobs that upon retirement their self-worth diminishes sharply.

Employment and retirement have had a different meaning for many of the poor black elderly. The Protestant work ethic, with its emphasis on the individual's productivity and contributions to society, has not always recognized and given status to the work roles of these old people. Black persons with few skills and limited education often have had the lowest paying and the dirtiest jobs. Although there are some older blacks who held jobs of higher status, a greater number had positions in laboring and service work, which have traditionally reflected a lower social status. Because they so often have an inadequate retirement income, more blacks are likely to be employed after the age of 65 than are whites (Dancy, 1977).

Retirement may be perceived as a privilege or as a threat. Persons who view it as a privilege are often those who have made realistic plans for retirement long before it actually occurs. Others who eagerly anticipate retirement may later find that their expectations were not realistic and that their planning was not adequate. Retirement is often seen as a welcome relief from the drudgery of a rigid schedule that was vital for financial survival. Streib and Scheider (1971) found that professional people are the least willing to retire. The most willing to retire are white-collar workers, followed by skilled workers, managers, and unskilled workers.

Adjustment may be particularly difficult for those who avoid retirement until they are forced to retire. Peretti and Wilson (1975) studied the psychologic effects of voluntary versus involuntary retirement. According to their findings, persons who had retired voluntarily had significantly greater emotional satisfaction, emotional stability, self-confidence, positive self-attitudes, and positive striving. This study also indicated that the voluntary retirees had greater feelings of usefulness and that persons who had been active and useful before retirement tended to follow a similar pattern after retiring.

The individual's self-perceptions and attitude towards work influence the acceptance of aging and retirement. Maddox (1970) has indicated that people who have problems with work also tend to have problems in retirement. Some persons who express a great dislike for their jobs find, after retirement, that their jobs regulated their daily lives. In some instances, the increased amount of leisure time available to the retiree leads to increased conflict with the spouse.

What appears to be a reaction to retirement might really be a reaction to aging. Some people deny their age throughout their middle years by taking great pride in looking and behaving younger than their chronologic age. Involuntary retirement often has a tremendous psychologic effect on these people, forcing them suddenly to face their age.

Beck's (1982) findings are similar to those reported by Atchley. Retirement was not found to significantly affect happiness. In a study of men, happiness with life was positively correlated with health and income and negatively correlated with loss of spouse. Those who expressed negative evaluations of retirement were more likely to have poor health, lower income, and an earlier-than-expected retirement.

There has been much debate regarding whether a satisfactory adjustment to retirement is related to disengagement or activity. Lehr and Dreher (1969) found that a temporary state of disengagement is often a means of coping with the problems of retirement. After the new retiree passes through a transition period, social activity increases. The retiree expresses strong feelings of being needed, along with a sense of increased life satisfaction and positive morale. Reichard, Livson, and Peterson (1968) have indicated that adjustment to retirement is dependent not on the degree of activity in retirement but on whether the activities are suited to the person's lifelong needs and interests. In their study they found well-adjusted persons who had disengaged.

In studying reactions to retirement, researchers must also consider the spouse of the retiree. A study by Fengler (1975) showed that some wives of retirees looked forward to their husbands' retirement, while others expressed grave reservations about it. Understanding the reaction of the spouse can be helpful in understanding the adjustment to retirement. Some nonemployed wives have trouble in adjusting to having their husbands around the home all day, possibly interfering with their established household routines.

In a study of retired teachers by Keating and Cole (1980) retired men and their wives were found to have higher morale than a group of preretired teachers. The women indicated that retirement of their spouses changed their roles as wives. About two-thirds perceived a need to plan socialization and household tasks to be done with a focus on the couple, rather than on the individual. Although most of the changes caused by retirement were perceived as being positive, the women indicated the negative effects to be loss of privacy, reduction in social network, and loss of independence. Now that more women are in the work force and because men in our society usually marry women younger than themselves, working couples may encounter stress when the husband retires while his wife is still employed full time.

A study by Cassels, Eckstein, and Fortinash (1981) found that the support of significant others was important for successful adjustment to retirement. In their study the group that had the most positive retirement experience was the same group that was the highest in evaluating the family as "a close family group."

Planning for Retirement

Retirement preparation is believed to aid in the preretirement and transition periods. In a study of the impact of preretirement programs Glamser (1981) found that prior to retiring almost 90 percent of the participants in his study expressed a desire for their company to sponsor a program to prepare workers for retirement. Many people who prepare themselves for other phases of their lives do not make adequate preparation for retirement.

Although preretirement planning may be initiated when a worker is first employed, most often planning for retirement occurs near the time when retirement is anticipated. During the early years of employment the focus of retirement counseling and planning is usually on financial concerns. In anticipation of retirement the worker may attend a series of retirement planning meetings sponsored by the employer or an organization in the community. Topics frequently discussed in retirement programs include:

- Knowledge about self
- Health
- Leisure activities
- Finances
- Place of residence
- Insurance
- Legal affairs

Classes that encourage people to learn more about themselves often ask the individual to identify past and present interests, talents, and achievements. Increasing the person's awareness of these things is intended to stimulate a new interest in them. Retirees are encouraged

to review their past accomplishments as an aid to increasing their self-esteem. Many programs assist individuals in examining present and past sources of frustration and their usual coping measures. These and other ways of helping retired people to understand themselves better are believed to enhance the adjustment to retirement.

Programs on health are largely concerned with primary prevention. The retirees are instructed about good health habits, accident prevention, and signs of impending health problems. At the same time, they are discouraged from becoming preoccupied with health-related problems.

Preretirement programs encourage individuals to plan for leisure activities according to their particular interests, talents, and resources. Opportunities for group interaction, volunteer activities, part-time employment, creative hobbies, sports, travel, and civic activities are presented.

Discussions concerning finances cover subjects such as budgeting, investments, and other ways of increasing income. Participants are informed about tax benefits, food and transportation programs, community services, and other areas where the elderly may benefit from reduced rates.

Retirement programs urge senior citizens to evaluate their present residence and to consider all aspects of other possible places of residence before making the decision to relocate. Factors of particular importance include the climate, community facilities and programs, transportation, nearness to significant others, and the availability of buildings with suitable physical facilities. Once the decision to relocate has been made, a trial or temporary move is suggested for most people (Fig. 7.3).

Usually, preretirement programs include a discussion of insurance and legal matters. The retiree is encouraged to evaluate the adequacy of health, life, and property insurance. Classes on legal matters cover such topics as wills, estates, and properties.

Retirement has a great influence not only on the work role but on many other aspects of a person's life. Because of many changes in lifestyle that may accompany retirement, prere-

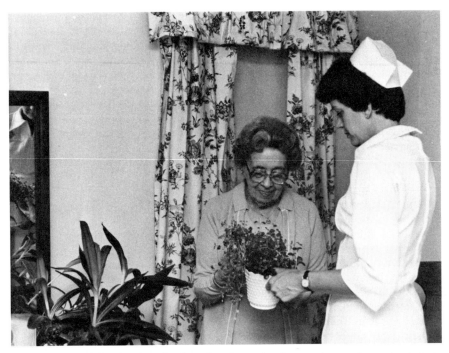

Figure 7.3. Adaptation to relocation is easier when valued possessions such as prized plants can be taken to the new environment. *(Photograph by Ed Spier, Murrysville, PA.)*

tirement planning is important in helping the individual adjust to his or her anticipated new role, that of retiree. In order for preretirement programs to be successful they must be realistic and individualized, and they must begin early enough. Employees should not be expected to perform a comprehensive and objective analysis of their anticipated retirement problems without assistance. Morrison (1975) recommends that companies hire trained personnel to obtain and analyze individualized data 5, 10, or 15 years prior to retirement. Since retirement may be viewed as a family process, Keating and Marshall (1980) suggest the development of educational programs for all of the family members.

The impact of preretirement programs may be most valued during the preretirement phase and during the period immediately after retirement. Glamser (1981) found that a substantial majority of participants in a retire-

ment planning program reported feeling better about retirement upon completion of the program. Nearly 90 percent indicated that they felt the program was helpful in preparation for retirement. Six years following completion of the program, when the participants had been retired an average of 3.7 years, the effects of the program were further evaluated. When compared with a group of retirees who did not have a preretirement planning program there was not any significant difference in the retirement experience in relation to the length of the adjustment period, the accuracy of expectations, the level of preparation, life satisfaction, attitude toward retirement, or job deprivation. Research is needed to determine the need for continuing retirement programs throughout the postretirement years. Keating and Marshall (1980) suggest that retirement planning programs be continued throughout the retirement period when individuals encounter needs such as those related to changes in socialization, income, and health status. Greene and Beutner (1981) suggest person-centered retirement planning, which would enable the retiree to deal with problems when they are encountered rather than attempting to provide specific answers to hypothetical problems. The goal is to enable the person "to respond independently, intelligently, and effectively to the challenges and problems which arise throughout retirement" (Greene and Beutner, 1981). The learning needs and priorities of retired persons are individualized and change over time.

Getting retirees and preretirees to attend retirement preparation programs can be a problem. As indicated by Glamser (1981), it is very possible that those with the greatest "need for preretirement education and counseling are often the ones who avoid participation." Robb (1978) attributes the problem to the tendency of today's retirees to be accustomed to being self-reliant and solving their own problems. Reluctance to use even the least threatening of health or welfare counseling services is not uncommon.

Retirement, including benefits and problems, needs to be further studied. Both older people and the larger society could benefit by encouraging the aged to remain at work longer. For the older person, knowledge that his talents and skills are needed and valued are likely to increase self-esteem. Both society and the aged person would benefit economically by postponing retirement. Society would benefit by having increased numbers paying into the system rather than taking from it. The number of persons receiving social security and pension benefits would decrease significantly. The older person would benefit from having a higher income for a longer period of time. As health care has improved more persons are living longer and are able to be productive members of society. With declining birth rates and earlier retirements the number of persons in the work force has greatly decreased. As indicated by Robinson (1981), with greater flexibility and more options for work and retirement combinations, more older people could continue to be employed. Older persons need more opportunities for part-time employment, flexitime, and incentives for employment rather than emphasis on retirement.

Leisure Activities

With retirement and other changes in responsibilities aged persons have more time to pursue leisure activities. Because of this opportunity, aged people's perceptions of leisure are of interest. Roadburg (1981) found that perceptions of leisure were influenced by whether or not retirement was voluntary. Aged persons who did not hold a remunerated job, such as housewives, and those who retired voluntarily perceived leisure in terms of "enjoyment/fun/fulfillment." Persons who were forced to retire defined leisure in terms of freedom. Changes in self-perception of leisure activities were determined by Bossé and Ekerdt (1981). In spite of having time available for leisure activities, recent retirees did not perceive themselves as being more involved in leisure activities than did their peers who continued to work. Prior to retiring, retirees overestimated the extent to which they would be involved with leisure activities upon retiring. Self-perception related to involvement in physical activity, social activity, solitary activity, and cultural activity were not markedly altered by retirement.

Moss and Lawton (1982) studied differences and similarities in the use of time among aged persons who lived in the community, who lived in public housing, who received social or health services from community agencies and who were on a waiting list for institutionalization. The groups were similar as to the amount of time spent alone, with family and with nonfamily members. Residents of public housing were found to spend the most time with friends. All four groups spent most of their time alone. Patterns of the four groups were consistent in time spent in religious activities, reading, listening to the radio, watching television, and in recreation. Of these activities, the most time consuming was watching television. All four groups spent an average of more than 3 hours a day watching television. The second most time-consuming activity for all four groups was "rest and relaxation." The groups living in the community and in public housing spent more time doing housework, cooking, shopping, and traveling than the other two groups. Persons waiting for institutionalization spent the most time in personal- or sick-care tasks, an average of 80 minutes daily. Moss and Lawton found that activities were enjoyed more by older persons who had higher behavioral competence and better psychologic well-being. Persons with impaired function were found to experience a greater proportion of all activities as routine. These routine activities were probably perceived more negatively because of greater difficulties encountered in performing them well.

Older people take part in a wide variety of leisure activities. Peppers (1976) indicates that although retirees tend to continue the same kinds of leisure activities as they did before retirement, they also tend to become involved in an increased number of activities. According to his study, life satisfaction was higher for persons who became more active after retirement than for those whose participation in activities decreased or remained unchanged. Life satisfaction was higher for those who were doing what they most enjoyed (Peppers, 1976).

Leisure activities that the aged participate in most often are watching television, reading, writing, participating in arts, crafts, cards, and other games (Roadburg, 1981). Other popular activities include walking, visiting with family and friends, gardening, and driving or other outings. In a study of morale in low-income blacks, fishing was found to be the most popular leisure activity (Gilson and Coats, 1980). Among 50 institutionalized aged women, meditation and worship was ranked as the most preferred activity, with watching television a close second (Lemmon and Pieper, 1980). Participants in the study indicated a preference for individual rather than group activities.

Membership in organizations and clubs varies in popularity. Cutler (1977) indicated that membership in organizations is probably lower among older adults than among younger adults because of financial differences. Further research by Cutler (1982) indicated that persons aged 65–74 may get much satisfaction from membership in voluntary associations. Satisfaction with life for the older old person does not appear to be affected by satisfaction with organizational involvements. Membership in organizations was found "to influence satisfaction with organizational involvement rather than with life satisfaction in general" (Cutler, 1982, p. 135).

Older adults can achieve self-fulfillment in a variety of ways. Some enjoy pursuing hobbies and interests in isolation, whereas others prefer group activities. Often rewards come through opportunities to use old skills in a new way. This may involve volunteer work or developing hobbies to such an extent that they become financially profitable. Many senior citizens join groups such as the American Association of Retired Persons. In addition to holding regularly scheduled meetings, this organization conducts informal classes, recreation, and social activities, plans group travel, and keeps its members informed of benefits and opportunities available to them. In recent years, the federal government has become more aware of the needs of retired persons and has sponsored several programs for their benefit. One such program is the Retired Senior Volunteer Program, which has helped many senior citizens to meet the expenses they encounter when doing volunteer work. Services that are provided by the senior volunteers vary according to the needs of the community. In the Pittsburgh area they include a school volunteer program; an advocacy service for individuals unable to speak for themselves to effect needed change; a multilingual service for persons in hospitals or nursing homes who cannot communicate in English; and a retired executive program. Volunteers in the retired executive program act as consultants for various businesses and organizations. Other federally sponsored programs pay older persons a small stipend for their various endeavors. An example is the Foster Grandparent Program, which pays elderly persons a small fee for providing love and emotional support to children living in institutional settings. These and other programs enable the retiree to have an increased feeling of productivity along with supplemental income.

The ways in which an older person uses time is a reflection of self-perceptions and the use of time throughout his life. As Ward (1982) indicates, there are many opportunities for the aged in relation to leisure, education, and service roles. If opportunities have not been taken for personal change and growth throughout one's younger years, persons will not be prepared "to explore the freedoms and options of old age, and their activities will become little more than playing out of those middle aged patterns that survive" (Ward, 1982, p. 181).

Maintaining Income

Elderly members of our society frequently encounter the problem of income maintenance. Normally, income increases steadily during an individual's working years. After retirement, however, income usually decreases in relation to expenses. In 1976, the median income for males over 65 was $4959; for females it was $2642. The United States Bureau of the Census reports that in 1978, 14.0 percent of persons 60 and 65 and over had incomes below the poverty level whereas in 1959, the figure was 35.2 percent. As noted in Table 7.1, since 1959 the percent of persons 65 years old and over below poverty level has steadily declined. Blacks continue to have the highest percent below poverty level. In a study by Gilson and Coats (1980), however, "lower income blacks did not indicate that they were unhappy with their lot in life."

Members of minority groups have been found to have greater problems related to income than do elderly whites. According to a study by Dowd and Bengtson (1978), the mean income of elderly blacks and Mexican-Ameri-

cans was significantly less than that of older whites. When the middle aged were compared with the aged, there was a greater decline in mean income among the minority groups than among the whites. The mean income among the blacks was found to decline 55 percent, the Mexican-American mean income decreased by 62 percent, and the income of older white persons decreased by 36 percent.

In 1970, 35.2 percent of white women 65 years and over and 24.7 percent in 1978 were below the poverty level. A lower percentage of black females 65 and over were found to be below poverty level—16.0 percent in 1970 and 14.3 percent in 1978 (Statistical Abstract, 1980). Women receive less income from government sources (such as Social Security), less from private pensions, and less from employment.

A study by Chatfield indicated that loss of income rather than loss of productivity was the primary reason for lower life satisfaction among recently retired persons. His data support the proposition that "higher income reduces the impact of health problems on life satisfaction" (Chatfield, 1977). Kreps (1976) attributes income problems to the low retirement benefits that early retirees receive, the small number of persons eligible for private pension benefits, and the increased length of the retirement period.

Cassels, Eckstein, and Fortinash (1981) found the upper, middle, and lower socioeconomic classes to have significant differences in their standard of living. Financial investments enabled the upper and part of the middle socioeconomic population to retain financial stability. Income for the lower socioeconomic group depended primarily on social security, pen-

TABLE 7.1 PERCENT OF PERSONS 65 YEARS OLD AND OVER BELOW POVERTY LEVEL 1959 TO 1978

	1959	1970	1975	1977	1978
Persons, 65 and over	35.2	24.6	15.3	14.1	14.0
White	33.1	22.6	13.4	11.9	12.1
Black	62.5	47.7	36.3	36.3	33.9
Spanish origin	(NA)	(NA)	32.6	21.9	23.1

(Source: U.S. Department of Commerce Bureau of the Census. Statistical Abstract of the United States 1980.)

sions, or both. All three groups were concerned about their "ability to adjust to a rapidly increasing cost of living" (Cassels, Eckstein, and Fortinash, 1981).

Inflation adds to the economic problems of the older person. As inflation occurs, salaries increase and the cost of living increases. Elderly people with fixed incomes often find that their financial resources will not permit them to maintain the life-style to which they have been accustomed. Inflation causes a steady increase in the cost of food, rent, utilities, transportation, clothing, and other necessities. Economic problems may prevent old persons from traveling, or from joining or maintaining membership in various organizations. Some find it difficult to accept the fact that they can no longer afford to give gifts to their family and friends (Fig. 7.4). Homeowners are likely to experience problems in retaining their homes as home maintenance costs rise and property taxes increase. Although most older persons are able to adjust their style of living and to find adequate financial resources as long as they remain healthy, the onset of major health problems may create a real financial crisis.

In an attempt to relieve older citizens of

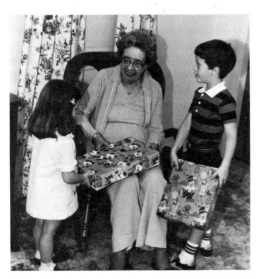

Figure 7.4. Continuing to give gifts to family members is often important for the aged person. *(Photograph by Ed Spier, Murrysville, PA.)*

some of their economic difficulties, the federal government has instituted benefits and programs for the elderly. These include nutrition and food programs, funds for transportation, Medicare and Medicaid, employment opportunities, stipends for volunteer work, primary health-care programs, and housing programs. In addition, the elderly also receive many tax benefits. Although old persons are entitled to these various benefits, they may not take advantage of them because of pride, location, or lack of information about programs available to them.

RELOCATION

Relocation is a life change experienced by many aged persons. Studies of the long-term effects of relocation on the mortality, health, and well-being of the aged person have produced conflicting results (Borup, Gallego, Heffernan, 1979, 1980). Making decisions in regard to relocation and the relocation process creates stress for some aged persons. Others realize that relocation is in their best interests and relocate with minimal difficulty. Being cognizant of factors leading to the decision to relocate and of considerations to be weighed in planning the relocation enables the nurse to be more effective in reducing stress and promoting adaptation to relocation (see Fig. 7.3).

Many older persons prefer not to relocate, but a variety of personal and environmental factors influence their decision to do so. Decreased mobility, and other health factors may necessitate moving more than once in the later years. For example, a person may move from a house to an apartment when home maintenance and repairs become a burden. Sometime later as the person's health declines it may be necessary to move to a facility that provides such services as meals, housekeeping, and health care. Declining health is one of several factors that may lead to relocation. In a study of relocation from metropolitan to nonmetropolitan areas, Clifford, Heaton, and Fuguitt (1982) noted moves of dependent type households are more frequently associated with crises such as loss of spouse, health problems, and decreased income. Moves in independent households are "more frequently associated with voluntary decisions to seek locations with more favorable climates and better recreational amenities and scenic living environments" (Clifford, Heaton, and Fuguitt, 1982, p. 154). In a study of persons who applied for community housing, Brody (1978) found that motivation to move was attributed to fear of crime, loneliness and isolation, and deteriorated housing. Reluctance to move was related to having an emotional attachment to one's home and neighborhood, lack of energy, health problems, an increased tolerance for stress, and unpreparedness for relocation.

One of the problems in elderly housing facilities is determining when the aged residents are no longer able to maintain independent housing. Bernstein (1982) reported that although such policies are not always clearly indicated the problem areas are usually related to safety, liability, and the inability to provide for one's own basic activities of daily living. Persons with problems of incontinence, mental confusion, emotional instability, substance abuse, and those who pose a safety hazard to themselves are usually considered individually.

Once it has been determined that the older person is experiencing difficulty in functioning in his or her present environment a variety of alternatives need to be considered. Before a decision is made, the positive and negative aspects of each alternative should be carefully considered. The individual and significant others should visit facilities being seriously considered for relocation before decisions are made.

One of the recent trends is to encourage the aged person to remain in the community as long as possible. In many locations support services are available to enable a person to avoid institutionalization. These include "meals on wheels," homemaking services, a variety of health services, home repair services, transportation services, and volunteers to prevent loneliness and to perform minor services. Nurses need to be more involved in assessing the aged person's living arrangements in order to identify needs for support services or relocation. Robertson and Rockwood (1982) found that in-

stitutionalization could be decreased by thorough assessment, rehabilitation, and support services for persons 85 years or older. Home-care services and a day-care hospital contributed to a decreased need for institutionalization. Hughes, Cordray, and Spiker (1981) also found that long-term home care reduced admission to nursing homes without increasing hospitalization or mortality rates.

Ability and willingness of the family to provide for needs of its aged members is an important factor in avoiding institutionalization. Families are not abandoning their elderly members. Brody (1978) indicated that more than twice as many severely disabled elderly reside at home as in institutions. Most older people receiving home care receive it from members of the household. An alternative to institutionalization of the aged person is living with a child or another family member. In a study of the morale of older adults living with children, Kivett and Learner (1982) found no differences in morale between older parents living with or apart from children. This finding conflicts with earlier beliefs that combined parent–child households contribute to lower morale of the older parents. Perhaps the better adjustment of the aged in the Kivett and Learner study can be attributed to the observation that most of the older people remained in their own homes, with the adult children moving into the parent's home. In such circumstances the older person probably has fewer problems with adjustment, losses, and misunderstanding over authority.

Although increased family involvement may prevent or delay institutionalization this involvement creates stress for the family. A follow-up study of aged persons who were not accepted for admission in a mental hospital revealed that the family provided most of the care, with the adult children providing most of the social support (Lindsey and Hughes, 1981). Family members who were providing the care expressed feelings of being overwhelmed and exhausted. According to Lindsey and Hughes institutionalization occurs when the family is not able to administer care, when there is a lack of a family support system, or when the family resources for care are depleted. In a study of life satisfaction of the primary care-giver in multigenerational households, Mindel and Wright (1982) found that the activity level of the elderly relative affected satisfaction. Lower satisfaction occurred when the elderly relative was more dependent, as measured by age, impairment, and activity and when a greater inconvenience in daily living occurred.

Although there are many supportive services that enable the older person to remain in the community, doing so is not necessarily in the best interests of the aged person or of the family. Options to be considered include high rises for the elderly, retirement communities, homes for the aged, boarding homes, nursing homes, day-care centers and facilities for respite care. These options are discussed in Chapter 6. When decisions are made the needs of the aged person, the needs of the family and the advantages and disadvantages of available resources should be carefully considered.

SIGNIFICANT OTHERS

Changing relationships with others comprise one of the life changes of aging. Changes may occur in the relationships with spouse, children, grandchildren, or any person who plays a significant role in the life of a particular individual. As a person ages, the number of people who are significant tends to decline. In many instances, the degree of significance of those people who are important to the old person seems to increase. The decline in the number of significant others is mainly due to the death and illness of friends and relatives, and to the decrease in the size of the individual's life space. Persons whose life space decreases are usually those who have problems with mobility. For these people, pictures, mail, and phone calls from significant others become increasingly important and meaningful.

Parent–Child Relationships
A study by Brown (1974) indicated that for most elderly persons relationships with their children tend to be more important than re-

lationships with friends. However, the elderly do maintain friendships, and most of them find the relationships gratifying. It was found that few elderly persons receive gratification from group contacts.

When groups of Mexican-Americans, blacks, and whites were asked if they felt that they saw their children, grandchildren, and other relatives frequently enough, the Mexican-Americans reported the highest satisfaction with the levels of contact. The whites consistently expressed the desire for more interaction. Although the responses of the blacks were somewhat in between, they more closely resembled the mean of the Mexican-Americans than that of the Anglos (Bengtson, 1976).

In many parent–child relationships, even when the children become adults and have children of their own, the parents continue to feel the need to protect and help their children in whatever ways they can. Frequently, parents and children establish a relationship in which they mutually help one another. They may help economically, with physical tasks, or in decision-making. It is especially important to the self-esteem of an older person who has suffered role loss for her to feel needed and helpful to those who are important to her. When parents and children are in close physical proximity, the opportunities to make physical contributions are greater. With the present trend toward small families and increased geographic mobility, opportunities to offer physical assistance have decreased in many instances. Some older persons are reluctant to ask for help when they need it, but will accept it when it is offered.

A study by Weeks and Cuellar (1981) found that "immigrants are more likely than native-born older people to have family members to turn to in time of need." Asians, with the exception of the Chinese, were found to be most likely to seek assistance from family members whereas the nonminority aged were less reliant upon family. In spite of having a large number of kin in the area, Hispanics were found to be less likely to seek help from family than the nonminority elders. In fact, Hispanics were more likely than any other group not to seek help at all when in need. When family members are not available the Chinese aged were found to be most likely to seek help from friends, and the nonminority aged more likely to seek professional help (Weeks and Cuellar, 1981).

According to Chang (1977), elderly Chinese do not feel uncomfortable about receiving financial support from their children. Instead, they are proud of their children and boast to others that their children are able to support them. In a study of Mexican-Americans, blacks, and whites, the whites responded most negatively when asked if they expected to live with their children when they were not able to live alone. All three groups indicated that they did not expect help from their families if they encountered financial difficulties (Bengtson, 1976).

Older persons often take pride in their ability to give something tangible to their significant others to remember them by. Many elderly people spend much time and energy in creating something special for each person who is important to them. Their creativity may involve food, poetry, artwork, needlecraft, or woodworking. These projects are often highly important to the older person, who may continue to work on them in spite of many difficulties. An example of this is the 84-year-old woman who is attempting to fulfill a promise that she would make a quilt for each of her seven grandchildren. After she had completed six quilts, arthritis and greatly impaired vision threatened her ability to finish the last one. In spite of her physical incapacities, her determination keeps her working on this project although it takes her hours to do what she was formerly able to accomplish in minutes.

Among Native Americans, there is typically a stronger identification with family, clan, or tribe than among the general American population. For the Native American, stronger loyalties are demanded and greater support is provided within the various social groupings. Instead of valuing change, Native Americans value traditional ways, and aged members of the community are highly respected (Rogers and Gallion, 1978).

A study of the Pueblo Indians showed that only 9 percent lived alone. The remainder lived either with a spouse or another family member. Although many of the younger persons have moved to more modern housing, the older, traditional homes lack running water, indoor plumbing, telephones, and electricity. Since 87 percent of the elderly studied indicated a preference for renovating their present homes rather than moving, there is often conflict between the younger and older generations. Some of the older Native Americans indicated that they would reject conveniences such as telephones even if they were provided (Rogers and Gallion, 1978).

Changes in family relationships occur when adult children are forced to assume increased responsibility for the care of aged parents. The family usually helps the older person in time of illness, whether or not the aged and relatives live under one roof. The important factor in the relationship is the emotional bond between the aged and younger family members (Shanas, 1979). Parent–child relations in later life are increasingly determined by factors such as "basic trust, respect, shared values and beliefs and genuine affection" (Hess and Waring, 1978).

When in need the aged usually turn for help "first to their families, then to neighbors, and finally to the bureaucratic replacements for families, social workers, ministers and community agencies" (Shanas, 1979, p. 174). The adult child or other responsible family member often encounters stress related to the additional responsibilities and when trying to determine the amount of assistance the older person needs. Robinson and Thurnher (1978) reported that stress from perceived mental deterioration of the parent generally resulted in negative portrayals of the parents by the children. Stress also resulted when the care-taking responsibilities infringed on the life-style of the adult child. With an increase in the number of divorces, remarriages, and women in the work force families encounter greater difficulties in providing for the needs of their aged members. Goldstein (1982) describes the plight of adult children as the "sandwich generation" when the aged parents become dependent on their children at a time when their own children are making increased emotional, physical, and financial demands. The aged parents experience a series of internal conflicts: loneliness versus a reluctance to impose; anger versus guilt; and fear of abandonment versus uncertainty and fear of being a "bother." The aged should be treated as adults with the preservation of their dignity, independence, self-worth, and purpose (Goldstein, 1982). Feelings of guilt may occur when the care-giver recognizes the needs of the aged member but realizes the inability to meet these needs. Being responsible for the care of an aged family member may create stress on all of the members of the family. Members of the health team should more readily recognize needs of the family as well as those of the older person and facilitate the use of support systems and support services.

Often those responsible for the care of an older person can themselves be classified as aged. This situation may occur when a person is responsible for a sibling, or a spouse, or when an aged parent is in the 80s or 90s. This latter situation is occurring more frequently, as more persons are living until their 80s or 90s. When aged persons are responsible for other aged persons the need for community services and support systems may be even greater.

Increased utilization of community services and supports may also be required by those who are childless. Kivitt and Learner (1980) found that childless people who experienced "poor health, death of a housing companion or inability to drive" had limited alternatives. For childless people support systems consist of siblings, more distant relatives, and neighbors. Marital status of childless people also has implications for well-being. Johnson and Catalano (1981) found in a group of childless elderly who had recently been discharged from a hospital that marital status was the "major determinant of the quality of support received and the patterns of adaptation to childlessness in later life." Unmarried childless aged persons were more active with friends and neighbors and were more socially involved with the church. Childless married couples were more isolated and tended to rely on each other. They had fewer other relatives for support than

did the unmarried childless. Friends were found to meet sociability needs and less likely to increase their involvement when health became impaired. Johnson and Catalano indicated that the unmarried childless elderly have an increased risk of institutionalization. Those who were married received continuous and committed care from a spouse. Childless unmarried persons were found to be distant in the degree of relationship with family and in the degree of emotional commitment. Widowed childless older women were found to have slightly lower psychologic well-being and were more lonely and dissatisfied with their lives than were widows with grown children (Beckman and Houser 1982). Well-being was found to be affected more by mental status, religion and social interaction than by childlessness. Physical capacity was found to predict well-being when a woman had neither children nor a spouse to provide assistance.

Grandparenting (Fig. 7.5)
Some persons eagerly anticipate the day when they will become grandparents. Others find themselves in the role before they are ready. A study by Neugarten and Weinstein (1964) showed that most grandparents found their role to be positive and satisfying. Those who expressed negative feelings related it to conflict in perceiving themselves as grandparents, conflict with the parents over child-rearing practices, or dismay about the caretaking responsibilities associated with grandparenting. Some of the positive feelings associated with being grandparents involved the feelings of youthfulness it provided, the knowledge that the family line or name would be continued, the opportunity to be a better grandparent than parent, and the satisfaction received from the ability to contribute to the needs of the grandchild.

Neugarten and Weinstein (1964) identified five "styles of grandparenting." The approaches they identified were the formal, the fun seeker, the surrogate parent, the reservoir of family wisdom, and the distant figure. Half of the grandparents they studied perceived themselves as being either the fun seeker or

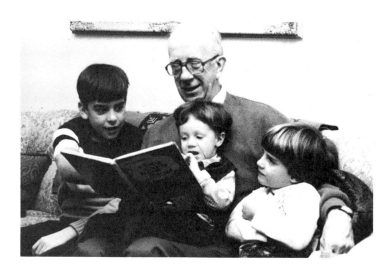

Figure 7.5. Interactions between grandparents and grandchildren are often rewarding for both generations. *(Photograph by Ed Spier, Murrysville, P.A.)*

the distant figure. It was pointed out that the issue of authority is minimal in these two styles of grandparenting. Grandparents who take the fun seeker role often express their delight in being able to have fun with their grandchildren without having the responsibilities associated with raising them.

The grandparent–grandchild relationship appears to be dependent upon the age and the developmental stage of the grandchild. Kahana and Kahana (1971) studied the ways children of different ages viewed their relationship with their grandparents. The age ranges they studied were 4 to 5, 8 to 9, and 11 to 12. They noted that young children valued the relationship with their grandparents for their giving of favors, gifts, and affection. Children from the middle group preferred grandparents who were more active and fun sharing. The oldest group tended to become distant toward doting grandparents. In a study of grandchildren ranging in age from 18 through 26, Robertson (1976) found that adult grandchildren expect little more from their grandparents than emotional gratification, some gift-giving, and information about family history and tradition. The grandchildren studied expressed the belief that they had responsibilities toward their grandparents, including providing emotional

support, tangible help, and visiting. The visiting with grandparents was found to be more qualitative than ritualistic.

In a study of the relationship between young adult children and grandparents, Hoffman (1979) found the adult grandchildren to be closer to maternal grandparents than to paternal grandparents. Emotionally they were the closest to the maternal grandmother. Involvement and emotional attachment to grandparents varied greatly among the young adult grandchildren.

Abuse

Abuse tends to occur to those who are the most vulnerable. When older persons become weak and dependent on others to meet their needs they are more likely to be victims of abuse. In a study of 39 abused persons by Lau and Kosberg (1979), 30 of the persons were women, 51 percent depended on another person, a walker, or a wheelchair for mobility, 10 percent had a visual or hearing impairment, 18 percent were incontinent, and 41 percent had a problem with confusion.

Abuse may be physical, psychologic, material, or a violation of a person's rights. Definitions of the categories of abuse by Lau and Kosberg (1979) are as follows:

Categories of Abuse by Lau and Kosberg

Physical abuse—beating; withholding personal care, food, and medical care; and lack of supervision.

Psychologic abuse—verbal assault and threats, provoking fear, and isolation.

Material abuse—monetary or material theft or misuse (money not being used to benefit the aged person).

Violation of rights—being forced out of one's dwelling or into another setting (most often a nursing home) (Lau and Kosberg, 1979, p. 12).

Examples of Abuse

Son of a 92-year-old woman beat her when she was incontinent. He regularly took her walker away and made her crawl to the bathroom.

A 75-year-old ambulatory female was confined to a room in her daughter's home. Whenever she left her room she was threatened that she would have to move elsewhere.

A 76-year-old female whose only relative was a grandson said, "The only time I see him is when he needs my money to buy drugs."

A 79-year-old female with mild mobility problems was taken "to visit" a nursing home. Without the woman's knowledge she was admitted to the home and her family disposed of her home and possessions.

Before abuse can be prevented, its causes need to be understood. The abuser may be the spouse, child, grandchild, another relative, friend, neighbor, or a paid care-giver. Frequently abuse is not intended, but it may occur when the abuser is experiencing stress. The stress may result from role conflict, financial pressures, lack of understanding of the problems and needs of the victim, and lack of knowledge about how to meet these needs or where to go for help. Abusers may be experiencing alcohol or drug addiction, retardation, or another type of mental or physical problem. The abuser may be young, immature, have a poor self-image, and have unmet dependency needs (Hooyman, 1981). Abuse may result from unresolved family conflict. Some families have a history of abusing the most vulnerable member. The victim may have been the abuser at one time, and vice versa. For example, a victim of wife abuse may abuse her spouse if he becomes physically disabled. Such abuses may be an attempt to get even. The abuser may not realize that abuse is occurring. Abusive behaviors may be perceived as protective actions. At times it is difficult to distinguish between abuse and protection, especially when the victim is experiencing cognitive changes. In some instances abuse may be intentional in order to preserve inheritance (Lau and Kosberg, 1981).

Sexuality

Our society has been slow to recognize that older persons have sexual needs. The older adult has been often thought of as an asexual being. Even a group of nursing students seemed quite startled when it was suggested that they consider what sexual problems their grandparents might be having. Most of the students indicated that they had never thought of sexual needs in relation to older people.

The sexual needs of any individual are both physiologic and psychosocial in nature. They incorporate the person's feelings about him or herself as well as the interactions with others. The sexual needs of older people are based on self-concept, past attitudes and beliefs, and on the opportunities available for meeting these needs. The aged vary greatly as to sexually related values, interests, and capabilities.

Psychosocial Aspects

Consider the question of self-concept. For some people their appearance is very important; for others, it is not. Those who have never attached much importance to their appearance will not suddenly value it when they become old. Yet there are many elderly people who take great pride in their appearance and make great efforts to remain attractive. Even on days when it is unlikely that they will have contact with others, some elderly women still wear attractive clothes, jewelry, and makeup. Even those with many physical problems have been known to continue their weekly trips to the hairdresser long after most other activities outside of the home have been given up.

Some old persons, especially women, have only limited opportunities for interactions with members of the opposite sex. First of all, there are fewer men to interact with. In addition, some widows are hesitant about developing relationships with men because of their own guilt feelings or because of reactions by their children. After an elderly person becomes institutionalized, there are only minimal opportunities for intimacy. Nursing homes and similar institutions rarely provide places where residents can be assured of privacy.

Economic problems may prevent some older persons from remarrying. Often remarriage reduces or eliminates benefits such as the pension of the former spouse. At times an elderly person will avoid remarriage in order to ensure passage of the estate to his or her children.

Sexual functioning is affected by the individual's long-standing attitudes and beliefs about sexuality. Those with negative attitudes may use old age as an excuse to avoid the physical aspects of sex. Others, whose religion views procreation as the primary purpose of sex, feel guilty about continuing to have coitus beyond the childbearing years. Older persons who view sex positively can continue to have coitus indefinitely, as long as there are not prolonged periods without sexual stimulation and as long as they have no physiologic condition that interferes with the functioning of their sexual organs.

Physiologic Changes

Several researchers have studied the sexual activity of aged persons. DeNicola and Peruzza (1974) studied 53 men and 32 women between the ages of 62 and 81. Persons 62 to 71 years of age were found to have coitus twice weekly, and those between 72 and 81 averaged three times a month.

Verwoerdt, Pfeiffer, and Wang (1969) studied the sexual activity and interests of a group of 254 persons who ranged in age from 60 to 94. Sexual activity was found to decline from a level of more than 50 percent during the early 60s to a level of 10 to 20 percent after age 80. Mild to moderate sexual interest persisted into the 80s. However, strong interest did not occur after age 75. Sexual interest in women was at its lowest during the early 70s. In men, activity and interest decreased during the mid-70s.

In a study of 50 couples who were married an average of 55.5 years, with an average individual age of 79 years, Roberts (1979) determined the following:

When 49 couples were asked if they continued to have intercourse, 1 couple reported having intercourse three times per week, 6 couples reported having it during the preceding month, 13 reported it had not been discontinued, and 15 couples said intercourse had been stopped within the last 5 years. Illness, loss of interest, and loss of potency of the husband were the reasons given for discontinuing intercourse (Roberts 1979).

Both functional and structural changes occur in the sexual organs of the aging person. Menopause, the cessation of menstrual functioning in women, generally occurs between the ages of 45 and 55. Most women have reached menopause by the age of 50. Usually ovulation

| | Sexual Feeling of 96 Persons | | | |
| | During Younger Years | | During Older Years | |
	Males	Females	Males	Females
Mid-strong	48	41	20	17
Weak or non-existent	1	6	29	30

ceases between the ages of 45 and 50. Although pregnancy is unusual after age 50, there is documentation on 26 women over 50 years of age who have had normal deliveries (Yeaworth and Friedeman, 1950).

Masters and Johnson (1966) have detailed the structural changes in the female sexual organs that result from a decrease in hormone levels following cessation of ovulation. There is a measurable loss in the amount and elasticity of breast tissue, so that the breasts tend to sag and become flat. There is also a loss of fatty tissue deposits, and of the elastic tissue of the labia majora. Later in the postmenopausal years the secretory activity of the Bartholin's glands is markedly reduced. While the vaginal walls of a woman with functioning ovaries appear reddish-purple, thickened, and well-corrugated, the vaginal walls of a postmenopausal woman become light pink and appear tissue-paper thin. The length and diameter of the vagina are also reduced. As the vaginal walls become thinner, the vagina loses some of its capacity for expansion. The uterus becomes smaller, so that 5 to 10 years after the production of ovarian steroids has ceased, the uterus and cervix are about equal in length.

In spite of the many changes in the female sexual organs, the older woman is fully capable of sexual performance at orgasmic response levels. However, regular sexual experience is essential for the elderly woman to maintain her sexual capacity and for effective sexual expression (Masters and Johnson, 1966).

Changes in the size of the vagina and in the consistency of the vaginal walls may cause dyspareunia (painful sexual intercourse) or burning on urination for a few hours after coitus. This is caused by the decrease in lubricating secretions from Bartholin's glands and the lack of protection for the bladder and urethra during active coitus. These problems are more likely to occur when sexual activity is infrequent.

The aging man also undergoes changes in the structure and functioning of the sexual organs. There is a significant loss in elasticity of the scrotal skin. This leads to increased relaxation, folding, and sagging of the scrotal tissue, and to a reduced scrotal vasocongestive response to sexual tensions (Masters and Johnson, 1966). The size and firmness of the testes are reduced, and the seminiferous tubules become thickened (Yeaworth and Friedeman, September, 1975). Although there is a decline in the level of testosterone, the male sex hormone, men may produce viable sperm into the tenth decade. However, considerably fewer sperm are produced (Weg, 1975).

Regardless of opportunity or of their partner's demands, most men over the age of 60 are satisfied with one or two ejaculations per week. Many older men are unable to have an erection during a 12- to 24-hour period after ejaculation. The time required to develop an erection is at least doubled and often tripled for the older male. The ability to maintain an erection for an extended period of time without ejaculation is associated with the aging process. This situation is often connected with a gradual seepage of seminal fluid rather than an expulsive ejaculation. The vasocongestive response of the older man is decreased in intensity, with a lowered ejaculatory pressure and sometimes an impairment of psychosexual pleasure during ejaculation (Masters and Johnson, 1966).

The sexual capacity and performance of the older man varies from individual to individual, and within the same individual from time to time. Acute and chronic health problems can influence sexual performance. One of the strongest influences, however, is the sociosexual environment that was present during the individual's formative years. For the older man, the single most important factor in maintaining effective sexual performance is consistency in active sexual expression. It is possible for a man to resume sexual activity if he has been sexually inactive for some physical or social reason. Men who continue to have coitus and who are free from acute and chronic physical incapacities can remain sexually active at least into their 80s (Masters and Johnson, 1966).

Six factors that commonly interfere with sexual performance in the older man have been identified by Masters and Johnson. One of these is monotony in the sexual relationship. The woman may no longer stimulate her partner, or both partners may take each other for granted and not work at their relationship. A second problem is preoccupation with career or economic pursuits, which may interfere with communications between husband and wife. There is usually more interest in sexual activity when the person has had a good day as opposed to a bad day. A third reason for sexual problems is mental or physical fatigue. Persons who do not regularly participate in physical activities may lose their sexual responsiveness for a day or two after excessive physical activity. Worry and mental fatigue have an even greater effect on sexual performance than does physical fatigue. A fourth factor that interferes with sexual activity is excessive drinking or eating. Alcohol tends to hinder a man's sexual performance at any age. A fifth reason for problems with sexual functioning is the physical or mental infirmity of either partner. If the condition is acute, the problem is usually only temporary. A sixth factor that might cause the man to avoid sexual activity is fear of failure. While Masters and Johnson emphasize the effect of these six factors on men, most of them can also interfere with sexual performance of the woman.

Medications can have an effect on sexuality. Drugs that affect the central or autonomic nervous systems may alter sexual function. Drugs that cause parasympathetic cholinergic stimulation may produce erections while drugs that interfere with parasympathetic impulses (anticholinergics, and ganglionic blockers) may prevent erections (Ball, 1980). Although antihypertensives frequently interfere with sexual functioning, using them may restore normal sexual behavior when depression subsides (Ball, 1980). L-Dopa, dopar, and other drugs used to treat Parkinson's Disease may be associated with increased sexual activity. The use of hormones and hormonal antagonists also may increase sexual functions.

For some older adults, discussion of sexually related topics has been taboo during most of their lifetimes. This, along with society's failure to recognize the sexual needs of the elderly, prevents many older persons from obtaining help for their sex problems. Lack of knowledge of the normal physiologic changes connected with aging, and hesitancy to admit

the existence of sexually related problems, causes many older persons to have unmet sexual needs. Sexual intercourse declines among the aged. Some older couples prefer to continue to have sexual intercourse, while others are satisfied with touch and physical closeness (Fig. 7.6).

CHANGES RELATED TO DEATH

Not only do changes in health exert a major influence over the life and well-being of the aged person, but stressors related to other life changes affect health. As indicated by Rahe and Arthur (1978), there is a relationship between recent life changes and the subsequent development of minor and major illnesses as well as the occurrence of death. Recent life-change experiences were strongly associated with subsequent levels of psychologic and physiologic symptoms. Since variations in health status are discussed throughout this text, they are not discussed here.

The last life change to be discussed is death.

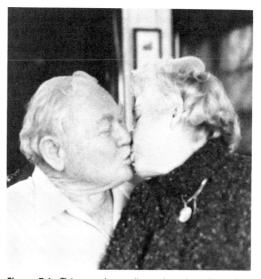

Figure 7.6. This couple continues to enjoy close physical contact which reflects their positive self-concept.

The older a person becomes, the closer he is to death. To the elderly, death is therefore more real than it is to persons in their middle or young years. Furthermore, society more readily accepts death of the aged than it accepts death of the young. The rationale for this attitude is that older people have had opportunities to fulfill their hopes, aspirations, and dreams, while a young or middle-aged person who dies is robbed of life before achieving this fulfillment.

Death has a different meaning for different individuals. For some, it simply means the end. For others, it means the end of physical existence and the beginning of an even better spiritual life. Some people fear death, while others welcome it. Those who fear death may be afraid of the unknown, or perhaps they relate death to punishment for sins. Persons who welcome death may view it as a relief from suffering, or they may believe that after death they will be reunited with loved ones who have died earlier. The aged person is confronted with the death of self and the death of significant others.

Death of Self

Individuals differ in their readiness for death. Many older persons, although they continue to live their lives to the fullest, have put their affairs in order, feel that they have achieved their major goals, and are ready for death when it occurs. These individuals would refrain from doing anything that might hasten death, but they prefer that measures not be taken to prolong their lives when death actually approaches. There are also a few old people who frequently verbalize the desire to die, talking and behaving as though they will die soon even though there are no physiologic indications that they are dying. This behavior may continue for weeks, months, or years. Such persons usually will not take actions to end their lives. However, they do not or cannot initiate measures to improve the quality of their lives. Unless someone intervenes, they are likely to spend the rest of their lives merely existing, rather than actually living. They may even die prematurely if nothing is done to provide for their basic health-care needs.

In a study of disengagement and awareness of finitude, Sill (1980) found that aged institutionalized persons who perceived themselves as being near death had a low level of activity and a decreased life space. The effects of physical incapacity or of age were not closely related to level of activity of the group studied.

Older persons who feel that they exist without purpose may take active measures to end their lives. Suicide rates are high among the elderly. According to Miller (1978), the only suicide rates that consistently increase with age are those of white males. The increased suicide rates for elderly men, as opposed to the rates for elderly women, may be related to the finding that widowers tend to be less self-sufficient and more socially isolated than widows (Barardo, 1967).

There are also a few individuals who deny the possibility that they can ever die. Such denial frequently constitutes a defense mechanism against a subconscious fear of death.

The majority of the elderly do not fear death. This was supported by the findings of Bengtson, Cuellar, and Ragan (1977). In a study of persons ranging in age from 45 to 74 years, they discovered that those from age 65 to 74 had the least fear of death. The greatest fear of death was expressed by subjects who were 45 to 54 years old. When elderly residents of a nursing home were asked if they feared death, only 16 percent indicated that they were fearful (Roberts, 1970). A study by Cooper and Simonin (1978) covering persons in the same age range confirmed that most elderly people do not fear death. Among the group from 65 to 74 years of age, 72.6 percent of blacks, 76.9 percent of Mexican-Americans, and 69.1 percent of whites who were surveyed were not afraid of death. Of the persons who were 45 to 54, 49.7 percent of blacks, 48.5 of Mexican-Americans, and 51.2 percent of whites indicated that they were not afraid of death. Persons with strong religious beliefs have been found to be less anxious about death than those who are not religious (Kalish, 1976).

Most old persons who express fears about death seem to be afraid of the process of dying, rather than of death itself. One of the greatest fears is the loss of control as death approaches.

In a study of healthy elderly, Beck and Cock-hill (1981) found that the aged in their study were prepared for death, did not fear it, but did fear incapacitation. Aged persons fear that they will lose the ability to meet their physiologic needs, they will become immobilized, that they will not be permitted to decide where they will die or the type and amount of care that they will receive before death, and that they will not be told the truth about their physical condition. Fear of being unable to obtain help when they need it is common among elderly persons who live alone. Some old people fear that their significant others will not be able to meet their needs and may abandon them by institutionalizing them. Many of the elderly prefer to die at home, rather than in an unfamiliar environment in the presence of people they do not know.

Once the individual becomes aware that death is approaching, time often becomes very important. Depending upon the person's physical abilities and the amount of time remaining, she may reflect upon her life, examine her goals, and set priorities for the tasks still unfinished. As with all developmental tasks, mastery of this last task of dying is affected by how the individual has mastered previous developmental tasks.

Five stages in the dying process have been identified by Elisabeth Kübler-Ross (1969). The first stage is that of denial and isolation. During this stage, the person expresses disbelief that she is dying, either verbally or through actions. The second stage is one of anger. The anger may be displaced, and the real source of the anger may not be understood by those in contact with the dying person. During the third stage of dying, the individual is believed to bargain. Most of these bargains are with God, for more time or for the chance to fulfill a particular wish. The fourth stage is evidenced by depression, resulting from the person's realization that she is actually dying. The depression may be related to the many losses that confront the person, as well as the realization that certain goals may not be achieved. The final stage of dying is that of acceptance. During this stage the person is at peace with what is to be (Kübler-Ross, 1969).

The stages identified by Kübler-Ross can also be seen in persons who are confronted with the loss of someone or something that they value. Individuals confronted with death or a loss move back and forth among the various stages. Evidence of several stages may be seen during a brief period of time. Not all persons reach the final stage of acceptance. When death is sudden or unexpected, there may be limited opportunity to go through the stages of dying, or none at all. When death has been anticipated, the significant others as well as the dying person may be able to proceed through the grieving process before death occurs (Kübler-Ross, 1969).

Observations and discussions involving the elderly have revealed that the majority value life. However, they are more concerned about the quality of their lives than they are about living as long as possible. Many have expressed satisfaction when they can be independent and in control of their lives, but show evidence of despair and readiness for death when these abilities are lost. The wish of most is to be comfortable until death and to be permitted to die with dignity when death does come.

Some old persons are unable to discuss their thoughts and wishes about their own deaths. Others are ready to discuss their desires concerning the final days of their lives and their wishes about the distribution of possessions, but find that their significant others are unable to discuss these subjects. Communication may be blocked by such phrases as, "Now, don't talk that way, you aren't going to die just yet." When the significant others convey the attitude that death is too painful to discuss, the elderly person may avoid further discussion of wishes in an attempt to protect loved ones. If they are never able to discuss death and related plans, the survivors are then left to guess what the person would have preferred. In an ideal situation, of course, people are able to discuss death and their related desires and plans.

Death of Significant Others

Reaction to the death of significant others depends upon many factors. These include the age of the person, the suddenness of the death, the amount of suffering experienced by the dying person, the state of health of the one who died, the person's state of affairs, and the adequacy of the support systems. Another important factor is the role or roles played by the person who died, and the amount and kind of changes that occur as a result of the person's death. For example, consider the changes that might occur in the economic situation. A couple with very meager savings might have been able to live comfortably on social security and pension benefits. If the pension benefits stop upon the death of one spouse, the survivor may have to make numerous adjustments in life-style. He or she may be forced to change his or her place of residence because of the reduction in income.

The degree of dependence on the person who died is also significant. Adjustment may be more difficult if the one who seemed to be the strongest and the healthiest was the one to die first.

When 100 older persons whose average age was 79 years were asked, "Given a choice, would you prefer to outlive your husband/wife?" Forty-four responded "yes," 34 said "no," 11 were undecided, and 11 others expressed the desire to die together. Those who wished to outlive their spouse indicated they felt better able to cope with grief, to take care of self, and to manage in general. Those who preferred to die first feared they would not be able to manage or to cope with loneliness or grief and expressed intense feelings of devotion and interdependence with their spouse (Roberts, 1979). The elderly appear to have more difficulty in accepting the death of a child than they do in accepting the death of other loved ones. In a study of adult bereavement reactions experienced upon death of a spouse, child, or parent, Sanders (1980) found grief to be at a significantly higher level of intensity among parents who survived their child's death. In Sander's study no differences were found in the intensity of bereavement between survivors whose significant other had died suddenly and survivors whose significant other had died following a chronic illness. The amount of compatibility between the survivor and the one who dies affects the reaction to death. Survivors who have strong feelings of guilt about the death of, or their previous re-

lationship with, the dead person have more difficulty in adjusting.

There is evidence that death often occurs at a time of great psychologic stress. This might be during the period of grieving for another, when it appears that something or someone of value is going to be lost, or on a particularly significant date, such as the anniversary date of the death of a loved one. Sudden unexpected death has been found to be related to highly significant events that cause a high degree of excitation or resignation. Such a reaction is proposed to cause a neurovegetative response, "involving both the flight–fight and conservation withdrawal system to lethal cardiac events." This type of death is believed to be more likely to strike individuals who have a history of cardiovascular disease (Engel, 1971).

In Sanders's (1980) study, bereaved adults were found to have more physiologic symptoms than did adults who had not experienced recent bereavement. Because the average lifespan is longer for females than it is for males, and the majority of men marry women who are the same age as themselves or younger, a large number of the older members of our society are widows. Only limited generalizations can be made about widowhood. Widowed people express feelings of being old and lonely more frequently than do married people of the same age (Atchley, 1975). Widowed people vary in the amount of assistance they need to adjust to the changes brought about by the loss of a spouse. Those who have good support systems, stability in environmental conditions, employment, and good health are less likely to need help (Silverman and Copperband, 1975). It has been found that widows adjust better when they are not the first of their group of friends to become widowed. They frequently need the support of others who understand. Many express feelings of increased discomfort in being without a spouse when in their old social groups. Many older widowed people need help to find a purpose in their lives and to become involved in new or old activities.

Clayton (1975) found the occurrence of depressive symptoms among widows and widowers to be caused by bereavement rather than the effects of loneliness and social isolation from living alone. The younger widows and widowers who did not live alone had more physical symptoms and more hospitalizations in the year following bereavement than did the control group or the older widows and widowers. Sanders (1981) found that spouses 63 years and younger initially manifested a greater intensity of grief than those 65 years and older. Eighteen months following the spouse's death there was a reverse in the trend, with the older group showing exacerbated grief reactions. That is, initially death of the spouse produced more of a shock for the younger group. Later the younger group was motivated by hope while the older group expressed feelings of hopelessness and helplessness. Older females expressed problems dealing with such things as house repairs and business transactions.

In a study of short-term and long-term adjustment to widowhood among those 62 or older, Barrett and Schneweis (1980) concluded that long after the death of the spouse, widowhood continues to be stressful. Long- and short-term widows and widowers are equally unhappy, impoverished, and lonely. No differences were found to exist in health status, visits by children, or in job opportunities between the two groups. Time is given too much credit as a healer. Health-care workers should be more aware that widows and widowers continue to have special needs, even when widowhood has occurred several years previously.

CONCLUSION

This chapter has emphasized the individuality of factors related to various life changes. To be effective in working with the older client, it is vital for the nurse to keep this in mind. The nurse must consider the interrelationship of all the life changes, as well as other aspects of the person's life. Important in the ability of the elderly to adapt to the life changes are the person's health and support systems.

The individual's state of health can be affected by life changes, or the reverse of this

sequence can occur. Physical conditions may limit independence, and at times may also limit the available alternatives for intervention.

For the elderly person, the environment can be a source either of additional stress or of support. Environmental support may come from a variety of sources, including government-sponsored programs, community organizations, or individuals. Stress, on the other hand, may be caused by changing environment, an unsafe environment, or an environment that lacks understanding of the problems of the elderly. A stable, supportive environment hastens adaptation to life changes; a stressful one may slow or prevent adaptation entirely.

If the individual's usual support systems are not adequate to permit adaptation to life changes, additional support systems may be needed, or changes may have to be made in the existing support systems. The number of existing support systems may decrease if friends and family members die or relocate, if the person moves from a familiar neighborhood, or if personal affiliations are reduced by such events as retirement.

Relationships with the support systems may change. These changes may be slight, or there can be a complete role reversal, as sometimes occurs in the parent–child relationship. At the beginning of the relationship, the parent provided for the child's physical, financial, and emotional needs. At the end of the relationship, the parent may become increasingly dependent on the child for these same needs.

It is important to keep in mind that the majority of older adults adapt well to life changes that occur. Their success depends on how well they have adapted to changes throughout their lives, on the amount of stress with which they are confronted, and on the sources of support which are available.

RECOMMENDED READINGS

Binstock, R.H., Shanas, E. Handbook of Aging and the Social Sciences. New York, Van Nostrand Reinhold, 1976. *A comprehensive discussion of all of the developmental tasks of aging is included. Contains significant in-depth research.*

Erikson, E. Growth and crises of the healthy personality. In Identity and the Life Cycle—Psychological Issues Vol. 1. New York, International Universities Press, 1950, pp. 50–100. *Discusses Erikson's theories of the normal developmental crises which occur throughout life.*

Kübler-Ross, E. On Death and Dying. New York, Macmillan, 1970. *Presents a detailed description of the stages of death, with excerpts of interviews which demonstrate the various stages.*

Masters, W.H., Johnson, V.E. Human Sexual Inadequacy. Boston, Little, Brown, 1970. *Discusses taking a sexual history and various sexual problems. Specific sections on sexual problems of the aging male and female are included.*

Neugarten, B.L. Middle Age and Aging: A Reader in Social Psychology. Chicago and London, University of Chicago Press, 1968. *Chapters on the significant issues of aging are presented by the experts in each area. Erikson, Peck, Neugarten and others present their developmental theories. Some of the early classical studies are included.*

REFERENCES CITED

Atchley, R.C. Adjustment to loss of job at retirement. International Journal of Aging and Human Development 6(1):17, 1975

Atchley, R.C. Dimensions of widowhood in later life. The Gerontologist 15(2):176, 1975

Atchley, R. The Social Forces in Later Life: An Introduction to Social Gerontology. Belmont, CA, Wadsworth, 1977

Ball, W.D. Drugs that affect sexuality, in Hogan R. (ed.), Human Sexuality—A Nursing Perspective. New York, Appleton-Century-Crofts, 1980

Barfield, M.A., Morgan, J.N. Trends in satisfaction with retirement. The Gerontologist 18(1):19, 1978

Barrett, C.J., Schneweis, K.M. An empirical search for stages of widowhood. Omega 11(2):97, 1980

Beaver, M.L. The decision making process and its relationship to relocation adjustment in old people. The Gerontologist 19(6):567, 1979

Beck, E., Cockhill, L. Ageism among the elderly: Attitudes of the Healthy Elderly Towards Old People, Aging, and Death. Paper presented at the meeting of the Gerontological Society, Toronto, November, 1981

Beck, S.H. Adjustment to and satisfaction with retirement. Journal of Gerontology 37(5):616, 1982

Beckman, L.J., Houser, B.B. The consequences of childlessness on the social-psychological well-being

of older woman. Journal of Gerontology 37(2):243, 1982

Bengtson, V.L. Families, Support Systems, and Ethnic Groups: Patterns of Contrast and Congruence. National Science Foundation and by UPS Foundation. Presented at the annual meeting of the Gerontological Society, New York, October, 1976

Bengtson, V.L., Cuellar, J.B., Ragan, P.K. Status contrasts and similarities in attitudes toward death. Journal of Gerontology 32(1):76, 1977

Bernardo, F.M. Social Adaptation to Widowhood Among a Rural–Urban Aged Population. Washington State University, Pullman College of Agriculture. Washington, D.C., Department of Agriculture, Bulletin No. 698, December 1967

Bernstein, J. Who leaves–who stays: Residency policy in housing for the elderly. The Gerontologist 22(3):305, 1982

Binstock, R.H., Shanas, E. Handbook of Aging and the Social Sciences. New York, Van Nostrand Reinhold, 1976

Blazer, D., Palmore, E. Religion and aging in a longitudinal panel. The Gerontologist 16(1):82, 1976

Borup, J.H., Gallego, D.T., Heffernan, P.G. Relocation: Its effect on health, functioning and mortality. The Gerontologist 20(4):468, 1980

Borup, J.H., Gallego, D.T., Heffernan, P.G. Relocation and its effect on mortality. The Gerontologist 19(2):135, 1979

Bossé, R., Ekerdt, D.J. Change in self-perception of leisure activities with retirement. The Gerontologist 21(6):650, 1981

Brody, E.M. Community housing for the elderly, the program, the people, the decision-making process, and the research. The Gerontologist 18(2):121, 1978

Brody, E.M. The aging of the family. The Annals of the American Academy of Political and Social Science 438:13, 1978

Brown, A. Satisfying relationships for the elderly and their patterns of disengagement. The Gerontologist 14(3):258, 1974

Butler, R., Lewis, M. Aging and Mental Health. St. Louis, Mosby, 1977

Cassels, C.S., Eckstein, A.M., Fortinash, K.M. Retirement: Aspects, response, and nursing implication. Journal of Gerontological Nursing 7(6):355, 1981

Chang, P. Working with the Elderly Asians, in Newsome, B.L. (ed.), Insights on the Minority Elderly. The National Center on Black Aged, Washington D.C., and the Institute of Gerontology, University of the District of Columbia, 1977

Chatfield, W. Economic and social factors influencing life satisfaction of the aged. Journal of Gerontology 32(5):593, 1977

Clayton, P.J. The effect of living alone on bereavement symptoms. The American Journal of Psychiatry 132(2):133, 1975

Clifford, W.B., Heaton, T., Fuguitt, G.V. Residential mobility and living arrangements among the elderly: Changing patterns in metropolitan and nonmetropolitan areas. International Journal of Aging and Human Development 14(2):139, 1981–82

Cooper, T., Simonin, M. Age and ethnic differences in attitudes toward death. Project Minority Aging and Social Policy Title IV-B Grant (No. 90-A-1297). Los Angeles, Andrus Gerontology Center, University of Southern California, 1978

Cutler, N.E. Voluntary association participation and life satisfaction: Replication, revision, and extension. International Journal of Aging and Human Development 14(2):127, 1981–82

Cutler, S.J. Aging and voluntary association participation. Journal of Gerontology 32(4):470, 1977

Dancy, J. The Black Elderly: A Guide for Practitioners. Institute of Gerontology, University of Michigan, 1977

Daum, M., Feeman, G., Canton, M.H. The Meaning of Work Among Older Adults. Paper presented at the meeting of the Gerontological Society, San Francisco, November, 1977

Davis, R. You can go home again. Geriatric Nursing 3(4):238, 1982

DeNicola, P., Peruzza, M. Sex in the aged. Journal of the American Geriatric Society 12(8):380, 1974

Dowd, J.J., Bengtson, V.L. Aging in minority populations: An examination of the double jeopardy hypothesis. Journal of Gerontology 33(3):427, 1978

Engel, G.L. Sudden and rapid death during psychological stress: Folklore or wisdom? Annual Internal Medicine 74:771, 1971

Erikson, E.H. Generativity and ego integrity, in Neugarten, B.L. (ed.), Middle Age and Aging. Chicago, University of Chicago Press, 1968

Erikson, E.H. Growth and crises of the healthy personality, in Erikson, E.H. (ed.), Identity and the Life Cycle, Psychological Issues. New York, International Universities Press, 1950

Erikson, E.H. Life History and the Historical Moment. New York, W.W. Norton, 1977

Fengler, A.P. Attitudinal orientation of wives toward their husbands' retirement. International Journal of Aging and Human Development 6(2):139, 1975

Fiske, M. Tasks and crises of the second half of life: The interrelationship of commitment, coping and adaptation, in Birren, J.E., Sloane, R.B. (eds.), Handbook of Mental Health and Aging. Englewood Cliffs, NJ, Prentice-Hall, 1980, pp 337–373

Gallagher, B.J., III. An empirical analysis of attitude

differences between three kin-related generations. Youth and Society 5(3):327, 1974

George, L.K. Role Transitions in Later Life. Belmont, CA, Wadsworth, 1980

George, L.K., Maddox, G.L. Subjective adaptation to loss of work role: A longitudinal study. Journal of Gerontology 32(4):456, 1977

Gilson, P., Coats, S. A study of morale in low income blacks. Journal of Gerontological Nursing 6(7):385, 1980

Glamser, F.D. Determinants of a positive attitude toward retirement. Journal of Gerontology 31(1):104, 1976

Glamser, F.D. The impact of preretirement programs on the retirement experience. Journal of Gerontology 36(2):244, 1981

Goldstein, S.E. Perspectives of grandparents and their children. Journal of the American Geriatrics Society 30(2):150, 1982

Greene, W., Beutner, G. Life Planning/Retirement: Expected Outcomes for Participants in a Person-Centered Program as Compared to Content-Centered Programs. Paper presented at the meeting of the Gerontological Society, Toronto, November, 1981

Hess, B.B., Waring, J.M. Changing patterns of aging and family bonds in later life. The Family Coordinator 27(4):303, 1978

Hoffman, E. Young adults' relations with their grandparents: An exploratory study. International Journal of Aging and Human Development 10(3):299, 1979–80

Hooyman, R.N. A Model for the Prevention, Detection, and Treatment of Elderly Abuse and Neglect. Paper presented at the meeting of the Gerontological Society, Toronto, November, 1981

Hughes, S.L., Cordray, D., Spiker, V.A. Impact of Long Term Home Care on Quality of Life. Paper presented at the meeting of the Gerontological Society, Toronto, November, 1981

Johnson, C.L., Catalano, D.J. Childless elderly and their family supports. The Gerontologist 21(6):610, 1981

Kahana, E., Kahana, B. Theoretical research perspectives on grandparenthood. Aging and Human Development 2:261, 1971

Kalt, N.C., Kohn, M.H. Pre-retirement counseling: Characteristics of programs and preferences of retirees. The Gerontologist 15(2):179, April, 1975

Kalish, R.A. Death and dying in a social context, in Binstock, R.H., Shanas, E. (eds.), Handbook of Aging and the Social Sciences. New York, Van Nostrand Reinhold, 1976, pp 483–507

Keating, N.C., Cole, P. What do I do with him 24

hours a day? Changes in the housewife role after retirement. The Gerontologist 20(1):84, 1980

Keating, N., Marshall, J. The process of retirement: The rural self employed. The Gerontologist 20(4):437, 1980

Kivett, V.R., Learner, R.M. Perspectives on the childless rural elderly: A comparative analysis. The Gerontologist 20(6):708, 1980

Kivett, V.R., Learner, R.M. Situational influences on the morale of older rural adults in child-shared housing: A comparative analysis. The Gerontologist 22(1):100, 1982

Kübler-Ross, E. On Death and Dying. New York, Macmillan, 1969

Lau, E.E., Kosberg, J.I. Abuse of the elderly by informal care providers. Aging 10:10, (No. 314), 1979

Lawton, M.P. An ecological view of living arrangements. The Gerontologist 21(1):59, 1981

Lehr, U., Dreher, G. Determinants of attitudes towards retirement, in Havighurst, R.J., Munnichs, J.M.A., Neugarten, R., Thomas, R. (eds.), Adjustment to Retirement: A Cross-National Study. Assen, The Netherlands, Koninklyke Van Gorcum, 1969, pp 116–137

Lemmon, D.K., Pieper, H.G. Leisure pursuits and their meaning for the institutionalized elderly population. Journal of Gerontological Nursing 6(2):74, 1980

Lewis, F. Factors to consider in selecting a nursing home. Nursing Homes 26(2):8, 1977

Lindsey, A.M., Hughes, E.M. Social support and alternatives to institutionalization for the at-risk elderly. Journal of the American Geriatrics Society 29(7):308, 1981

Locher, R., Rublin, A.K. The Roles of the Geriatric Day Program in the Spectrum of Services for Older Adults. Paper presented at the meeting of the Gerontological Society, Toronto, November, 1981

Maddox, G.L. Themes and issues in sociological theories of human aging. Human Development 13:17, 1970

Masters, W.J., Johnson, V.E. Human Sexual Response. Boston, Little, Brown, 1966

Miller, M. Geriatric Suicide: The Arizona study. The Gerontologist 18(6):488, 1978

Mindel, C.H., Wright, R. Satisfaction in multigenerational households. Journal of Gerontology 37(4):483, 1982

Moberg, D.O. Religion in old age. Geriatrics 20(1):977, 1965

Morrison, M.H. The myth of employee planning for retirement. Industrial Gerontology 135, Spring 1975

Moss, M.S., Lawton, M.P. Time budgets of older people: A window on four lifestyles. Journal of Gerontology 37(1):115, 1982

Neugarten, B.L. Time, age, and the life cycle. The American Journal of Psychiatry 136(7):887, 1979

Neugarten, B.L., Weinstein, K.K. The changing American grandparent. Journal of Marriage and the Family 26(2):199, 1964

Peck, R.C. Psychological developments in the second half of life, in Neugarten, B.L. (ed.), Middle Age and Aging. Chicago, University of Chicago Press, 1968, pp 88–92

Peppers, L.G. Patterns of leisure and adjustment to retirement. The Gerontologist 16(5):441, 1976

Peretti, P.O., Wilson, C. Voluntary and involuntary retirement of aged males and their effects on emotional satisfaction, usefulness, self-image, emotional stability and interpersonal relationships. International Journal of Aging and Human Development 6(2):131, 1975

Quinn, J.F. The extent and correlates of partial retirement. The Gerontologist 21(6):634, 1981

Ragan, P.K. Ethnic and Racial Variations in Aging: Implications for Social Policy and Service Delivery. Andrus Gerontology Center, University of Southern California. Paper presented at the 105th Annual Forum of the National Conference of Social Welfare, Los Angeles, CA, May, 1978

Rahe, R.H., Arthur, R.J. Life change and illness studies: Past history and future directions. Journal of Human Stress 4:3, 1978

Regnier, V., Gelwicks, L.E. Preferred supportive services for middle to higher income retirement housing. The Gerontologist 21(1):54, 1981

Reichard, S., Livson, F., Petersen, P.G. Adjustment to Retirement, in Neugarten, B.L. (ed.), Middle Age and Aging. Chicago, University of Chicago Press, 1968, pp 178–180

Roadburg, A. Perceptions of work and leisure among the elderly. The Gerontologist 21(2):142, 1981

Robb, S.S. The nurse's role in retirement preparation. Journal of Gerontological Nursing 4(1):25, 1978

Roberts, J.L. How aged in nursing homes view dying and death. Geriatrics 25(4):115, 1970.

Roberts, W.L. Significant elements in the relationship of long-married couples. International Journal of Aging and Human Development 10(3):265, 1979

Robertson, J.F. Significance of grandparents' perceptions of young adult grandchildren. The Gerontologist 16(2):137, 1976

Robertson, D., Rockwood, K. Outcome of hospital admission of the very elderly. Journal of the American Geriatrics Society 30(2):101, 1982

Robertson, P.K. NPC on Employment and Retirement. Paper presented at the meeting of the Gerontological Society, Toronto, November, 1981

Robinson, R., Thurnher, M. Taking care of aged parents: A family cycle transition. The Gerontologist 19(6):586, 1979

Roger, C.J., Gallion, T.E. Characteristics of elderly Pueblo Indians in New Mexico. The Gerontologist 18(5):482, 1978

Sanders, C.M. A comparison of adult bereavement in the death of a spouse, child, and parent. Omega 10(4):303, 1980

Sanders, C.M. Comparison of younger and older spouses in bereavement outcome. Omega 11(3):217, 1981

Schulz, J.H. Income distribution and the aging, in Binstock, R.N., Shanas E (eds.), Handbook of Aging and the Social Sciences. New York, Van Nostrand Reinhold, 1976, pp 561–591

Shanas, E. The family as a social support system in old age. The Gerontologist 19(2):169, 1979

Sill, J.S. Disengagement reconsidered: Awareness of finitude. The Gerontologist 20(4):457, 1980

Silverman, P.R., Cooperband, A. On widowhood: Mutual help and the elderly widow. Journal of Geriatric Psychiatry 8(1):9, 1975

Strieb, G.F. Retirement Roles and Activities: Background Issues. In White House Conference on Aging. Washington D.C., U.S. Government Printing Office, February, 1971

Streib, G.F., Schneider, C.J. Retirement in American Society, Impact and Process. Ithaca, Cornell University Press, 1971

Uhlenberg, P. Older women: The growing challenge to design constructive roles. The Gerontologist 19(3):236, 1979

U.S. Bureau of the Census: Statistical Abstract of the United States 1976, 97th Annual Edition. Washington D.C., U.S. Department of Commerce, July, 1976

U.S. Department of Health and Human Services, Office of Human Development Services, Administration on Aging. Elder Abuse. Philadelphia, Franklin Research Center, Contract No. HEW 105-79-3010, May, 1980

Verwoerdt, A., Preiffer, E., Wang, H.S. Sexual behavior in senescence: Patterns of sexual activity and interest. Geriatrics 24(2):137, 1969

Ward, R.A. Aging, the use of time, and social change. International Journal of Aging and Human Development 14(3):177, 1981–82

Weeks, J.R., Cuellar, J.B. The role of family members in the helping networks of older people. The Gerontologist 21(4):388, 1981

Weg, R.B. Physiology and sexuality in aging, in Burnside, I.M. (ed.), Sexuality and Nursing. The Ethel Percy Andrus Gerontology Center, University of Southern California, 1975

Yeaworth, R.C., Friedeman, J.S. Sexuality in later life, Nursing Clinics of North American 10(3):565, 1975

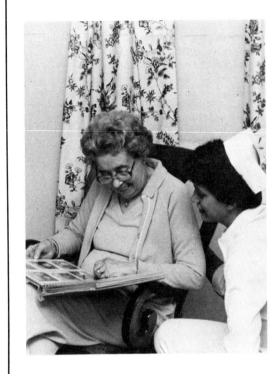

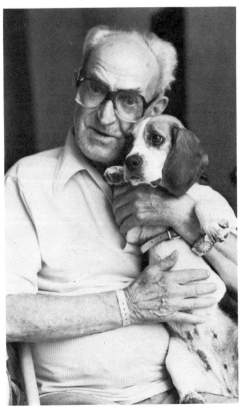

Part 2

The Nursing Process as Applied to the Adaptive Experience of the Aged

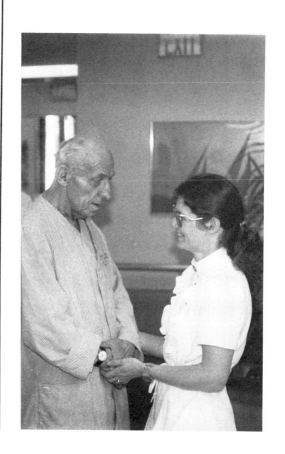

8

The Nursing Process as Applied to the Life Changes of the Aged

Barbara Elliott Spier

Reading this chapter will enable the individual to

1. Identify components of an assessment of life changes, self-concept, and coping mechanisms of the aged person
2. Discuss measures to promote self-esteem of the aged person
3. Promote optimal client–family interaction
4. Describe nursing interventions related to life changes

As discussed in Chapter 7, life changes that may be significant for the aged include those related to productivity, role, leisure activities, income, housing, relationships with others, sexuality, and death. Most aged persons adapt well to these changes and do not need nursing intervention. As they encounter problems, the majority of the elderly successfully utilize the coping mechanisms that have evolved during their younger years. Some, however, find that these coping mechanisms are no longer adequate. These are often persons who are confronted by multiple problems, who have diminished support systems, and who are also coping with health problems.

Since nurses are often the first to encounter those who need help, and are usually the health-team members in closest contact with clients experiencing problems, the role of the nurse is very important. Health problems may create or necessitate additional life changes; therefore, it is important for nurses to assess and intervene in areas where there is a potential for psychosocial problems even when the presenting problem is physical in nature. Better coping is often achieved through a realistic preparation for life changes and through optimal affiliations with others. Nursing assessments include determining the usual coping mechanisms, their availability, and their effectiveness. Life changes or health problems may have an effect on the self-concept of the aged person. Intervention related to life changes of the aged is very individualized, depending on the needs of the aged person and his or her support systems. As family members become increasingly involved in providing for the needs of their older members, they as well as the older person benefit from nursing intervention.

The purpose of this chapter is to present guidelines for assessing and intervening in those areas directly and indirectly related to common life changes of the aged. Since life changes may alter self-perceptions and self-esteem the nurse's role in these areas is discussed. Nursing intervention to increase self-esteem is emphasized, as increased self-esteem may enhance coping with life changes. When coping mechanisms are not effective, it may be necessary to implement measures to promote behavioral change. A method of promoting behavioral change is included in this chapter.

Since families have a role in the aged person's adaptation to life changes, nursing intervention related to the family of the aged is discussed.

ASSESSMENT OF LIFE CHANGES, SELF-CONCEPT, AND COPING MEASURES

The depth of the assessment depends on the nurse's role, the purpose of the assessment, and the problems the client is experiencing. Table 8.1 is a guide that can help the nurse in gathering information about frequently occurring life changes, self-concept, and coping mechanisms. The client may be reluctant to share some of this personal information. The nurse should be alert to verbal and nonverbal clues that the individual does not wish to discuss a particular problem. Continued attempts to pursue a problem when the client clearly does not wish to discuss it can be considered prying and an invasion of privacy. On the other hand, nurses should also be perceptive to clues that the client has problems and would welcome the opportunity to discuss them. Some elderly persons develop the attitude that no one cares about their problems. Others are embarrassed by their difficulties and do not realize that sources of help are available. These people may try to hide their problems from family and friends, but may be willing to discuss them with a member of the health team. Occasionally the older person or a family member may exaggerate or misinterpret the problem or situa-

---

TABLE 8.1 GUIDE FOR ASSESSING LIFE CHANGES, SELF-CONCEPT, AND COPING MECHANISMS

Information About the Following Can Be Determined

Roles/Occupation
Types of employment and/or other responsibilities
  Past
  Present
  Physical activity involved
  Presence of occupational hazards
    Noise pollution
    Air pollution
    Radiation
    Safety hazards
  Satisfaction with
Potential changes
  Retirement readiness
  Retirement plans
  Recent or projected change in responsibilities
  Desire for role changes

Activities
Patterns of activities
Time of day for optimal activity
Preferred activities
Use of leisure time
Hobbies
Organization membership and participation
Interests
Dislikes
Degree of independence
Satisfaction with independence
Volunteer activities
Boredom
Activity pattern for a 24-hour day

TABLE 8.1 (Continued)

Economic Status
Sources
  Social security
  Supplemental security income
  Pension plan
  Veteran's benefits
  Governmental assistance
Perceptions of adequacy of income
  Present
  Anticipated
Health insurance
  Medicare
  Extended coverage
Management of cost of health care
  Medications
  Supplies
  Transportation to health care
  Medical services
  Health Insurance costs
Ability to pay for leisure activities
  Dues for membership in organizations
  Transportation or automobile expenses
  Materials for pursuit of hobbies
  Expenses for alcohol or tobacco
Ability to pay for housing expenses
  Needed repairs
  Needed improvements
  Taxes
  Rent or mortgage
  Utilities
Ability to pay for groceries
Measures taken to decrease expenses
Use of opportunities for reduced costs to aged
Budgeting

Housing
Type
Location
Ownership or rent status
Distance from significant others
Management of maintenance and repairs
Size in relation to need
Accessibility to and mobility within
Safety features
Transportation
  Public or private
  Access to grocery store, bank, beauty or barber shop, health facility, pharmacy, friends, family, leisure
    activities
Adequacy of heating, lighting, ventilation, water, and bathrooms
Feelings of security and safety in home, neighborhood, and community
Anticipated change
Satisfaction with
Other people and/or pets in living environment
Adequacy of privacy

(continued)

TABLE 8.1 (Continued)

Housing (Continued)
Health hazards
Important objects in environment

Family Profile and Significant Others
Significant others and family members (parents, siblings, spouse, children, grandchildren)
Age
Health status or cause of death
Relationship with family and/or significant others
Amount of contact
Satisfaction with amount of contact
Satisfaction with relationships
Most important people in the Immediate environment
Sources of conflict
Important pets

Religious Affiliations
Desire to follow religious practices
Opportunity to attend religious services
Contact with clergy
Significance of religious articles
Observance of religious holidays

Ethnicity
Ethnic influence on health practices
Recognition of need for health care
Kinds of health care sought
Folk medicine practices
Ethnic foods
Ethnic influence of family concerns for elderly members

Self-Concept
Perceptions of self:
As a male or female
In relation to age
Of self-appearance
Changes in appearance
Importance of appearance
Changes in grooming or style of dress

Sexuality
Relationship with members of same sex
Relationship of members of opposite sex
Ability to maintain sexual activity
Desire to maintain sexual activity
Discomfort of genitalia
Change in sexual habits
Change in pattern of urinating
Post-menopausal or climacteric difficulties
Presence of discharge or bleeding
Other sexually related problems
Use of oral or topical hormone preparations
Douching
Frequency
Solution used
Frequency of examinations of:
Breasts
Vagina with Papanicolaou smear
Prostate

TABLE 8.1 (Continued)

Sexuality (Continued)
Illness, surgery, or medications related to sexual organs or sexual functioning
Difficult childbirths

Health Resources
Frequency of health assessments
Facilities used
Knowledge of available resources
Access to
Availability of support services

Death Preparation
Presence of a will
Arrangements for funeral and burial
Communication with significant others in regard to desires concerning death, funeral arrangements, and
    distribution of belongings
Thoughts and fears about dying

Additional Information
Satisfaction with life
Fears
Plans for future
Usual mood
Factors which affect mood
Does time
    Pass quickly
    Drag

Self-Perceptions
Ask the person to answer *yes* or *no* to the following:
Do you see yourself as being:

Happy_____	Easily angered_____	Demanding_____
Cooperative_____	Frustrated_____	Restless_____
Friendly_____	Helpless_____	Irritable_____
Outgoing_____	Depressed_____	Critical_____
Trustful_____	Worried_____	Withdrawn_____
Attractive_____	Annoying_____	Moody_____
Active_____	Discouraged_____	
Productive_____	Lonely_____	
Useful_____		
A private person_____		
Quiet_____		
Energetic_____		
Bored_____		

Then ask the person to discuss as appropriate.

Coping Mechanism
Are problems usually anticipated?
Describe behavior when a problem:
    Is anticipated
    Occurs
    Has occurred

Reaction to Stress
Usual behavior when problems are encountered
    Confrontation
    Avoidance
    Discussion
    Crying

(continued)

TABLE 8.1 (Continued)

Reaction to Stress (Continued)

Praying
Laughing
Seeks presence of others
Avoids presence of others
Smokes
Eats
Drinks alcohol
Uses medication
Activity increases
Activity decreases
Other

Physical Examination

Sexuality
Breasts
Vagina
Papanicolaou smear
Male genitalia

tion. Throughout the assessment the nurse must be alert for inconsistencies. When inconsistencies are apparent it may be necessary to obtain data from additional sources.

Some clients prefer not to discuss their most pressing problems during their initial contact with a health-care worker. Mrs. M was an example of this. Mrs. M initially made an appointment with the nurse practitioner at a senior-citizen center for a physical examination. During their first interview, Mrs. M indicated that she is very independent and outgoing, and that she had no problems she was unable to handle. However, the nurse noted that she was reluctant to discuss certain areas of the health assessment. Mrs. M agreed to return the following week to discuss a minor health problem. As she was leaving after the second visit, she indicated that she would like to return to discuss ways in which she could get her husband to become more active. On the third visit, Mrs. M was very open about her problems, which included an alcoholic husband with whom her relationship had deteriorated over the last 5 years to the point that they were no longer speaking. While tearfully discussing these problems, she revealed that she had been putting up a front for 2 years. Even her family was not aware of the situation. After Mrs. M

was able to admit the problem, the nurse succeeded in convincing her to accept help from other health-team workers. They worked together in assisting Mrs. M to cope with her situation and to improve it.

When clients are suspected of having problems that they are hesitant to discuss, the nurse should attempt to establish rapport and to keep the lines of communication open. The client should be told that the nurse will be available in the future in case new problems arise or if the person wishes to discuss the current problems to any further extent. The client should be told how to contact other members of the health team who might be of assistance.

Specific Areas to be Assessed

Role or Occupation

Information about the client's roles increases the nurse's understanding of the individual's needs and abilities. The significance attached to past and present roles may be important. Pertinent data to be obtained includes specific information related to the type of occupation, the person's satisfaction with the occupation, and his degree of readiness to retire. The information obtained should be kept in mind by the nurse when giving guidance about further employment, volunteer work, or leisure activities.

Responsibilities associated with multiple or particularly demanding roles may result in the person neglecting or not being able to meet his or her own personal needs. An example is when the older person assumes responsibility for an ill family member. Aged persons who have experienced a decline in roles may have decreased feelings of self-worth.

Activities

Assessment of the amount and kind of activity is not sufficient. It is even more important for the nurse to determine the person's satisfaction with these activities. Nonverbal clues often add to the client's verbal communication. Signs of comfort, happiness, and satisfaction during periods of both activity and inactivity should be noted. Although all persons need some periods of relative inactivity, there is wide variation in the amount needed and desired by different individuals.

Economic Status

Most people consider the exact amount of their income to be a personal matter, and the nurse should not pursue this information. However, it is important to determine whether the income is adequate for the client's needs. Of particular concern is the person's ability to pay for health care, including the cost of medications and other supplies, transportation to health-care facilities, and payment for medical services and health insurance. For some clients, the nurse might use a statement such as the following to obtain clues to the person's priorities: "I'll bet you'd rather have a (six-pack of beer, or a pack of cigarettes) than this medicine." Many older people who own their own homes experience difficulties in paying their taxes and in paying for the cost of utilities and for home maintenance. Those on a fixed income who must pay rent may encounter financial problems when their rents are increased. Although inadequate income is a major problem among the elderly, many are reluctant to admit this. Some older persons are too proud to take advantage of opportunities for reducing their expenses.

Housing

Housing is another area in which many people are reluctant to admit difficulty. Often this is because they fear that they will be urged to relocate. During assessment of housing, the nurse should consider the client's physiologic, psychologic, and sociologic needs. Failure to consider these three areas decreases the chances that the person will achieve the highest possible level of wellness.

Significant Others

Assessment related to significant others is dependent upon the situation. When clients are able to provide for their own needs with minimal assistance from others, usually all that is necessary is information from the client pertaining to his relationships with others, his preferences, and whether or not he perceives problems in affiliations with others. Discrepancies in the information provided by the client or clues to problems that are not adequately explained should alert the nurse to the need for additional data. Other sources of information are significant others and members of the health team who are knowledgeable about the client. The information obtained from these three sources does not always agree. For example, one person may feel that there are problems in the relationship whereas the other may either not perceive the problems or may be reluctant to admit that they exist. All of the data obtained need to be carefully analyzed in order to perceive the situation accurately.

Health changes of older individuals may necessitate that significant others become very involved in providing for the aged person's needs. In such instances data pertaining to the needs and concerns of those assuming most of the responsibilities should be obtained. Pertinent data include identifying the willingness of significant others to become involved and determining if there are problems that may interfere with providing for the needs of the client. Common problems include role overload, health problems, and financial problems of the major care provider. The care provider's view of the client's physical, psychologic, and sociologic problems, abilities, and expectations should be assessed. Identification of the care provider's perceptions of his own role, and of his support systems is important (Hooyman, 1981).

Sexuality

Clients are often reluctant to discuss sexually related topics and may decline an examination of their genitalia. The elderly may be even more hesitant than younger clients to discuss sexuality, partly because our society tends to view the old person as sexless and partly because sexually related topics have only recently been brought out in the open. The nurse should respect the client's wishes not to discuss the subject, and should maintain a matter-of-fact attitude during any discussion of sexuality.

Cancer is the second leading cause of death in males and females aged 55–74 and males 75 and over. For females 75 and over cancer is the third leading cause of death. In females aged 55–74 cancer most often occurs in the breast. For this age group cancer of the ovary is the fourth most common site and the uterus the fifth most common site. For females over 75 cancer of the breast is the second most common site (Vital Statistics, 1977). Many older women are reluctant to have breast examinations. Women should be urged to have annual breast examinations by a nurse or a physician and to do self-breast examinations monthly. Low-dose mammography is recommended for all women over 50 (Cancer of the breast, 1980). Annual bimanual gynecologic examinations are recommended, as ovarian cancer is asymptomatic in the early stages. There is a significant decline in the incidence of cancer of the ovary in those 75 and over. Cancer of the uterus is the fifth leading site for cancer in this age group (Vital Statistics, 1977). There is much controversy in regard to the recommended frequency for Papanicolaou (Pap) smears. In 1980 the American Cancer Society recommended that Pap smears be done once a year for two years in women who are or who have been sexually active and who do not have a history of cancer. After two normal examinations Pap smears are recommended every one to three years until age 60. Few cytologic abnormalities have been found in asymptomatic women over age 60. The need to do Pap smears in this group is debatable (Wingate, 1982). Many gynecologists recommend Pap smears annually for all women after the age of 40. Postmenopausal bleeding indicates the need for an immediate gynecologic examination. Annual rectal examinations are recommended for both males and females. The digital rectal examination has been found to be the most efficient screening test for cancer of the prostate (Guinan et al., 1981). The testes are not a leading site for cancer in males over 75 (Vital Statistics, 1977).

Members of the health team should be more aware of the age-related changes in the genitalia of the older woman. Because of thinning of the vaginal walls and lining, the older woman is more likely than a younger one to be uncomfortable during a vaginal examination. The nurse can take measures such as encouraging slow, deep mouth breathing, or continuing casual conversation with the client, in an attempt to help her to relax during the examination. The reduction in length and diameter of the vagina often calls for the use of a smaller-sized vaginal speculum in examination of the older woman.

Recently, The Gravlee Jet Washer has been used to collect cells to detect uterine cancer as an alternative to the Pap smear (Austin et al., 1983). The Gravlee Jet Washer collects cells for examination in a reservoir attached to the Jet after washing the uterine cavity with normal saline solution. Contraindications for the test include severe cervical stenosis, a history of blood dyscrasias, anticoagulant therapy, cardiac conditions, open heart surgery, petechial hemorrhage, severe hypertension, and a vaginal infection within 45 days. The procedure should not be used when there is evidence of the influence of alcohol, other stimulants or the use of phenobarbital, amphetamines, or marijuana. Following the procedure, vaginal bleeding or spotting can be expected. During the procedure slightly to moderately severe painful contractions may be experienced. The procedure may have to be repeated in postmenopausal women due to absence of endometrial cells.

Death Preparation

The nurse should be sensitive to problems the client may have with regard to death preparation. However, there is no need to obtain specific details about death preparations which have already occurred. Persons having problems related to death preparation may welcome an opportunity to discuss it with the nurse, since their family members may be avoiding discussions of this subject.

Self-Perceptions and Coping Mechanisms

There is great variation in the way the elderly perceive themselves. As with all age groups, some persons have a positive self-concept and others have a negative self-concept. A study by Lee (1976) supported the belief that the many individual differences in self-image cannot be attributed to differences in age. Although a person's self-image is influenced by the environment and by life changes, most of the elderly are the same people when they are old as they were when they were young.

Among the changes that affect an individual's self-concept are those connected with health, income, environment, and role change. Larson has reported that state of health exerts the greatest influence on the old person's feelings of well-being. Next in importance are socioeconomic factors and the degree of social interaction. Marital status and living situations were also found to influence the well-being of the individual. There appeared to be no correlation between well-being and the person's age, sex, race, and employment (Larson, 1978).

Self-concept is closely associated with the role identities that have been acquired throughout life (Lemon, Bengtson, and Peterson, 1976). With life changes, role changes occur. Most people are able to cope effectively with these changes and thus maintain their general self-concept. Feedback from those in the environment influences both self-concept and coping ability. Not only are support systems significant in maintaining a person's self-concept, but so too is the importance of the role that has

changed and whether or not a substitute role can be found.

An individual's self-perceptions and view of his coping mechanisms may differ from the perceptions of others in the environment. Some people are unaware or only partially aware of their coping mechanisms. The pattern of an individual's coping mechanisms may vary according to the circumstances. The mechanisms utilized by certain people may be annoying or unacceptable to others in the environment. Although this is not usually the case, when it does occur it can affect the person's relations with others.

Life Satisfaction Indexes

In most situations, the nurse will not need to use a standardized assessment tool. Various tools are available, depending upon the focus of the assessment. Examples include the Life Satisfaction Index A and the Life Satisfaction Index B. These two indexes, which have been validated, are brief and can be used to measure the psychologic well-being of persons over the age of 65 (Neugarten, Havighurst, and Tobin, 1961).

One advantage of using a standardized tool is that comparison between groups of individuals is more meaningful. Standardized tools may be helpful in determining the effectiveness of a particular nursing intervention. In such instances the tools can be administered prior to the intervention and again after the intervention has been in effect for a period of time.

PLANNING AND INTERVENTION

Even if careful analysis of the data collected reveals that the client has no problems related to the life changes of aging, the nurse still has an important role in prevention of future problems. Although most people are able to cope effectively with the various life changes, the nurse's contact with the client often occurs at times when the person is most vulnerable to problems, such as during illness. The nurse whose plans include the client's significant

TABLE 8.2 NURSING-CENTERED GOALS RELATED TO LIFE CHANGES

To promote a high level of self-esteem
To promote optimal client–family Interaction
To promote effective coping in relation to life changes

others will be more effective than the nurse who focuses only on the individual.

Three broad nurse-centered goals are indicated in Table 8.2. Implementation of measures to achieve these goals will enable the nurse to prevent problems, as well as to deal with problems that may be faced by the client and the client's significant others. The nurse should plan and collaborate with the client, the client's significant others, and with the various members of the health team in order to increase the probability of achieving the goals.

Promotion of Self-Esteem (Fig. 8.1)

A factor essential for successful aging is maintenance of self-esteem or a positive self-concept (Schwartz, 1975). Self-concept is the individual's perceptions of himself and his behavior

and his opinion of how others view him. Self-esteem is defined by Elder (1968) as feelings of personal worth that are influenced by performance, abilities, appearance, and the judgments of significant others. Calhoun and Morse (1977) indicate that "high esteem means worth, value and high regard" (p. 320). Self-esteem is the person's satisfaction with the self-concept (Calhoun, Warren, and Kurfiss, 1976). The elderly have greater problems in coping with the various life changes when they have become habitually dependent, when they have poor affiliations with others, and when they lack social initiative (Abrahams and Patterson, 1978).

To maintain a high level of self-esteem the individual must have his identity acknowledged, must have hope, must have control over his own life, must have a sense of self-worth, and must have affiliations with others. People with low levels of self-esteem tend to exist rather than to live. Life becomes meaningless, and feelings of hopelessness and helplessness tend to take over. Such a person may withdraw from the environment and express the wish to die. The nurse's role is to prevent withdrawal by using measures to increase the person's self-esteem.

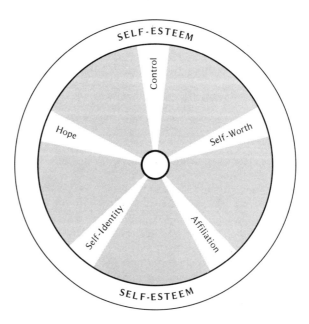

Figure 8.1. Self-identity, hope, control, self-worth and affiliations are important in promoting self-esteem.

Self-Identity

Nurses can promote self-esteem by recognizing the older person as an individual. Too often nurses focus on the client as he or she is today with a particular physical disability. Instead time must be taken to learn about the "person" being cared for. If the 80-year-old in 213 is treated like an old man with a fractured hip, that is how he will respond. Once his roles, accomplishments, needs, and desires have been identified, they should be acknowledged.

The first step in promoting identity is in determining how the person wishes to be addressed. Dignified older persons may be highly insulted if they are referred to as "Honey," "Granny," "Rosie," and so on. Respect is communicated when nurses use Miss, Mrs., or Mr. when addressing clients. If another manner of address is preferred, clients usually communicate this to the nurse.

Self-esteem can be promoted by increasing the individual's awareness of both present and past achievements. The person can be reminded of his positive attributes by placing pictures and meaningful symbols of success in the person's environment. Butler (1982) indicates that familiar objects and possessions provide a sense of continuity, aid the memory, and provide comfort, security, and satisfaction. When aged persons relocate, even if it is to an institution, they should be permitted to take with them as many of their significant furnishings and belongings as is possible. Having important belongings from the past in their environment helps to preserve the person's identity. Frequently aged persons need assistance in deciding what can be taken along and in disposing of treasured belongings that cannot be taken. Nurses can enhance a person's self-esteem by commenting on articles in the environment that the individual perceives as important. Older persons usually enjoy telling stories related to the items over and over. Reminiscing with the client may result in identification of past successes and of what the client perceives as being significant. Reminiscing often reminds people of their own identity and increases their feelings of self-worth and self-meaning.

Once a client's successes have been identified and appropriate symbols of those successes have been selected and placed in the environment, the person's self-esteem is further increased when others notice the symbols and provide positive feedback. Along with emphasizing the client's achievements, the nurse should deemphasize the negative attributes. Individuals should not be reminded of their failures and misfortunes, since these cannot be changed.

Hope

Emphasizing the client's past accomplishments is not enough. A person must also be able to hope for future achievements and for the resolution of present problems. Hope for the future is important for self-esteem. As Stotland (1969) indicated, hope is essential for action. Without hope, people become apathetic and inactive. The old-old may become overwhelmed by their problems. Feelings of helplessness and hopelessness tend to increase as problem-solving abilities diminish and new problems are encountered. Nurses can intervene not only to prevent apathy but to assist the apathetic person in establishing goals. The apathetic individual usually has no goals.

The nurse should remember that people will not work toward goals unless the goals are important to them. For this reason the nurse needs to know the client's problems and what changes are desired. Once this has been determined, the nurse can help the client to establish goals that are not only important but also realistic. Setting unattainable goals merely increases the person's anxiety and leads to further frustration. Hope of achieving a realistic goal or of improving the present situation increases the individual's feelings of well-being and provides motivation for effort.

Once the goals are clear the nurse needs to determine the amount of assistance that the client needs to achieve them. What needs to be done to reach the goals may be viewed by the older person as insurmountable. Nurses may need to assist the person in either achieving the goal or in approaching significant others or members of the health team who can provide step-by-step support. Frequent reminders should be given to take one step at a time. As each step is achieved the progress needs to be pointed out and appropriate praise given. Hope increases as the client recognizes movement toward the goal.

Control

For individuals to maintain self-esteem, they must have maximum control over their lives. Too often significant others or persons in the environment make decisions for the older person. The nurse can provide help in decision-making by increasing the client's understanding of the various alternatives, and the advantages and disadvantages of each. Whenever possible, however, the final decision should be made by the client.

Psychologic well-being is influenced by the degree of control an individual believes he has over life events. In a study of senior citizens, Ried and Ziegler (1980) found better adjustment among those who felt more in control of everyday events that were important to them.

Two studies by Reid, Haas, and Hawkings (1977) indicate that there is a relationship between low self-control and a negative self-concept. Those persons with a negative self-concept were found to be less content and less happy. The relationship between a low sense of control and a negative self-concept was particularly high among men living in homes for the aged. Reid et al. speculated that feeling a sense of control is more relevant to the adjustment of males than to females and that this relationship is amplified in institutional settings where opportunities for personal control are more limited.

Lack of privacy is another problem experienced by many aged persons. It has been shown that privacy is important to the self-esteem of the elderly (Aloia, 1974). Loss of privacy is more of a problem for persons who enter the health-care delivery system, particularly those who are institutionalized. A person's privacy may be invaded by the many personal questions that are asked and by the records that are kept. When a client is sharing personal information with one member of the health team, she may

not realize that the information is going to be recorded on her medical record for many others to read. For the institutionalized client, simply getting a chance to be alone often becomes a problem. Clients may find it impossible to have a private conversation with their significant others. It may even be difficult to have a few minutes alone with one's spouse. Privacy is also important for releasing emotional tension. It enables a person to deal with self and to have the freedom to behave in a particular manner by the removal of certain social constraints (Tate, 1980). Nurses must become more aware of the client's need for, and right to, privacy. Nurses need to be sensitive to clues that a person is reluctant to answer certain questions. People who are institutionalized should have places where they can go if they wish to be alone. The furniture in rooms and lounges should be arranged to enable a small casual grouping of chairs. A large lounge not near the person's room is more of a public space than a social space. Plants, bookcases, and tables can be used to create dividers in large rooms. The nurse's role includes discussing with institutionalized persons their need for privacy. Plan with the person times during the day when privacy can be provided (Tate, 1980). Although it is necessary at times for the nurse to invade the client's privacy, these instances should be kept to a minimum. In deciding whether or not to impinge upon a person's privacy, the nurse must consider what is best for the client's welfare.

In order for clients to have maximum control over their lives, they must be treated with respect and recognized as individuals with varying needs. Clients should be encouraged to be independent and given as much freedom of choice as possible. Institutions must become more flexible, eliminating rigid hours, rules, and procedures to the greatest extent possible, and residents should be encouraged to assume more responsibilities. Older persons in institutions should choose their own activities, decide what is right for them, and be encouraged to run their own institution through a board of residents (Bengtson, 1973).

Most clients are capable of deciding what

to eat, the décor of their environment, and when they will participate in what activities. In too many instances, clients who have lost independence do not even decide what they will wear. Those who are accustomed to having others make decisions for them can be expected to have difficulty in making decisions when given the opportunity. Such persons should be given choices, but it may take a certain amount of time before they are able to do more than choose between two alternatives. As these clients regain control over their lives, they can be expected to have a more positive self-concept.

Self-Worth

When people believe that they can make contributions to others or to society, their self-esteem is enhanced. The individual's sense of self-worth is increased by the satisfaction of helping others and from the recognition by others of such contributions. As productivity increases, so do sources for gratification.

Younger persons often lower their expectations for the elderly, tending to protect them rather than encouraging them to function to their potential. This may decrease the older person's feelings of self-worth. Old people may feel that their services are no longer needed or wanted, or, even worse, that they are no longer capable of providing them. This is not to say that the elderly can continue to function exactly as they did when they were younger. Instead, they should be encouraged to do what they want to do and what they are capable of doing. Frequently, old people do not realize that their services are wanted or needed.

Government and community programs provide the elderly with opportunities for volunteer work (Fig. 8.2). In many instances, those who perform volunteer services at a distance from their homes are provided with transportation and meals. In some cases, they are given a small stipend. Typical of such programs are the Foster Grandparent programs, which pay senior citizens a nominal fee to serve as foster grandparents to underprivileged or mentally retarded children. The children in these programs benefit from the love and individual attention they receive from the foster grandparents. In return, the self-esteem of the elderly volunteers increases as a result of the love they receive from the children and their increased feelings of self-worth.

Many volunteer programs have been established in which the elderly can perform a wide range of activities, depending upon their abilities, interests, and needs. Payne (1977) describes a program in which senior volunteers can develop new skills and maintain old ones. This program develops social independence and interdependence, as well as providing feedback about each person's social effectiveness and self-worth. An example of how an individual can use prior skills in a volunteer role is the retired executive who served as chairman of the board of the program center. This person also became a staff coordinator of the Meals-on-Wheels program, delivering some meals himself. Delivering meals was a new service skill which he combined with his former managerial and community organization skills (Payne, 1977).

In addition to volunteer programs, there are many other ways for the elderly to make contributions. One is by assisting other people in their environments. For example, an exchange of services might be set up in which a woman does some cooking or baking for a male acquaintance, who in return performs some maintenance work for the woman. Residents in long-term care facilities may benefit from helping one another and from assisting with various tasks in the facility, according to their interests and abilities and according to the need.

The matter of asking residents in long-term care institutions to assist one another has become an issue without an answer. Work laws, and the possibility of this practice being interpreted as coercion, can be a problem. Past abuses have given rise to rules and regulations that severely curtail such activities, although they may have therapeutic value. The nurse who wishes to promote therapeutic work activities may thus be constrained by agency or other regulations. Possible tasks which might be assumed by residents in homes for the elderly include keeping the reality boards up to date and orientation of new residents. Persons

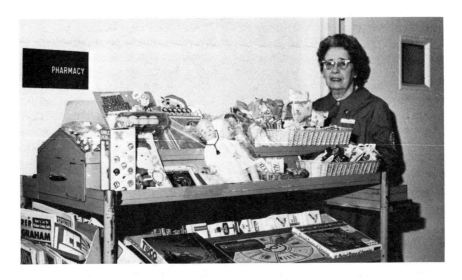

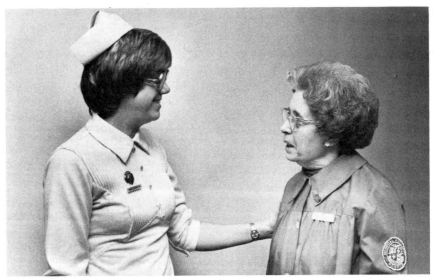

Figure 8.2. An elderly woman whose self-esteem is increased through her work as a hospital volunteer. *(Photographs by Ed Spier, Murrysville, PA.)*

who are immobile could take part in telephone activities, such as the many community programs in which people living alone are called each day to make sure they are all right and to provide a few minutes of socialization.

Many old people experience increased self-esteem as a result of the recognition they receive in pursuing their hobbies, such as playing bridge, gardening, or handicrafts (Fig. 8.3). Further satisfaction may come from selling or

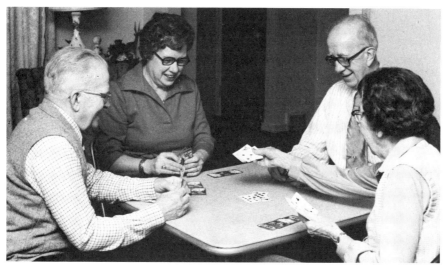

Figure 8.3. Card playing provides opportunities for increased self-esteem and increased affiliations. *(Photograph by Ed Spier, Murrysville, PA.)*

giving away the products of their hobbies. When a person's efforts are recognized and praised, feelings of self-worth are enhanced.

Affiliation

Self-esteem is also promoted by positive affiliations with others. An individual's self-concept is more positive when she knows that someone cares about her and needs her. Nursing intervention to encourage affiliation includes measures to promote the client's feelings of being cared about and needed, and measures to promote behavioral change. Such measures may enable the client to form more positive affiliations, which, in turn, leads to an increased level of self-esteem.

Feeling Cared About and Needed. The nurse should encourage clients to continue their relationships with friends and family, as well as their usual roles (Black, 1973). When this is not possible, then the nurse must look for appropriate substitutions. The finding of significant others has been discussed in greater depth in Chapter 4. In order for persons to maintain their relationships and roles, problems must be anticipated and dealt with. As a decline in

mobility leads to increased dependence, the elderly may come to rely more strongly on the phone or mail for communication.

When it is no longer possible for an elderly client to maintain old contacts, it may be appropriate for the nurse to initiate contact with a friendly visitor. Many communities have friendly visiting programs, which match a volunteer with a person who needs a friend. The friendly visitor visits the person regularly and helps the person to feel that someone cares. The activities of the visitor depend upon the elderly person's needs and on the abilities, interests, and willingness of the visitor. Friendly visitor programs can increase the self-esteem of both the visitor and the person being visited. A study by Mulligan and Bennett (1977–1978) supports the view that such programs are therapeutic.

Some elderly persons may be hesitant to form new relationships. In some instances, lack of self-confidence and of energy prevents new relationships from being formed. The person may have not needed to make new friends for a long time and fear lack of acceptance. Some older persons may not have the energy to entertain new friends and to participate in activities as they did in the years gone by. Carter and Galliano (1981) indicate that because of fear of loss the aged tend "to become isolated in an effort to defend and protect themselves against the pain of loss" (p. 349).

A study by Dudley and Hillery (1977) found that in a comparison of all types of institutions, residents of homes for the elderly were the most alienated and the second most deprived of freedom. Significant others should be encouraged to help alleviate these problems, by visiting often and taking part in the activities of the institution. According to a study by Greene and Monaham (1982), nursing home residents who are visited more frequently experience lower levels of psychosocial impairment. They suggested that visiting has a significant therapeutic influence on patient well-being. Contrary to this, Lee and Ellithorpe (1982) found that interaction with relatives had no desirable effect on the emotional well-being of the elderly. More effort needs to be made to improve the quality of relationships between the aged and their family members. Frequency of interactions does not assure quality. Nurses need to assume a more active role in promoting more effective communications between the aged and their significant others.

Affiliation can be promoted by visiting regulations with no restrictions on the length of stay or on who may visit the person. Children of all ages should be encouraged to visit. Guidelines should also be established to allow visits by the client's favorite pets. Policies must be set that enable visitors to have meals with the client and to attend various social functions.

Getting elderly residents of nursing homes back into the community was found to be more significant in increasing morale than was the number of visitors (Kahana, 1973). Families should be encouraged to take aged family members into the community for meals, shopping, visits with friends, and special events as much as possible. Since many elderly residents have neither friends nor families, the nurse must often consider other approaches. For example, efforts might be made to involve nursing home residents or those isolated in the community in activities at a gerontology center.

Hirsch (1977) describes a program that encourages institutionalized old persons to become members in a senior center. The project has been successful in providing the nursing home residents with social and intellectual stimuli through interaction with members residing in the community.

Most of the elderly benefit greatly from having children in their environment (Fig. 8.4). Children frequently remind them of their happier days and are often very stimulating. Old people who interact passively with adults may be very active in interacting with a young child. To cite an example, a 2-year-old boy named Bradley was taken to visit a nursing home. Many residents who had not smiled for months grinned broadly when this toddler approached them. They frequently followed his activities with their eyes. When Bradley neared them, they reached out to touch him and made motions and sounds to attract his attention. Older children are also usually welcomed by the aged. Frequently the elderly enjoy reminiscing with

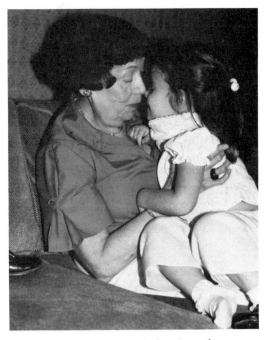

Figure 8.4. The warmth and closeness of a young child helps to communicate love. *(Photograph by Ed Spier, Murrysville, PA.)*

the young, and are interested in the activities, ideas, and customs of today's youth. Children of all ages often help the older person to laugh and to relax.

As discussed in Chapter 4, pets, especially dogs and cats, are sources of love and companionship for the elderly. These animals readily reciprocate with affection for the care they receive. Since pets depend on their masters for their care, they can increase a person's feelings of being needed. Elderly clients are often motivated to be more active than they would be otherwise by the need to maintain and provide for their pets. Pets should be selected according to the individual's interests, needs, and ability to provide for them physically and financially (Levinson, 1969).

Although not as emotionally rewarding as having a pet, some elderly residents derive satisfaction from caring for plants of their own (Fig. 8.5). Plants are easy to maintain and add visual interest and individuality to a room. Some elderly persons may bring a cherished plant with them when they come to the extended-care facility; others may respond favorably to the idea when it is suggested by a nurse.

Significance of Religion

Research has produced conflicting findings in regard to the significance of religion for the aged person (Devine, 1980). Whenever possible, interested clients should be enabled to attend religious services and to participate in religious activities, according to individual preference. When attendance is not possible, the nurse should provide the client with opportunities to listen to services on radio, television, or even on tape recordings. Prayers and visits by church members or the clergy may enable the person to cope better with problems. When a member of the clergy cannot visit as needed, it may be helpful to determine if the client desires to have a person of similar beliefs visit.

Some elderly people continue to observe religious laws and practices that are no longer adhered to by the current majority membership of their religion. The person's beliefs should be respected, and no attempt should be made to change them.

Religious services often provide opportunities for quiet personal meditation and reflection. Through religion, many persons learn to

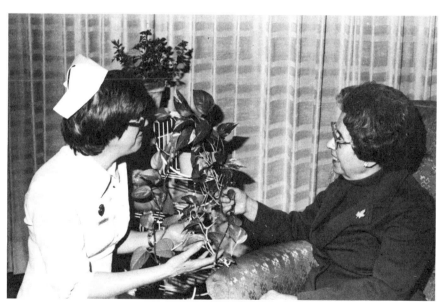

Figure 8.5. Nurse admires woman's plants. *(Photograph by Ed Spier, Murrysville, PA.)*

accept themselves and to face the problems that they encounter. The recognition an individual receives from his church for services and contributions often helps to increase that person's self-esteem. A person may also be honored by the religious congregation because of age, regular attendance, or talents. Religious affiliations may provide the individual with a sense of belonging and with opportunities to serve others, as well as to receive comfort and other services when they are needed (Staser and Staser, 1976).

This section has focused on ways the nurse can help to promote self-esteem through measures that increase the older person's feelings of being cared about and needed. The healthy aged are usually able to meet these needs without intervention from the nurse. When health problems result in isolation and increased dependence the role of the nurse in providing for these needs becomes increasingly important.

Aged persons are needed and have much to contribute to others. Research by Banhoff (1983) has revealed that aged parents were the most crucial source of support when their daughters were recently widowed. Large amounts of support from others, such as the daughter's own children, were found to be virtually ineffective. Nor is support provided by the aged just limited to their families. Frequently older persons are effective in providing support to other aged, to young people, and to numerous groups and organizations within the community. Nurses can enhance the aged person's self-esteem by showing recognition of the contributions he or she has made to others.

Promotion of Optimal Client–Family Interaction

The role of the nurse in promoting optimal client–family interactions includes identifying relationships that are not optimal, identifying sources of stress, and facilitating improved communication and understanding between the aged and significant others. Such actions by the nurse help to improve the self-esteem of the aged and the significant other and help to prevent abuse.

It is important to remain objective in determining appropriate intervention for the aged and their family members. Incomplete data result in premature conclusions and ineffective intervention. Adult children may have views differing from their aged parents on the importance or priority of problems experienced by the aged parents and in regard to the types of services that should be sought. Nurses have an important role in clarifying and in resolving the differences. Discussion groups composed of adult children, aged parents, or children and parents together may be helpful in meeting the needs of both (Cicirelli, 1981).

Reduction of Stress of the Adult Care Provider

The amount of stress created by being responsible for an older family member or friend varies greatly. The extent of the stress is affected by the amount and type of care needed, the other responsibilities and roles of the care provider, the support systems available to the care provider, and the effectiveness of the coping mechanisms of the care provider. The past and present relationship between the older person and the care provider also affects the amount of stress. For some there is minimal stress; for others it is extensive. In some instances no matter how much time and care is given, the older person demands more. On the other hand, stress may result from the demands and attitude of the care provider rather than by the aged person.

Nurses have an important role in counseling and in providing support when working with the client's significant others. Helping families cope with the stress related to responsibilities for an older person can help to prevent abuse. Families may feel that they should be able to cope with their own problems and be reluctant to seek assistance. The stress being experienced may not be apparent until the responsible family member experiences a stress-related physical problem. Even then the source of the stress may not be recognized. Family members directly involved in providing care for the elderly often need help in identifying their own physiologic, psychologic, and sociologic needs. Ignoring these needs can reduce their effectiveness in providing for the needs of elderly family members or negatively affect their functioning in other roles.

Frequently individual family members experience feelings of guilt when it becomes impossible to meet numerous demands placed on him or her. These are often particularly troublesome when families find it necessary to place an aged member in a nursing home or another facility for the aged. The role of the nurse includes assisting the aged person and the adult child to determine if the expectations of either are unrealistic. If they are, assistance is usually needed in identifying specific ways to set limits and to determine resources in the family or community that may be useful.

David (1977) suggested the following guidelines to help a person to distinguish between reasonable and unreasonable demands:

1. A person should not expect to remain always patient and even-tempered toward those they love
2. Although it is inevitable to direct anger towards those we love, it should be controlled and discharged harmlessly
3. Responsibilities to aged parents may be fewer than those that are self-imposed
4. A person should do what is right for him or her
5. Perfection is unrealistic
6. Mistakes that have been made need to be accepted and forgotten

When either aged persons or family members experience guilt, it may be helpful if nurses help them to accept the above guidelines.

A nurse in an outpatient setting discovered the following situation. Mrs. G, an 80-year-old widow, asked her daughter to come to her apartment two or three times daily. In order to avoid guilt feelings the daughter usually went as requested, a 30-minute trip each way. After the daughter described how the situation was interfering with her role as a wife and mother, as well as affecting her physically, the nurse worked with the daughter in resolving the problem. The daughter learned to anticipate her mother's requests and to plan for her needs. Through the nurse's efforts the daugh-

ter succeeded in persuading her brother to assume responsibility for their mother 3 days a week. The daughter was able to limit her visits to once daily, 4 days a week. As a result of the changes her stress level decreased, the relationship with her mother, husband, and children improved, and her physiologic symptoms were alleviated.

Many times family members expect the aged person to function as the person did when he or she was 30 or 40 years younger. Significant others often need help in understanding the changes that have occurred and continue to occur in the life of the older person. Nurses can help them to understand and cope with these various changes. Families frequently need help in promoting an optimal level of self-esteem in their older relative. It is particularly important that the families encourage the older person to maintain as much control over his own life as possible. Counseling with families may increase their awareness of what to expect from the aged member, how to communicate more effectively with him, how to set limits on demands that may be made, how to deal with the behavioral and physical changes inevitable in aging, and how to better provide for the needs of the aged family member.

Although some significant others may wish to help but not know how, others are reluctant to get involved and leave most of the responsibilities to one or two people. Nurses may have to be very specific in helping those not involved to show them how they can become more involved.

Sometimes lack of involvement is due to feelings of inadequacy or to earlier conflicts with the older person. Sometimes professional counseling is needed to help the adult child "to resolve conflicts and issues of earlier years which may influence their reaction to their parents, to gain a more mature perspective, and to learn to deal with dependent parents more effectively" (Cicirelli, 1981, p. 177).

Major care-givers may need help in understanding the value of getting away from the situation on a regular basis. Respite care for themselves results in emotional relief (Hartford and Parsons, 1982) and makes it possible to gain a better perspective of their situation. The care-giver needs brief respite periods a couple of times a week and for extended periods no less than annually.

Group counseling sessions for persons with aged family members or friends are becoming popular in both institutions and communities. Such groups provide information and emotional support as well as opportunities to ventilate frustrations and to learn about other available services and resources. Persons attending such support groups can learn from one another and more effectively deal with role changes. The group may enable the person to laugh at incidents in their own situations that were frustrating when they occurred. The role of the nurse in such groups can include that of facilitator, educator, and counselor.

Abuse by Significant Others

Assessment
Health team members working with older clients need to be alert for signs of abuse, especially when the aged person becomes increasingly dependent on others. Since abuse is frequently denied the term "abuse" should be avoided. Instead, when trying to determine if abuse is a problem information should be obtained about the aged person's relationship with significant others; he should be encouraged to discuss areas that may be a problem. The abused person may be inconsistent in his or her willingness to discuss the problem.

Signs of abuse include undue fear of the care-giver or undue compliance (Phillips, 1980). Observe for angry verbal interaction, derogatory comments, withdrawal, remarks designed to provoke guilt, and self-abuse with alcohol, cigarettes, or medication (Fulmer, 1980). Abuse may be suspected when the person is brought for treatment of an injury by someone other than the care-giver and when there is a prolonged interval between occurrence of the injury and presentation for medical care (Hooyman, 1981). The abuser may be reluctant to give information, may make far-fetched contradictory remarks, be overly critical of the person, respond inappropriately to the seriousness of the condition, and may have minimal interactions with the client (Fulmer, 1980).

When abuse is suspected the client should be interviewed alone and observed for signs of physical abuse. Bruises, burns, and various other sores that may be untreated are signs of physical abuse. Other indications of abuse include poor hygiene and grooming, malnutrition, and dehydration without a physical cause. Bruises on the upper arms may have resulted from the person having been shaken, shoved, or held. The presence of old and new bruises at the same time are evidence of repeated injury. When bruises are clustered on the trunk the client may have been struck or hit (Hooyman, 1981). A complete description of the bruises, their location, and the circumstances should be recorded.

Table 8.3 identifies data that should be obtained when the nurse suspects that a client is being abused. Many times it is very difficult to determine if abuse has occurred. Clients may be unable to admit, even to themselves that they are being abused. Even when a person realizes that abuse is occurring he or she may be reluctant to admit it for the reasons described in Chapter 7, page 259. Inconsistencies between the stories of the care provider and the care receiver make it difficult to decide what data are accurate. The cognitive status of both needs to be taken into consideration. Data from others and the nurse's observations of interaction between the care provider and the care receiver may provide significant information.

Common reactions to abuse are denial and resignation. The victim may or may not realize that abuse is occurring. The realization that one's child or other loved one is mistreating the person is often too overwhelming to face. The victim may be ashamed of the problem and fear retaliation if the incidents of abuse are reported. Resignation occurs when the abused person believes that there are no other alternatives.

Nurses need to be more active in identifying cases of abuse, in preventing abuse, and in seeking help for the abused and the abuser.

TABLE 8.3 ASSESSMENT TO DETERMINE POSSIBLE ABUSE

Physical Abuse

Interview
  Amount of care perceived necessary
  Type of care provided
  Identification of care provided
  Identification of care providers
  Frequency of care
  Identify if medications, food and care are withheld and reason for
  Determine amount of time left alone in relation to need
  Provision for care when alone
  Obtain complete information about bruises, burns, fractures, and malnutrition
  Determine reason if someone other than care-giver did not bring for care
Observations
  Hygiene
    Body odors, care of nails, and mouth and hair cleanliness
  State of nutrition
    Emaciation
    Dehydration
  Integrity of skin
    Burns
    Decubitus ulcers
    Bruises
      Note if clustered on trunk, or present on upper arms
      Note of evidence of old and new bruises

Psychologic Abuse

Interview
  Determine amount of contact with others
  Determine amount of time spent alone
  Identify relatives, friends, and health-care team members with whom there is regular contact
  Determine how disagreements are handled
  Determine what the care receiver would like the care-giver to do differently
  Identify fears of the aged person
Observations
  Fearfulness of care-giver
  Undue compliance and agreement with care-giver
  Interactions indicative of anger and guilt
  Evidence of unrealistic expectations
  Lack of interaction

Material Abuse

Interview
  Determine if gifts are received for special occasions—such as birthday or Christmas
  Determine if the aged person is satisfied with the use and care of money and possessions
Observations
  Condition and adequacy of clothes and possessions

(continued)

TABLE 8.3 (Continued)

Violation of Rights

Interview
  Determine the degree of involvement in decision-making
  Satisfaction with amount of control over events directly affecting the person
  Awareness of plans for the day, immediate future, and for change
Observe
  If opinion is sought
  If choices are given
  If continual demands are made for inconsistent requests

Intervention

The best intervention for abuse is prevention. Reducing the stress of the adult care-giver is necessary to prevent abuse. (Refer to page 292.)

When abuse has occurred both the care-giver and the aged person need to be aware of the specific problem and of factors that have contributed to the problem. Both need to be aware of sources for help. Help is more likely to be sought if specific agencies, contact persons, and phone numbers are provided. At times it is advisable to make appointments as needed.

The failure to seek help by both the abused and the abuser is a major problem in reducing the incidence of abuse. Problems that have been admitted on one occasion may be denied on the next. Attempts should be made to minimize feelings of guilt and to give both parties a sense of hope that the problem can be alleviated.

Both the care-giver and aged person should be interviewed separately as well as together. There may be times when the aged person perceives the actions of the care-giver as being abusive when they are not. The care-giver's actions may be a justified attempt to protect the older person. This is especially likely when the aged person is not mentally competent. An example was when Mrs. J reported that her daughter had taken all of her money. Additional data revealed that the daughter had been given power of attorney, as the mother was no longer able to manage her financial affairs. The woman was given more than an adequate amount of money to spend as she wished. She was not able to comprehend what had occurred,

and repeatedly told acquaintences that her daughter had taken all of her money.

Promoting Behavioral Change. Occasionally a nurse encounters clients whose behaviors interfere with their relationships and communications with others. These persons usually need help in changing their behavior to enable them to form more positive relationships. If the nurse makes no attempt to change the client's behavior in a positive way, she may influence the behavior in a negative way without realizing it. For example, consider a person in an institution, such as a hospital or nursing home, who frequently annoys others by loud calls and outbursts. If this client gets attention only when he is being noisy, his behavior is reinforced by the resulting attention. On the other hand, if the client is provided with attention at times other than when he is being noisy, the noisy behavior will cease to be necessary.

Behavior therapy techniques are measures that nurses can utilize in a variety of circumstances to promote change in specific behaviors. Although behavior therapy may incorporate other forms of intervention, in this discussion the term refers to measures that promote desirable or effective behaviors and discourage behaviors that are undesirable or ineffective. Ineffective behaviors include those that disrupt the environment or interfere with relationships because they annoy others. Behavior therapy techniques can be applied to most cases in which a change in behavior is desired. These techniques can also be used to promote affiliation and independence.

Without even realizing it, health-team members and others in the environment often encourage behaviors that are not in the client's best interest. Before evaluating the client's abilities or needs, health-care workers have been known to encourage dependency. For example, a member of the nursing team might automatically begin to bathe a client or might say, "You can take it easy today, I'll do it for you." Both parties may receive rewards from this behavior. The health-care worker may complete the task in less time, and the client is rewarded by attention from the health-care worker. However, this is not in the client's best interests.

Behavior therapy requires a careful assessment of both the client's behaviors and of related factors. For behaviors that present a problem, the nurse needs a description of current factors related to the behaviors. The assessment should include a complete description of the problem behavior, the events that preceded the behavior, the consequences of the behavior, the benefits the client derives from the behavior, and the variables that are related to the behavior. The nurse should also determine how other persons in the environment are related to the behavior. Are they reinforcing the behavior? How would they be affected if the behavior were changed? Alternatives to the behavior (and their possible consequences) should be determined. The client's desires, views, and preferences are a very important consideration. Successful approaches to behavior therapy are dependent upon an adequate assessment (Gambrill, 1977).

Reinforcers are used to change behavior, and should be implemented immediately after a behavior has occurred. Positive reinforcers are measures that are taken to encourage a behavior. For a reinforcer to be positive, the client must perceive it as positive. What is positive for one client is not necessarily positive for another. Praise, food, and attention can all be positive reinforcers if they are provided after a desirable behavior has occurred. The removal of undesirable circumstances in re-

sponse to a desirable behavior can also be a positive reinforcer. Measures that are used to discourage behavior are negative reinforcers. A negative reinforcer might be the removal of something which the client desires, or the provision of something that the client would like to avoid. Behavior therapy can incorporate the use of both positive and negative reinforcers.

Initiation of behavior therapy requires a specific description of the behavior to be changed and of the reinforcer that is to be used (Leitenberg, 1972). Throughout the therapy, the nurse must have specific descriptions of what the client did or did not do in order to evaluate the therapy's effectiveness and to determine what modifications need to be made. "Mr. A was angry" is an inadequate description of behavior, because it is subjective and does not indicate an action. The record should describe not the nurse's conclusion, but what was observed that led to the conclusion. For example: "Mr. A threw the book on the floor and shouted, '_____'." Other information related to the incident should be included in the description. Conditions can be arranged to encourage performance of a desirable behavior. These include the use of instruction, audiovisual aids, and demonstrations. Behaviors can also be encouraged by reinforcing, in sequence, steps that lead to the performance of the desired behavior (Leitenberg, 1972).

After the desired behaviors are generated, a schedule of reinforcement should be established. If the reinforcer is suddenly withdrawn, the client may revert to previous behavior patterns. Continuation of the desired behaviors can be promoted by intermittent reinforcement. The behavior will be likely to continue if reinforcement is received from significant others or from society (Leitenberg, 1972).

Evaluation of behavior therapy provides important guidelines for the continuation of the therapy. Before initiating the therapy, the nurse should determine the client's baseline of behaviors. The number of times the behavior occurred prior to the therapy should be compared with the number of times it occurs during the therapy. Graphs and charts are helpful for recording behaviors and determining if change is occurring. The extent of the recording necessary depends upon the problem and the factors that influence it. Keep in mind that the record of a behavior must be specific. It should indicate actions as the therapy progresses.

Behavior therapy is a controversial form of intervention. Some persons regard it as a form of manipulation in which subjects are punished or bribed. As long as behavior therapy is performed with the consent of the client or an advocate for the client, it is not manipulation. The nurse should establish good rapport with the client, and both client and nurse should be working toward the same goals. If a client does not agree to behavior therapy, the nurse can explain how the treatment contributes to the goals. If client and nurse continue to disagree, the goals should be reviewed and revised as necessary. Behavior therapy is thus similar to other forms of intervention that require the client's cooperation in order to achieve the established goals. Much of human behavior is determined by the gains received, the consequences of the behavior, and by rules and norms of society. Just as wages are the reward for employment, reinforcement is the reward for behavioral change. On the other hand, bribery is a reward for unlawful behavior (Berni and Fordyce, 1973). There are times when negative reinforcement may seem like punishment. However, if the goals set are the client's goals and the behavior becomes more effective, then the client usually receives the benefits associated with achievement of the established goals.

For an example of applied behavior therapy, consider the case of Mrs. D, a 74-year-old nursing home resident. Mrs. D complained to the nurse assigned to her that no one cared about her. She said that her family hardly ever visited and that the other nursing home residents would not talk to her. Further assessment revealed that Mrs. D's two daughters each visited their mother once a month. It was true that the daughters, other residents, and health-care workers avoided talking to Mrs. D because of her constant complaining. Those who tried to converse with her reported that she never had anything positive to say. During a team conference, the nurse assigned to Mrs. D agreed to confront Mrs. D about the problem and try to determine whether she was interested in changing this annoying behavior. When approached, Mrs. D indicated that she was not aware of having complained so much, but after much discussion she seemed to understand the problem and indicated a willingness to change. Mrs. D was pleased at the prospect of increased interactions with others if she would quit complaining. She was reassured that they really cared about her, but was also told that everyone involved would have to follow the agreed plan while she was in the process of changing her behavior.

Mrs. D, her daughters, and the nurses assigned to her agreed on a plan. The daughters and the nurses would spend more time conversing with Mrs. D, but they would leave her for at least 5 minutes every time she started to complain. Each of Mrs. D's daughters agreed to visit her at least twice a week. During the first few days after the plan was initiated the nurses and her daughters told Mrs. D why they were leaving when she began to complain. At first she tried to argue that she was not complaining. Rather than argue, the nurses or her daughters simply told her that they knew that she was trying and that they would be back later. After the explanation, they would then leave.

Gradually, Mrs. D began to talk about varied topics for increasing periods of time. The nurses and the daughters provided positive reinforcement during these periods by telling Mrs. D how much they enjoyed conversing with her. As the behavior therapy continued to succeed, reinforcement became more subtle; only smiles and positive head nods were necessary. As Mrs. D's complaints became more infrequent she learned to change the subject upon the cue of hearing the listener clear her throat. Mrs. D was pleased with the success of the therapy, especially once rapport was reestablished with her daughters and with the other residents of the nursing home. Once again, her daughters found themselves enjoying their visits with their mother, and no longer visited out of a sense of obligation.

Behavior therapy techniques can be very

helpful in assisting clients to improve their relationships with others. Nurses should become more aware of which behaviors they are reinforcing. Without even realizing it, they may be encouraging clients to withdraw and to isolate themselves, rather than to establish positive and meaningful relationships.

Promoting Effective Coping in Relation to Life Changes

Since many of the elderly who require intervention in relation to the various developmental tasks are also experiencing health-related problems, the nurse's role is particularly important. It includes helping the client to recognize and deal effectively with present and potential problems. The client and/or the client's family may find it difficult to recognize that a problem exists or to view the problem objectively. Persons whose stress levels are high, or who are experiencing great feelings of fear, guilt, or love, may develop a skewed view of their situation. All members of the health team should work together to help client and family examine the present problems, as well as to recognize potential future problems. If such problems are anticipated and dealt with, a crisis can often be prevented.

Once problems have been identified, clients should be given ample time to make decisions about how to accept and deal with them. Decisions made during times of great stress are often not the best decisions. The nurse can help the client to accept the problem by providing opportunities for client and family to express their feelings. When the person is ready, members of the health team should work together in helping the client to see the various alternatives and the advantages and disadvantages of each. Once the client and his family have decided how to deal with the problem, the nurse may be able to assist in implementing the plan, while providing emotional support during the process. Depending on the situation and the problem, details of the plan may be implemented by the social worker. At times the nurse's role is to identify the agency or agencies that are best able to meet the person's needs. Nurses should be aware of the services

available in their own communities. City, county, and federal agencies, as well as various religious organizations, should be considered.

The nurse also has an important role in promoting the client's health and safety. Clients confronted with stress may neglect their health and be unaware of hazards present in their environment. The nurse should assess the client's health status and attempt to make the client aware of both potential problems and measures that can be taken to prevent them. Many of the approaches previously discussed with regard to promoting self-esteem are also helpful in promoting effective coping with developmental tasks.

Relocation

The nurse's role may include helping clients and their families to determine whether the client should relocate for reasons of health and safety. This is often a difficult decision for both client and family. A client who wishes to remain in his familiar environment should be encouraged to do so if it is at all possible. The client's physical, psychologic, and sociologic needs and the available support services should be carefully evaluated. Home services from a nurse, a home health aide, a homemaker, a physical therapist, or from Meals-On-Wheels may enable the client to remain in his own home. Too often it is decided to institutionalize a client before other alternatives are considered. No one should be placed in an institution until it is clear that such a move is appropriate.

A study by Morris (1975) found that persons whose move to an institution was considered to be clinically appropriate did not react negatively as they progressed upward on a waiting list. Negative reactions were found among those for whom institutionalization was considered less appropriate.

The needs of the client's family must also be considered. Sometimes families have strong negative reactions to the idea of institutionalization. This may lead the family to move the client into their home before considering fully the implications of such a move. Take, for example, the H family's experience. On the surface, it seemed like a good idea for Mr. H's mother to move into their home. They had always gotten along well with her, although a distance of 300 miles had limited the amount of contact. When the senior Mrs. H moved into their home, all of her furniture was sold and her apartment given up. Since the H's did not have a spare bedroom, it was necessary for their 15-year-old son to give up his bedroom and move in with his younger brother. At first the family reacted positively to the move. It was nice to have Grandma with them, it helped to ease their financial pressures, and it alleviated worries about having her so far away.

After a couple of weeks, problems started to appear. The entire family seemed to suffer from lack of privacy. The boys began to resent having to share a room, and the daughter-in-law felt as though she was no longer in charge of her household. The senior Mrs. H, in turn, was unhappy away from her friends, and felt that she was becoming too dependent on her son's family. She said, "I appreciate my son and his family taking me in, but I feel as though I'm no longer able to lead a life of my own." When the visiting nurse was called to the home because old Mrs. H was having problems related to diabetes, she became aware of these difficulties. The nurse contacted a social worker; together, they evaluated the situation and considered the alternatives. The problem was resolved when Mrs. H. and her son agreed that the best alternative was for her to move to an apartment building for the elderly, which was located nearby.

Whenever possible, the client should make the final decision about relocation. Involuntary relocation affects the person's adjustment, and may also affect her health. A study of 75 institutionalized old people showed that those who were relocated involuntarily expressed greater life dissatisfaction than those who had made their own decision to move into the nursing home. Life dissatisfaction was also correlated with poor health, limited social interactions, and financial dependence (Smith and Brand, 1975).

Clients and their families should be encouraged to visit several facilities when it appears that a move to a nursing home will be necessary. They should be urged to consider the following when trying to select a nursing home:

- Public transportation
- Nearness to significant others
- Ease of entering and leaving the facility
- Décor
- Adequacy of lighting and heating
- Opportunity for social interaction
- Absence of safety hazards
- Opportunities to be out-of-doors
- Planned activities
- Support for individual activities
- Quantity, quality, and type of food
- Nursing personnel
    Adequacy of staffing
    Level of preparation
    Friendliness and use of touch
- Satisfaction of present residents
- Interaction among residents
- Restrictions and regulations
- Opportunities for privacy
- Facilities for personal belongings
- Care provided for personal belongings
- Cleanliness
- Support services available

Both the client and the family need support when the aged person is moving to an institution. Both should be helped to understand the necessity for the move, and should have an opportunity to express their feelings about the change. The client needs to feel that she is still loved, not that she is being abandoned. The family should be given opportunities to express any guilt they may feel, and should be encouraged to interact with the client as much as is feasible in the future. The staff of the nursing home should help the client to feel as though she belongs, introducing her to other residents who can help her to adjust. A special effort should be made to include the new resident in the various activities. She should not be expected to remember many new things all at once, but should be helped by repeated explanations and demonstrations, as well as written information. During the first few days in a new environment, the client's stress levels can be expected to be high, and interfere with her perceptions of the new environment.

Sexuality

Still another important role for the nurse is to promote recognition of the sexual needs of elderly persons, and to encourage them to meet such needs. What does this role involve? First, the nurse should recognize that there are wide variations in sexual needs among individuals. Such needs may be related to appearance, togetherness, touch, or genital contact.

In the future, nurses may play an important part in promoting a sexual "revolution" among the elderly. The goals of this revolution might include the following:

- To recognize that the elderly have sexually related needs
- To be aware of the great variation in sexual needs among elderly individuals
- To promote increased comfort for older persons with regard to their individual sexual needs
- To prevent and alleviate sexually related problems among the elderly

The sexual revolution should begin with sex education classes, not only for the caretakers of the elderly but for old people themselves. First, the elderly need to be instructed about prevention of sexually related problems. Instruction might start with an examination of the genitalia during each annual physical examination. Cancer of the breast, ovaries and uterus most often occur in women between the ages of 55 to 74. Cancer of the prostate occurs most often in men 75 and over (Vital Statistics, 1977). The older person needs to be informed of the increased risks occurring with age when being urged to have annual examinations and to perform regular self-examination. Women who experience any of the following should know that they have an increased risk for cancer of the breast:

- History of breast cancer
- History of certain other cancer such as uterine cancer
- A family history of breast cancer
- The absence of a full-term pregnancy before the age of 35
- Menarche at an early age
- Exposure to ionizing radiation (Seracci, 1980)

In addition to having an annual rectal exam to detect prostate problems, older men should be advised to see a urologist if any urinary problems such as urgency or a slow stream is experienced. These signs may be indicative of enlargement of the prostate since the urethra of the male passes through the prostate. Older men are prone to prostate enlargement.

The elderly should be informed about the normal physiologic changes that accompany aging and how these changes may affect their sexuality. It should be stressed that even though these changes occur, old persons are still sexual beings, with normal sexual needs that are a direct outgrowth of the sexual needs and feelings of their younger years.

Classes in sex education should help the elderly to feel comfortable about expressing their sexual needs and seeking help when problems are encountered. Women should be taught to seek medical help if vaginal bleeding or vaginal drainage occurs. Vaginal bleeding may indicate a malignancy. Vaginal drainage often indicates infection. The increased vaginal pH levels that occur with aging appear to predispose toward vaginal infections (Schiff and Wilson, 1978).

Older women experiencing dyspareunia, which was discussed in Chapter 7, may be too embarrassed by this condition to seek medical attention. A water-soluble lubricant is usually more helpful than a petroleum lubricant. If this does not alleviate the problem, the client should be urged to seek medical advice regarding the use of an estrogen cream (Schiff and Wilson, 1978). Although such creams are highly effective, use of them is controversial because of possible side effects. In addition to relieving the problems associated with atrophy of vaginal tissue, estrogen replacement therapy has been useful in controlling the "hot flashes" associated with menopause, in retarding or arresting osteoporosis, and may protect women against atherosclerotic heart disease and heart attacks (News Update, 1983). Women using estrogens for more than a year in the postmenopausal period have an increased risk of endometrial cancer. The risk is believed to decrease after estrogen use has been discontinued. Those who have had a total hysterectomy are not at risk for developing endometrial cancer. Other possible dangers of estrogen therapy include the development of gallbladder disease and cancers of the breast, vagina, or liver. Estrogens should be used with great caution and only if severe symptoms of menopause are present in persons who have had a myocardial infarction, angina pectoris, or a cerebral vascular accident (Ayerst, 1979). "Estrogens should be used only for responsive indications in the smallest effective dose, and for the shortest period that satisfies therapeutic need" (News Update, 1983, p. 303). Women using estrogen ointment and creams to vaginal tissues should be examined every 6 to 12 months.

Sex education classes should also include information on surgical procedures and medical conditions that can affect sexual functioning. Persons who are taking medications should learn if and how the medications may affect their sexuality. Examples of such medications include the ganglionic blocking agents and the Rauwolfia compounds (Vemireddi, 1978). Even modest amounts of alcohol may interfere with sexual functioning. Men are more vulnerable to the effects of drugs, because drugs, including alcohol, may interfere with their ability to have or to maintain an erection.

Other factors that interfere with the ability to have an erection include antihypertensive medications, stress, fear, diabetes, or surgery of the urogenital system. Sex education classes should include a discussion of possible alternatives to the elderly person's accustomed ways of meeting sexual needs. A presentation of the pros and cons of alternative methods may help individuals to better accept certain practices. For example, although masturbation is not acceptable to most old persons (Wasow and Loeb, 1974), it may be accepted more readily by those who have been told about the relationship between regular sexual stimulation and effective functioning of the sexual organs. As noted in Chapter 7, Masters and Johnson (1966) have indicated that consistency of active sexual expression is the most important factor in maintaining effective sexuality in the elderly of both sexes. In addition to preserving

potency in men and maintaining the Bartholin's gland function in women, masturbation helps to release tension, stimulates the sexual appetite and, as a result, contributes to the person's general well-being (Weg, 1975).

Fear of failure, which can cause impotence in the male, frequently can be attributed to lack of knowledge about the normal parameters of sexual function for older men (Sander, 1976). The elderly man who has difficulty in performing might do better if sexual activity takes place early in the day, when hormonal and energy levels tend to be higher (Weg, 1975). Increasing both knowledge and self-esteem in the older man may alleviate impotency. When these measures are not effective, the client should be referred to a physician, ideally to a urologist.

Persons with coronary artery disease may fear loss of ability to have sexual intercourse. Rossman (1978) indicates except for those "who are left with severe myocardial insufficiency or congestive failure," patients are encouraged to resume as nearly a normal life as is possible. According to Rossman, following recovery from a myocardial infarction, anyone able to climb two flights of stairs without symptomatology is usually able to resume sexual activity.

Members of the health team should become more cognizant of the importance of sexual needs among the elderly and should take more initiative in helping elderly clients to meet these needs. The nurse can often assist by encouraging the individual to take greater pride in his appearance. When clients appear attractive their appearance should be praised, as this helps to increase self-esteem. A study by Kaas (1978) supports the importance of encouraging the aged to remain attractive. The study also showed that there is a difference between the attitudes of the staff and the attitudes of residents of nursing homes with regard to sexual expression in the elderly. Although residents considered that their major mode of sexual expression was the attempt to remain physically attractive, the majority of them also indicated that they no longer felt sexually attractive.

When considering sexual needs, it is important to remember that many older persons need and respond positively to touch and to closeness. Health-care workers have found that touch is often helpful in establishing rapport with an elderly client (Pfeiffer, 1977). Older persons can often be seen to reach out and touch others, especially children. This is not meant to imply that all aged persons like to be touched; in fact, some of them decidedly do not. Even individuals who do like this expression of closeness vary as to when they wish to be touched and by whom they wish to be touched. When group sessions are conducted strategies that provide for opportunities for touching should be included.

Institutions for the elderly should make efforts to provide for the sexual needs of their residents. Residents of institutions should be provided with areas in which they can have privacy. Personnel should recognize the right to privacy by respecting closed doors and by providing "Do not disturb" signs. Clients should be encouraged to interact with members of the opposite sex, through such activities as dancing. Finally, segregation of the sexes in institutions for the elderly should be halted.

In the past, society has encouraged older persons to repress their sexual needs and feelings (Sander, 1976). It is to be hoped that in the future a better-educated society will understand the sexual needs of the elderly and will take measures to meet those needs.

Preparation for Health Emergencies

Older persons, especially those living alone, should be urged to have a plan for communicating important information regarding their health status in case an emergency occurs. A popular means for communicating information is the Vial of Life. This program was initiated in Detroit by the Wayne County Public Health Service. Many drugstores across the country sell the Vial of Life. The vial is a plastic container that comes with a health information data sheet and Vial of Life labels. When completed, the data sheet should be placed in the vial, which is then stored on the upper shelf of the refrigerator on the side where the door opens. Red and white Vial of Life stickers, which indicate that important medical information is stored in the refrigerator, are to be placed at

eye level on the outside of the refrigerator and on the doors to the home. (Refer to Figure 8.7)

Many older persons living alone fear that they will have a health emergency and will not be able to obtain help. These fears may be intensified at night. Such apprehensions can be decreased when arrangements have been made for a friend or family member to phone the older person the first thing every morning. Aged persons should be urged to have emergency phone numbers clearly visible by each of their telephones.

Death

Nursing intervention related to death may involve any or all of three areas. These include planning for death, intervention for the dying person, and intervention with regard to the death of significant others.

Planning for death is often difficult, both for the person who is doing the planning and for the significant others. It requires everyone involved to recognize the inevitable—that life is not infinite. Planning for death should take place while the person is still healthy. If planning is delayed until illness strikes, the individual may have neither the energy nor clarity of mind to devise the plans or to complete them. There is also the risk that death may occur suddenly, before planning has even been considered. Persons who have made careful plans in advance may be comforted by the knowledge that their significant others know how to proceed in the event of their death, and that they have made provisions for the disposal of their estate.

Preparation for death should include details about funeral arrangements, including burial or cremation. The person should have an up-to-date will that has been drawn up by a competent lawyer. Wills should be reviewed periodically, and revised if changes occur in the family structure. Changes may also be necessary if persons move to another state, if they are unable to locate the witnesses to the will, or if laws change. If there is no will, the person's estate may not be distributed according to his wishes, and estate taxes and legal fees are likely to be higher (Otten and Shelley, 1976). With the aid of a lawyer, most persons can

To My Family, My Physician, My Lawyer, and All Others Whom It May Concern

Death is as much a reality as birth, growth, maturity, and old age—it is the one certainty of life. If the time comes when I can no longer take part in decisions for my own future, let this statement stand as an expression of my wishes and directions, while I am still of sound mind.

If at such a time the situation should arise in which there is no reasonable expectation of my recovery from extreme physical or mental disability, I direct that I be allowed to die and not be kept alive by medications, artifical means or "heroic measures." I do, however, ask that medication be mercifully administered to me to alleviate suffering even though this may shorten my remaining life.

This statement is made after careful consideration and is in accordance with my strong convictions and beliefs. I want the wishes and directions here expressed carried out to the extent permitted by law. Insofar as they are not legally enforceable, I hope that those to whom this Will is addressed will regard themselves as morally bound by these provisions.

Signed _____

Date _____
Witness_____
Witness_____
Copies of this request have been given to _____

_____

_____

_____

Figure 8.6. The Living Will. *(Reprinted with permission of Concern for Dying, 250 West 57th St., New York, New York 10107.)*

ensure that their estates are distributed exactly as they had intended. This can be done by setting up trust funds or by giving monetary gifts annually, up to the amount which is permitted tax-free.

Nurses may or may not play a role in helping a client plan for death. When the person wishes to discuss such plans, the nurse should be willing to listen, and may be able to help identify areas which present potential problems. Nurses may be able to help the client to realize the importance of consulting a lawyer in making plans or updating them. The nurse may also assist the client in discussing plans with the family, especially if the family is reluctant to approach the subject of death. At least one family member should know the location of the will, bank books, valuable articles, and important documents such as insurance policies. The family should also know how to contact the person's attorney or community legal services. It is best if special instructions and important information is written.

Intervention for the dying person varies according to individual need. As indicated in Chapter 4 most old persons do not fear death itself, but instead fear the process of dying or loss of control. The nurse can help by giving the client as much control as possible over his life and circumstances. Some persons may be interested in signing a "Living Will" (Fig. 8.6.) Although most states do not consider the "Living Will" legally binding, those who complete it may be comforted by the knowledge that they have made their wishes known, and can hope that their family and the medical team will respect their wishes. In 1977, California passed the Natural Death Act, enabling adults to make legal decisions about their medical care. Adult California residents can now direct physicians not to use "artificial extraordinary life-sustaining supports under certain terminal conditions" (Gonda, 1977).

Many nurses need to become more aware of their own feelings about death. Some find it very difficult to respect the client's wish to die

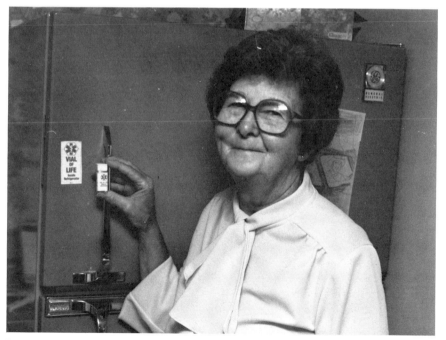

Figure 8.7. The Vial of Life communicates important information in the case of a medical emergency. *(Photograph by Ed Spier, Murrysville, PA.)*

with dignity. For example, instead of following the dying person's request to be permitted to die, the nurse may feel it necessary to institute cardiopulmonary resuscitation measures. This action raises two questions. First, is the nurse meeting her own needs or the client's needs? Second, is the nurse preserving life or is she merely postponing death?

The nurse has an important role in communicating with the dying person. Many people fear that they will be left alone when they are dying. Nurses must be knowledgeable about the normal behaviors associated with various stages of the grieving process. If people in the client's environment do not anticipate normal reactions such as denial and anger, they may feel threatened by such behavior and withdraw from the client, rather than showing acceptance and understanding.

It is important to understand that when death is approaching, both the client and his or her significant others proceed through the stages detailed by Kübler-Ross, discussed in Chapter 7. However, these stages do not necessarily coincide and, as noted earlier, persons normally move back and forth through the stages. In such cases, the nurse can act as a catalyst between client and family. For example, if the client has reached the stage of depression while family members are still alternating between denial and anger, conflicts are almost inevitable. The nurse, however, can view such a situation objectively and can assist all the persons involved in expressing their feelings. An alternate problem might arise if the significant others, long aware of the client's terminal illness, arrive at the stage of depression or acceptance while the client is at the stage of denial or anger. In either of the cases described, there is bound to be lack of understanding on all sides. The nurse's role is that of listener and counselor, and the goal to be achieved is emotional support for both client and family.

Whenever possible, the nurse should help the dying client to fulfill any last important wishes. As the person reaches the stage of acceptance, sincerity becomes particularly important. During this stage, the client may wish to have contact only with those who are very close to him. The nurse can help to limit visitors to those few very special people and can explain to them how important their presence is to the dying person. At this time, the closeness of the client's significant others is far more important than words (Kübler-Ross, 1971).

Nursing intervention for significant others of the dying person is particularly important when the grieving person is alone. According to Megerle (1983) courage may be what is holding the grieving person together. Nurses are advised to be hopeful, but not overly sympathetic. When the dying process occurs over an extended period of time, family members may need to be reminded to provide for their own health. The grieving person is more likely to leave for meals, sleep, bathing, or hair care when the nurse assures the person that she will look in on the client often.

Family members may not recognize the signs when death is imminent. After the person is told what is happening the role of the nurse includes determining if the person wishes to have a clergyman, a friend, or another family member contacted ((Megerle, 1983).

EVALUATION OF INTERVENTION

Evaluation of intervention is highly individualized, according to the developmental problems experienced by a particular client and the goals established in relation to these problems. The evaluation should follow the criteria that were identified when the goals were established. Following is a list of general guidelines to consider when determining the effectiveness of nursing intervention.

Determine verbal and nonverbal cues which indicate change in the person's self-perceptions with regard to

Self-satisfaction	Role
Control	Environment
Hope	Finances
Self-worth	Health
Feelings of	Appearance
belonging	

Determine changes in the adequacy of housing with regard to

- Health
- Safety
- Security
- Interaction with others
- Mobility within the housing
- Mobility outside of the housing
- Maintenance

Determine changes in affiliations with regard to the satisfaction received, the amount of contact, the type of contact, and whether an active or a passive role is assumed. Consider the above in relationships with

Spouse	Members of the
Children	health team
Friends	Others
Neighbors	

Determine changes in activities with regard to

- Size of life space
- Degree of independence
- Patterns
- Group activities
- Participation in hobbies and other activities

General considerations. Determine changes with regard to

- Expression of emotions
- Evidence of happiness
- Degree of cooperation
- Trust
- Coping mechanisms
- Appearance

Determine effectiveness of specific supportive services

- Evaluate approaches as they pertain to significant others.
- Determine evidence of change in significant others as it pertains to:

Feelings about the client
Feelings about the relationship with the client
Expression of guilt
Amount, type, and quality of contact with the client
Satisfaction received from contact with client

CONCLUSION

In order to intervene with regard to a client's developmental problems the nurse must assess the interrelationship between the various life changes, the person's coping mechanisms and their effectiveness, and the person's support systems. Although most persons are able to resolve their development problems, nurses often become involved when a health-related problem presents an additional stress. In addition to helping the client with specific developmental problems, the nurse must also help the person to prevent problems. Persons who have a high level of self-esteem and who have optimal affiliations with others are more likely to be able to resolve problems related to life changes.

Nurses should keep in mind that other members of the health team can also help the client. The various members of the health team should work together to resolve the problems and to help the client utilize the community resources that are available.

RECOMMENDED READINGS

Agras, W.S. Behavior Modification: Principles and Clinical Applications. Boston, Little, Brown, 1972. *A detailed explanation of the principles of behavior therapy, with examples of their application. This book is helpful for those who wish to develop skill in the use of behavior therapy techniques.*

Berni, R., Fordyce, W.E. Behavior Modification and the Nursing Process. St. Louis, Mosby, 1977. *Gives specific examples of the use of behavior modification in nursing.*

Neugarten B.L., Havighurst R.J., Tobin S.S. The measure of life satisfaction. Journal of Gerontology 16(1):134, 1961. *Presents the Life Satisfaction*

Indexes A and Z and discusses their validity and reliability. The Life Satisfaction Indexes are short, easy to administer instruments which were devised to measure successful aging.
Otten J., Shelley F.D. When Your Parents Grow Old. New York, Funk and Wagnalls, 1976. *Although written for those who have older parents, this book contains many practical suggestions which the older person might find useful. Discusses all of the developmental issues of aging.*
Stotland E. The Psychology of Hope. San Francisco, Jossey-Bass, 1969. *Emphasizes the importance of hope and how to maintain hope. Excellent guidelines for establishing goals.*

REFERENCES CITED

Abrahams, R.B., Patterson R.D. Psychological distress among the community elderly: Prevalence, characteristics and implications for service. International Journal of Aging and Human Development 9(1):1, 1978–1979
Agras, W.S. Behavior Modification: Principles and Clinical Applications. Boston, Little, Brown, 1972
Aloia, A.J. Relationships between perceived privacy options, self-esteem and internal control among aged people. Dissertation Abstracts International 34(10-B):5180, April, 1974
Austin, J.M., Cain, M.G., Hicks, J., Wolf, F.S. The Gravlee Method an alternative to the Pap smear? American Journal of Nursing: 1057, 83(7) 1983
Ayerst, information for the patient. Ayerst Laboratories, Inc. New York: 315, September, 1979
Bankoff, E.A. Aged parents and their widowed daughters: A support relationship. Journal of Gerontology 38(2):226, 1983
Bengtson, V.L. Self-determination: A social-psychologic perspective on helping the aged. Geriatrics 28(12):118, 1973
Berni, R., Fordyce, W.E. Behavior Modification and the Nursing Process. St. Louis, Mosby, 1973
Black, Sr, K. Social isolation and the nursing process. Nursing Clinics of North America 8(4):575, 1973
Butler, R.N., Lewis, M.I. Aging and Mental Health; Positive Psychosocial and Biomedical Approaches. St. Louis, Mosby, 1982
Calhoun, G., Morse, W.C. Self-concept and self-esteem: Another perspective. Psychology in the Schools 14(3):318, 1977
Calhoun, G., Warren, P., Kurfiss, J. A comparison of the self-concept and self-esteem of black and white boy scouts. Clearing House 50:131, 1976

Cancer of the breast. Ca—A Cancer Journal of Clinicians 30(4):224, 1980
Carter, C., Galliano, D. Fear of loss and attachment a major dynamic in the social isolation of the institutionalized aged. Journal of Gerontological Nursing 7(6):342, 1981
Cicirelli, V.G. Helping Elderly Parents: The Role of Adult Children. Boston, Auburn House, 1981
David, L. The many faces of guilt. Family Health/Today's Health 9(7):22, 1977
Devine, B.A. Attitudes of the elderly toward religion. Journal of Gerontological Nursing 6(11):679, 1980
Dudley, C.J., Hillery, G.A. Freedom and alienation in homes for the aged. The Gerontologist 17(2):140, 1977
Elder, G.H. Adolescent socialization and development, in Bogatta, E.F., Lambert, W.W. (eds), Handbook of Personality Theory and Research. Chicago, Rand McNally, 1968
Fulmer, T.T. Elder abuse in the family: The hidden victim. Aging and Leisure Living 3(5):9, 1980
Gambrill, E.D. Behavior Modification: Handbook of Assessment, Intervention, and Evaluation. San Francisco, Jossey-Bass, 1977
Gonda, T.A. Coping with dying and death. Geriatrics 32(9):71, 1977
Greene, V.L., Monahan, D.J. The impact of visitation on patient well-being in nursing homes. The Gerontologist 22(3):418, 1982
Guinan, P., Gilham, N., Nagubadi, S.R., Bush, I., Rhee, H., McKiel, C. What is the best test to detect prostate cancer? Ca—A Cancer Journal of Clinicians 31(3):141, 1981
Gusberg, S.B. An approach to the control of carcinoma of the endometrium. Ca—A Cancer Journal of Clinicians 30(1):16, 1980
Hartford, M.E., Parsons, R. Groups with relatives of dependent older adults. The Gerontologist 22(3):394, 1982
Hirsch, C.S. Integrating the nursing home resident into a senior citizens' center. The Gerontologist 17(3):227, 1977
Hooyman, N.R. A Model for the Prevention, Detection, and Treatment of Elderly Abuse and Neglect. Paper presented at the meeting of the Gerontological Society, Toronto, November, 1981
Kaas, M.J. Sexual expression of the elderly in nursing homes. The Gerontologist 18(4):372, 1978
Kahana, E. The humane treatment of old people in institutions. The Gerontologist 13(3):282, 1973
Kübler-Ross, E. What is it like to be dying? American Journal of Nursing 71(1):54, 1971
Larson, R. Thirty years of research on the subjective well-being of older Americans. Journal of Gerontology 33(1):109, 1978

Lee, R. Self images of the elderly. Nursing Clinics of North America 11(1):119, 1976

Lee, G.R., Ellithorpe, E. Intergenerational exchange and subjective well-being among the elderly. Journal of Marriage and the Family 44(1):217, 1982

Leitenberg, H. Positive reinforcement and extinction procedures, in Agras, W.S. (ed), Behavior Modification: Principles and Clinical Applications. Boston, Little, Brown, 1972, pp 27–37

Lemon, B.W., Bengtson, V.L., Patterson, J.A. An exploration of the activity theory of aging: Activity types and life satisfaction among inmovers to a retirement community, in Bell, D.B., Erdman, P. (eds), Contemporary Social Gerontology: Significant Developments in the Field of Aging. Springfield, IL, C.C. Thomas; 1976, pp 51–62

Levinson, B.M. Pets and old age. Mental Hygiene 58(3):364, 1969

Megerle, J.A.S. Surviving. American Journal of Nursing 83(6):892, 1983

Morris, J.N. Changes in morale experienced by elderly institutional applicants along the institutional path. The Gerontologist 15(4):345, 1975

Mulligan, Sr, M.A., Bennett, R. Assessment of mental health and social problems during multiple friendly visits: Development and evaluation of a friendly visiting program for the isolated elderly. International Journal of Aging and Human Development 8(1):43, 1977–78

Mutran, E., Reitzes, D.C. Retirement, identity and well-being: Realignment of role relationships. Journal of Gerontology 36(6):733, 1981

Neugarten, B.L., Havighurst, R.J., Tobin, S.S. The measure of life satisfaction. Journal of Gerontology 16(1):134, 1961

News Update. Estrogen replacement carries cautions. Journal of Gerontological Nursing 9(5):303, 1983

Otten, J., Shelley, F.D. When Your Parents Grow Old. New York, Funk and Wagnalls, 1976

Payne, B.P. The older volunteer: Social role continuity and development. The Gerontologist 17(4):355, 1977

Pfeiffer, E. Psychopathology and social pathology, in Birren, J., Schaie, K.W. (eds), Handbook of the Psychology of Aging. New York, Van Nostrand Reinhold, 1977, pp 650–671

Phillips, L.R. Elder abuse—What is it? Who says so? Geriatric Nursing 4(3):167, 1983

Phillips, L.R. The Relationship of Social Supports and Physical Status to Maltreatment of Frail Elderly Adults. Paper presented at the Nursing Research Conference at the University of Arizona, Tucson, September, 1980

Reid, D.W., Haas, G., Harkings, D. Locus of desired control and positive self-concept of the elderly. Journal of Gerontology 32(4):441, 1977

Reid, D.W., Ziegler, M. Validity and stability of a new desired control measure pertaining to psychological adjustment of the elderly. Journal of Gerontology 35(3):395, 1980

Rossman, I. Sexuality and aging: An internists's perspective, in Solnick, R.L. (ed), Sexuality and Aging. The University of Southern California, The Ethel Percy Andrus Gerontology Center, 1978

Sander, F. Aspects of sexual counseling with the aged. Social Casework 504, October, 1976

Schiff, I., Wilson, E. Clinical aspects of aging of the female reproductive system, in Schneider, E.L. (ed), Aging: The Aging Reproductive System. New York, Raven, 1978, pp 8–28

Schwartz, A.N. An observation on self-esteem as the linchpin of quality of life for the aged. An essay. The Gerontologist 15(5):470, 1975

Seracci, R., Repetto, F. Epidemiology of breast cancer. Seminars in Oncology 5:342, 1980

Smith, R.T., Brand, F.N. Effects of enforced relocation on life adjustment in a nursing home. International Journal of Aging and Human Development 6(3):249, 1975

Staser, C.W., Staser, H.T. Organized religion: Communication considerations, in Oyer, H.J., Oyer, J. (eds), Aging and Communication. Baltimore, University Park Press, 1976, pp 225–237

Stotland, E. The Psychology of Hope. San Francisco, Jossey-Bass, 1969

Tate, J.W. The need for personal space in institutions for the elderly. Journal of Gerontological Nursing. 6(8):439, 1980

Vemireddi, N.K. Sexual counseling for chronically disabled patients. Geriatrics 33(7):65, 1978

Vial of Life instruction sheet. Health Enterprises, Inc., North Attleboro, MA

Vital Statistics of the United States 1977

Wasow, M., Loeb, M.B. Sexuality in nursing homes. Journal of the American Geriatric Society 27(2):73, 1979

Weg, R. Sexual inadequacy in the elderly, in Goldman, R., Rockstein, M. (eds), The Physiology and Pathology of Human Aging. New York, Academic, 1975, pp 203–227

Wingate, M.B. Geriatric gynecology. Primary Care 9(1):53, 1982

9

The Nursing Process as Applied to the Cognitive Aspects of Aging

Barbara Elliott Spier

Reading this chapter will enable the individual to:

1. Identify changes in the cognitive functioning of the aged person
2. Assess the cognitive status of the aged person
3. Promote memory development
4. Promote sensory stimulation
5. Prevent sensory overload
6. Reduce depression

Before the nursing process can be applied to the cognitive aspects of the older person, the nurse must understand the various cognitive changes that accompany the aging process. *Cognitive* changes are those that affect thinking ability or mental processes. Too often the elderly are viewed as senile "old folks" who spend most of their time in rocking chairs. Although this is true of some old people, it is not an accurate assessment of the majority, nor does it take into consideration the changes that result from the normal effects of aging on the cognitive processes.

COGNITION AND THE AGING PROCESS

A decline in cognitive functioning may not be seen before a person reaches 50 or 60, and, even then, decline may be minimal. For activities in which speed of response is required, decline may be apparent earlier in life (Botwinick, 1977). Few generalizations can be made about the cognitive changes that occur with aging. For the most part, the changes are highly individualized. The two disturbances in cognitive functioning that nurses are most likely to encounter are brain failure and depression.

Structural Changes

Certain structural changes take place in the cerebrum as a person ages. Cerebral atrophy occurs, with a decrease in cerebral weight and a decrease in the number of functioning neurons. From the 20s to the 80s, brain weight decreases about 200 grams from an average adult weight of 1300 grams (Knox, 1977).

Aged persons who were living independently and able to cope with their environment until death have been found to have minimal cerebral atrophy if male and almost non-existent atrophy if female. Certain conditions, such as those which cause trauma, change the cerebral metabolic rate, or interfere with the circulation to the cerebrum, are believed to decrease the number of neurons over time. As the neurons die they are replaced by neuroglia, which is the supporting structure of nervous tissue. Instead of a generalized loss of neurons, there appears to be a decrease in selected regional associated neurons and a neuroglial increase. Loss of neurons is not a reliable index of aging. In certain areas of the cerebrum, accumulations of lipofuscin, a fatty pigment, have been found to be an indicator of chronologic age (Bondareff, 1977).

Cerebral changes become more pronounced during the seventh and eighth decade of life. Brains of persons in their seventh decade show an increase in the amount of senile plaque and in neurofibrillary tangles (Bondareff, 1977). Throughout life, changes occur in the gray and the white matter. Usually, both increase in amount until the mid-70s, after which both tend to decrease (Knox, 1977).

A considerable number of senile plaques and neurons with neurofibrillary changes and granulovascular degeneration have been found in persons with severe brain failure when compared with aged persons with unimpaired cognitive functioning. Adams (1980) concluded that in persons with severe brain failure "either vascular lesions or plaque-fibrillary abnormality or both are usually present and severe" (p. 158).

The cerebral changes that accompany aging are not well understood. More research must be undertaken to determine the relationship between structural and functional changes. Little is known thus far about the effects of physiologic changes in the cerebrum on the behavior of the older person.

Intelligence

Certain variables within the older population lead to difficulty in determining changes in intelligence related to aging. These include health problems, differences in education, and slowness of response. Eisdorfer has reported that a great deal of evidence supports the belief that the quality of intellectual functioning is affected by the presence of disease, by predisease conditions, and by stress that the individual is experiencing. These conditions are believed to affect cognitive functioning independent of aging (Eisdorfer, 1977).

Older persons tend to become fatigued more easily than younger persons. Thus they may not perform as well on tests that are administered over an extended period of time. Another consideration is that both the type and the amount of education provided to young people today are very different from the education experienced by most of the elderly population. It is thus difficult to compare groups of young persons with groups of aged persons because the educational preparation of the groups is not the same. Whether or not the individual has had recent educational experience is another factor to consider.

If these factors are not allowed for when assessing the intelligence of older persons, the determinations will not be valid. Although many studies have attempted to determine what changes occur in intelligence as individuals age, many of these studies were culturally biased and so did not provide accurate results.

Changes in intellectual capacity connected with aging are related more to changes in specific functions rather than to alterations in intelligence itself. In particular, these changes usually involve memory, speed of response, and perceptual integrative functions. Studies of persons ranging in age from 60 to 75 indicate, however, that there may be a general decline in intelligence very late in life (Botwinick, 1977).

Although an individual's creative potential is believed to peak between the ages of 35 and 40, this varies according to the person's profession. In some professions the peak occurs only after a considerable amount of experience (Riegel, 1977). Knowlege and skills continue to improve until the person has applied his basic knowledge under a variety of conditions and has gained new knowledge and skill in the process. Motivation and creativity, however, are greater during the period when the individual is learning. Motivation tends to decrease in those who believe they fully understand a subject.

The elderly are often more hesitant to take risks than are younger persons. This cautiousness interferes with measurement of the older person's intelligence. Many old people tend not to answer questions when they fear that they may be wrong. More research should be done to determine whether fear of failure replaces the elderly person's need to achieve (Marsh and Thompson, 1977).

Reaction Time

It is well known that the amount of time required for response to stimuli increases with age. This is not to say that the young respond faster than the elderly. Speed of response is highly individualized, and some older people are faster than many young people. Performance of psychomotor tasks undergoes a greater decrease than the performance of verbal functions.

Beginning at age 46 to 50 and continuing until approximately 66 to 70, there is a decline in speed of performance (Botwinick, 1977). This is believed to be largely due to changes in the central nervous system. Because response speed continues to be slower even when the intensity of sensory stimulation is increased, this problem is probably not related to changes in sensory functions. Peripheral neuromuscular mechanisms are also not likely to be involved, since impulse conduction by the peripheral nerves is too rapid to explain the increase in time of response (Botwinick, 1973).

Aged persons take longer to make decisions. As the complexity of the decision increases, the amount of time required for response increases disproportionately to the time required for response to a simple choice (Birren and Renner, 1977). An older person will take much longer to perform a task if the instructions contain unnecessary detail and explanation. The amount of time required to respond also increases when the response involves multiple choices (Botwinick, 1973). The nurse who keeps these points in mind when assessing and instructing the elderly will be more efficient and more effective in her interactions with the aged.

Reaction time can be decreased through increased motivation, practice, or experience. Studies have shown that older subjects take less time to respond when they are motivated to do so in order to avoid electrical shocks (Botwinick, 1973). According to other researchers, practice also increases the speed of response for a particular activity, and sometimes for other

activities as well (Hoyer, Labouvie, and Baltes, 1973).

Learning

It is unclear whether the older person's capacity to learn declines, as was once believed. Botwinick stresses the importance of distinguishing between learning and performance. Learning occurs internally and cannot be seen, but it can be measured by observable changes in performance. There is general agreement that performance ability does diminish with age (Botwinick, 1973).

Older persons not only take longer to respond, they also take longer to assimilate new information. This may be partially due to the tendency of the elderly to pay attention to irrelevant stimuli. Younger learners, on the other hand, can more readily select the points significant to comprehension when multiple distractors are present. Older learners tend to be easily distracted by extraneous factors (Kausler and Kleim, 1978).

Motivation is important in learning. If tasks are not meaningful to the elderly, they will not be likely to learn them. In order for learning to occur, the individual must believe that there is something worthwhile to be learned (Frey, 1977). Much of the research into learning ability in the older person has involved the learning of meaningless information. Lack of motivation to learn such material might, therefore, have been interpreted as inability to learn. Older persons may also be reluctant to learn because new information may pose a threat to firmly held beliefs and habits. In some instances, motivation to learn is decreased by fear of inability to learn. Older persons find it more difficult to organize information than younger persons and experience disproportionate difficulties when information must be recalled and reorganized. They also have problems with interference if items have not been fully registered in their short-term memory (Craik, 1977).

Memory

Memory involves the three processes of acquiring, storing, and recalling information. For information to be acquired it must be registered in the person's mind. The information may then be stored for seconds, minutes, or years. Recall is the retrieval of stored information. As discussed above, older people have difficulty in acquiring new information, and they are more easily affected by interference than are younger persons. When the delay in recall is increased, the older person becomes increasingly vulnerable to interference (Botwinick, 1973).

Young people are often amazed at the older person's ability to remember details of events that happened decades ago, while having forgotten something that happened very recently. Recall of memories from the past is not impaired, whereas memory of recent events often is. Botwinick suggests that this may be attributed to the greater importance of the past events and to the fact that the old person frequently rehearses them mentally (Botwinick, 1973).

Problem-Solving

Elderly persons are less effective at problem-solving than are younger adults. This can be attributed both to the differences in educational experience and to the many changes in the cognitive processes of the elderly. Problem-solving abilities are taught and emphasized in current educational practice. However, this is a very recent development. Most of today's old people received no formal preparation with regard to problem-solving. The age-related changes such as those involving memory, acquisition of information, and attention to irrelevant stimuli all contribute to the problem-solving difficulties the elderly often encounter.

Part of this diminished effectiveness in solving problems is attributable to the fact that aged persons tend to think in concrete terms more frequently than do younger people. As the educational background of the older person increases, however, so does the preference for abstract thought (Botwinick, 1973).

For the elderly, identifying relevant data is one of the greatest difficulties encountered during problem-solving. Older people tend to gather data that are irrelevant and repetitious. They often find it hard to distinguish between essential data and data that are unrelated to the problem. At times, they dwell on concepts

and strategies that were effective in the past, but have no bearing on the present task (Knox, 1977). Part of the problem in gathering data may be due to difficulties in setting appropriate goals (Botwinick, 1973). Sources conflict on the question of whether or not rigidity interferes with the problem-solving abilities of the elderly. Often older persons ask redundant questions when obtaining information. They seem to have difficulty in utilizing an organized approach for gathering data and in organizing the data obtained.

The elderly find it more difficult to solve novel problems than those that are related to their past experiences. On the other hand, they are often more effective than younger people when a problem can be solved by a solution that has been effective in the past (Knox, 1977). Old people tend to be less creative than young people, so they have more difficulty in formulating solutions to problems not previously experienced. Creativity, however, varies with the individual, and many creative contributions have been made by elderly persons (Botwinick, 1977).

Although much research has been done into the cognitive changes that accompany the aging process, relatively little is known about them. Table 9.1 provides a summary of the changes that are currently believed to occur. As newer research techniques are utilized and age-related biases are eliminated, more will be understood about the changes that take place in the cognitive processes of aging persons.

DISTURBANCES IN COGNITIVE FUNCTIONING

The two most common disturbances of cognitive functioning that nurses are likely to encounter in the elderly are brain failure and depression. Although research into these two subjects has been extensive, understanding of their causes and of the related pathophysiology is minimal. Of course, the nurse's primary concern is not with the pathophysiologic basis of these problems but with identifying their effects on various individuals and with intervening to improve the quality of life for the

TABLE 9.1 CHANGES IN THE COGNITIVE STATUS OF THE AGED

Structural changes	Decreased cerebral weight
	Decreased number of neurons
Reaction time	Increased reaction time
	Decreased speed of performance
Intelligence	Little general decline until very late in life
Learning	Fatigues more readily
	Diminished performance abilities
	Increased response time
	More readily distracted by irrelevant stimuli
	Increased difficulty in organization of information
Memory	Vivid recall of some long-past events
	Impaired recall of recent events
	Increasingly vulnerable to interference with delays in recall
Problem-solving	More concrete thinking
	Redundancy in gathering data
	Difficulty in distinguishing between relevant and irrelevant data
	Decreased creativity
	Increased difficulty in solving new problems

affected client. Nevertheless, some background knowledge of these two problems is of value.

Brain Failure

There has been much confusion related to classification and naming of conditions that are related to brain disorders. Any person having problems related to orientation or other aspects of cognitive functioning may be said to be experiencing brain failure. This term incorporates conditions that may be acute or chronic, reversible or irreversible. Utilization of the term "brain failure" or "cognitive impairment" falls within nursing diagnosis and should relieve the nurse of problems caused by the misuse of terms such as dementia, senile dementia, acute brain syndrome, and chronic brain syndrome. The medical profession has not been consistent in use of these terms and presently tends to lump them together as "organic brain syndrome." Persons have been and continue to be diagnosed as having chronic brain failure or senile dementia, both of which refer to irreversible brain damage, and months or years later it has been discovered that this was not their problem. In such instances, once the correct diagnosis is made and treatment begun, the person may be found to have a reversible condition. Fox et al. (1975) reported a study in which 5 out of 40 persons diagnosed as having senile dementia were found to have potentially treatable conditions.

Wolanin (1981) indicates that confusion may be caused by systemic problems related to brain cell metabolism, mechanical problems that obstruct the flow in the vascular system, or presenile irreversible dementias. Systemic problems that may cause brain failure include hypoxia, hypoglycemia, hyperglycemia, dehydration, electrolyte imbalance, endocrine dysfunction, hypo- or hyperthermia, hypotension, stress, medications, pellagra, or pernicious anemia. According to Wolanin the mechanical problems that cause confusion are obstruction to cerebral blood flow, increased intracranial pressure, and loss of brain cells.

The presenile irreversible dementias that cause confusion are Alzheimer's disease, Pick's disease, and Jakob–Creutzfeldt disease (Wolanin, 1981).

Environmental factors also contribute to cognitive impairment or may worsen it if the condition has existed previously. Most of the environmental factors can be attributed to overstimulation or understimulation. As the speed of response declines, aged persons are more likely to experience sensory overload. The problem may progress to the point where trying to sort stimuli becomes such an overwhelming task that the person withdraws from the environment.

Many cognitive changes have been known to result from a lack of stimulation to the senses. Research has examined the cognitive changes that have affected sailors, astronauts, patients confined to critical-care units, and older people who have experienced sensory deprivation. Persons deprived of sensory stimulation have displayed impaired judgment, inability to solve problems, disorientation, and even hallucinations and delusions. According to Oster, sensory deprivation in the elderly is believed to accelerate the normal degenerative changes associated with aging. He indicates that sensory deprivation "enhances the loss of functional cells in the central nervous system" (Oster, 1976).

In recent years many persons have been mislabeled as having Alzheimer's disease. Of 75 patients who were referred to the VA center and UCLA with the diagnosis of Alzheimer's disease, it was found that only 19 actually had Alzheimer's (Alzheimer's That Isn't, 1983). In this disease there is a progressive, irreversible decline that usually results in death within 2–12 years. Brain failure in this condition results from degeneration of cortical neurons. Signs of Alzheimer's disease include memory impairment, inability to reproduce simple drawings, such as that of a circle; difficulty in interpreting proverbs; inability in maintaining a coherent conversation; and impairment of spatial orientation. Late in the disease bilateral motor abnormalities tend to develop (Alzheimer's That Isn't, 1983). The nurse's role is not to diagnose the cause of brain failure, but to keep the physician, family, and others informed of pertinent data and changes in the client's status.

In addition to assessment of mental status (page 322) a variety of diagnostic tests are used to determine the cause of brain failure. Blood chemistry and urine tests can be performed to determine the presence of many of the conditions mentioned previously. Other tests include an electroencephalogram (EEG), a brain scan, a computed tomography (CT) or computerized axial tomography (CAT) scan, and cerebral angiography. An EEG is the application of electrodes to the scalp to record cortical electrical activity. A brain scan is the counting of radioactivity following the parenteral injection of a radioactive isotope (Billings and Stokes, 1982). A CAT scan is the simultaneous scanning of two planes of the brain with the use of a computer and an x-ray machine and without the use of isotopes. CAT scans are especially efficient in detecting cerebrovascular lesions and brain neoplasia (Phipps, Long, and Woods, 1979). According to a study by Ford and Winter (1981) CAT scan findings of cortical atrophy is not related to brain failure. Ventricular enlargement was found to be correlated with brain failure.

The term *brain failure* does not apply to persons who are experiencing normal age-related changes in cognitive processes. These changes are not considered pathologic. Sometimes, however, the line between "normal" and "pathologic" is very fine. There is a wide variation both in the degree of brain failure and in the clinical manifestations it produces. Table 9.2 compares behavioral changes for three persons. Mr. A's behaviors do not indicate impairment of cognitive functioning whereas Mr. B's indicate a mild degree of brain failure; and Mrs. C's are indicative of a severe degree of brain failure. Nurses need not be concerned with distinguishing the degree of brain failure. Their role is to recognize the manifestations of this syndrome and to plan and intervene accordingly.

There is a great deal of variety in the severity or extent of brain failure, depending on the rapidity of onset, the effectiveness of the person's environment, and on the personality resources possessed by the affected individual (Pfeiffer, 1977). When impairment is severe and onset rapid, it is usually easy to recognize brain failure. When onset is gradual, which is usually the case, and impairment is slight, brain failure may have begun months or years before it is recognized by persons in the environment. Most individuals with brain failure are able to remain in their home settings.

Persons experiencing brain failure typically have problems with particular aspects of cognitive functioning. One common problem is difficulty in remembering recent events. This is generally followed by a loss of orientation to time. Usually, the person first has difficulty in

TABLE 9.2 A COMPARISON OF THE BEHAVIORS OF THREE DIFFERENT LEVELS OF COGNITIVE FUNCTIONING

	Mr. A Unimpaired Cognitive Function	Mr. B Mild Brain Failure	Mrs. C Severe Brain Failure
Age	75	75	75
Residence	Lives alone in home.	Lives with wife in duplex.	Lives in an institution.
Mobility	Drives a car distances under varied conditions. Prefers to avoid night driving.	Drives a car short distances during the day, in light traffic.	Walks with assistance. Remains where placed.
Independence and intellectual functioning	Maintains self, home, and personal affairs independently.	Indecisive. Needs some direction and reminders to maintain house and self (to cut the grass, to wear clean clothes).	Will not bathe self unless handed the equipment and given instructions for each step.
Personality and interaction with others	Initiates communication with others. Actively participates in groups.	Occasional outbursts of anger. Makes increased errors, then denies them. Inconsistent in attempts to accommodate others when interacting with them.	Loses train of thought in middle of sentence. Hallucinates and rambles to self.
Orientation	Complete orientation to time, person, and place. Occasionally forgets the names of recent acquaintances.	Is oriented to frequently visited places. Has difficulty in finding way in new environments. Forgets the names of most recent acquaintances. Occasionally forgets appointments and commitments.	Knows name. Does not recognize children. Does not recognize belongings or room. Is not aware of time of day, month, or year.

recalling days or dates, then the month, and finally the year. Smaller units of time may be forgotten more readily because the individual has had a shorter period in which to learn and use them. Next, there tend to be problems with orientation to place, and then orientation to person (Glickman and Friedman, 1976). In all three areas of orientation, the greatest difficulty lies in recalling recent events that have not been well rehearsed in the person's mind.

Intellectual functioning becomes impaired with brain failure. Usually the highest level of intellectual functioning, the capacity for ab-

stract thought, is impaired first. As brain failure progresses, impairment affects the ability to learn, to adapt to change, to perform activities that involve a series of sequential steps, and the ability to make accurate judgments. Brain failure may also include disturbances in visual–motor coordination (Pfeiffer, 1977). In the case of more severe intellectual impairments, the person is no longer safe. Persons with severe brain failure are unable to care for themselves and cannot make decisions concerning their own welfare.

In some persons, the first indications of

brain failure involve personality changes. The individual may become irritable and have social outbursts. At times there may be a loss of interest in activities, manifested by a decrease in participation and sometimes progressing to withdrawal. Denial is frequently used as a defense mechanism by persons with brain dysfunction. Changes in cognitive abilities are often denied. Pfeiffer states that denial protects the individual from depression which might occur if he were aware of his deficits (Pfeiffer, 1975).

According to a study by Snyder et al. (1978), persons who wander are more likely to have brain dysfunction. For their study, wandering was defined as the "tendency to move about, either in a seemingly aimless or disoriented fashion, or in pursuit of an indefinable or unobtainable goal." Wanderers were found to spend about 32 percent of their time wandering. Such persons also called out and screamed more often than did nonwanderers. These researchers believe that the tendency to wander is influenced by an earlier pattern of walking to relieve stress, and by searching for previous work or previous sources of security (Snyder et al., 1978).

Depression

The incidence of depression is believed to be high among the aged. Most authorities attribute depression to the impact of losses and to the lack of adequate support systems to help the individual cope with the losses. Glickman and Friedman (1976) indicated that depression is most often related to the loss of a significant other, frequently a spouse or a child. Loss of physical health is also a major factor in the development of depression in the aged (Verwoerdt, 1981). Physical losses and the fear of loss of function, along with loss of support systems, lead to decreased self-esteem. As self-esteem decreases and feelings of hopelessness increase, depression occurs (Salzman and Shader, 1978).

Biologic factors, such as increased production of monoamine oxidase (MAO), may also be connected with the increased incidence of depression among the elderly. The levels of MAO, an enzyme that is related to norepinephrine metabolism, are believed to increase with advancing age. This is especially true in women, as there is an inverse relationship between levels of estrogen and those of MAO (Grauer, 1977). Old persons tend to sleep less and to have fewer periods of REM sleep. Research has indicated that deprivation of REM sleep leads to depression (Grauer, 1977). According to Jarvik (1976), many depressed persons have actually experienced depression when they were younger, but were better able to cope with it because of supportive resources, such as family and job security. Jarvik further indicates that if the family has forgotten such depressive episodes, they might not be a part of the client's history.

The primary symptoms of depression are a depressive mood and reduced behavior (Sternback, 1980). Adjectives frequently used to describe a depressive mood include sad, dejected, listless, guilty, unworthy, lonely, fatigued, apathetic, helpless, and hopeless. Reduced activity encompasses apathy and "can be considered 'given-up' behavior, subsequent to loss and failure at adaptation" (Sternback, 1980, p. 618). Sternback perceives reduced activity as the external manifestation of lowered self-esteem, helplessness, and hopelessness.

Secondary symptoms of depression include a variety of somatic and cognitive disturbances. Common somatic symptoms of depression in the aged are insomnia, anorexia, fatigue, and weight loss. Hypochondriasis and gastrointestinal and urinary disorders may be attributed to depression in the aged (Hussian, 1981). Depression in late life has been found to be more flat, monotonic, and less self-blaming. Older depressed persons tend to have an increase in somatic complaints (Sternbeck, 1980). Hussian indicates that the main behavior of depression that occurs in the elderly and not in the younger age groups is the apparent confusion or cloudiness of cognitive functioning. Affect and intellectual functioning may be dulled and moderate levels of disorientation may occur. Less attention may be paid to personal appearance and hygiene (Hussian, 1981). Depression may be worsened by strong feelings of guilt in those persons with a strong conviction about their own responsibility for their lives. Those who typically blame others direct aggressiveness toward the environment. This increases feelings of loneliness and bitterness. The anxiety of depression is a part of the pessimistic outlook and hopelessness (Sternbach, 1980).

Since depression may be readily denied assessment is particularly important in identification of the problem. The most important nursing intervention in dealing with depression includes those measures that improve the client's self-esteem and the support system, as was discussed in detail in Chapter 7. Nurses have a role in assisting depressed clients to receive psychologic counseling.

ASSESSMENT OF COGNITIVE FUNCTIONING

In most instances, nurses can assess their client's cognitive status without the use of a standardized test. Most elderly persons do not have problems related to cognition, and a lengthy assessment is therefore unnecessary. For those experiencing problems, more data must be collected according to the client's areas of difficulty. Nurses should maximize the use of their observation skills, rather than routinely bombard their clients with questions. When gathering data, the nurse must be sensitive to clues that the client is becoming tired. Such clues include restlessness, decreased attention span, and easy distraction by environmental factors. Older clients tire more readily. Fatigue interferes with the reliability of the data that a client provides.

The nurse can obtain more useful information if she sets priorities in gathering data. This is particularly helpful when only part of the data can be obtained in one session with the client. The greater the client's degree of confusion, the shorter is the usual attention span. For an in-depth assessment of a confused client, the nurse may find it necessary to provide a period of rest and obtain additional information at another time.

When obtaining data for a total assessment, it is wise to assess the client's cognitive status first, as this will provide clues on how to proceed. The status of the person's memory and orientation is an indicator of the reliability of other information which may be obtained. Data related to the person's intelligence level enable the nurse to ask questions and provide instructions according to the individual's level of understanding. Since denial is often used as a defense mechanism by persons with brain dysfunction, the nurse may have to rely more heavily than usual on obtaining data from persons in such a client's environment. Significant others naturally tend to be reluctant to provide information about brain dysfunction in the presence of the affected person, so the nurse should make an opportunity to interview the significant other alone. Privacy is essential, since brain dysfunction is a sensitive subject and people may often attempt to cover up information or try to protect a family member from embarrassment if privacy is not maintained. Both the client and the family may be distressed when cognitive impairment interferes with the person's ability to answer questions and to perform tasks. Although an accurate and reliable assessment is needed, clients should not be repeatedly asked to perform functions beyond the person's ability. Measures such as praising the client's efforts should be taken to prevent frustration.

The nurse should keep in mind the elderly person's increased time of response and tendency to be distracted by irrelevant stimuli. Data should not be collected when either the interviewer or the interviewee is rushed. Questions should be brief, clear, and concise, and each question should contain only one thought. Look for clues that the client has either lost sight of what was being asked or else does not understand what was being asked, and rephrase the question if necessary. Hearing and vision impairments may interfere with the client's responses.

When there is evidence of brain dysfunction in any area, some general points should be determined. First, how consistently does the impairment occur? Some problems may be present only when the person is overtired, in an unfamiliar environment, or at a certain time of the day. Next, was the onset of the problem sudden or gradual? Has evidence of the problem existed for days, months, or years? The nurse should also determine the client's degree of awareness of the problems, which may range from total denial to a more or less complete understanding. Changes that have occurred in the cognitive status are a very significant part of the assessment. However, testing the cognitive status should not be repeated unnecessarily. Failures in specific areas of cognitive functioning may be very stressful for either the client and/or family members. Encouragement and positive reinforcement need to be offered as much as possible. Providing opportunities for success are useful to promote self-esteem.

Specific Areas to Be Assessed

Level of Consciousness

Since the person's level of consciousness is of primary importance, it should be assessed first. The person who is conscious is alert and responsive to stimuli. Refer to Table 9.3 for a description of altered states of consciousness.

Orientation

Assessing clients' orientation determines the extent of their awareness of person, place, and time. Assessment of person may be done at the beginning of the interview by asking the client to state his or her full name and to indicate the name of the individual who brought him

or her for the examination. If the nurse suspects a problem with disorientation, persons in the client's environment, such as family or staff, should be asked if the client has difficulty distinguishing persons in the environment. To determine the client's orientation to place, ask, "What is the name of this place?" If the person is institutionalized, determine if he knows his floor and room number. (A client who is confined to his or her room is less likely to know this.) Some persons may be able to find their room, but may not know the room number.

The nurse should next determine if the person can find places of significance to him or her and then return to his or her place of residence. For the institutionalized person, such places might include the bathroom or the dining room. For the person in the community, they might be the grocery store or the health-care center. Assessment of orientation to time should determine the client's awareness of the month, day, and year. Knowledge of the month and year are more significant than knowledge of the day, since persons can lose track of the days if they have no reason for remembering them. Those who give incorrect responses to other aspects of orientation should be asked to indicate the time of day, i.e., morning, afternoon, evening, or night.

TABLE 9.3 VARIED STATES OF CONSCIOUSNESS

State	Behavior	Example of Observation
Conscious	Responds appropriately to stimuli.	Answers questions without hesitation.
Lethargy	Sleeps or dozes inappropriately. Can be aroused by stimuli.	Drifts into sleep when visitors are present. Answers when name is called.
Stuporous	Slowed response or incomplete response to stimuli. Response is not sustained. May be restless. Reflexes usually present.	Opens eyes momentarily and looks in direction of nurse who calls by first name.
Semiconscious	Responds to painful stimuli. Reflexes may be present but the plantar reflexes are often extensor (Luckmann, p. 418, 1974).	Moves hand away in reaction to a pinprick.
Unconscious	No response to painful stimuli. Reflexes absent or minimal. Extremities flaccid.	Pupils unresponsive to light. Does not move when jabbed by a pin.

Memory

To assess a client's recent memory, ask her to tell you her phone number, who is president, or what she ate at her last meal. To measure retention and recall the nurse may give the client an address or three numbers or objects to remember. Two to 5 minutes later the person is asked to recall the material given.

To determine the status of the client's long-term memory, ask her date of birth, including the day, month, and year. To further test memory and orientation, also ask her how old she is. Pfeiffer suggests asking the person, "What was your mother's maiden name?" (Pfeiffer, 1975).

Intellectual Functioning

When the nurse is asssessing a client's intellectual functioning, the individual's educational background should be determined before other aspects of intellect are evaluated, so that the interviewer will have an idea of what to expect and will be able to gear questions to the individual. Intellectual functions include the person's ability to think abstractly. One means of determining this is to ask the client to tell you the meaning of a familiar proverb. For example: "What does the expression, 'The grass is always greener on the other side of the fence' mean?" Another measure is to ask the client to subtract 7 from 100 and to continue to subtract 7 from each new number until told to stop. The nurse should be alert to feedback from the client that may indicate the inability to think in abstract terms.

Some insight into the person's ability to conceptualize or to make associations can be obtained by asking the person to tell how two objects in a class of objects are alike. For example: "How are an apple and a peach alike?" "Fruit" is an abstract response. It indicates a higher level of thinking than a concrete response, such as that both can be eaten, or that both grow on trees.

Information can also be obtained in relation to performing a sequence of actions. The client can be told to touch her knees, to close and open her eyes, then to fold her hands. Having her perform such a series of activities may uncover difficulties the nurse is likely to encounter when giving the client instructions or in teaching her to perform psychomotor activities.

For persons with brain dysfunction, data should be gathered to determine if the cognitive changes have interfered with their performance of activities of daily living. If physically able, can the person maintain himself safely in his environment? This includes activities related to the preparation of meals, eating, grooming, dressing, and even bowel and bladder control. If the client lives alone, is the person able to manage financial affairs, such as paying bills?

The nurse can also do a brief evaluation of the person's reading and writing skills. In some instances, the client may be asked simply to write her name. Reading and writing skills may be further assessed by having the person complete a brief form, or asking her to read a sentence or a short paragraph. Assessment of comprehension would require the person to explain what she had read.

Personality

The client may or may not be aware of any personality changes that have occurred. Data about such changes can be obtained from persons in the client's environment, significant others, and health-care workers. Personality features are considered to be problems when they interfere with the functioning of the client or others. Some personality changes are disruptive and may be very stressful for those in the environment.

Since denial is the most basic defense mechanism, it may be adaptive for the older person as a mechanism to deal with physiologic changes that are occurring. Use of denial is not a problem unless it is utilized excessively and results in failure to seek medical or other help. If the problems become worse and effective coping mechanisms are not found, then denial is not an effective coping mechanism (Salzman and Shader, 1978).

Assessments of cognitive status should include assessment of the stimulation in the environment. This is particularly important when the person's life space has been decreased, limiting activities to a particular community, building, or room. As a life space decreases there is an increased danger that the individual will experience sensory deprivation.

Because the elderly are more likely to experience sensory deprivation than are younger persons, assessment of environmental stimulation is important. It should include the person's interpersonal contacts, the clues to reality that are present in the environment, and the degree of environmental stimulation to vision, hearing, taste, smell, and touch.

It is not enough simply to describe the sources of environmental stimulation. Unless the client perceives these stimuli as meaningful, they are of little value. In analyzing the data related to cognitive status, the nurse should determine whether the person is experiencing either sensory deprivation from too little stimulation or sensory overload from too much stimulation. These problems can have a damaging effect on the cognitive processes of the older person.

Refer to Table 9.4 for an assessment guide. Keep in mind, however, that this is merely a guide; it is not meant to be a valid and a reliable tool. The purpose of the guide is to provide a general outline for nurses who are assessing a client's cognitive status. Many of the questions are unnecessary for the person who has no brain dysfunction. For those clients who are suspected of having brain dysfunction, additional observations may be necessary.

Many persons feel threatened by a cognitive assessment. As indicated by Comfort, much information about cognitive status can be obtained very subtly during the first few minutes of an interview, by asking the client her "name, address, age, year of birth, date of birth, name of next-of-kin, past or present occupation, and the time of her scheduled appointment" (Comfort, 1978). This information will give the nurse clues as to how the remainder of the cognitive examination should be conducted.

An objective and comprehensive analysis of the data obtained is essential for nursing effectiveness. There are several reasons for this. First of all, the problems related to cognitive status are often not recognized by the client or her significant others until they become overt. If they are recognized, they may be denied because of the stigma frequently associated with problems related to brain dysfunction. A second reason for the importance of analysis is that problems related to cognitive status may interfere with the collection of data. The client

TABLE 9.4 GUIDE FOR ASSESSMENT OF COGNITIVE STATUS

Subjective Data (History)

Determine client's and/or family's awareness of the present status and of changes in any of the following
  areas:
  Affect:
    Personality
    Usual mood
    Attitudes
  Cognitive:
    Memory (recent or past)
    Remembering names, dates or places
    Ability to complete usual tasks
    Ability to participate in usual activities
    Interests
    Problem solving
  Communication:
    Hearing or understanding people
    Expressing ideas to others
    Relationships with others

(continued)

TABLE 9.4 (Continued)

Subjective Data (Continued)

Self-concept:
 Feelings about self
 Dependence, independence
 Health
Refer to Table 8.1 for guide for assessing self-perceptions, coping mechanisms and reactions to stress.
Educational background:
 Years of formal education
 Highest education degree received
 Describe education beyond high school
 When last received formal education
 Interest in continued learning
Medications:
 Prescribed or over the counter medications
 Length of time taking each medication
 Changes in dose, time or type of medication
 Occurrence of behavior changes since medication changed

Objective Data (Physical Exam)

Level of consciousness
 Determine the level and observations which support conclusion. Example: Alert—readily responds to questions and initiates verbal communication.

Orientation	If confusion occurs note the patterns and precipitating factors.
To person:	What is your full name?
	What is the name of the person who brought you here?
	(Determine if people in the environment are appropriately identified.)
To place:	What is the name of this place?
	(If institutionalized) What is your room number?
	(If at home) What is your address?
	Observe if difficulties are encountered in locating places of significance and then returning to room.)
To time:	What is the month, day and year?
	What time of day is it? (Morning, afternoon, evening, or night)
Memory	
Recent memory:	Who is president of the United States? or,
	What is your phone number? or,
	What did you have to eat for _____?
	(most recent meal)
Long-term memory:	In what month, day or year, were you born?
	How old are you? or,
	What was your mother's maiden name?
	(Pfeiffer, 1975)
Intellect	What health problems do you have?
	(Determine the client's understanding of the health problem, its limitations, and of what can be done or is being done for the problem.)
	Observe the length of attention span.
	Describe evidence of tiring during the interview.
	Describe comprehension of questions.

(continued)

TABLE 9.4 (Continued)

Objective Data (Continued)

Observe evidence of excessive distraction by irrelevant stimuli?
Note if excessive time is required to respond to questions?
Assess data related to evidence of problem solving ability.
Have interpret the expression "The grass is always greener on the other side of the road."
Ask to subtract 7 from 100 and continue to subtract 7 from each new number until told to stop.
Ask "How an apple and a peach are alike."
Have perform three successive tasks such as: "Touch your knees, close and open your eyes, then fold your hands."
Assess performance of activities of daily living, as affected by cognitive functioning (household tasks, food preparation, feeding and bathing self, and bladder and bowel control).
Instruct the person to write his or her name.
Instruct the person to read a sentence or a short paragraph.

Personality

Observe for the following behaviors:
Agitation
Aggression
Undue anxiety
Frequent demands
Hallucinations
Delusions
Indecisiveness
Observe for signs of depression
Withdrawal
Disinterest
Apathy
Change in sleep, eating, or sexual habits
Crying spells
Expression of powerlessness
Expression of hopelessness
Exaggeration of problems and of physical complaints
Note defense mechanisms used.

Environmental stimulation

Interaction with others, observe
Opportunities for interaction
Initiation of interaction
Response to interaction
Frequency of interaction
Meaningfulness of interaction
Environmental clues to reality
Clues provided by others
Presence of clues to time, place and person
Describe the variety, the intensity, the pattern, the meaningfulness of stimulation to:
Vision
Hearing
Taste
Smell
Touch
Describe factors interfering with perception of stimuli.
Describe reaction to environmental stimuli.

may be confused and therefore provide inaccurate information, or the nurse may question her beyond her tolerance and cause problems of sensory overload. If the nurse is aware of these potential problems, measures can be taken to avoid them. Since nurses usually spend more time with clients than physicians do, a nurse may have information that the physician is unaware of that could affect the plan of care. The nurse is sometimes the first to identify a problem, and often is able to obtain information that may lead to reconsideration of the diagnosis.

PLANNING AND INTERVENTION

The broad goal of planning and intervention is to enable the client to attain a maximum level of cognitive functioning. Achievement of this goal takes time, planning, and cooperation from everyone in the client's environment.

Too often the physical needs of the elderly are met while cognitive problems are ignored. This is the result of several factors: the lack of emphasis placed on cognitive skills over the years; the amount of skill, tact, and patience required to minister to a client's cognitive needs; and the frequently greater rewards received from performance of physical tasks. Most persons can be trained to perform physical tasks in a relatively short period of time, but the development of interpersonal skills takes much more time and effort. When a physical task has been completed, the results are visible, and the task can then be forgotten until it is time to repeat it. Interpersonal skills, on the other hand, must be used continuously in interactions with the client, and they are not readily visible during their use.

Effective use of interpersonal skills is only one way of helping clients to reach a maximum level of cognitive function. The nurse must also consider the individual client's problems and must work with the client, his significant others, and various health-care workers to set appropriate goals and plan approaches.

Four goals have been identified to enable clients to attain a maximum level of cognitive functioning:

- To promote memory development
- To promote sensory stimulation
- To prevent sensory overload
- To reduce depression

Usually nursing measures will be directed toward a combination of these goals rather than toward a single one, in isolation from the others. For example, when a nurse approaches a cognitively impaired person and says, "Good morning Mrs. Hartman, I'm Jill, the nurse who will be assisting you today," she has promoted orientation. With one statement she has reminded the woman of her own identity, the time of day, who she is, and of her role. Although Mrs. Hartman may not comprehend all that has been said, the nurse has promoted memory development. Jill can promote sensory stimulation by encouraging Mrs. Hartman to make simple decisions and to actively participate in her care whenever possible. For example, Jill could say, "Mrs. Hartman, which would you like to eat first, your cereal or your egg?" In this instance Jill has stimulated Mrs. Hartman's thinking in addition to increasing the amount of control Mrs. Hartman has over her activities. Jill has used a positive approach by asking which item Mrs. Hartman preferred to eat first. If she asks, "Which would you like to eat?," the implication could be that both items are not expected to be eaten.

In some situations it may be appropriate to take measures related to all four of the goals that have been identified. In others the focus of the nursing care may be directed toward one of the goals. To be most effective the goals selected and the approaches utilized should be determined according to the client's needs.

Nursing Measures to Promote Memory Development
Memory development can be defined as manipulation of the physical and social environment in order to improve mental function in persons experiencing brain failure. It may be promoted through the use of objects, individual interactions, or group sessions. In many instances all three of these approaches are used in promoting cognitive functioning. However, some may be more effective than others for a

particular client. Memory development includes measures to promote orientation to time, person, and place. Since motivation is an important factor in the achievement of goals, the nurse should determine which aspect of orientation is most important to the client. If the client associates no importance with knowing the days of the month, then it is a waste of time to try to orient the client in this direction. Either the person should be motivated to care about the days of the month, or the nurse should emphasize another aspect of orientation that is more meaningful.

Objects are very useful in promoting memory development and in improving orientation to time, person, and place. However, objects in the environment are useless unless the client perceives them. The nurse should take this into consideration when determining the size, color, and placement of objects. First, they should be large enough that they can be easily seen. Numbers and letters, in particular, must be clear and distinct as necessitated by the client's visual status. In some cases, objects should be three-dimensional, so that they can be felt. Colors should usually be vivid and contrasting, in order to increase visibility.

Objects should be placed where they can often be seen, and at an appropriate height. For example, if the client spends most of the time sitting in a particular chair, then there is no point in placing an important object behind the chair. Instead, it should be placed at eye level where the client is most likely to notice it.

Orientation to time can be promoted through the use of calendars, clocks, and watches. Calendars should show the year clearly. Time can be made more meaningful to the client by marking on the calendar significant future events. These events might include appointments, visits, favorite television programs, or perhaps days on which special foods are served. It is important that sources of orientation are reliable. Calendar pages must be turned, and clocks and watches must be accurately set and regularly wound. Clients may need help with this from reliable persons in the environment. If the client is in an institution a roommate might take over this task,

or could at least remind the person to do it. Decorations related to seasons, holidays, or religious festivals are sources of orientation to time. The use of lights may contribute to one's orientation. Bright lights left on during the night may be a source of confusion, although a soft light left on at night may aid persons in remembering where they are. Orientation to time may be promoted by encouraging the person to listen to news broadcasts or to read newspapers and magazines.

When orienting a person to place, the nurse should consider the need for orientation to the extended environment as well as the immediate environment. The individual's life space usually determines the extent of orientation required. A person in the community may need help in learning to travel from his place of residence to various significant places in the community, such as a store or health center. Persons in institutions may need assistance in finding their way to the bathroom or to the dining room. Large, clear signs should be posted to identify particular locations for persons who are confused as to place. In helping an individual with orientation to place, the nurse should refer to clues in the environment that are not likely to be changed. For example, instead of instructing someone to turn down the hall opposite a certain picture, instruct the person to turn down the first hall past the water fountain. The fountain is a more permanent fixture than the picture.

A person will be oriented more readily if contrast in the environment is provided. Decorating each floor of an institution with a different color will help to promote orientation to place. Rooms are easier to identify if there is a picture of the occupant on the door, if a different picture is painted on each door, or if the color of each room is different. Reality orientation and individualization are promoted when each resident is permitted to have his own furniture and personal objects in the environment to make *his* room his own (Fig. 9.1). Although it may not be feasible for individuals to have their own beds in an institution, they might be able to have such personal belongings as bedspreads, chairs, and pictures.

The use of signs to identify places and in-

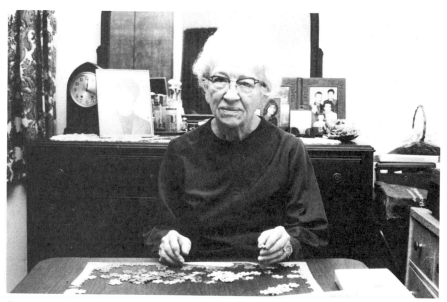

Figure 9.1. Orientation is promoted when persons are permitted to have their own furniture, pictures, and other items of significance in their environment. Activities such as putting puzzles together stimulate the cognitive processes. *(Photograph by Ed Spier, Murrysville, PA.)*

dicate directions is important in promoting memory development. The name of the resident occupying each room, and the names of employees occupying offices, should be indicated on the doors, in letters large enough to be easily read. Signs with arrows should be posted to direct residents to frequently utilized places. Directories should appear both inside and outside of elevators. Hallways and floors should be clearly identified with signs. Some clients may need memory cues to recall the name of the institution, which should appear on elevator directories, bulletin boards, and reality boards.

Stability in the environment is highly important to the individual with brain dysfunction. A change in location is disruptive, even if the change is within the same room. The greater the change, the greater the effect on the person and the longer it takes to adapt to the change. When a client must be relocated, the nurse should plan a program for orienting the person to the new environment.

The last aspect of orientation an individual loses is self-identification. More recent ac-

quaintances in the person's environment are forgotten first. A woman experiencing severe dysfunction may not recall her married name. Orientation to person can be promoted by calling the individual by name and by placing a name card at his place of residence. It is important that each person be called by an appropriate name, not by a nickname such as "grandma." Addressing an individual by names to which he is not accustomed contributes to the loss of self-identity. Instead of assuming that a client wishes to be called by his first name or surname, confer with the person and determine what he prefers to be called.

Health-care workers should identify themselves verbally at the onset of each interaction, in addition to wearing a large-lettered name tag. They should not assume that a client remembers who people are or what their functions are. A disoriented person may be too embarrassed to admit that he does not remember someone, or may mistakenly identify a person.

Orientation of a person is increased when those coming in contact with the confused person wear identification tags indicating name and status. All unnecessary information should be eliminated. The identification tag will be most helpful if the person's name is printed exactly as the person wishes to be addressed and if status is indicated as it is significant to the client.

Individuals can be assisted in maintaining their self-identity if they are encouraged to dress according to their own style unless physical conditions impose limitations. Some women will feel comfortable wearing housedresses, some will prefer slacks, and others may wear dressy clothes with matching jewelry. Many aged women enjoy wearing makeup (Fig. 9.2). The range of attire among the men may vary from sports clothes to suits and ties.

In institutions, reality orientation boards placed in strategic locations can be used to promote orientation and to stimulate thinking. Reality boards, such as the one shown in Figure 9.3, indicate the place, the date, and a variety of other things which might include the weather, the season, the next holiday, and the day of the week. The boards can be made of any materials which permit easy changing of dates and events. Flannel boards and materials with Velcro backing are often used. A reliable resident can be delegated the task of keeping the reality board up-to-date.

Reality orientation therapy was shown to improve the mental status of elderly institutionalized persons in a study by Nodhturft and Sweeney (1982). Over the 10-week period participants in their study attended half-hour group reality orientation classes and received reinforcement of reality orientation concepts from the staff. Compared with a group of aged persons who did not participate in reality orientation therapy, there was a significant improvement in the mental status scores of the participants. In some studies reality orientation did not produce a significant decrease in the level of confusion (Voelkel, 1978; Hogstel, 1979). The lack of success of certain reality orientation programs could be related to the absence of a reinforcer that is significant to the

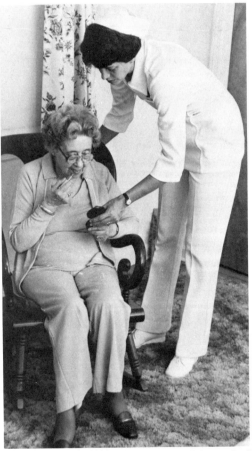

Figure 9.2. Applying makeup daily is an important activity for some aged women. *(Photograph by Ed Spier, Murrysville, PA.)*

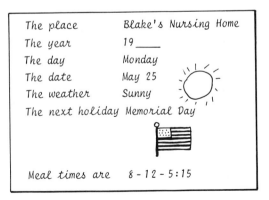

The place   Blake's Nursing Home
The year   19____
The day   Monday
The date   May 25
The weather   Sunny
The next holiday Memorial Day

Meal times are   8 - 12 - 5:15

Figure 9.3. Specific up-to-date reality boards help the aged to orient themselves to time and place.

client when a desired behavior is exhibited (Langston, 1981). The role of the nurse includes determining which reinforcers are appropriate for each client. Langston indicates that reality orientation should be on a 24-hour program with one-to-one sessions to enable the immediate application of appropriate reinforcers. Use of the reinforcer should be combined with positive statements such as "very good." The extent of reality orientation that is appropriate varies from client to client.

Interpersonal interactions are important in memory development. During interactions, the client should be stimulated to think and be an active participant, rather than a passive listener. One of the most effective ways to stimulate thinking in the older person is reminiscence. People who are depressed or who are experiencing brain failure often are happiest when they are talking about vivid memories from the past rather than the painful realities of the present (Fig. 9.4). Ryden (1981) indicated that reminiscence therapy bolsters the self-esteem, primarily for persons who find that old age "has little to offer in experiences with mastery, achievement, and control" (p. 462). Healthy old persons, free from cognitive problems, also benefit from reminiscence, as do those with varying degrees of brain dysfunction. Reminiscing enables the elderly to find meaning and worth in their lives.

Even persons with more severe brain dysfunction have been known to benefit from reminiscence. An example of this was Mrs. D, an 88-year-old former schoolteacher institutionalized because of severe brain dysfunction. Frequently, Mrs. D could be heard calling out to her students as though she were in the classroom with them. When repeated efforts to orient her to reality failed, an attempt was made at reminiscence therapy. At the onset of the therapy, conversation with Mrs. D was impossible because her attention span was less than 30 seconds. Through repeated interactions, during which she was asked about her students, her beliefs about teaching, and her methods of handling various classroom problems, Mrs D's attention span gradually increased. Eventually she was able to discuss subjects other than teaching.

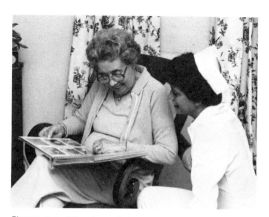

Figure 9.4. Viewing pictures from the past encourages reminiscence. *(Photograph by Ed Spier, Murrysville, PA.)*

Reminiscence therapy requires much time and patience. However, the results are usually worth the effort if the timing and the selection of topics are right for the individual. The nurse can evaluate the effectiveness of reminiscence therapy by noting the client's facial expression and verbal response. Through listening to a client's hallucinations the nurse can identify appropriate topics. If the person is tired or has been overstimulated, the therapy will not be successful. Sessions should be conducted when the client is well rested and not distracted by activities in the environment.

For persons who readily reminisce, one of the problems is boredom on the part of the listener. People hearing a story for the first time react more positively than those who have heard the same story over and over. By using a variety of changing objects in the environment and by changing topics of conversation, the nurse can stimulate reminiscence about a greater variety of topics, or can expand discussion of the client's favorite topics.

Persons in the environment of elderly clients experiencing brain failure should serve as sources of reality. Hallucinations and delusions should not be supported. Clients with severe disorders may believe that a health-care worker or another person in the environment is a significant other, who has died. For example, a roommate may be mistaken for the client's mother. The client should be told that her mother has died and that this is Jenny, her roommate. The extent of explanation necessary varies according to the client's level of comprehension, attention span, and environment. The nurse correcting a person's delusions or hallucinations should do so firmly, but in a calm, sincere, and friendly manner. Elderly persons should be treated as adults, and not as children (Lehman, 1974). When an aged person repeatedly asks about his or her mother, who has been dead for many years, the person may be expressing feelings of being lost and fear of inability to provide for self-care (Mace and Rabins, 1981, p. 103). In such instances the person needs to be reminded as to who will take care of him and of the provisions that have been made for the person's care. Usually a detailed explanation is inappropriate.

Consistency of behavior toward the person suffering from brain dysfunction is important. It must be extremely disconcerting to an already confused individual if some persons in the environment are promoting memory development and others are not. All of those in contact with the client should take part in the effort. Some people, such as family members and nonprofessional staff, may not understand their role in promoting memory development. The nurse can do much to help these persons in understanding and implementing the concept.

Orientation is not promoted by segregating confused persons from those whose cognitive functions are intact. They should be integrated and encouraged to assist one another. Both parties can benefit from this. For example, consider Mr. H, whose cognitive functioning is intact, although he is relatively immobile. His self-esteem is increased from knowing he is helping his disoriented roommate by reminding him of important things. In return, Mr. H's roommate assists him with problems related to his immobility.

Persons in the environment can promote orientation by encouraging clients to participate in their own care to the fullest extent possible. Those who have not participated in their own care for a long time may have to be reminded of each step and handed the equipment necessary. Others may only need to have the equipment placed in front of them and then be told to proceed. Some clients may be able to carry out certain functions, but may not know when to do them or may not remember if they have done them already. Reminder cards, check-off systems, and consistent daily routines may help these persons to function. When clients respond correctly or show improvement in functioning, they should be told. Rewards, such as praise, touch, or smiles, are important motivators (Scarbrough, 1974).

The primary group activity to promote cognitive functioning is the reality orientation class. Such classes can be conducted formally or informally, and ideally, should contain no more than five people. It is difficult to maintain the attention span of groups larger than this. Members of each group should be compatible with one another. Classes usually begin with the members identifying themselves. Frequently the leader utilizes a reality board to indicate the place, the day, and the date. Other clues to orientation should be present and referred to. Activities in reality orientation classes often include physical activities, such as singing, exercises, games with a ball, or other action games. Many focus on activities that appeal to the senses. For example, a class might concentrate on fruit, thereby stimulating touch, taste, and sight. When objects are used, their physical qualities should be emphasized. The length of a class depends on the attention span of the members of the group. Often 20 or 30 minutes is all that is possible. The classes should never last longer than an hour.

Nursing Measures to Promote Sensory Stimulation

Sensory deprivation is a common problem among elderly clients. Deprivation may result from a decreased life space or a decrease in the amount or variety of environmental stimuli. In other instances, the problem may be related to body changes that interfere with the reception or perception of stimuli.

Sensory deprivation itself causes additional problems that can lead to further diminishment of cognitive functioning. According to Chodil and Williams (1970), persons who experience sensory deprivation have difficulties related to boredom, incoherent thinking, and inability to concentrate. There may be regression, emotional lability, and hallucinations. Black (1973) states that persons become preoccupied with needs at a lower level when they have no opportunity to fulfill needs at a higher level. Schultz (1965, p. 31) reports that an optimal range or optimal level of external stimulation is necessary in order for a person to function effectively. Stimuli below or beyond this range interfere with learning and "disrupt learned responses."

Presenting a variety of stimuli is important when promoting sensory stimulation. Perception is influenced by the intensity, the variation, the patterning, and the size of stimuli. The intensity of stimuli often must be increased for the aged. However, there should also be variation in the intensity of stimuli within the environment. Overstimulation and increased problems with organization and discrimination may occur if the number and intensity of environmental stimuli are too great.

Repetition of stimuli is useful to a point, in that regularly repeated stimuli are more likely to be received than are stimuli that are repeated infrequently. However, there is a limit to the effectiveness of repetition. After a period of time, change is perceived more readily than continued repetition (Chodil and Williams, 1970). For example, when the same type of music is heard continuously at the same volume, persons in the environment may not even be aware of its presence. Size of stimuli is also a factor, in that the larger of two visual stimuli is perceived more readily, assuming all other factors are equal (Chodil and Williams, 1970). Features in the environment should be designed to appeal to more than one sense, while at the same time avoiding overload.

To prevent stimuli from becoming monotonous, efforts need to be made to vary the stimuli. Music, for instance, is more readily perceived when the volume is varied, when the type of music changes at intervals, and when there are periods without music. Materials in the environment should be varied in temperature, texture, and degree of firmness, to stimulate the tactile senses. Merely viewing these materials is not enough; clients should have opportunities to handle them. Outdoor activities often promote sensory stimulation (Fig. 9.5).

Institutions should make special efforts to prevent serving bland food. Serving a variety of foods helps stimulate taste. Some institutions serve ethnic foods one day each week or month. Others now permit alcoholic beverages to be served at certain events. A study was performed by Burrell, McCourt, and Cutter (1974) regarding the effects of beer consumption on social responsiveness. The study showed that persons drinking beer during a group session did not become more sociable than those who were given soda to drink. It did reveal, however, that everyone became more sociable during group interactions. On the other hand, a study by Carroll (1978) indicated that socialization was significantly increased when whiskey, gin, vodka, and wine were available during a social hour. Unless contraindicated for specific individuals, alcoholic beverages should be available during social events for those who prefer them.

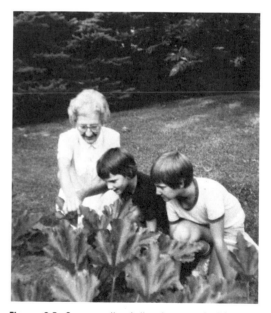

Figure 9.5. Sensory stimulation is promoted by encouraging interest in outdoor activities.

Flowers and different soaps, perfumes, and deodorizers can be used to stimulate the sense of smell. Vision can be stimulated by encouraging individuals to observe objects at different distances—for example, events taking place outside of their windows. It may be helpful to rotate pictures within the immediate environment and to change the contents of the bulletin board periodically.

Research has shown that colors can be used to create certain moods or feelings. Although there is not complete agreement among the findings of the various researchers, it is evident that there is a relationship between colors and emotions. Nurses should keep this in mind when trying to promote or prevent certain emotions or feelings among clients. Table 9.5 is a guide for nurses who are attempting to use color in promoting or decreasing sensory stimulation. If a client tends to become easily agitated, orange, black, and red should be avoided in favor of blues and greens. For a client suffering from depression, brown and black in the environment should be minimized, while yellow or red may be helpful. This, of course, depends on the stage of depression and what the colors mean to the client.

The significance of particular colors may be related to biologic factors, cultural background, and individual experience. What is right for one person is not necessarily right for the next. The individual's responses to colors should be determined before they can be effectively utilized to promote certain moods. The effects of particular colors should be considered in the selection of room decoration and the color of clothing. The shades and vividness of colors will also influence the degree of reaction.

Mood and feeling tones are affected by a variety of factors: physical comfort; environmental temperature, noise and odors; and aesthetic pleasantness of the colors. A dilemma confronting many nurses and family members is determining the amount of life space that is appropriate for a particular aged person. Sensory stimulation for many individuals is promoted by extending the person's life space. Aged persons who are experiencing brain failure may need to have their life space restricted to promote safety or to prevent sensory overload.

TABLE 9.5 COLOR AND MOOD-TONE RELATIONSHIPS IDENTIFIED BY WEXNER*

Color	Mood-Tones
Blue	Secure, comforting Tender, soothing Calm, peaceful, serene
Black	Despondent, dejected, unhappy, melancholy Distressed, disturbed, upset Dignified, stately Defiant, contrary, hostile Powerful, strong, masterful
Brown	Secure, comforting Protective, defending Despondent, dejected, unhappy, melancholy
Green	Secure, comforting Tender, soothing Calm, peaceful, serene
Orange	Distressed, disturbed, upset Defiant, contrary, hostile Exciting, stimulating†
Purple	Dignified, stately
Red	Protective, defending Exciting, stimulating Cheerful, jovial, joyful Defiant, contrary, masterful Powerful, strong, masterful
Yellow	Cheerful, jovial, joyful

*Mood-tone and color associations included in this report are only those to which more than 15 out of 94 who were interviewed indicated the relationships.
†Schaie, 1961.
(Adapted from Wexner, L. The degree to which colors (hues) are associated with Mood-Tones. J App Psych, 1954, 38(6):432, 1954.)

Increases in life space are particularly beneficial for those whose mobility has been limited for reasons other than brain failure. This can be done by taking the person for walks, to restaurants, to shopping centers, cultural centers, and to various forms of appropriate entertainment. The family may wish to do these things but may not know how to cope with the client's physical problems. The nurse can help by anticipating difficulties and preparing the family and client to deal with them or to avoid them.

Deciding the optimal amount of life space for persons experiencing brain failure is often a difficult decision. Freedom to move about in one's environment is essential to the person's physical, psychologic, and sociologic health. Brain failure may interfere with a person's ability to protect him- or herself from environmental hazards. Although physical restraints may be necessary at times they should be avoided whenever possible and only used for short periods of time. Some individuals with brain failure are wanderers. Robb and Monsour (1980) found that institutionalized wanderers had experienced a greater number of stressful events and had participated in social and leisure activities that required more physical energy than nonwanderers. Restricting movement of a person leads to agitation and may result in aggression. Wandering may occur to relieve tension and may be a sign of boredom (Burnside, 1981). Although wanderers need to be provided with a safe environment to enable them to move about, they need to be protected from hazards such as getting lost or being run over by a vehicle.

In some instances, sensory stimulation can be increased by encouraging the client to form social relationships with others. The nurse may need to introduce the person to neighbors or to others in the environment, and may also be able to help him form new relationships or revive old ones. This can be done through identifying common interests and experiences, or through involvement in group activities.

The initial interaction with a group is important because it influences future interactions (Snyder, 1978). A single bad experience may make a person reluctant to attend other group activities. Often clients do not participate in group activities because of lack of information about the activity, lack of transportation, or fear of joining a new group. Nurses can help with all of these problems. Promoting interaction between clients at social events may make a big difference in whether or not the person feels a part of the group and decides to attend future group functions. Simply taking the client to a function is not enough. Planning

must be done to prevent any embarrassment to clients during group activities. They should not be asked or expected to do things beyond their abilities. Special efforts should be made to provide for physical needs at group functions. This includes preventing incontinence and providing food for those on restricted diets, if refreshments are a part of the activity.

Physical exercise may be helpful in stimulating cognitive functioning. Powell (1974) compared the effects of exercise therapy with those of social therapy and found that after a 12-week period the group that had participated in exercise therapy showed significant improvement in cognitive functioning. Exercise also promotes sleep, and it is known that lack of sleep interferes with cognitive functioning. The amount and type of exercise, of course, will vary according to the physical limitations of the client.

For some individuals, music therapy is effective in improving cognitive functioning. According to Beavers (1969), the study and practice of music promote improved concentration, memory, and attention span. Kartman (1977) has reported on the use of music therapy to reengage older clients. Self-identity and socialization improved among members of the group who participated in music therapy.

Remotivation groups to promote sensory stimulation can be formed either in the community or in the institution. These groups are designed to reactivate individual interests, abilities, and activities, and they provide opportunities for socializing, stimulating thinking, imagining, remembering, and making choices (Needler and Baer, 1982). Although providing opportunities and reinforcing participation is likely to have a positive effect, the success of remotivation programs for a particular individual is largely influenced by the person's previous interests, degree of enthusiasm, and the satisfaction he or she has received from being involved in similar activities in the past. When forming remotivation groups, it is important to bring together persons who are compatible with one another, and to keep the group small enough to permit recognition and acceptance of each person at every session. Individuals should be given reinforcement both for attendance and for the contributions they make to the group. At the same time, the leader should be careful not to reinforce undesirable behaviors. Although members of the group should be encouraged to participate, the leader must avoid making excessive demands on any individual. Ideas for topics of the meetings can come from current events, common experiences, and past interests and hobbies. Older people often enjoy comparing and contrasting today with yesterday.

Toepfer, Bicknell, and Shaw (1974) suggest utilizing props in remotivation groups. Props should include pictures, maps, or objects relevant to the topic being discussed. Participants should be encouraged to bring articles related to the subject under discussion.

Nursing Measures to Prevent Sensory Overload

Excessive stimulation interferes with learning and comprehension. To understand this, try to recall a time when you experienced an excessive amount of stimulation. Perhaps it was your first few days at a new school or college. Think about how difficult it was to find your room, the cafeteria, or to remember when you were supposed to be where and for which class. If you, who have not experienced the cognitive changes of aging, felt overwhelmed, try to imagine how an older person might feel in a totally new environment, such as a nursing home.

The degree of stimulation considered to be excessive varies tremendously among individuals. For Mrs. E, excessive stimulation was receiving more than one item at a time on her meal tray. If only one dish, such as a bowl of cereal, was placed in front of her, she could feed herself without difficulty. If her tray contained several items, such as eggs, toast, juice, coffee, and cereal, she became completely immobilized and was unable to feed herself anything. Nurses should be alert for cues that a client is receiving too much stimulation, such as confusion, bewilderment, or lack of response. Persons who are experiencing sensory overload related to brain failure may become aggressive in order to defend themselves. Invading what the institutionalized aged

person perceives as his or her personal space or territory may result in physical aggressiveness. Aggressiveness often occurs when the person feels threatened because of an inability to control his environment (Maagdenberg, 1983). In many instances a violent action is a defensive response to an invasion of what is perceived as personal and private area. Nurses can reduce the chances of violence by explaining their purpose and plans prior to invading a person's territory.

It is best to prevent excessive stimulation before it occurs. Usually, it can be avoided by taking one thing at a time. In obtaining information, phrase questions so that only one thought is being asked. Remember that the older person takes longer to react and longer to comprehend. If a second question is asked before the first one is answered, the person may not answer either. A delayed response may indicate that the individual did not understand the question. Conversely, it may indicate that he understood the question but is simply taking a while to formulate a response.

When teaching a client something, teach only one step at a time. Do not assume that the person grasped the first step; obtain feedback, such as return demonstration, to confirm that the first step was understood. The process of obtaining feedback enhances learning, as learning is an active process. The more actively an individual tries to comprehend something, the more likely that he will retain what is being taught. Because recall and practice also enhance learning, opportunities for recall should be provided soon after learning has occurred, and at appropriate intervals thereafter.

Another means of preventing excessive stimulation is to eliminate irrelevant stimuli, which are more distracting to the elderly than to younger persons. When trying to obtain information from a client and when providing directions or instructions, communications should be brief, concise, and to the point. For example, if you are instructing the client to go to the hematology lab, brief, concise instructions would be: "Turn down the second hall to the right. The hematology lab is the third door on the left." Directions containing irrelevant stimuli might be: "Walk past the beauty shop and the gift shop. Then you will come to the corridor that leads to the pharmacy. Keep going until you pass inhalation therapy, then turn down the first hall to the right. You will see signs for many labs. Walk past the cytology and the biochemistry lab. The next one is hematology, where you are to go." The first set of instructions is more likely to be retained, as they are simple, brief, and to the point. The second set of instructions is complex, unclear, and contains much irrelevant information.

Memory reminders help the individual to cope with excessive stimuli. These are usually brief notes or instruction cards that enable a person to follow directions, function more independently, or develop routines. Memory reminders should be well organized and concise. Using pictures, both when communicating verbally and in the written instructions, promotes comprehension. Cues can be used to help persons recall information. Usually it is easier for people to recognize information than to recall it. Recognition can be encouraged by giving persons a choice of responses when asking questions (Carroll and Gray-Fliss, 1978).

Feedback is important in memory training. Feedback should be immediate, whether it is for an appropriate or an inappropriate response. However, the nurse must take care to be tactful when providing feedback for inappropriate responses. If the client feels humiliated he may withdraw from further participation. Positive feedback must be perceived by the client as being positive, and should motivate the person to continue participation.

Sensory overload can be minimized through optimal usage of things familiar to the client. This includes use of terminology that the client understands, use of equipment with which he is familiar, and the utilization of previous experiences. Equipment should be the same as that which will be used by the client in his own environment. Whenever possible, it is best to instruct the client in that environment or in one similar to it.

If more than one person is involved in a teaching plan, communication among personnel is important. All should take part in formulating the plan and should know what has been taught. Knowledge should be shared in identifying difficulties and in revising the plan. It is best to keep a written account of what is being taught for each individual, to increase consistency among the personnel involved in the teaching.

Factors that interfere with learning include fatigue and excessive anxiety. In order to avoid fatigue during the teaching–learning process, teaching should take place when the person is well rested and not troubled by other problems. Sensory overload causes fatigue. Once it has occurred, teaching should be discontinued until the person has had a chance to rest. Since excessive anxiety also interferes with learning, teaching should be delayed if the person's stress level is high.

To be successful, the teaching goals must be the client's learning goals. The client should be involved in deciding what should be taught, when teaching will occur, and how teaching should take place. If the material to be taught is not meaningful to the person, it will not be retained.

When sensory overload is a problem, measures need to be taken to assure that the person does not assume responsibilities beyond his or her capabilities. Doing so may be hazardous to the older person or others in the environment. Health team or family members may have to intervene when it is no longer safe for the person to operate machinery such as a motor vehicle. Activities such as driving require good vision, good hearing, quick reaction time, ability to make appropriate decisions without hesitation, good coordination, and alertness to environmental factors (Mace and Rabins, 1981). Giving up driving may have an effect on self-esteem and independence as well as lead to depression. The problem must be approached with much tact and understanding. Telling somebody that he is a terrible driver is likely to provoke resentment and anger, whereas observing that lately he seems to be having difficulty with driving will elicit a more favorable response. When it is necessary for the person to quit driving, alternatives should be presented to enable the person to continue his or her activities. If the person refuses to quit driving the support of the physician or attorney may be necessary. In some states the Department of Motor Vehicles will suspend a license or investigate if a written statement from the physician indicates that the person's health makes him or her an unsafe driver (Mace and Rabins, 1981).

Nursing Measures to Reduce Depression

The role of the nurse in reducing depression is primarily related to those measures that increase self-esteem (see Chapter 8) and in the measures to promote sensory stimulation (p. 330). Intervention should be focused on utilizing the person's remaining assets. In order to prevent a fixation on withdrawal the person needs to be directed toward new interests, contacts, and activities. Measures need to be taken to increase social contacts and to prevent or to reduce sensory deprivation (Verwoerdt, 1981). Establishing a hopeful attitude is helpful in regaining self-esteem. Assistance is needed in accepting what cannot be changed, in forgetting failures, and in developing stimulating but realistic goals (Sternback, 1980). For some, group involvement is helpful.

Cognitive Functioning and Drugs

Medications can either interfere with or improve the cognitive functioning of the elderly. Old persons tend to be more susceptible to the side effects of drugs which affect cognition. When there is a deterioration of cognitive processes, it should be determined whether the problems are related to the side effects of a medication or whether they are caused by interactions between drugs the person is taking. Drug categories such as hypnotics, tranquilizers, and antidepressants frequently cause daytime drowsiness, vertigo, and confusion in older persons. The two most common categories of psychotropic drugs used to treat cognitive problems in the elderly are tranquilizers and antidepressants.

Because a number of hazards are associated with the use of psychotropic drugs, efforts should be made to minimize their use. A therapeutic environment in which nursing approaches are utilized effectively may eliminate or reduce the need for such drugs. When it is necessary to administer psychotropic drugs, the smallest possible dosage to obtain a therapeutic effect should be given. It is important to remember that the elderly excrete drugs more slowly than younger adults. Initially, old persons usually receive one-quarter to one-half of the usual adult dosage of psychotropic drugs. The dosage is then gradually increased until the symptoms are controlled. Finally, the dosage is slowly reduced until the symptoms return or until the dose is zero. Usually, spontaneous remission of symptoms takes place. It is rare for persons who have functioned in the community until old age to require maintenance on psychotropic drugs until death (Glickman and Friedman, 1976).

Nurses have an important role in determining whether a particular medication has been effective, in identifying side effects, and in teaching the person receiving drugs. Both client and family should be told to watch for decreased levels of alertness, especially when the drug is administered initially. During this period, the person should avoid driving and operating potentially hazardous equipment. The physician should be notified if stupor develops.

Because individuals may become tolerant to tranquilizers, they should be warned against increasing the dosage on their own. Antidepressants can cause cardiac arrhythmias. Both tranquilizers and antidepressants can cause postural hypotension. The client should be told to move from a lying to a sitting position and from a sitting to a standing position slowly, to avoid dizziness, and to hold on to something when changing positions. Problems with hypotension usually disappear about 10 days after the dosage has been stabilized. They are usually most pronounced initially and when the dosage is being increased (Glickman and Friedman, 1976). Anticholinergic side effects may also occur. The more common problems include dry mouth, constipation, blurred vision, and urinary retention.

Major tranquilizers can cause extrapyramidal symptoms during the first few weeks of administration. These symptoms include insomnia and restlessness, numbness and muscle weakness, spastic muscle movements, muscle rigidity, and tremors. All except the restlessness and insomnia tend to appear within the first 2 weeks, and usually disappear within

2 to 16 weeks (Newton, Godbey, Newton, and Godbey, 1978).

Cerebral vasodilators have long been used for treatment of brain dysfunction. However, there appears to be little justification for their use. This is indicated in a study by Branconnier and Cole (1977).

Little has been written on the problem of alcoholism and the aged. Segal has indicated that the craving for alcohol is less intense in the aged, but at the same time old people seem to display a decreased tolerance for alcohol (Segal, 1977). Alcoholism in the elderly frequently leads to brain failure and other neurologic problems.

Alcoholism is a definite problem among the aged. Many elderly alcoholics have a past history of alcohol abuse. Persons who become alcoholics during old age, however, are usually those who find it difficult to cope with various problems and resort to alcohol as a means of escape. In a study by Brown (1982), professionals attributed drug and alcohol abuse among the elderly to loss of productive social roles or functions, loneliness, lack of supportive social relationships, or acquiring a drinking habit during earlier years. The aged need to be cautioned about mixing alcohol with drugs. More needs to be known about the problem, prevention, and treatment of alcoholism among the elderly.

EVALUATION OF INTERVENTION

The effectiveness of approaches should be measured against the criteria that have been established for specific client-centered goals. Since criteria are specific for each individual, only general guidelines can be given here. The following indicates items which can be considered in the evaluation of nursing measures.

Evaluation of measures to promote orientation to the environment

- Determine evidence of gains and losses with regard to
  Awareness of time
  Interest in time
  Awareness of the identities and functions of persons in the environment

  Independence in movement about life space
  Size of life space
  Awareness of sources of orientation
- Determine if sources of orientation are
  Reliable
  Of significance to the client

Evaluation of measures to promote sensory stimulation

- Determine whether sources of stimulation are
  Perceivable according to client's sensory status
  In accordance with client's interests and tastes
  Available according to need
  Perceived
  Effective in eliciting a positive response
  Varied to an optimal degree
- Determine evidence of client's
  Response to intervention
  Attitude toward stimulation

Evaluation of measures to prevent sensory overload

- Determine evidence of changes in
  Attention span
  Appropriateness of responses
  Progress toward learning goals
  Orientation
  Comprehension
  Attentiveness to relevant stimuli
  Occurrence of fatigue

Evaluation of measures to reduce depression

- Determine evidence of changes in
  Degree of self-esteem
  Involvement in activities
  Interaction with others
  Establishment of goals
  Amount of focus on past
  Views of future

General evaluation considerations

- Determine evidence of
  Consistency of client's response to implementation
  Response and understanding of significant others to implementation
  Response and understanding of health team members to implementation

Change in client's independence of functioning

Change in interest and attitude

Change in physiologic complaints

Environmental variables affecting response

Pattern of response to implementation

Client's desire to change

Support from significant others

The need to re-evaluate goals and priorities

CONCLUSION

It is hoped that the cognitive status of the elderly will be improved through increased understanding of the problems and appropriate treatment. Nurses should become more involved in teaching health-care workers and families ways in which they can better assist clients. More emphasis needs to be placed on the importance of intervention to improve the client's cognitive status. Nurses should assume a more active role in researching various methods of implementation with regard to improving cognitive status.

RECOMMENDED READINGS

Birren, J.E., Schaie, K.W. Handbook of the Psychology of Aging. New York, Van Nostrand Reinhold, 1977. *A comprehensive discussion of the physiological and environmental influences on the behavior of the aged person. Contains in-depth significant research.*

Birren, J.E., Sloane, R.B. Handbook of Mental Health and Aging. Englewood Cliffs, NJ, Prentice-Hall, 1980. *A comprehensive presentation of the latest findings and concepts related to the mental health of the aged. Included is content related to the physiological, behavioral and social sciences. Normal change pathology, treatment and prevention are covered.*

Mace, N.L., Rabins, P.V. The 36 Hour Day: A Family Guide to Caring for Persons with Alzheimer's Disease, Related Dementing Illnesses, and Memory Loss in Later Life. Baltimore, The Johns Hopkins University Press, 1981. *An excellent guide for families and nurses who are providing care for aged persons who are experiencing brain failure. Contains many practical suggestions.*

Wolanin, M.O., Phillips, L.R.F. Confusion Prevention and Care. St. Louis, Mosby, 1981. *A comprehensive presentation on the role of nurses in assessing and intervening for clients experiencing confusion.*

REFERENCES CITED

Adams, R.D. The morphological aspects of aging in the human nervous system, in Birren, J., Sloane, R.B. (eds), Handbook of Mental Health and Aging. Englewood Cliffs, NJ, Prentice-Hall, 1980, pp 149–160

Alzeheimer's that isn't. Transition 1(3):16, 1983

Arenberg, D. Cognition and aging: Verbal learning, learning, memory, and problem solving, in Eisdorfer, C., Lawton, M.P. (eds), The Psychology of Adult Development and Aging. Washington, D.C., American Psychiatric Association, 1973

Arenberg, D., Robertson-Tchabo, E.A. Learning and aging, in Birren, J.E., Schaie, K.W. (eds), Handbook of the Psychology of Aging. New York, Van Nostrand Reinhold, 1977

Beavers, V. Music therapy. American Journal of Nursing 69(1):89, 1969

Bellak, L. Psychological aspects of normal aging, in Bellak, L., Karasu, T.B. (eds), Geriatric Psychiatry: A Handbook for Psychiatrists and Primary Care Physicians. New York, Grune and Stratton, 1976

Billing, D.M., Stokes, L.G. Medical–Surgical Nursing. St. Louis, Mosby, 1982

Birren, J.E., Renner, V.J. Research on the psychology of aging: Principles and experimentation, in Birren, J.E., Schaie, K.W. (eds), Handbook of the Psychology of Aging. New York, Van Nostrand Reinhold, 1977, pp 3–38

Black, Sr, K. Social isolation and the nursing process. Nursing Clinics of North America 8(4):575, 1973

Bondareff, W. The neural basis of aging, in Birren, J.E., Schaie, K.W., (eds) Handbook of the Psychology of Aging. New York, Van Nostrand Reinhold, 1977, pp 157–176

Botwinick, J. Aging and Behavior: A Comprehensive Integration of Research Findings. New York, Springer, 1973

Botwinick, J. Intellectual abilities, in Birren, J.E., Schaie, K.W. (eds), Handbook of the Psychology of Aging. New York, Van Nostrand Reinhold, 1977, pp 580–605

Branconnier, R., Cole, O. Senile dementia and drug therapy, in Nandy, K., Sherion, I. (eds), The Aging

Brain and Senile Dementia Advances in Behavioral Biology. New York, Plenum, 1977, pp 271–283

Brown, B.B. Professionals' perceptions of drug and alcohol abuse among the elderly. The Gerontologist 22(6):519, 1982

Burnside, I.M. Psychosocial issues in nursing care of the aged. Journal of Gerontological Nursing 7(11):689, 1981

Burrill, R., McCourt, J.F., Cutter, H.S.G. Beer: A social facilitator for FMI patients? The Gerontologist 14(5):430, 1974

Butler, R.N., Lewis, M.I. Aging and Mental Health. St. Louis, Mosby, 1977

Carroll, K., Gray-Fliss, K. Memory Development. Prepared through the Human Development in Aging Project, NIMH Grant No. 23924, Minneapolis, Ebenezer Society, 1978

Carroll, P.J. The social hour for geropsychiatric patients. Journal of the American Geriatric Society 26(1):32, 1978

Chodil, J., Williams, B. The concept of sensory deprivation. Nursing Clinics of North America 5(3):453, 1970

Comfort, A. Non-threatening mental testing of the elderly. Journal of the American Geriatric Society 26(6):261, 1978

Craik, F.I. Age differences in human memory, in Birren, J.E., Schaie, K.W. (eds), Handbook of the Psychology of Aging. New York, Van Nostrand Reinhold, 1977, pp 384–420

Eisdorfer, C., Wilkie, F. Disease, aging and behavior, in Birren, J.E., Schaie, K.W. (eds), Handbook of the Psychology of Aging, New York, Van Nostrand Reinhold, 1977, pp 251–275

Elias, M.F., Elias P.K. Motivation and activity, in Birren, J.E., Schaie, K.W. (eds), Handbook of the Psychology of Aging. New York, Van Nostrand Reinhold, 1977, pp 357–383

Fishback, D.B. Mental status questionnaire of organic brain syndrome, with a new visual counting test. Journal of the American Geriatric Society 25(4):167, 1977

Ford, C.V., Winter, J. Computerized axial tomograma and dementia in elderly persons. Journal of Gerontology 36(2):164, 1981

Fox, J.H., Topel, J.L., Huckman, M.S. Dementia in the elderly—a search for treatable illnesses. Journal of Gerontology 30(5):557, 1975

Frey, L.A. Education and consultation on mental health in long-term care facilities: Problems, pitfalls and solutions. Learning and teaching with adults—with special reference to long-term care training. Geriatric Psychiatry 10(2):137, 1977

Glickman, L., Friedman, S. Changes in behavior, mood, or thinking in the elderly: Diagnosis and management. Medical Clinics of North America 60(6):1297, 1976

Goga, J.A., Hambacher, W.D. Psychologic and behavioral assessment of patients: A review. Journal of the American Geriatric Society 25(5):232, 1977

Grauer, H. Depression in the aged: Theoretical concepts. Journal of the American Geriatric Society 25(10):447, 1977

Hogstel, M.O. Use of reality orientation with aging confused patients. Nursing Research 28(3):161, 1979

Hoyer, W.J., Labouvie, G.V., Baltes, P.B. Modification of response speed deficits and intellectual performance in the elderly. Human Development 16(3):233, 1973

Hussian, R.A. Geriatric Psychology: A Behavioral Perspective. New York, Van Nostrand Reinhold, 1981

Jarvik, L.F. Aging and depression: Some unanswered questions. Journal of Gerontology 31(3):324, 1976

Kartman, L.L. The use of music as a program tool with regressed geriatric patients. Journal of Gerontological Nursing 3(4):38, 1977

Kausler, D.H., Kleim, D.M. Age differences in processing relevant versus irrelevant stimuli in multiple-item recognition learning. Journal of Gerontology 33(1):87, 1978

Kinney, M. Neurologic assessment, in Phipps, W.J., Loog, B.C., Woods, N.F. (eds), Medical Surgical Nursing. St. Louis, Mosby, 1979

Knox, A.B. Adult development and learning. San Francisco, Jossey-Bass, 1977, p 679

Langston, N.F. Reality orientation and effective reinforcement. Journal of Gerontological Nursing 7(4):224, 1981

Lawson, J.S., Rodenburg, M., Dykes, J.A. A dementia rating scale for use with psychogeriatric patients. Journal of Gerontology 32(2):153, 1977

Lehman, E. Reality orientation: Doing it better. Nursing '74 3:61, 1974

Luckmann, J., Sorensen, K.C. Medical-Surgical Nursing: A Psychophysiologic Approach. Philadelphia, Saunders, 1974

Maagdenberg, A.M. The "violent" patient. American Journal of Nursing 83(3):402, 1983

Mace, N.L., Rabins, P.V. The 36-Hour Day: A Family Guide to Caring for Persons with Alzheimer's Disease, Related Dementing Illnesses, and Memory Loss in Later Life. Baltimore, The John Hopkins University Press, 1981

Marsh, G.R., Thompson, L.W. Psychophysiology of aging, in Birren, J.E., Schaie, K.W. (eds), Handbook of the Psychology of Aging. New York, Van Nostrand Reinhold, 1977, pp 219–248

Mattis, S. Mental status examination for organic mental syndrome in the elderly patient, in Bellak, L., Karasu, T.B. (eds), Geriatric Psychiatry: A Handbook for Psychiatrists and Primary Care Physicians. New York, Grune and Stratton, 1976, pp 77–121

Needler, W., Baer, M.A. Movement, music, and re-motivation with the regressed elderly. Journal of Gerontological Nursing 8(9):497–503, 1982

Newton, M., Godbey, K.L., Newton, D.W., Godbey, A.L. How you can improve the effectiveness of psychotropic drug therapy. Nursing '78 8(7):46, 1978

Nodhturft, V.L., Sweeney, N.M. Reality orientation therapy for the institutionalized elderly. Journal of Gerontological Nursing 8(7):396, 1982

Onter, C. Sensory deprivation in geriatric patients. Journal of the American Geriatric Society 24(10):461, 1976

Pfeiffer, E. A short portable mental status questionnaire for the assessment of organic brain deficit in elderly patients. Journal of the American Geriatric Society 23(10):433, 1975

Pfeiffer, E. Psychopathology and social pathology, in Birren, J., Schaie, K.W. (eds), Handbook of the Psychology of Aging. New York, Van Nostrand Reinhold, 1977, pp 650–671

Powell, R.R. Psychological effects of exercise therapy upon institutionalized geriatric mental patients. Journal of Gerontology 29(2):157, 1974

Riegel, K.F. History of psychological gerontology, in Birren, J., Schaie, K.W. (eds), Handbook of the Psychology of Aging. New York, Van Nostrand Reinhold, 1977, pp 70–102

Robb, S.S., Monsour, N. Wandering Behavior in Old Age: A Psychosocial Exploration. Paper presented at the meeting of the Gerontological Society, San Diego, California, November, 1980

Rosin, A.J. The physical and behavioral complex dementia. Gerontology 23(1):37, 1977

Ryden, M.B. Nursing intervention in support of reminiscence. Journal of Gerontological Nursing 7(8):462, 1981

Salzman, C., Shader, R.I. Depression in the elderly. I: Relationship between depression, psychologic defense mechanisms and physical illness. Journal of the American Geriatric Society 26(6):253, 1978

Scarbrough, D. Speaking out reality orientation: A new approach to an old problem. Nursing '74 4(11):12, 1974

Schaie, K.W. Scaling the association between colors and mood tones. American Journal of Psychology 74(2):266, 1961

Schultz, D.P. Sensory Restriction Effects on Behavior. New York, Academic, 1965

Segal, B.M. The effect of the age factor on alcoholism, in Seixas, F.A. (ed), Currents in Alcoholism. New York, Grune and Stratton, 1977, vol II

Smith, J.M., Oswald, W.T., Waterman, L.J. Relationship between the Geriatric Interpersonal Evaluation Scale and the WAIS Verbal Scale. Perceptual and Motor Skills 44:571, 1977

Snyder, L.H. Environmental changes for socialization. Journal of Nursing Administration 8(1):44, 1978

Snyder, L.H., Rupprecht, P., Pyrek, J., Brekhus, S., Moss, T. Wandering. The Gerontologist 18(3):272, 1978

Sternbach, A. Depression and suicidal behavior in old age, in Birren, J.E., Sloane, R.B. (eds), Handbook of Mental Health and Aging. Englewood Cliffs, NJ, Prentice-Hall, 1980

Storandt, M. Psychologic Aspect, in Steinberg, F.U. (ed), Cowdry's The Care of the Geriatric Patient. St. Louis, Mosby, 1976, pp 321–333

Toepfer, C.T., Bicknell, A.T., Shaw, D.C. Remotivation as behavior therapy. The Gerontologist 10:451, 1974

Verwoerdt, A. Clinical Geropsychiatry. Baltimore, Williams & Wilkins, 1981

Voelkel, D. A study of reality orientation and resocialization groups with confused elderly. Journal of Gerontological Nursing 4(3):13, 1978

Vogel, F.S. The brain and time, in Busse, E.W., Pfeiffer, E. (eds), Behavior and Adaptation in Late Life. Boston, Little, Brown, 1977, pp 228–239

Wershow, H.J. Reality orientation for gerontologists: Some thoughts about senility. The Gerontologist 17(4):297, 1977

Wexner, L.B. The degree to which colors (hues) are associated with mood-tones. Journal of Applied Psychology 38(6):432, 1954

Wolanin, M.O., Phillips, L.R.L. Confusion prevention and care. St. Louis, Mosby, 1981

Zung, W.K., Richards, C., Short, M.J. Self-rating depression scale in an outpatient clinic. Archives of General Psychiatry 13(6):508, 1965

10

Sensory Experiences of the Elderly Person

Ann Gera Yurick

Reading this chapter will enable the individual to:

1. Appreciate the interrelationship of sensory functioning and behavior
2. Assess taste, touch, and smell sensitivity of the elderly person
3. Know the nursing interventions for age-related changes in touch
4. Know the nursing interventions for the elderly person who experiences pain
5. Know the nursing interventions for age-related changes in smell
6. Know the nursing interventions for age-related changes in taste

The functional ability of the elderly person's senses has a marked influence on his perceptions of the world, and can influence both his behavior and the behavior of others toward him. Basic to the individual's relationship with other people and with the environment is the ability to sense and perceive within the living environment. Sensory detection and perception are complex feedback systems. These systems involve the sensory organs as well as the interactions of several hormones, neurotransmitters, and the nervous system.

Perception includes the evaluation of information gathered by the senses and the meaning that is attached to it. Each person moving through a world of constant external and internal stimulation is affected by objects, events, and other people in the environment. These are interpreted in terms of the individual's past experience, and behavior is modified according to this interpretation. Perception is thus characterized by constant interaction with the environment and the associated mental processes of interpreting external events.

When exposed to many external stimuli, each person recognizes and gives priority to messages that have personal meaning or that are necessary for continued survival. The individual's response to a stimulus can be affected by the intensity, size, change, or repetition of that stimulus (Chodel and Williams, 1970). The effect of the stimulus should be considered. High-intensity stimulation, such as loud music or a cloyingly heavy perfume, can provoke unpleasant feelings, whereas softer music or a delicate fragrance are usually perceived as pleasant.

The individual's perception of a stimulus is highly dependent upon the context of the situation and on past experience (Marks, 1974), which influences the way stimuli are symbolically organized. A person's behavior is regulated by the external environment and the biopsychosociocultural background, because all of these factors influence the information upon which a response is based (Auger, 1976). In health, all senses work together to enhance the meaning of the information received.

As aging occurs, sensory changes usually develop. These changes occur gradually. The rate of change varies with the individual person as well as with each sensory organ. These changes can affect the reception of stimuli, thus altering the person's perception of his or her internal and external environment. A highly developed area of research is concerned with age-related changes in sensory function. The study of the direct relationship between the specific properties of the physical stimulus and the perceived quality experienced by the individual is called *psychophysics* (Auger, 1976). A fundamental tenet of psychophysics is the view that under certain conditions, people can make meaningful evaluations of the magnitude of their sensory experiences (Marks, 1974). These experiences include the interrelationships among visual, auditory, and olfactory processes, as well as taste and the tactile senses. Both the intensity and the quality of sensation are studied. The affective aspects of sensory experience are also included. Corso (1971, 1981) provides a review of experimental studies that have attempted to determine exactly the kind and amount of change that takes place over time in the sensory functions of adults.

The nurse can take part in research into age-related sensory changes, and is also a consumer of research findings in directing intervention toward compensating for these changes. Elderly people can be maintained in a healthy state even though sensory changes develop. The sensory changes present in most older persons vary in degree and do not necessarily imply dysfunction. A person who is considered "elderly" does not necessarily have to sense and perceive the environment in a dysfunctional manner. The nurse should determine which sensory processes are altered and the degree of alterations. Because alterations in sensory reception can lead to behavioral changes, it is important that the nurse consider both the person's behavior and the behaviors of others toward that person. The remaining senses can continue to function to receive information. One of the nurse's major concerns, therefore, is the adequacy of the old person's adaptation to sensory changes. The nurse can help the elderly client to determine sensory assets so that compensation can be made for any deficits present, and can assist the client's adjustment to sensory changes. Adjustment in this sense refers to the use of behaviors that enable the individual to function in the environment in which he lives.

The nurse must give particular consideration to the old person's environment. A decrease in sensory adequacy has a major influence on the world in which the elderly person lives. Therefore, the nurse should try to understand what effect a given sensory deficit has on the client's self-image, social relations, and ability to function in the physical environment. Changes in sensory functioning may cause changes in the person's territorial claims, so that the territory becomes more limited.

Because people interact with their environment through sensation and perception, the nurse should remember that the environment can become functionally different when a client's sensory and perceptual processes are altered. Understanding the elderly person's relationship to the environment is crucial to understanding the person's behavior, as well as the interventions that relate to this behavior. Carefully planned environmental modifications can support adaptation to sensory changes, facilitate self-sufficiency, and make life more meaningful for the elderly person. In many instances, the filtering effects of sensory changes can be decreased by increasing the amount and intensity of environmental stimulation and impact. Because the mind experiences the internal and external world through the senses, the person needs to have knowledge of that environment in order to adapt to and interact with the environment. The nurse needs to consider the sensory stimulation that is available in the environment of the elderly client (Fig. 10.1.)

Sensory deprivation can occur as a result of the sensory changes connected with the aging process. The next three chapters will discuss the age-related changes that affect hearing, vision, taste, smell, and touch. These changes in reception, in turn, affect the individual's sensory perceptions. The major focus of discussion will be the nurse's role in assessing the elderly client's sensory status and planning with the client for most effective use of the senses. With some elderly clients, systematic sensory assessment may be limited by physical or mental health problems. However, valuable sensory assessment data can be obtained through observation during physical activities and at mealtime, and from verbal and

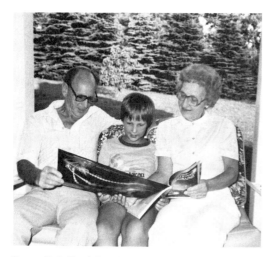

Figure 10.1. The interrelationship of the person's senses can add to the enjoyment of life.

nonverbal responses during communication. Facilitators to sensory assessment include the presence of significant others, a familiar setting, and a time of day when energy levels are higher. The person should also understand and agree with the value of the sensory assessment process. A change or loss of one of the senses can affect the functioning of the other senses.

The purposes of the assessment of sensory functioning include the early detection of sensory changes, the prevention of adaptation problems resulting from sensory changes, and the promotion of the most efficient use of the remaining sensory functions. The assets of the client as well as changes experienced by the client need to be determined. Sensory assessment provides a basis for planning and implementing care directed toward promotion and maintenance of the client's health.

THE ELDERLY PERSON'S SENSE OF TOUCH AND BODY SENSITIVITY: ASSESSMENT BASE

Tactile Sensitivity

Changes in sensitivity to touch often accompany the aging process. However, the degree of change varies among individuals. In some cases, there are losses that are related to neuropathy caused by pathologies, injury, or circulatory insufficiency. Changes in touch sensitivity among the elderly population have not been studied as extensively as other sensory areas. However, research indicates that there may be a change in sensitivity of the skin on the palm of the hand and the sole of the foot, but not of hairy skin (Kenshalo, 1977). This may be caused by degenerative changes in the Meissner corpuscles, believed to be the receptors responsible for sensitivity to light touch. Meissner corpuscles may exhibit changes in size, shape, and relationship to the epidermis.

Decreased acuity in the sense of touch can affect the elderly person's ability to localize stimuli and can also reduce the speed of reaction to tactile stimulation. For example, an old person may have difficulty differentiating between coins, fastening buttons, or grasping small items as a result of difficulty in sharply localizing stimuli. The decrease in speed of reaction to tactile stimulation may lead to injury because the stimulus is not perceived as quickly. An example might be trauma to the foot from the pressure of a tight shoe. The slower response to noxious agents (such as chemical irritants) or to temperature extremes can cause greater trauma to the elderly person than to a younger one, because the old person takes longer to become aware of a harmful stimulus.

Touch

The elderly person's freedom to touch others and the comfort in being touched by others frequently can be related to the person's cultural and social history. In a study of nursing home patients' perceptions of touch by nurses, deWever (1977) found that patient's feelings about affective touch developed by his or her socialization. Another consideration is the freedom and comfort health-care providers experience in touching the elderly. Barnett (1972) found that in the hospital setting, the age group receiving the least frequent amount of touch by health personnel was the 66- to 100-year-old group. Huss (1977) observed that the lack of meaningful touch with others compounds the elderly person's diminished sensorium. To-

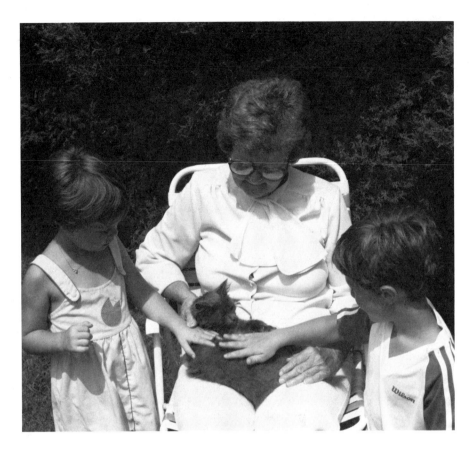

Figure 10.2. This elderly person's tactile sensitivity is enhanced through contact with a variety of textures and through touching another person. *(Photograph by Ed Spier, Pittsburgh, PA.)*

biason (1981) reported that nursing students were unsure of their feelings about touching the aged or were unable to express their feelings. Nursing students experienced more anxiety in anticipating than actually touching the elderly. Experience is needed in interacting with and touching older people in order for the nurse to feel comfortable with a therapeutic level of interaction.

Further study of touch sensitivity of the elderly is needed. It may be that with the generalized thinning of epidermal skin layers, some elderly may experience an increase in touch sensitivity in some areas of the body.

Thermal Sensitivity

The temperature-regulating system of the elderly person may display impaired ability to cope with extreme environmental temperatures, especially low temperature (Kenshalo, 1977). With aging there is a degeneration of papillary capillaries. These capillaries are close to the body surface and are responsible for skin nourishment and heat dissipation. This change in vascular circulation as well as loss of subcutaneous tissue predisposes an elderly person to feeling cold. Institutional settings, air conditioned for the comfort of the employees, may cause the elderly client to be very uncomfortable. On days that seem quite warm to a younger person, an elderly person may find it necessary to wear a sweater. Corso (1981), however, reported that some researchers suggest that older people do not experience cold as intensely as young people. As a result, they may not avoid or alter cold environments. Watts (1971) found that elderly people with low mouth temperature have a greater risk of developing hypothermia because there is no safety margin for additional heat loss.

Pain Sensitivity

Pain responses can be elicited by a wide variety of mechanical, chemical, thermal, and electrical stimuli. Pain receptors are not specialized to react to a single form of energy (Corso, 1981). The elderly person often displays decreased sensitivity to pain. This may be due to degenerative changes in the receptors and peripheral nervous system. However, information gathered by studies of the pain threshold and pain tolerance in the elderly is conflicting. The subjective definition of pain is a variable that seems difficult to control. Pain is an individual and unique experience. The experience of pain and the way the individual reports it seem to be closely related to personality and cultural background. As a result of life experiences, the elderly person may have learned to cope with pain, especially pain that is chronic. Differences in skin thickness and elasticity may also affect pain sensitivity. It is important for the nurse to remember that the fact that an elderly person may demonstrate decreased pain sensitivity does not make it any easier for the individual to cope with the pain that is experienced.

Pain can increase the elderly person's anxiety and increase the sense of helplessness. Pain can be a lonely experience for elderly persons who have experienced many losses in their support systems. With decreased sensitivity to pain, the elderly person may not be as aware of warnings indicating pathologies accompanied by the inflammatory process. Abdominal or cardiac problems may not be accurately diagnosed because the elderly person may not experience the severity of pain experienced by a younger person. Another concern relating to pain is the elderly person's response to analgesics. As a result of changes in the metabolism and excretion of drugs, some elderly persons may become confused or have problems with maintaining equilibrium when some pain medications are given. In addition to altered mental states, toxic accumulation of analgesics can lead to respiratory depression and cardiac irritability. Meinhart and McCaffery (1983) reported that complaints of pain in the elderly may be related to factors such as loneliness, boredom, depression, and the desire to conceal a problem that is not acceptable such as memory loss.

Vibratory Sensitivity

Changes in the elderly person's sensitivity to vibrating stimuli are sometimes connected with nervous system disorders. However, clinical and experimental measurements have demonstrated that there is a definite loss of sensitivity to vibration in a significant proportion of old people in whom no pathologies have been detected. The loss of vibratory sensitivity seems to begin at about age 50, and tends to be more severe in the lower than in the upper extremities (Kenshalo, 1977). This may be due to undetected changes in the microcirculation of the legs or the lower spinal cord.

Stereognosis

Stereognosis is defined as the person's ability to recognize an object by touching and manipulating it. Deficits in this area for the elderly person may involve identification of more complex designs. When such deficits occur, they appear to be connected with impairment of central neurologic processes (Kenshalo, 1977).

NURSING ASSESSMENT OF TOUCH AND PAIN

Assessment of Light Touch

Sensitivity to light touch is assessed by touching the skin with a wisp of cotton. Instruct the client to close both eyes, to eliminate visual cueing. The skin itself should be tested, rather than the hair on the skin. The client is then asked to tell the nurse when the cotton is felt and to point to the spot where he or she was touched. In performing this assessment the nurse should apply only light pressure, because actual depression of the skin may stimulate the deep touch receptors.

Assessment of Thermal Sensitivity

Thermal sensitivity can be assessed by filling one test tube with cold water and one with warm water. Extremes of water temperature should be avoided. While the client closes both eyes, a test tube is applied to the skin. The client is directed to indicate whether this tube is perceived as warm or cold.

Assessment of Pain Sensitivity

A safety pin is used to assess pain sensitivity. While the person closes both eyes, the nurse touches the skin in such a way that the client will respond to sharpness rather than to pressure. Deep or heavy touch sensation is transmitted through different tracts from those of pain sensation. At intervals, skin should therefore be touched with the dull end of the safety pin, in order to determine the client's ability to distinguish between sharp and dull.

Because the elderly person tends to experience decreased sensitivity to pain, close assessment of other client responses is necessary. As an example, the elderly client may not complain about acute pain when other objective data indicating inflammation may be present. This can include an elevated temperature and an increased pulse rate. Objective data can be more significant than subjective data when the elderly person does not indicate the presence of pain. When pain is present, the elderly person may talk about hurting, aching, or being sore. They may feel that these are aches that accompany the process of getting old.

In the assessment of the pain experience, the nurse should determine the cause of pain, onset of pain and the duration of pain, differentiating constant from intermittent pain and chronic from acute pain. The location of the pain as well as the manner in which the elderly

TABLE 10.1 GUIDE FOR ASSESSING TOUCH

Tactile sensitivity
  Response to light touch
  Response to sharpness and dullness
  Identification of objects through touch
Thermal sensitivity
  Response to cold
  Response to heat
  Appropriateness of clothing to environmental
    temperatures
Pain sensitivity
  Precipitators of pain
  Responses to pain
  Intensity of pain
  Location of pain
  Radiation of pain
  Duration of pain
  Treatment used to relieve pain
Vibratory sensitivity
  Response of extremities to vibratory stimuli
Touch as a means of communication
  Use of touch in communicating
  Response to touch

person expresses it need to be determined. The limitation caused by the pain on functional activities should be assessed. The history of the client's management of pain needs to be determined. This includes the pain medication patterns. The client's methods of coping with pain can give evidence of beliefs about pain and appropriate responses to pain. Cultural values and beliefs will affect the pain response.

Assessment of Vibratory Sensitivity

A tuning fork is used to assess vibratory sensitivity. While the client closes both eyes, the nurse applies the vibrating tuning fork to bony prominences such as the elbows, knees, fingers, or toes. The client is asked to indicate when vibrations are felt and when they stop. In some cases the nurse may wish to plug the person's ears with cotton, to insure that the client is responding to the vibration and not to the sound. At intervals, a nonvibrating tuning fork is applied instead, to prevent the client from reacting to the sound of striking the fork to begin the vibration. In the elderly person, vibratory sensitivity may show a marked decrease in the lower extremities.

Assessment of Stereognosis

To assess stereognosis, the nurse has the client close both eyes. A familiar object, such as a coin, key, paper clip, or cotton ball, is placed in the client's hands. The client is then asked to identify the object.

Client History

In some cases, the client may be aware of changes in touch sensitivity and may mention areas of tingling or numbness. The nurse should ask the person about reactions to extremes in environmental temperature, especially to cold weather. The client's history of experience with pain should also be discussed. The manner in which a painful experience is described often provides clues about the client's reactions to pain and methods of coping with it. The elderly person may be able to evaluate the manner in which he or she has been able to tolerate pain, and in some instances can describe measures that seem to be effective in managing pain when it does occur. Client history can include touch that the person enjoys such as the smoothness of a silk-like fabric or the coarseness of a heavy fabric like wool.

Assessment of Client's Reaction to Touch

The nurse can observe the client's ability to manipulate and hold on to objects. The client can also be presented with objects of different textures and asked to identify the textures. Reaction to varying temperatures should be observed. The way a client dresses in relationship to the environmental temperature may give the nurse clues to the person's reactions to heat and cold.

Another significant component of touch is the way in which it is used as a communication tool. The nurse should observe the client's use of touch in relating to others, as well as his or her reactions to the touch of others. This information can be used to determine whether touch is an acceptable strategy in intervening with a particular client.

PLANNING AND INTERVENTION FOR TOUCH AND PAIN SENSITIVITY

In establishing goals with the client in relation to touch, two components of touch must be considered: the touch sensitivity of the client and the use of touch for communication. Goals can be established with regard to the client's ability to experience light touch, temperature, pain, and vibration. Nursing interventions with the elderly can be planned to include touch.

Compensation for Tactile Sensitivity Changes

If a deficit is found in the elderly person's tactile sensitivity, nursing goals can involve use of the other senses to compensate for the changes. Variation among textures can be used to compensate for losses in tactile sensitivity. For example, rough textures can be used on utensils and for hall handrails and stair rails. The client's security through tactile environmental cues should be enhanced by the use of varying textiles. Plastic forks and spoons should be avoided. Heavy utensils are preferable because the old person is more aware of weight and can use the sense of touch more effectively. A variety of textured materials can be used for clothing, bedding, decoration of the environment. Textures with which the client is familiar are preferable to synthetic materials such as plastics and paper.

Goals should also relate to protection of the elderly person's extremities. Because the discomfort of tight shoes may not be obvious to the client, new shoes should first be worn only for short periods. Adequate covering of the hands and feet during cold weather is another protective measure.

Pain Prevention and Management

The elderly person's subjective response to pain comes from a lifetime of experience. Nursing interventions for prevention or relief of pain experienced by the elderly client can focus on the client's response to pain. Effective methods for pain control used by the client in the past should be encouraged. Interventions can be directed toward decreasing anxiety and fear, which can aggravate the pain response. Even though analgesic medication may be necessary, the nurse can assist the client to potentiate the effect of the medication. The nurse can assist with general comfort measures such as positioning. The elderly person can be taught relaxation techniques and the use of rhythmic breathing. These techniques can be practiced when the person does not experience pain. The nurse can use cutaneous stimulation. Stimulation of the skin is believed to stimulate the production of endorphins. These measures will convey to the elderly person the nurse's confidence in the role of the client in pain control. Wachter-Shikora and Perez (1982) described the advisability of adding foods that contain l-tryptophan, a precursor to serotonin. Some foods that contain l-tryptophan include yogurt, milk, poultry, beef, bananas, and pineapple. These foods are important in the descending inhibition of pain and contribute to the person's sense of well-being.

Through an examination of the pain experience, the elderly person can be helped to assimilate this experience. For example, the person can discuss concerns about the pain, the impact of the pain on functional abilities, and the successes experienced in coping with the pain.

The nurse needs to have an awareness of personal reactions to the elderly client's pain experience. This includes beliefs about medications for pain relief, the role of the elderly person as an active participant in care and decision-making, the role of the nurse in listening to and understanding the elderly person, and personal comfort in being with the elderly person while pain is experienced. The nurse must take seriously the pain experience of the elderly person and not assume that aches and pains are an expected part of the aging process.

Touch as a Way to Communicate

Before nurse and client can establish goals with regard to the use of touch as a communication tool, the nurse should be aware of his or her own feelings about touching the elderly person.

A nurse who reacts adversely to the apparent skin changes of old people may find it difficult to touch a client. The nurse's reluctance, in turn, communicates a negative message to the elderly person. Old people need tactile stimulation even though they may be reluctant to express this need openly. The need for tactile stimulation increases when sensory changes occur, since touch then becomes an important method of communication.

The nurse can gain greater sensitivity to the touch loss experienced by the client by taking part in a simulation experience. The nurse's fingers can be covered with a heavy substance, or plastic gloves can be worn. Then, to add to the sense of frustration experienced by those who have lost touch sensitivity, the nurse can try to thread a needle.

Copstead (1980) found that the nurse can effectively use touch to foster positive client self-appraisal among institutionalized elderly. deWever (1977) found that a nurse putting his or her arm around a client's shoulders was the touching behavior perceived as uncomfortable by the greatest number of elderly in her sample. A nurse placing his or her hand on the elderly client's arm was the touching behavior perceived as comfortable by the greatest number of elderly. Touching an elderly client's face also was perceived as comfortable. The use of touch by the nurse helps to establish and to maintain a nurse–client relationship and to help clients remain responsive to their environment.

EVALUATION OF TOUCH SENSITIVITY

By observing the client's use of aids in the environment that stimulate touch, such as rough-textured stair rails, the nurse can determine how well the client is able to utilize such aids, and the extent to which they compensate for loss or change in tactile sensitivity. Greater security in ambulation can be achieved through environmental modifications and aids for the person with reduced touch sensitivity who also experiences visual changes. The degree of client safety achieved by prevention of accidents that might occur because of reduced tactile sensitivity is part of the evaluation of the effectiveness of intervention.

The elderly person's degree of comfort within the environment can be measured by whether clothing appropriate to the weather is worn. For example, if temperature-regulating mechanisms are working normally, a sweater is not needed on hot summer days. Environmental temperatures can also affect the activity levels of the client. Losses in touch sensitivity are not likely to be regained. However, interventions can promote the use of what sensitivity remains, and can compensate for irreversible losses through environmental modifications.

In conclusion, changes in touch sensitivity connected with the aging process are not as obvious as certain other sensory changes, such as those in vision and hearing. The necessity for heavier reliance on touch becomes magnified when visual losses occur. Goals should relate to intensification of environmental clues, to allow for reduced tactile sensitivity or the increased need to use touch to compensate for other sensory changes and losses.

THE ELDERLY PERSON'S ABILITY TO SMELL: ASSESSMENT BASE

There is a close association between the sense of smell and human behavior. Research has demonstrated that behavior changes in response to olfactory input. For example, consider the emotions that can be aroused in response to the presence or recall of particular odors. Other functions of olfaction include protection of the individual by warning of danger in the air, such as smoke or gas fumes; assistance in digestion; and facilitation of recollections (Farber, 1978). The olfactory system connects with structures in the limbic system, thus permitting olfactory stimuli to affect behavior and emotion (Farber, 1978). An individual's

response to a given odor seems to be affected by age, sex, ethnic background, and previous experience with that odor. Schamper, Voss, and Cain (1981) found that the elderly person has a reduced sense of smell as well as cognitive tools for odor identification. Young persons are better able to name odors spontaneously. Garg (1981) found that demented elderly people have a severe decrement in their ability to identify and discriminate food odors.

Much of the research into olfaction has used classic psychophysical methods of measuring the ability to detect differences in the odors of a variety of substances. Studies done to determine the effects of the aging process on the sense of smell have utilized these methods. More recently, new studies have considered the effect of odors on the person's behavior. The degree of an odor's pleasantness, and the desire to smell it, probably become highly significant as the acuity of smell diminishes. The desire for food as well as the enjoyment of food are affected by smell acuity. Research is continuing in this area. The current literature indicates that olfactory sensitivity does show a decline with advancing age.

Olfactory Sensitivity

Smell is provoked by chemical stimuli, in the form of rapidly diffusing molecules of volatile substances that initiate activity when they contact olfactory receptor cells in the nasal cavity (Auger, 1976). A person can develop smell adaptation with continuous exposure to an odor. Research into the effects of aging on the acuity of the olfactory sense indicates that the sense of smell is not seriously affected by age alone, but probably by other factors associated with age (Engen, 1977). There is wide variation among individuals in the ability to smell.

Change in olfactory sensitivity seems to be affected by health, and alterations in health may be the reason for the change in smell sensitivity some old people experience. Research indicates, however, that healthy elderly people may show little, if any, deficit in the olfactory acuity. Observed changes in the sense of smell with age may also be caused by occupational odors, airborne toxic agents, and smoking (Corso, 1971). However, continued research will be needed to establish with certainty the effects of aging on olfaction. Odor preferences seem to be influenced by maturation and learning, rather than by aging. More emphasis should be placed on measuring these preferences. Even though some researchers report no change in olfactory acuity with age, those who believe that there is an age-related decrement of sensitivity base their views on the anatomic and physiologic changes that can accompany the aging process.

Degenerative Changes in Olfactory Structures

Research has shown that fiber loss in the olfactory bulb increases steadily with age, and that although there is wide variability, about three-fourths of the olfactory fibers are absent by the time a person reaches 80 or 90 years of age (Ruben, 1971). Degeneration of these nerve fibers may occur as a result of inhaling pollutants. Diseases of the respiratory system may also affect the ability to smell, by causing alterations in nasal anatomy and physiology. Some researchers hypothesize that age-related changes in the sense of smell may be due to cellular degeneration in the parietal lobe at the foot of the postcentral gyrus in the brain (Goldman, 1979).

Sex of the Client

In general, women have greater olfactory acuity than men. This is especially true with regard to biologic odors, such as the smell of urine or perspiration. However, postmenopausal women exhibit decreased ability to smell, since estrogen levels appear to affect odor perception in women (Farber, 1978).

NURSING ASSESSMENT OF THE CLIENT'S ABILITY TO SMELL (TABLE 10-2)

In assessing a client's sense of smell, the nurse should remember that the nasal mucosa can be stimulated by touch, as produced by the im-

TABLE 10.2 GUIDE FOR ASSESSING SMELL

History
Upper respiratory problems
Allergy problems
Epistaxis
Nasal discharges
Nasal polyps
Smoking history
Responses to odors
  Odors enjoyed
  Odors found repulsive
Weight loss

Physical assessment
Nose: symmetry
Nasal mucosa: color, swelling
Nasal turbinates
Responses to specific odors (coffee, spices, etc.)

Environment
Heating system
Exposure to industrial pollution
Safety measures: smoke detectors, gasline protectors, etc.
Toxic cleaning substance odors
Living alone or with others

pact of a gush of air or by forceful inhalation; by cold, as caused by evaporating menthol; and by pressure, heat, and pain. The most efficient olfactory stimulus is obtained by placing an odorous substance beneath the nostril and having the client sniff.

In assessing smell, the nurse may encounter some difficulty in controlling environmental factors—temperature, humidity, and air flow—that can affect perception of an odor. The duration of exposure to the odor and the concentration of the odorous substance must also be considered. The client's reactions to odor can be assessed by observing facial expressions and evaluating verbal responses.

Assessment of Olfactory Sensitivity

The threshold of smell is the point at which a person first perceives an odor, even though it cannot yet be identified. Identification of odors is highly dependent upon sociocultural background and previous experience with odors. For example, odors can be mentally associated with holidays or religious services. The smells of

Christmas are familiar to many people. Specific ethnic groups experience the smells of particular foods prepared in the home. Exposure to a familiar odor can lead to an emotional experience sparked by the memory of events associated with the odor.

In the assessment of smells, the nurse should avoid use of substances that can irritate the nasal mucosa, such as ammonia or vinegar. Extremely foul odors may affect the regularity and depth of respirations. During the assessment, the client is requested to close his or her eyes while identifying the substance. Each nostril can be tested separately by pressing one nostril closed. A cotton applicator is saturated with a solution that produces a strong and familiar aromatic odor, such as coffee, oil of spearmint, soap, or tobacco. If the client cannot identify the odors presented, the nurse should ask whether the difficulty is with identification or with detection of the odor. Problems with immediate memory can affect the identification of the odor.

Health History
The health history is significant to the assessment of olfactory sensitivity. The sense of smell can be affected by respiratory problems, epistaxis, nasal discharges, or nasal polyps. The client's work history is also significant, particularly if it includes exposure to noxious industrial odors. The quality of the environmental air to which the person has been exposed may be important. The person may have lived in an industrial area or in a rural area for many years. The client's history of smoking should be determined. There is a need to determine a history of weight loss because changes in olfaction can affect the person's desire to eat.

Assessment of Nasal Structures
The nose and nasal mucosa are inspected for symmetry and color. A nasal speculum can be used to separate the nares for this inspection. Abnormalities, such as a deviated septum, enlarged turbinates, or the presence of polyps may interfere with olfactory acuity. Nasal discharge may indicate a respiratory problem that affects the ability to smell.

PLANNING AND INTERVENTION FOR SMELL

In planning and intervention related to the sense of smell, the nurse and client can enhance odors or suppress them to add to the client's enjoyment and pleasure obtained from the environment and from food.

Enhancement of Odors
Perfumes and deodorizers can enhance the pleasantness of the environment. The person who is institutionalized can be exposed to familiar odors, such as spices, fresh flowers, or after shave lotion. It is important to alternate odors in order to provide a stimulating effect. Familiarity and acceptability are also important considerations. Some people dislike the smells of perfume and smoke, whereas others enjoy them. The smell of a cigar or pipe can elicit intense pleasure in one individual and extreme aversion in another. In group living situations (such as long-term care settings) odors should be chosen for general appeal.

Pleasant and familiar odors, such as the smell of fresh bread baking, may be used to evoke pleasant memories. In order to detect the flavor of a food, the person must also be able to smell it. Foods may, therefore, seem tasteless to the elderly person whose sense of smell is impaired. For the person with an olfactory impairment, hot foods will usually produce more pleasant aromas than foods that have become cold.

Suppression of Odors
Some unpleasant odors in the environment can be suppressed by improving hygiene. For example, the elderly person may not be aware of body odor which is offensive to others. Deodorants, as well as regular baths and changes of clothing, can eliminate this potential source of unpleasant odors. Odors in the home environment of the elderly may also be offensive, if food has been allowed to spoil because the odor of decay was not detected. Eating such spoiled food can lead to the further problem of gastrointestinal disturbances. Room deodorizers can be used to suppress unpleasant en-

vironmental odors. However, the better alternative is to determine the source of the unpleasant odor and eliminate it if this is possible. Living in an institution setting can deprive the person of familiar home odors. In many of these settings the sense of smell tends to be depressed rather than stimulated. Many of the familiar home odors can be re-created in the institutional setting. The elderly person should be exposed to kitchen and food preparation odors.

Safety in the Environment

The old person's safety can be endangered by a change in olfactory functioning, which normally can warn the individual of such dangers as smoke and gas. The elderly person who lives alone is even at a greater risk. Smoke detectors with loud buzzers should be installed in the home of the elderly person. Accidental gas poisoning can result from leaking gas lines, a gas stove that has been turned on but not ignited, or a gas flame that has accidentally gone out. Spring safety caps are available for the gas jets of a stove. It may be advisable to replace the gas stove with an electric one if the elderly person with an olfactory impairment lives alone. The person may also be unaware of toxic odors from cleaning agents, such as ammonia. Elderly individuals may be safer wearing clothing of flame-resistant or low-flammability materials. Items such as kitchen utensils should not be placed where an elderly person may have to lean over an open flame to reach them.

The elderly person with an olfactory loss may not define his or her territory as confidently. Many rooms, such as the kitchen, can be identified by odor. This can be an especial problem if the old person also experiences some loss of vision.

EVALUATION

Because the sense of smell is so closely related to behavior, the elderly client's behavior can indicate both the adequacy of the sense of smell and the effect of nursing interventions designed to enhance it. Sudden lack of interest in food may signal a change in olfactory sen-

sitivity. Interventions should include enhancing the smells of food and insuring that hot foods are served. For the client who has been made aware of changes in smell sensitivity after assessment, the nurse could expect to see modifications in the home environment. The client's recognition of changes in smell might be demonstrated by smoke detectors in the home and precautions aimed at preventing gas leakages.

In conclusion, the assessment of the sense of smell may at first appear valueless to the nurse. The roles of other senses, especially vision and hearing, seem so much more important. Even the person who has experienced a temporary decrease in ability to smell because of an acute upper respiratory infection tends to take the sense of smell for granted once it is fully regained. The nurse should give careful consideration to the number of messages about the environment a person receives through the ability to smell. For an elderly person who has other sensory losses, the impairment caused by changes in the ability to smell can be major.

THE ELDERLY PERSON'S ABILITY TO TASTE: ASSESSMENT BASE

The senses of smell and vision are closely related to the sense of taste. The individual's perception of taste can be either enhanced or diminished by the sight and smell of food. The social situation in which food is consumed may also affect the person's perception of its taste.

Four primary sensations of taste are perceived by the taste buds on the tongue—bitter, salty, sweet, and sour. Many combinations of these primary sensations can be perceived by most adults. Sweet tastes are perceived by the anterior surface of the tip of the tongue, bitter tastes by the posterior surface of the tongue, and sour tastes by the lateral edges of the tongue. Salty taste is perceived by all parts of the tongue by the receptors on the surface of the taste buds. The flavors of a substance may be detected by the sense of smell. Other factors that affect the perceived taste of a substance, particularly food, include appearance, temperature, consistency, and texture. There may even be a pain component associated with taste, as when foods are described as being "hot and spicy."

Research indicates that taste sensitivity decreases with age (Corso, 1977). Even though there is no agreement on the cause of this change, it is known that the number of taste buds decreases with age. The review of research done by Corso (1981) suggests that the combined loss of functioning taste buds and progressive neuron reduction in taste centers, including the cortical area in the parietal lobe, may account for changes in taste with aging.

Although taste buds have the power to regenerate, regeneration does not keep pace with the rate of loss. Age-related changes in taste acuity are thought to be small. Some researchers hypothesize that the decline in taste sensitivity may be related to smoking or illness states in the elderly person. Pipe smokers, especially, may demonstrate marked changes in taste sensitivity (Goldman, 1979). Other age-related changes that may affect the taste of foods include changes in the elasticity of the mouth and lips, a decrease in the flow of saliva, changes in oral secretions, increased incidence of gingivitis and periodontitis, and the presence of fissures of the tongue. These mouth problems may be associated with malodorous volatile compounds that cause an unpleasant taste and smell sensation. These unpleasant sensations can affect the perceived taste of food. The progression of diabetic neuropathy can diminish taste acuity (Abbasi, 1981). Hypertension appears to increase the salt threshold (Corso, 1981). With an increased threshold, the elderly person needs to use more salt for taste, which has the potential of increasing the hypertensive problem. Significant changes in taste related to aging are unlikely to occur before the age of 70 (Shore, 1976). The elderly person seems to have increased sensitivity to bitterness and decreased sensitivity to sweetness and saltiness. The taste buds at the front of the tongue, which are responsible for identifying sweet and salty tastes, are the first to atrophy, while those responsible for the sensitivity to bitter and sour tastes continue to function more effectively. These changes may be responsible

for complaints by elderly people that their food tastes bitter or sour (Shore, 1976). Most studies of taste sensitivity indicate that with age there is an increased aversion to bitterness. However, this is an area that needs to be investigated further. The influence of procedural variables can affect studies of taste acuity. Corso (1981) indicates that because the adequate stimulus for taste is not completely known, much research in this area has been directed toward the correlation of chemical structures of gustatory stimuli and qualitative taste response. It is known that the stimuli for taste are substances in liquid form, in aqueous solution or readily soluble in saliva.

The elderly person may be able to compensate for altered taste sensitivity. Along with taste and factors related to taste sensation, habit tends to influence food selection. Taste preference appears to be connected with some mechanism in the central nervous system rather than with the taste buds themselves. Previous experiences with tastes apparently determine whether the individual perceives them as pleasant or unpleasant. Highly seasoned foods are enjoyed by some people and disliked by others. Garlic is very pleasant to many, and may have a mental association with certain holiday foods. Relating food tastes to happy events, such as holidays, enhances the pleasure derived from these foods.

NURSING ASSESSMENT OF TASTE (TABLE 10.3)

Sensory scales of taste intensity have been derived by Stevens (1969). Each of these tastes relates to a different chemical substance including sucrose or an artificial sweetener (for sweet), sodium chloride (for salt), lemon juice (for sour), and quinine sulfate (for bitter). Experiments were controlled for the percent of the solute, molarity of a solution, and the normality of a solution. In addition to determining the detection of sweet, salt, sour, and bitter, the degree of sensitivity, differential thresholds, blends and mixture, and hedonic properties can be determined (Corso, 1981). Complex tastes are produced by odorous constituents

TABLE 10.3 GUIDE FOR ASSESSING TASTE

Health history
  Medications
  Tobacco use
  Weight loss patterns
  Wearing of dentures
Taste sensitivity
  Sweet
  Salt
  Sour
  Bitter
Reactions to food and mealtime
  Patterns of interaction at mealtime
  Tastes preferred
  Tastes disliked
  Participation in food selection
  Participation in food preparation
Inspection of tongue and mouth
  Color
  Smoothness
Environment
  Odors
  Dining area
  Food preparation facilities
  Food storage areas

in the stimuli. Because the sense of taste is affected by the sight and smell of a substance, these cues must be avoided when the function of the taste buds is assessed. Four substances that the nurse can use to assess taste sensitivity are sugar for testing sweetness; salt; lemon juice for assessing sensitivity to sourness;,and quinine for testing sensitivity to bitterness. An applicator dipped in a solution of any of these can be applied to the lateral aspect of both sides of the tongue, the anterior aspect, and the posterior aspect. The tongue should be brushed before beginning the assessment. The client should rinse his or her mouth between applications of the substance. The preferred solution for rinsing the mouth is distilled water. The sugar and salt should be dissolved in distilled water. The concentration of the solution should progress from a less concentrated to a greater concentrated solution. During the testing, distilled water, without any substance, can be used at random. The solution should be held in the mouth for 15 to 30 seconds and should be ex-

pectorated into a container rather than swallowed. The detection threshold is the lowest concentration of the test solution that can be distinguished from the distilled water. The mouth should be rinsed with distilled water before the client tastes another solution. It is advisable to wait to assess taste sensation at least 1 hour after the elderly person has eaten.

Health History

The nurse can assess the client's reactions to the taste of foods by observing him during mealtimes. Social interactions during mealtime may affect the way food tastes and the pleasantness or unpleasantness associated with it. If there is a history of family conflicts erupting during mealtimes, a person may remember them as unpleasant. Mealtimes that include the company of family or friends and the opportunity to communicate tend to evoke more pleasant feelings. In long-term settings, the nurse may not be fully aware of an elderly resident's need to sit in his "own seat" at his "own table." Sitting with a different group of people at each meal may detract from the enjoyment of mealtime and the food itself. In taking a client's history the nurse can ask questions about taste preferences and reactions to tastes. The past associations that the client has had with specific foods can be determined during this history. Other assessment areas include medication intake and tobacco use, including pipe smoking, cigar smoking, and chewing tobacco. The condition of the teeth as well as the wearing of dentures are included in the assessment. Weight patterns also need to be considered. Antihypertensive medications can increase the person's salt taste threshold.

Assessment of the Client's Mouth

The dorsum of the tongue should be inspected for color, the appearance of the papillae, the degree of smoothness, and presence or absence of fissures or ulcerations. The gums and teeth should be inspected at this time, since irritations or lesions in the mouth can affect taste. Some clients may describe a generally bitter taste in the mouth. The amount of salivation should also be considered, since a very dry mouth may cause the client to complain of dry, taste-less food. A malodorous mouth can cause un-pleasant taste sensations that affect the per-ceived flavor of food. The presence of noxious stimuli in the nose can adversely affect taste.

PLANNING AND INTERVENTION

To be able to find pleasure in food while main-taining optimal nutrition and weight is an ap-propriate goal to be set by the client who ex-periences decreased taste sensitivity. The nurse may need to assist the client whose cardiovas-cular status limits the amount and kind of sea-sonings that can be used. Because of dimin-ished taste sensitivity, the old person may prefer more highly seasoned food. However, addition of large amounts of salt to improve the taste of foods may create problems with fluid reten-tion. Lemon juice, herbs, and other seasonings can be used to replace part of the salt. Elderly people who are experiencing increased sensi-tivity to bitter tastes may not wish to use salt or sugar substitutes. The client can be en-couraged to try substitutes that enhance the taste of foods without a bitter taste. The client also needs to experiment with the appropriate amounts of the substitute needed to enhance taste without bitterness.

The nurse can help the client or family members to recognize other factors that can enhance taste. These include the appearance of food, its temperature and texture, the set-ting in which it is served, and the social in-teractions that occur at mealtime. Maximizing use of the client's senses of smell and vision may help to compensate for reduced taste sen-sitivity. Participation in food preparation may enhance taste, as the client can gain the full advantage of smell while food is being pre-pared. Encouraging or assisting the client to maintain oral hygiene practices is also ad-vised, since a clean, moist mouth often en-hances the taste of foods.

The likelihood of eating food that is not spoiled is enhanced by the sense of smell. The client with diminished smell or taste may not be aware that food is spoiled; he or she needs to be encouraged to smell foods prior to tasting them. The amount of time and method in which food is stored should be discussed with the el-derly client. Shopping for or preparing smaller quantities of food may be indicated to reduce spoilage potential.

A major role of the nurse is to encourage effective oral hygiene practices to remove de-bris that might cause unpleasant taste sen-sations. Mouth care that includes careful brushing of the teeth and thorough rinsing of

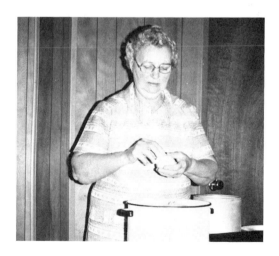 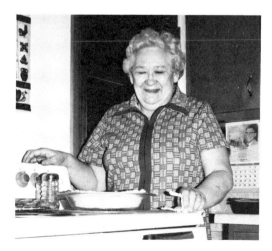

Figure 10.3. Participation in food preparation enhances the sense of taste. *(Photographs by Eugene Mizikar.)*

the mouth can promote the fuller use of taste sensitivity. Dental care needs to be encouraged, even when the person wears dentures. Treatment of gingivitis and periodontitis can reduce the microorganisms that cause unpleasant tastes and thus affect the flavor and enjoyment of food. To provide foods that the person can chew can increase the pleasure of eating.

EVALUATION

The degree to which the client appears to enjoy food and mealtimes is part of the evaluation of the person's ability to compensate for decreases in taste sensitivity. The client's weight pattern can also indicate the level of compensation. However, many other factors can affect weight patterns. The client may be deriving too much pleasure from food as a way of compensating for other age-related losses. A more extensive consideration of nutrition and the elderly person is presented in Chapter 13.

In conclusion, taste and smell have a strong influence on the individual's reactions to food. Food flavors are experienced through smell. Both taste and smell can trigger a person's emotional responses. Complaining about the taste of food may be a socially acceptable way for the resident of a nursing home to express unhappy feelings about being in this setting. The greater the elderly person's degree of involvement in the selection, preparation, and serving of foods, the greater the possibility for optimal use of taste.

RECOMMENDED READINGS

Auger, J.R. Behavioral Systems and Nursing. Englewood Cliffs, NJ, Prentice-Hall, 1976. *Provides an assessment base relating to the significance of sensory perceptions. Sensory stimulus and response are discussed.*

Corso, J.F. Aging Sensory Systems and Perception. New York, Praeger, 1981. *A complete discussion of all sensory changes that are part of the aging process. Provides a base for assessment.*

Engen, T. Taste and smell, in Birren, J.E., Schaie, K.W. (eds), Handbook of the Psychology of Aging.

New York, Van Nostrand Reinhold, 1977. *A comprehensive report of significant research relating to taste and smell. Provides an assessment base.*

Farber, S.D. Olfaction in health and disease. Journal of Occupational Therapy 32:155, 1978. *Assessment and interventions are discussed as these relate to the olfactory sensitivity of the client.*

Grzegorczyk, P.B., Jones, S.W., and Mistretta, C.M. Age-related differences in salt taste acuity. Journal of Gerontology 34(6):834, 1979. *A description of the control needed for accurate assessment of taste.*

Kenshalo, D.R. Age changes in touch, vibration, temperature, kinesthesis, and pain sensitivity, in Birren, J. F., Schaie, K.W. (eds), Handbook of the Psychology of Aging. New York, Van Nostrand Reinhold, 1977. *A comprehensive report of research into changes in touch, vibration, temperature, kinesthesis, and pain sensitivity with the aging process. Provides a foundation for assessment.*

Marks, L. Sensory Processes. New York, Academic, 1974. *The relationship of perception to sensory processes is the focus of this book. The individuality of sensory processes is stressed.*

Meinhart, N.T., McCaffery, M. Pain: A Nursing Approach to Assessment and Analysis. Norwalk, CT, Appleton-Century-Crofts, 1983. *A complete reference on pain, including age-related pain perception.*

Montagu, A. Touching, 2nd ed. New York, Harper and Row, 1977. *Provides an assessment base for the significance of touch as a way to communicate.*

Shore, H. Designing a training program for understanding sensory loss in aging. The Gerontologist 16:157, 1976. *The focus of this article is on gaining empathy toward the person with sensory losses. Intervention with persons experiencing sensory changes is supported.*

REFERENCES CITED

Abbasi, A. Diabetes: Diagnostic and therapeutic significance of taste impairment. Geriatrics 36(12):73, 1981

Auger, J.R. Behavioral Systems and Nursing. Englewood Cliffs, NJ, Prentice-Hall, 1976

Barnett, K. A theoretical construct of the concepts of touch as they relate to nursing. Nursing Research 21(2):102, 1972

Chodel, J., Williams, B. The concept of sensory deprivation. Nursing Clinics of North America 5:453, 1970

Copstead, L. Effects of touch on self-appraisal and interaction appraisal for permanently institutionalized older adults. Journal of Gerontological Nursing 6(12):747, 1980

Corso, J.F. Aging Sensory Systems and Perception. New York, Praeger, 1981

Corso, J.F. Sensory process and effects in normal adults. Journal of Gerontology 26(1):90, 1971

deWever, M.K. Nursing home patients' perceptions of nurses' affective touching. Journal of Psychology 96:163, 1977

Engen, T. Taste and smell, in Birren, J.E., Schaie, K.W. (eds.), Handbook of the Psychology of Aging. New York, Van Nostrand Reinhold, 1977

Farber, S.D. Olfaction in health and disease. Journal of Occupational Therapy 32:155, 1978

Garg, M. Olfactory Identification and Discrimination in Depressed and Demented Patients. Paper presented at the meeting of the Gerontological Society, Toronto, November, 1981

Goldman, R. Decline in organ function with aging, in Rossman, I. (ed.), Clinical Geriatrics, 2nd ed. Philadelphia, Lippincott, 1979

Huss, A.J. Touch with care or a caring touch. American Journal of Occupational Therapy 31:12, 1977

Kenshalo, D.R. Age changes in touch, vibration, temperature, kinesthesis, and pain sensitivity, in Birren, J.E., Schaie, K.W. (eds), Handbook of the Psychology of Aging. New York, Van Nostrand Reinhold, 1977

Marks, L. Sensory Processes. New York, Academic, 1974

Meinhart, N.T., McCaffery, M. Pain, A Nursing Approach to Assessment and Analysis. Norwalk, CT, Appleton-Century-Crofts, 1983

Montague, A. Touching, 2nd ed. New York, Harper and Row, 1977

Ruben, R. Aging and hearing, in Rossman, I. (ed.), Clinical Geriatrics. Philadelphia, Lippincott, 1971

Schemper, T., Voss, S., Cain, W.S. Odor identification in young and elderly persons: Sensory and cognitive limitations. Journal of Gerontology 36(4):446, 1981

Shore, H. Designing a training program for understanding sensory loss in aging. The Gerontologist 16:157, 1976

Stevens, S.S. Sensory scales of taste intensity. Perception and Psychophysics 6(5):302, 1969

Tobiason, S.J. Touching is for everyone. American Journal of Nursing 81(4):728, 1981

Wachter-Shikora, N., Perez, S. Unmasking pain. Geriatric Nursing 3(6):392, 1982

Watts, A.J. Hypothermia in the aged: A study of the role of cold-sensitivity. Environmental Research 5:119, 1971

BIBLIOGRAPHY

Bozian, M.W., Clark, H.M. Counteracting sensory changes in the aging. American Journal of Nursing 80(3):473, 1980

Godykoontz, I. Touch: Attitudes and practice. Nursing Forum 18:11, 1979

Grzegorczyk, P.B., Jones, S.W., Mistretta, C.M. Age-related differences in salt taste acuity. Journal of Gerontology 34(6):834, 1979

Hayter, J. Modifying the environment to help older persons. Nursing and Health Care 4(5):265, 1983

Hollinger, L.M. Perception of touch in the elderly. Journal of Gerontological Nursing 6(12):741, 1980

Langland, R. Effects of touch on communication with elderly confused clients. Journal of Gerontological Nursing 8(3):152, 1982

Monroe, C.H. Adjustment services for the blind. Journal of Rehabilitation 44(1):30, 1978

Moore, L.M., Nielson, C.R., Mistretta, C.M. Sucrose taste thresholds: Age-related differences. Journal of Gerontology 37(1):64, 1982

Ramos, L. Oral hygiene for the elderly. American Journal of Nursing 81(8):1468, 1981

Seaman, L. Affective nursing touch. Geriatric Nursing 3(3):162, 1982

Thornbury, J.M., Mistretta, C.M. Tactile sensitivity as a function of age. Journal of Gerontology 36(1):34, 1981

Weiss, S.J. The language of touch. Nursing Research 28(2):76, 1979

Wiffenbach, J.M., Baum, S.J., Burghauser, R. Taste thresholds: Quality specific variations with human aging. Journal of Gerontology 37(3):372, 1982

11

Vision in the Elderly Person and the Nursing Process

Ann Gera Yurick

Reading this chapter will enable the individual to:

1. Know the normal changes in vision that accompany the aging process
2. Know the common eye pathologies that can affect the elderly
3. Recognize environmental barriers to optimal visual functioning
4. Assess the eyes and vision of the elderly
5. Know the interventions to maximize the visual functioning of the elderly person
6. Promote the safety of elderly people with visual impairments

Vision has an impact on the total functional ability of the elderly person. For most people, the aging process leads to a slow but steady decrease in visual efficiency. Even though age-related physical changes within the eye are believed to be inevitable, their degree varies among individuals, and seems to depend upon the amount of optical or neuronal change. Many of these changes are distinct physiologic processes. Some, however, are manifestations of tissue changes in other parts of the body caused by the aging process. Both heredity and environment can influence the clinical course of eye changes in the elderly individual. The person's psychologic status can modify reactions to visual changes. The way a person copes with diminishing vision is affected by prior life experience, feelings of self-worth, and their interpersonal relationships. This chapter will focus on the effects of normal aging on vision. Common pathologic changes affecting the eye of the elderly person will be included.

The nurse has a role in preventing the blindness that can occur when pathologic eye problems go unrecognized or untreated. By recognizing normal eye changes, the nurse can help the elderly client adapt to these changes and conserve vision to the greatest degree possible. The old person may need assistance in compensating for visual changes. Vision has been linked to mental function and social interaction (Snyder, 1978). Gradually changing vision may be the reason behind gradually decreasing mobility, changes in orientation, or the occurrence of frightening visual impressions. The effects of socioeconomic problems common to the elderly tend to multiply when they are experienced by a visually impaired old person. These problems include isolation, low income, loss of status and public understanding, and reduction of independence (Facts About Aging and Blindness, American Foundation for the Blind). Because eye changes in the elderly vary so widely, the degree of visual impairment, if any, is also variable. The nurse's primary concern is with how well the elderly person can function with visual changes. It must be determined to what degree these changes affect or alter the client's accustomed way of life. *Functional vision* is that level of vision that enables a person to perform tasks essential to maintenance of the person's routine life-style. Functional vision for the individual changes along a continuum throughout the life cycle (Mini-White House Conference on Vision and Aging, 1981). Functional vision refers to how a person makes use of vision.

Severe visual impairment is defined as inability to see or to read ordinary newspaper print, even with visual correction. A person is considered to be *legally blind* if central visual acuity is less than an angle of 20° (Facts About Blindness, American Foundation for the Blind). All definitions of blindness refer to how well the person can see with the best corrective lenses. According to most definitions, more than 75 percent of blind persons have some usable vision. *Low vision* describes people who are partially sighted. Low vision is a state of imperfect vision that cannot be improved by medical or surgical means or by refraction. Low vision can include people who are legally blind or those who have a severe visual impairment. The American Foundation for the Blind recommends reserving the term "blindness" for complete loss of sight. Of those persons in this country who are legally blind or who function as if they were legally blind, about 65 percent are 65 years of age or older—a total of more than 1 million persons (Facts About Blindness, American Foundation for the Blind).

Because definitions of blindness and visual impairment vary, the nursing assessment is vital in determining the elderly client's ability to see and the effect of any impairment on his or her way of life. Along with data obtained by the nurse, the assessment will utilize data obtained by other health team members. The nurse must be cautious in making assumptions about the client's visual abilities, especially when the person is labeled as being blind. For example, goals established with the "blind" client who is able to detect light will be different from those established with the client who cannot detect light. The American Foundation for the Blind defines "visual ability" as the degree to which a person can use whatever vision exists. Together the nurse and the elderly client can establish goals related to the use of this visual ability.

The visual functions that will be discussed in this chapter include visual acuity, accommodation, visual field, light sensitivity, color discrimination, and visual spatial ability. These functions will be related to the daily living tasks of the elderly person. As the nurse assesses, plans, implements, and evaluates in working with the elderly client, it is necessary to protect, maintain, and maximize these visual functions.

ASSESSMENT BASE

In the course of the aging process, structural changes in the eye have various effects on visual functions. Vision depends not only on eye structures but upon nerve pathways from the eye to the brain and the receptor area in the occipital lobe of the brain. Research findings indicate that marked changes in visual perception can accompany advanced age (Corso, 1971). Visual perception refers to the processes involved in sensing, interpreting, and responding to visual information (Fozard et al., 1977). It is important to assess both physiologic factors, which affect vision, and psychologic factors, which relate response bias to perceptual judgments. Even though some workers with the elderly feel that a dysfunction in the central nervous system contributes to perceptual slowing with increasing age, no complete theory has yet described the underlying psychologic or physiologic processes behind visual perception in the elderly person (Corso, 1971).

Light Sensitivity
The physical stimulus for the visual experience is light (Auger, 1976). The quality of the retinal image is largely determined by the amount of illumination falling on the retina (Fozard et al., 1977). Age-related changes in the structure of the eye determine how the eye is able to manage the light stimulus. The visual functions associated with light sensitivity include lumination needs, contrast sensitivity, dark adaptation, and reaction to glare (Cristarella, 1977). Degenerative changes in the posterior endothelial layer of the cornea can contribute to scattering of light in the eye (Fozard et al., 1977). With aging, the lens tends to yellow and to increase in size (Fozard et al., 1977), reduc-

ing the amount of light which reaches the retina and changing its spectral distribution. Because the lens refracts light in addition to transmitting it, changes in the lens modify the eye's ability to produce a sharp image on the retina.

The amount of light reaching the retina also is affected by the size of the pupil. A decrease in pupillary size with age is referred to as *senile miosis*. The smaller pupil is caused by changes in the iris, stemming from increases in connective tissue and in the hyalinization and sclerotic changes in the iris vasculature, all of which may make the iris more rigid (Reichel, 1978). Other researchers argue that the decrease in pupillary size cannot be explained by sclerosis of iridal tissues. The muscles that control pupil dilation weaken more rapidly than the sphincter muscles that control contraction of the pupil. It appears that senile miosis and immobility of the iris cannot be attributed to any single mechanical cause (Weale, 1963). Though a variety of causes are possible, the effect of smaller pupil size in limiting the amount of light that reaches the retina depends on the eye's ability to adapt (Fozard et al., 1977).

Adaptation to the Dark
Dark adaptation is the process by which the eye becomes more visually sensitive after remaining in darkness for a period of time. After a certain length of time in the dark, outlines of objects become more discernible (Cristarella, 1977).

The minimum amount of light to which the eye can respond is determined by the region of the retina that is stimulated, the intensity and duration of the stimulus, the wavelength of the light, and the time spent in the dark. The retina contains two types of light-sensitive cells, the rods and the cones. A light stimulus causes these cells to respond by translating the input into nerve impulses that are transmitted over optic pathways to the visual cortex of the brain (Murch, 1973).

The periphery of the retina contains mostly rods, which are sensitive to very low light intensities and relatively insensitive to detail. The central retina, on the other hand, contains

a great number of cones, which provide information on detail if the level of light intensity is great enough. The cones are the first analyzers of color, brightness, and contour (Murch, 1973). There are several age-related decrements in retinal metabolism. The supply of oxygen to the retina is believed to diminish with age as a result of vascular changes. This is pronounced especially in the rod-dense area that responds to low levels of illumination. This change is thought to affect the efficiency of dark adaptation in the elderly person. Even though it is agreed that the dark adaptation threshold decreases as a function of age, evidence about the relationship between age and rate of dark adaptation seems to vary among researchers (Corso, 1971).

As discussed previously, the pupil of the eye becomes smaller in diameter as part of the aging process. Even if the eye undergoes no other changes, the diminution of the pupil will allow less light to reach the retina (Weale, 1963). With age there is fibrosis of the iris, which leads to reduced response to mydriatics. Also, the smaller pupil size of the elderly person is compounded when miotic drops are used to control glaucoma. When assessing a client's ability to adapt vision to darkness, the nurse should consider the length of time it takes to develop maximum seeing ability and the level to which seeing is reached in the darkened area (Botwinick, 1973). Thus, dark adaptation is assessed in terms of both the speed and the adequacy of adjustment.

Reaction to Glare
For the old person, problems with vision can result from too much illumination as well as too little. Elderly people often have increased susceptibility to visual glare, the dazzling effect associated with light of apparent high brightness (Hatton, 1977). Glare is the sensory response that is produced by light entering the eye in such a manner as to inhibit distinct vision (Corso, 1981). Simultaneous glare can occur when the peripheral field is at a lower luminance than the central field of vision. Successive glare is perceived when the eye moves from an area of lower level illumination, to which it has become adapted, to an area of

much higher illumination (Hatton, 1977). The effects of glare can create problems if there is an altered state of retinal adaptation or if other eye changes cause scattering of light. Increasing opacity of the lens is believed to be a primary cause of increased glare sensitivity, since such opacity diffuses incoming light and thus makes the eyes more sensitive to glare. Turbidity of the vitreous can contribute to the sensation of glare. It can also be caused by irritation or changes in the cornea (Fozard et al., 1977).

Contrast Sensitivity

Contrast sensitivity involves the ability to detect differences in luminances between neighboring regions of a visual field. The brightness of one region may be perceived as less bright if the surrounding area has a greater amount of light. Conversely, the same region may seem brighter if the surrounding area has a lesser amount of light. The ability to discriminate among degrees of brightness appears to decrease with age. This differential sensitivity was found to be most pronounced in persons in their 60s and 70s (Fozard et al., 1977). An increase in light scatter due to age-related eye changes also seems to affect contrast sensitivity (Weale, 1963). More research, however, is needed in the entire field of sensitivity to changes in light intensity (Fozard et al., 1977).

Lumination Needs

The lumination requirements of an elderly person are increased. As a result of miosis and yellowing of the lens, the retina of a 60-year-old individual receives only about one-third of the amount of light that reaches the retina of a 20-year-old (Weale, 1963), regardless of whether the person's eye is light- or dark-adapted. The light requirements of the retina rise as the size of the pupil decreases. The lens acts as a light filter. Because a yellowed lens is believed to absorb light, more light must be received by the eye in order to stimulate the retina. When these eye changes take place, the elderly person requires a higher level of illumination than a younger person. This requirement, however, varies according to the task being performed. Simply increasing the level

of illumination is not the complete answer, because the potential problem of glare must be kept in mind.

Visual Acuity

Visual acuity is the ability to discriminate the fine details of objects within a visual field (Riggs, 1966). Research findings indicate that there is a marked downward trend in visual acuity beginning with the sixth decade, even though the degree of variability in visual acuity among elderly persons does increase with age (Corso, 1971). By age 70, unless visual correction has been achieved, low vision seems to be the rule (Botwinick, 1973). Visual acuity is expressed as a ratio between what a person *should* see at 20 feet and what the person *can* see at 20 feet. Low vision in an elderly person is defined as visual acuity of 20/70 to 20/100 (Smith and Pyrek, 1978). The change in visual acuity with the aging process is probably caused by alterations in the lens and vitreous humor. Any eye changes that interfere with the normal transmission of light produce a scattering of light, which blurs the retinal image. Blurred vision also may be a result of a change in the curvature of the cornea, which often flattens as a person ages (Fozard et al., 1977).

Visual Fields

The visual field boundaries are determined by the positions at which a person, while fixing the eyes on a central point, first detects a target light moved from the light-insensitive area to the light-sensitive area of the retina (Fozard et al., 1977). Changes in the retina, especially in the peripheral area, have an effect on the visual field (Weale, 1963). Research also indicates that a decrease in retinal metabolism in persons over the age of 60 is connected with alterations in the visual field (Fozard et al., 1977). With loss of orbital fat, the mechanical displacement of the eyeball can alter the field of vision.

Accommodation

Accommodation is the ability of the eye to focus sharp images on the retina, independent of object distance (Weale, 1963). The decrease in this ability that often accompanies aging is referred to as *presbyopia*. It is caused by the diminished capacity of the lens to increase in thickness and curvature in order to focus on nearby objects. The expression frequently used by a person beginning to experience accommodation changes is, "My arms are not long enough any more." This refers to the difficulty that this person is experiencing with small print or small detail unless the object is held at a distance. Loss of accommodation is gradual. Bifocal lenses minimize the need for the lens of the eye to change shape.

Accommodation involves an adjustment of the ciliary muscle, which alters the focal length of the lens. Ciliary muscle atrophy is thought to contribute to age-related changes in accommodation (Corso, 1971). There are also indications that loss of accommodation is associated with a decrease in the elasticity of the lenticular capsule. Because the lens grows throughout life, this growth leads to a decrease in its accommodative power (Fozard et al., 1977).

Color Discrimination

Changes in the lens affect the ability to differentiate among colors, known as *color sensitivity* or *color discrimination*. Studies indicate that as aging occurs there is loss of color discrimination at the blue end of the color spectrum and loss of sensitivity over the entire spectrum (Fozard et al., 1977). Light pastel colors, such as beige and pink, may become difficult to distinguish. Optimal lighting may be needed to distinguish dark shades such as brown, navy, and black. The ability to discriminate between blue and green shows the greatest rate of decline with aging (Corso, 1971). Reds and yellows can be discriminated most readily. Even though the lessening of ability to discriminate between colors seems to be related to the yellowing of the lens, which causes a filter effect, it has been demonstrated that this cannot completely account for changes in color discrimination. *Aphakia* is the absence of the lens of the eye. When young and elderly aphakic clients were tested, changes in color sensitivity similar to those of senescence were found (Fozard et al., 1977).

Visual Spatial Ability

The ability to perceive the position of objects in visual space is referred to as *visual spatial ability*. Environmental cues that provide information about the relative position of objects in visual space include object size, position, overlap, shadows and highlighting, and relative motion of the object. *Depth perception* is the ability to estimate the relative distance and relief of objects. Since the quality of stereopsis depends on brightness and contrast, eye changes or environmental conditions that reduce illumination of the retina thus decrease the binocular depth perception (Fozard et al., 1977). Loss of depth perception occurs with the loss of vision in one eye. Judging the height of steps as well as realizing when the last step has been reached is a problem when depth perception is altered. The elderly person may also misjudge the height of a curb when walking outdoors.

Body-Image Changes Relating to Vision

Changes in vision have the potential to influence the person's body image. Anyone who wears glasses probably remembers the impact on his or her body image when they were first worn. The wish to maintain the same body image provides motivation for the many people who use contact lenses. Many people can relate body-image alterations to the first pair of bifocals worn for correction of the "too-short arm" problem connected with changes in accommodation. Changes in the appearance of eye structures or surrounding structures may signal eye-related changes. Loss of orbital adipose tissue and elastic connective tissue and fat under the skin surrounding the eye may give the eyes a sunken appearance. Advancing age may be accompanied by the appearance of wrinkles around the eye and loss of muscle tone in the eyelids. When changes occur in the muscle tone of the eyelids, the eyes may seem to tear. Because the lower eyelid margin can turn outward, the opening of the lacrimal duct (punctum) may also be oriented in an outward direction. This interferes with the normal exit of tears. As a result, the elderly person may appear to have an excessive production of tears, when there is actually a decreased tear secretion. High levels of air pollution seem to cause greater irritation to the eyes of an elderly person with decreased tear production, who is less able to cope with the ocular irritants present (Reichel, 1978). Another eye change may be observed in the iris, which appears to fade as pigment diffuses to its periphery.

A vision problem that can distress the elderly client is the appearance of vitreous floaters. Floaters are the result of any thickening within the vitreous cavity that blocks incoming light rays and casts a shadow on the retina. These opacities may be experienced as transient flashes of light, dots, lines, or webs floating in front of the eyes. Often this problem is caused by a hemorrhage of a retinal blood vessel into the vitreous humor, resulting from detachment of the vitreous from its natural connections to the retina (Reichel, 1978). The normally semisolid gel of the vitreous body commonly shrinks after the fifth or sixth decades of life. This especially occurs in the myopic eye, which is a larger eye. Because the vitreous functions as a tampon to support the retina, with shrinkage a posterior detachment of the vitreous can occur. Complaints of flashes of light may occur when the person turns suddenly. Sudden massive showers or floating opacities can occur with a retinal hemorrhage and may signal the likelihood of a retinal detachment (Kenney and Kenney, 1980).

Some pathologic eye problems demonstrate a high degree of correlation with age. These common problems are discussed in this chapter as part of the assessment base, in order to alert the nurse to eye changes that may indicate pathologies. This does not mean that the nurse makes the medical diagnosis of the pathologic problem. Instead, the nurse makes an appropriate referral for definitive medical diagnosis and necessary therapy. For example, when decreased visual fields are assessed, the plan of care should include a referral for testing the intraocular pressure of the client's eyes. If the nurse has acquired the skill of intraocular pressure testing, this may be included as part of the assessment. In addition to planning and implementing care for the client's problem, the nurse should be aware of the need to conserve vision by referring the client for prompt medical treatment.

Nursing Considerations of Eye Pathologies of the Elderly Person

In this chapter, discussion of the nurse's role in conserving vision and maximizing the remaining vision focuses on glaucoma, cataracts, macular degeneration, and diabetic retinopathy, listed by the American Foundation for the Blind as four of the five leading causes of blindness. (The remaining cause is prenatal influences.) The chances of becoming blind from all except prenatal causes increases with age. The National Society for the Prevention of Blindness reports that half of all blindness that will occur could have been prevented. The nurse has a vital role in this prevention.

Cataract

The most prevalent ocular pathology of old age is cataract (Marmor, 1977). The vision problem created by a cataract cannot be corrected by eyeglasses. Even though cataracts occur to some degree in more than 95 percent of those over 65 years of age, only a small percentage of these people have significant visual impairment (Reichel, 1978). The extent to which a cataract affects vision depends on its position and density. Opacity of the lens occurs as a result of thickening and sclerosis. Because transmission of light is reduced, cloudy, smoky vision is experienced. The elderly person may have the impression that there is a film over the eyes. The most commonly reported alteration is progressive unilateral or bilateral painless decrease in vision. The person may complain also of headache and eye fatigue. Upon examination, a white spot may be detected in the normally black pupil area.

Cataract is one of the most easily and successfully remedied ocular problems (Reichel, 1978). Medical therapy, consisting of extraction of the lens, is recommended when the opacity interferes with the person's daily activities. There are several types of surgery for cataract removal. One specific cataract extraction procedure is phacoemulsification. An ultrasonic instrument with high-frequency vibrations emulsifies the cataract. The disintegrated cataract is removed by aspiration. The incision with this surgery is small and tends to heal faster. The recovery period after cataract surgery varies with the individual. There may be some eye discomfort during the healing period. A scratching sensation may be due to the presence of sutures. Rubbing and touching the eye should be avoided.

The healing wound of the eye must be protected. While the client is sleeping or napping, a patch or a light protective shield should be worn to prevent accidental injury. The client should not sleep on the operative side. When an eyepatch is worn, depth perception is lost. As a result, the client may need assistance. Care should be used when putting on and removing eyeglasses to prevent the temple pieces from touching the eye.

Following cataract surgery, eyedrops are ordered to decrease inflammation. The use of these drops is continued for a prescribed period following surgery. Prior to instilling eyedrops, the person's hands should be washed thoroughly and the eyes should be cleansed gently with moist cotton balls to remove accumulated secretions. Pressure should not be exerted on the eye. The tip of the dropper should not touch the eyeball at any time. The medication should be placed into the conjunctival sac rather than directly onto the eye.

Certain activities can inhibit the healing process by increased strain or pressure on the operative eye. The person is advised to move slowly to avoid bumping into objects or falling down. Caution is especially advised when walking up and down stairs. Watching television or reading usually are acceptable as long as the client avoids eye fatigue. Other examples of precautions to avoid strain on the operative eye and to avoid increasing intraocular pressure include the avoidance of bending; avoidance of squeezing the eyelids together since this places pressure on the eye; avoidance of coughing, sneezing, vomiting, straining on elimination, and lifting; and avoidance of bumping or jostling while riding. Showers and bathing are permitted with caution to avoid slipping or falling. Shaving or brushing the teeth are permitted. Hair should be brushed or combed very gently. Advisability of shampoo-

ing hair will vary with the healing process of the eye and the manner in which shampooing is done. The client's head should not be lowered. These instructions should be started prior to surgery. Adequacy of home care should be investigated. Complete healing of the eye usually takes several months. The removal of a cataract creates aphakia. With aphakia, even though visual acuity may be 20/20, mobility and visual comfort may be affected because the aphakic eye has no focusing mechanisms. Glasses designed for the aphakic individual limit the visual field and can cause magnification of images, which can be confusing to the elderly person (Marmor, 1977). Objects appear closer than they really are. Because of the magnifying effect of cataract lenses, the person needs to be especially careful when ascending or descending stairs or when sitting down on a chair. They need to be directed to feel the chair at the back of the legs before sitting. The person needs to turn his head to see objects at the side rather than seeing them out of the corner of the glasses. However, more recent aspheric lenses with thinner edges widen the field of vision and produce less magnification. It is important to keep cataract lenses properly adjusted and aligned. Because the power of the thick lenses varies with their distance from the eye, when these glasses slide down the nose or are closer to the face, the clarity of the focus can be markedly altered. If the optical center of the lens does not coincide with the pupil, distortion and displacement of objects in space can occur.

Contact lenses seem to provide better vision for the aphakic person. However, inserting and removing the contact lens may be difficult for the elderly person suffering from arthritis or hand tremors. Use of soft and hard contact lenses requires finger dexterity and eye-and-hand coordination. Continued improvements in extended-wear contact lenses will lessen the frequency of insertion and removal. For some suitable individuals, intraocular implantation of an artificial lens can be performed at the time of surgery. Lens implantation is being done with increasing frequency. With an intraocular lens (IOL), the lens may move or slip inside the eye. This can cause

A Photographic Essay on Partial Sight

The material on these pages is reproduced with permission from a pamphlet prepared by the Lighthouse Low Vision Service, copyright 1976, The New York Association for the Blind. The photograph on the right shows how a person with normal or 20/20 vision sees this street scene. The photographs are presented as if the right eye were the camera.

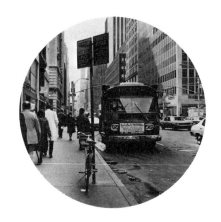

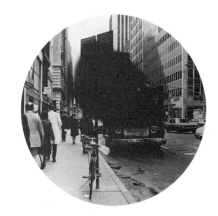

Macular degeneration: The most prevalent eye disease. The photograph shows the area of decreased central vision called a *central scotoma.* The peripheral or traveling vision remains unaffected.

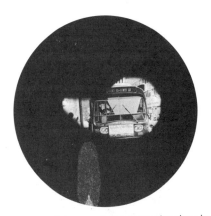

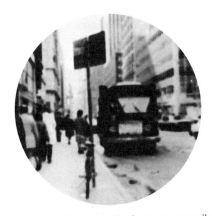

Glaucoma: Advanced glaucoma involves loss of peripheral vision, but the individual still retains most of his or her central vision. Early detection and cooperation with good medical care will prevent this drastic loss of vision.

Cataract: Diminished acuity from an opacity of the lens. The field of vision is unaffected. There is no scotoma, but the person has an overall haziness of the view, particularly in glaring light conditions.

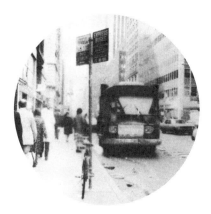

Corneal pathology: When the cells of the cornea are damaged or injured, the image becomes distorted or clouded so that the clear detail is no longer discernible. The field of vision is normal.

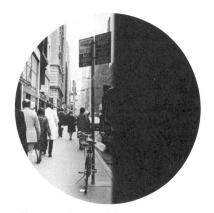

Hemianopia: A defect in the optic pathways between the eye and the brain. Vision is lost in half of a field. The most common defect occurs in the right field of vision, which causes reading impairment, *right homonymous hemianopia.*

Hemianopia: This defect can also occur on both halves of the field vision. When the defect is an inferior hemianopia, there may be interference with traveling and reading. When the visual defect is in the upper half it is called a *superior hemianopia.*

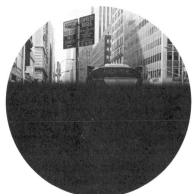

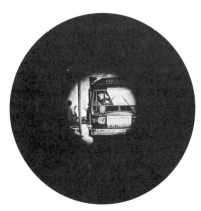

Retinitis pigmentosa: Commonly called "tunnel vision." Only a small area of central vision remains in these cases and traveling is difficult without side vision.

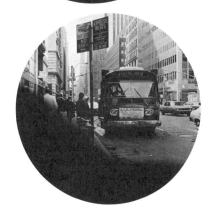

Retinal detachment: Shown here is the active stage. There are many causes for detachment, but the hole or tear allows fluid to lift the retina from its normal position. This elevated retina causes a field of vision defect, seen as a dark shadow in the peripheral field. It may be above or, as illustrated, below.

blurred vision, discomfort, problems with the cornea, or glaucoma. However, the intraocular lens usually provides excellent vision while avoiding the inconvenience of contact lenses and glasses. With an intraocular lens implant, miotic eyedrops may be ordered to constrict the pupil and to reduce the risk of lens displacement.

The nurse should be able to compare the status of the client's visual functioning before and after removal of the cataract. The client's adjustment to the replacement lens should be determined, whether it is an implanted lens, contact lens, or eyeglasses. The nurse can provide an opportunity for the client to express concerns about the cataract extraction, as well as feelings about adaptation following the extraction.

Glaucoma

Glaucoma is another major cause of visual impairment among the elderly. With glaucoma there is an elevation of intraocular pressure that can lead to optic nerve damage. Glaucoma can be acute or chronic. Irreversible visual field loss can occur if the increased pressure is not prevented or controlled. Although there are different forms of glaucoma with different causes, all forms involve some impairment in the outflow of aqueous humor from the eye (Smith, 1976). The type of glaucoma most often associated with aging is open-angle glaucoma. The drainage angle in the eye can become obstructed by the periphery of the iris. Elevated ocular pressure is connected with changes in and around the anterior chamber angle of the eye, which cause a decrease in the normal outflow of aqueous humor. Because the lens increases in thickness with age, there is a progressive shallowing of the anterior chamber. The efficiency of the mechanism for reabsorption of intraocular fluid decreases (Goldman, 1979). As the aqueous humor continues to be produced at a normal rate, the high intraocular pressure can occlude the blood supply to the retina, resulting in damage to the retinal nerve cells.

Vision can be damaged without warning, since glaucoma is painless. Peripheral vision is affected first. The visual field assessment is thus a vital aspect of the visual functioning

assessment of the elderly client. The elderly person may complain of blurred or foggy vision that is not corrected by eyeglasses. The blurred vision may be intermittent. It occurs when the increase in pressure damages the inner lining of the cornea and allows fluid to seep into its inner layer. The person is looking through a swollen cornea instead of a clear cornea. Another frequently mentioned symptom is the appearance of a halo effect, or colored rings around lights. The elderly person may complain of early morning headaches. The final stage of glaucoma may be tunnel vision, followed by blindness. Tunnel vision can create serious safety problems for the elderly person, who can easily trip over unseen objects in the environment.

Miotic drops to control glaucoma compound the reduced light access through the already smaller pupil size resulting from age-related fibrosis of the iris. Therefore, the person may have more difficulty seeing early in the morning or at dusk. Night driving may be especially difficult. A more recent drug, timolol, a beta-adrenergic blocker, results in suppression of aqueous formation. It is helpful in the elderly who have some degree of cataract formation and a contracted pupil since this medication does not cause pupillary contraction or accommodative spasm (Kornzweig, 1980). When this medication is administered, the punctum should be occluded. Systemic absorption may cause a mild slowing of the pulse. When eyedrops are not effective, oral carbonic anhydrase inhibitors will reduce aqueous production enough to control intraocular pressure. Frequently, glaucoma can be controlled by medication. Treatment for glaucoma needs to continue throughout life to maintain the controlled state. This needs to be stressed with the client. For the person with glaucoma, it is suggested that this person learn to administer the eyedrops himself. The time intervals between drops should be equally divided over the waking hours.

Dilation of the pupil resulting from sitting in the dark or the use of mydriatic medications can evoke an acute reaction, with severe eye pain. A hard and congested eye can cause a dramatic impairment in vision. Anticholinergic medications such as atropine should not be given to a person with glaucoma. It is important to reduce emotional stress situations that stimulate the autonomic nervous system and cause pupil dilation. Developing lasar technology is being used for iridectomies and to promote drainage for aqueous humor in the treatment of glaucoma.

Macular Degeneration

Another source of visual impairment in the elderly is macular degeneration. This is a serious problem, with an uncertain prognosis, since there is no specific treatment for macular degeneration. The macula is a small area of the retina responsible for distinct central vision, such as that needed to read a newspaper. The macula is vulnerable to age-related sclerotic changes. Persons with macular degeneration see only a gray shadow in the center of the visual field, and therefore find it difficult to determine what is straight ahead. Macular degeneration does not lead to total blindness. Mobility probably will continue because the person experiencing macular degeneration continues to have peripheral vision.

The exact cause of macular degeneration is not known. However, there seems to be a familial tendency, which may have a metabolic basis or could involve a disturbance in retinal circulation. It is believed that sclerosis of the choroidal vessels leads to a reduction in the amount of nutrients that reach the macula and fovea (Reichel, 1978). Some clients have been helped by photocoagulation with the laser beam. Low-vision aids, such as magnifiers and telescopic lenses, may also be helpful. The nurse can assist the elderly client with goals relating to the use of low-vision aids. The nurse's role in vision assessment is important in case-finding. Laser beam treatment may prevent or postpone severe visual loss from neovascular senile macular degeneration but early detection is essential before irreparable damage occurs.

An assessment technique that can be used to instruct elderly clients is to have the person at regular intervals of time cover one eye at a time while looking at a straight object like a door frame. With one eye covered, the door frame should look straight. If it appears bent, distorted, or has a blank spot, an ophthalmologist

should be consulted. This will allow for earlier detection of changes in vision.

Diabetic Retinopathy

Persons with diabetes now survive longer, and thus comprise an increasing percentage of the population. As a result, there is an increased frequency of diabetic retinopathy, in which the retina displays microaneurysms and small hemorrhages. New vessels form and grow out into the vitreous humor. Changes in the visual field can occur. Laser photocoagulation has been used to treat some clients with this problem. Even though photocoagulation can slow down the progression of retinopathy, it cannot restore vision and, thus, is not a cure for this problem. The nurse should stress the importance of periodic eye examinations to the client with diabetes. A determination of the client's need for health education should be one of the nurse's goals.

NURSING ASSESSMENT OF THE VISUAL FUNCTIONING OF AN ELDERLY PERSON

The nursing assessment of the elderly client's visual status should take into consideration the age-related changes in vision, the person's methods of adapting to these changes, and the visual assets that the person does possess. The environments in which the client functions must also be considered. The nurse should exchange visual status assessment data with other members of the health team, so that the client does not have to be unnecessarily subjected to repetition of the same assessment processes.

The goal of this assessment is to determine the level and adequacy of visual functioning in relation to the client's daily living needs, as a base for planning and intervening to promote optimal visual health. (For a summary, see Table 11.1.) When the nurse detects deviations that might indicate a pathologic condition, the client should be referred to the appropriate member of the health team. Eye changes in the elderly client may stem from an expected part of the aging process, eye pathologies, or systemic pathologies. The concern of the nurse is to determine the adequacy of visual functioning in relation to the daily living needs of the elderly client. Client behaviors that may indicate a vision problem include fatigue, loss of attention, frequent shifts of body position, lack of interest in the environment, and high levels of anxiety (Cristarella, 1977). In the visual assessment, the client's health history is significant because systemic health problems, such as diabetes or vascular disorders, can affect vision. The medication history also is important.

It is felt generally that the elderly do not receive adequate care for vision impairments. In institutional settings, in particular, there appears to be a lack of understanding of the importance of vision to the overall functioning of the elderly person (Pyrek and Smith, 1976). Progress continues with the use of computerized instrumentation for assessing such areas as acuity and intraocular pressure. Accurate assessment of vision is important, especially for the elderly person who continues to drive a car. Low vision can be the cause of automobile accidents.

Assessment of Light Sensitivity

Assessment of Reactions to Glare
In light sensitivity, the nurse should consider the elderly person's reactions to the lighting or sources of glare in the environment. Individual variations related to light scattering by the ocular structures will influence the optimal level of light preferred by each person. Because glare can affect the adequacy of visual functioning and can cause client discomfort, sources of glare must be identified. For example, a white ceiling can cause an overhead ceiling light to glare. In the attempt to provide adequate lighting, much glass has been used in the construction of residences and nursing homes for the elderly. However, a window that is not shaded on a bright sunny day can be another source of glare. Still other sources can include chrome furniture, glass-covered furniture, mirrors, and highly polished furniture.

The nurse observes the client in the environment to determine the area that the individual tends to choose while performing tasks or communicating with others. If an area in the environment receives a large amount of sunlight, does the client choose or avoid this area? If the sunny area is chosen, the nurse can next observe the client's activities. The client may like to sit in the sun with eyes closed, in order to enjoy its warmth. The nurse can obtain additional data about the person's light sensitivity through interviews. The client should be asked about his or her relative eye comfort in different degrees of brightness. The person may have felt varying degrees of comfort in the environment but did not realize that this was related to the lighting or glare present. The nurse can also ask the client about outdoor activity on sunny days, to determine whether he or she avoids the outdoors on bright days.

Assessment of Reactions to Dark
The elderly person's reaction to darkness is part of the light sensitivity assessment. The nurse should observe the client's mobility and ability to discriminate between objects in a darkened environment. Clues to the person's reaction to a darkened outside environment can be obtained by asking about evening activities, the mode of transportation to these activities, and reactions to being outdoors at night. The client can also be questioned about reactions to night driving. Some elderly persons may seem reluctant to discuss eye changes that affect dark adaptation and night driving because they fear losing their driver's license. Perhaps because of esteem needs, the old person who has difficulty with driving is often reluctant to accept transportation from another source. Other excuses, however, may be given for declining evening activities.

Assessment of Sensitivity to Contrasts
The nurse should assess the old person's ability to distinguish objects within varying degrees of contrast. For example, to what degree can the client distinguish a white water pitcher placed on a white tablecloth, as compared to a colored water pitcher on a white tablecloth? The elderly client may display more difficulty in detecting a darkly colored stepstool on a dark floor, as compared to a brightly colored stepstool on the dark floor. Besides using such

color contrasts to determine the ability to distinguish objects, the nurse can also try to find out which particular contrasts make objects most easily distinguishable to the client.

Assessment of Lumination Needs

The elderly person's contrast sensitivity can be affected by lumination levels. Even though eye changes can alter lumination needs, the nurse should remember that these changes and the resulting needs vary among individuals. The client can be taught ways of assessing his or her own lumination requirements and thus be able to provide for them. Often lumination needs are determined by specific tasks performed.

Assessment of Visual Acuity

The assessment of visual acuity is an important and easily performed test. It should take place in an area where lighting can be controlled. Appropriate lighting is important in determining the person's visual capabilities. Both near and far visual acuity should be assessed. A gross assessment of near visual acuity can be done by observing the client reading printed material. Print in a magazine or a book is darker than newspaper print and should be seen more readily. However, glare can be a problem if the print is on high-gloss paper. The nurse cannot always assume that the elderly person is literate, however, as some of the elderly have not had the opportunity for formal education. Recognition of familiar objects is another gross assessment technique, especially valuable in the absence of literacy. During the assessment of acuity, the client may wear corrective lenses if he has them. The nurse should be sure that the lenses are clean and properly centered on the client for a more accurate assessment of acuity. In reading printed material, the client should be asked to cover one eye with an opaque card and read several sentences. Print of different sizes can be used in this assessment. The eyes should be assessed separately and then together. Another test for near visual acuity uses reading cards. One such test is Jaegar test type, which consists of cards printed in different sizes of ordinary type. The smallest type is numbered 1, and successively

higher numbers indicate larger type. The cards are held at a distance of about 14 inches from the eye.

Another technique for assessing visual acuity is to have the client count the nurse's raised fingers. This can be used to determine both near and far vision. The distance at which the fingers are counted should be measured. The nurse can assess the client's ability to read print on television at varying distances and to read printed materials on bulletin boards.

A standardized chart can be used to assess visual acuity for distance. The Snellen chart, with various sizes of letters, is most commonly used for assessing distance vision. In using this chart, one eye should be assessed at a time, with and without corrective lenses. The client should be instructed to stand 20 feet away from the chart. Visual acuity is expressed as a ratio of what a person should see at 20 feet as compared to what the person is able to see at 20 feet. The client is asked to read the smallest line he can see. If the majority of the letters on a given line are read correctly, the person is credited with this line of vision (one or two letters may be missed). For clients with vision so impaired that they cannot see even the largest letter or symbol on a chart, additional acuity tests include counting fingers, perceiving hand movements, and perceiving light. The nurse should remember that the Snellen chart provides an assessment of recognition acuity. An illiterate client may say that he cannot see the chart, rather than admit the inability to recognize letters or words. Charts with easily recognizable symbols are available for use with illiterate persons. Kenney and Kenney (1980) strongly recommend testing visual acuity with familiar running text that the client ordinarily uses rather than unrelated letters. They also encourage flexibility in the use of distances, positions, and lighting. Even though 20 feet is a standardized simulation of distance, the elderly person may need to assume his own preferred distance for the test of near vision.

In tests of resolution acuity, the client responds to the separation between elements of a pattern. For example, vertical and horizontal bars can be used, with space between the bars varied until the client can no longer divide the bars and spaces. The client may see the area as a gray patch, or may be able to detect and count the bars. The assessment of visual acuity indicates the adequacy of central vision and the functioning of the macular area of the retina. It is important to realize that visual acuity does not exactly predict visual performance. The individual's personality is a key factor in the ability to use visual assets.

Assessment of Accommodation

Before assessing accommodation, the nurse must determine whether the client is aphakic as a result of cataract extraction. If the person is aphakic, the nurse should determine the type of replacement lens the client uses and how often the lenses are used. Clients who have not had a lens extraction can be requested to read printed material without corrective lenses. The nurse may find that the client is able to read print only from a distance, but does not have bifocal lenses to correct this change in accommodation. The client may compensate by avoiding print materials and fine detail work.

To assess the accommodative response of the pupil, the nurse can hold one fingertip about 4 inches away but directly in front of the eye being tested. The person is asked to look at the fingertip, then at the far wall directly beyond the fingertip. In this way the client utilizes both near and far vision. The pupils should constrict as the glance is shifted from a distant object to a near object. This is part of the eye's adaptive mechanism for focusing on distant, then on close objects. The time needed for this response to occur varies among individuals, but the presence of the response and the equality of response in both pupils are significant. In assessing accommodation, the nurse can ask the client about reactions to work requiring near vision and his or her responses to corrective lenses.

Assessment of Visual Fields

Assessment of the visual fields provides a measurement of the retina's ability to receive peripheral stimuli. To perform a gross assessment of peripheral vision, the nurse sits opposite the client at a distance of about 2 feet. (It is assumed that the nurse performing the as-

sessment has normal peripheral vision.) The client covers one eye with an opaque card. The nurse covers his or her eye that is opposite the client's covered eye. Each looks directly toward the other's open eye. The nurse holds a small object beyond the field of vision and gradually moves the object toward the center of the field. The object should be moved horizontally, superiorly, and inferiorly during this assessment. The client and the nurse should be able to visualize the object at the same time. More accurate ophthalmic measurements can be utilized to determine visual fields if this gross assessment indicates limited peripheral vision. The position of the client may affect the visual fields. The loss of orbital fat can cause some recession of the eye. This can result in a deepening of the upper lid fold and a slight obstructive reduction in the peripheral visual field. This recession is greater when the elderly person is in a supine position.

The nurse should also observe the client for the presence of visual spatial neglect, in which a person appears to ignore objects and people in half of the environment. For example, the person may eat food from only one side of the plate, or may bump into objects on a specific side. This problem may exist in persons who have a history of cerebrovascular accident with resulting hemianopsia. As part of this assessment, the nurse places a newspaper or magazine in a midline position in front of the client. The client is asked to read this material, starting at the upper left-hand corner and continuing across the entire page. The client may also be asked to identify objects placed horizontally on a table. A person with decreased visual fields may also display problems with mobility, such as the tendency to bump into or trip over objects in the environment.

As mentioned earlier, assessment of peripheral vision is significant in detecting the possibility of glaucoma. If further medical testing, including a test of ocular tension, leads to a diagnosis of glaucoma, appropriate treatment can be initiated. There is a strong possibility that treatment can prevent further visual loss. Two nursing students, as part of their clinical training, were performing a sensory assessment of their clients in an acute-care setting. They detected decreased visual fields in two elderly clients. These individuals were referred for further diagnostic study, which revealed the presence of glaucoma. Both of these persons were not aware of any visual impairment prior to the sensory assessment performed by the nursing students. This demonstrates the nurse's important role in preventing further visual impairment.

A sudden curtain-like loss of the visual field from any direction may indicate the likelihood of a retinal detachment, especially if floaters and flashing lights before the eyes have been experienced in the preceding days or weeks. The person needs to be cautioned against strenuous or abrupt physical activities.

The loss of vision in one eye, whether due to pathology, trauma, or eyepatching, results in the loss of the full visual field.

Assessment of Color Discrimination
In assessing the ability to discriminate colors, the level of illumination is important, because color can change in appearance as illumination changes. Color depends on the reflective characteristics of the colored material and the distribution of the illumination. Color contrasts are also significant. For example, a white area surrounded by yellow may appear to be tinged with blue.

The elderly person may not be aware of difficulty in discriminating colors. Clothing color combinations that appear inappropriate may indicate problems with color discrimination. Elderly women who use hair dyes may be unaware that their hair has taken on a blue-gray color. Standard tests, such as the Holmgren test, can be used to determine color discrimination. During this test, the client is given a set of pieces of yarn. The colors of the yarn include the three primary colors, with derivative shades of each. The client is asked to match the yarn according to colors. Similar tests can include matching colored paper or other colored material.

Assessment of Visual Spatial Ability
To assess visual spatial ability in the elderly client, cues in the environment can be utilized. The person can be asked to describe the size,

distance, and position of objects placed at varying distances. The objects chosen can also be illuminated to varying degrees, to allow for the effects of shadows and highlights. An object chosen may overlap another object. Assessment of the client's visual spatial ability can include depth perception, which determines the ability to estimate relative distances and relief. Depth perception is distinguished from the spatial ability needed to estimate the height and width of an object. The client's ability to determine the relative motion of an object is also a part of this assessment. Problems with visual spatial ability can affect the person's perception of long hallways, which may appear to be endless. This, in turn, can affect the person's degree of motivation to move about in an area with many long hallways.

Assessment of Ocular Structures

Eyelashes and Eyebrows
As part of the external examination of eye structures, the eyelashes and eyebrows should be inspected. The eyebrows are assessed for quantity, distribution, and color of brow hair. The eyebrow should be inspected for loss of support and sagging that may compound upper lid ptosis. The underlying skin also should be inspected for irritation or scaling. Although greying seems to proceed at the same rate over the aging body, there is preservation of melanin in the eyelashes and, to a lesser extent, the eyebrows. The eyelashes act as tactile organs, and both eyebrows and eyelashes have a protective function. The nurse can assess the tactile sensitivity of the eyelashes and the direction in which the lashes turn. Inward turning of an eyelash can lead to corneal irritation. The eyelashes should be evenly distributed.

Eyelids
The eyelids should be assessed for their ability to close and the degree to which they are able to open. With the loss of orbital fat there is a deepening of the upper lid fold. Loss of elasticity in the skin of the eyelids can cause them to become wrinkled, while loss of subcutaneous fat can increase their transparent appearance. The assessment of the elderly person's eyelids

should include the ability to open and close both eyelids equally. A cotton-tipped applicator can be used to evert the eyelids for inspection of the palpebral conjunctiva. The tissues underlying the conjunctiva should be inspected for color, smoothness, and the presence of secretions. In the elderly person, the conjunctiva may appear yellow as the result of fat deposits in subconjunctival layers.

Old persons who have lost eyelid muscle tone may experience a sagging or eversion of the lower lid. This condition, known as ectropion, can cause chronic conjunctivitis or a problem with overflow of tears, since it interferes with normal tear drainage. An in-rolling or inversion of the lower eyelid, called entropion, can also occur. This problem can lead to corneal irritation as a result of the lower lashes rubbing the cornea. In addition, as the skin of the eyelids undergo thinning and relaxation with age, a redundant fold from the lower lid can fall onto the lashes. This can cause an awning-like restriction of the upper visual fields. The weight of the upper lid fold may cause an upper lid ptosis. Relaxation of the eyelids may be more apparent when the elderly person leans forward in the reading position. Besides the irritating effects of eyelid changes, the elderly person may experience an altered body image because of altered cosmetic appearance. Drooping or wrinkled eyelids, as well as entropion or ectropion of the lids, can cause a distinct change in facial appearance. The nurse should also palpate the eyelids gently for smoothness and sensitivity. The presence of crusting, which can cause irritation, may indicate abnormal secretions or problems with eye hygiene.

Lacrimal Functioning

The lacrimal functioning of the eye is part of the eye assessment. Tear secretion may decrease with age, even though the eye may appear to be wet. Normally, as the tears wash across the eye, they drain through the puncta, which are located on the nasal end of both upper and lower eyelids. Stenosis of the puncta or eversion of the lower lid can interfere with the passageway of the tears. If lower lid relaxation has resulted in the forward rotation of the puncta, there will be inadequate tear si-

phoning. Also, the sphincter-like lacrimal papilla may relax. This, too, interferes with the efficient siphon of tears. Tears spilling into the lower eyelid of the elderly person can cause reddening and irritation. Whether the supply of tears is adequate should also be considered, as some elderly persons secrete only scanty amounts of lacrimal fluid. A deficiency can lead to corneal irritation, because tears have both cleansing and lubricating functions. There tends to be a slight physiologic reduction in tear secretion with advancing age. Deficient tear secretion can result in an uncomfortable gritty sensation of the eye.

Conjunctiva

An assessment of the palpebral conjunctiva was included in the discussion of the eyelids. The palpebral portion of the conjunctiva lines the eyelids and covers their vascular structures. It is continuous with the bulbar conjunctiva which lies over the sclera. The conjunctiva merges with the cornea at the limbus. The bulbar portion contains many small blood vessels. Reddening of conjunctiva may be due to vascular proliferation. The bulbar conjunctiva thins with age, probably because of a loss in conjunctival elasticity (Weale, 1963). The bulbar conjunctiva of the elderly person may contain calcareous deposits embedded in the subepithelial tissues. These deposits are a source of irritation. Atrophic changes of the conjunctiva can cause conjunctivitis, often accompanied by a profuse shedding of tears. To assess the conjunctiva and sclera, have the client look up as the lower lid is depressed with the thumb.

Sclera

The sclera of the elderly person's eyes may exhibit a yellowish tinge as a result of lipid deposits. There may be increased rigidity of the sclera, and the blood vessels may appear to be tortuous (Weale, 1963). Moderate changes in the vessels of the sclera in the elderly person are not considered to be pathologic.

Cornea

Brightness of the cornea can indicate tear flow adequacy. Spotty or extensive corneal dullness may indicate subnormal tear flow. In the assessment of the cornea of the old person, the arcus senilis or gerontoxon may be observed. This is a demarcatory circle between the iris and sclera, produced by the fatty invasion of the corneal margin. The cornea may appear flattened in the elderly person, and degenerative changes may be observed in the corneal epithelium. The cornea should be inspected for opacities. In the elderly person, it may have less lustre. The sensitivity of the cornea tends to decrease with age (Fozard, 1977), and there is loss of corneal endothelial cells. Pigment deposits may be also seen on the posterior corneal surface.

The nurse can test the corneal reflex of the elderly person by gently touching the cornea with a wisp of cotton. The nurse should bring the wisp of cotton from the lateral side of the eye before brushing the cotton across the cornea. The client should react by closing both eyelids to protect the cornea. Tearing should occur when the cornea is touched.

Iris

In assessing the iris of the elderly person, a decrease in pigmentation may be observed, especially around the pupillary margin. In this assessment, the nurse can compare the color of the iris in both eyes. The client may also be questioned about the perception of the color of his or her eyes.

Pupil

The pupil of each eye should be assessed for size, shape, reaction to light, and accommodation, and the results compared. A penlight is used to assess pupillary reflexes. To assess the response to light, the light beam is brought in from the side and directed at one eye at a time. The eye toward which the light is directed is observed for constriction, while the other eye also is observed. While performing this assessment, it is advisable to have the room darkened.

Retina

In order to assess the retina, an ophthalmoscope is needed. Opacities of the lens and of the vitreous humor may be observed in the elderly person. The number and degree of these opacities will determine the degree of visibility of the retina. Structures to observe on the retina include the optic disc, the four sets of retinal vessels, the macular area, and the retinal background. The eyes of the elderly person may reveal a thickened choroid, dilated retinal veins, yellowish-white spots (known as Drusen or Bruck's membrane), and high transparency of the retina in the most central region. There may be vitreous and peripheral retinal detachments (Fozard et al., 1977).

Assessment of Ocular Movements

To assess the functioning of the eye muscles, the nurse should ask the client to move his or her eyes through the six cardinal positions of gaze, while following an object such as a pencil or the nurse's finger. The nurse moves the object laterally to either side along a horizontal axis, then along two oblique axes that make a 60° angle to the horizontal axis. The nurse observes the client's ability to move both eyes together, as well as the movements of the eye when the gaze is transferred to a lateral position. This movement should appear as a smooth process.

Nystagmus is the fine, rhythmic involuntary movement of the eyes that occurs when the gaze is transferred to a lateral position. In testing for nystagmus, extreme lateral fixation points should be avoided. A study of gaze measurements in elderly clients demonstrated that there were no age differences in lower limits of gaze, but changes were noted in upward gaze among the elderly. The explanation given was that the elevator muscle of the eyeball atrophies with age due to disease (Fozard et al., 1977).

Assessment of Reactions to Visual Changes

Visual changes in the elderly person may first be detected by the nurse or by another member of the health team. The individual may or may not be aware of any changes in visual function. Because these changes tend to occur gradually, the elderly person may not recognize a vision problem until it has progressed to the point of affecting activities of daily living. Old persons may experience changes in eye comfort, in the form of eye strain or fatigue. The individual may eliminate reading because of such discomfort.

If visual change progresses to the point of impairing normal functioning, the elderly person often feels handicapped, and may need to grieve for the visual losses that are impairing personal and social activities. The grieving process may be especially evident in those who have experienced sudden severe vision impairment or blindness. Changes in the ability to see can threaten an individual's feelings of wholeness. The person may feel a loss of power and control. This is especially significant in the elderly person who is experiencing loss of power and control in other areas at the same time. There tends to be resistance to giving up sight-oriented activities. A major loss is experienced when vision problems force the elderly person to stop driving a car.

In the assessment, the nurse must determine the elderly person's degree of acceptance of any visual impairment present, as well as the degree of anxiety connected with visual changes that are viewed as handicapping. Visual impairment often intensifies the person's feelings of dependency and inadequacy. The nurse should determine how these changes have affected both the person's physical and psychologic independence. The visually impaired person's freedom of mobility should be assessed. Hesitant movements may indicate the need for mobility training or mobility aids. The elderly individual's reluctance to move about in the environment may indicate a need for help with environmental orientation. The effect of the visual impairment on the person's self-concept must also be considered, and will be strongly influenced by the person's self-concept prior to the visual change or loss of vision.

The elderly person may have transient attacks of blindness. It is important to determine when these attacks occur, how long they last, and the amount of vision involved. The person may lose half of the right or left fields of vision in both eyes, or there may be intermittent bilateral blurred vision. Both of these situations call for further medical cerebrocirculatory diagnostic study. These changes may cause high levels of anxiety in the client, who should be encouraged to discuss them with the nurse.

The elderly person may experience changes in vision as a result of medications. The nurse should find out what medication the client is taking and whether it has the potential to cause vision changes. The nurse can share this information with the client and should also provide appropriate follow-up reports on any vision changes. It is possible that changes can be made in the medication. Alternatively, the nurse may plan approaches with the elderly person to reduce the disturbing effects and anxiety caused by the medication. It is important for the nurse to understand what effect vision changes experienced by the elderly person have on self-image, social relationships, and ability to function in the physical environment.

Social relationships may be hampered markedly with the elderly person whose visual functioning interferes with accurate interpretation of the environment. Inappropriate behavior may occur, thus further alienating the elderly person, who may then be labeled as confused, further reducing social interaction. This in turn increases the sensory deprivation of the person, adversely affecting mental functioning.

Reactions of the Nurse to the Elderly Person with Changes in Vision

To gain a better understanding of the age-related changes in vision, nurses should assess their present level of knowledge and degree of empathy toward persons with visual changes. In this introspective process, the nurse must consider various questions. To what degree does the nurse feel comfortable in assessing the elderly person's vision? What does the nurse do with the assessment data obtained? What community services are available to the client experiencing changes that lead to visual impairment? Does the nurse label as confused the person who misinterprets the environment?

To increase empathy with the elderly client experiencing vision changes, the nurse can experience these changes through simulation. For example, a pair of glasses can be covered with wrinkled plastic wrap, or a lubricant can be placed on the glasses to blur the image. A nurse who wears corrective lenses can remove these and attempt to function in the environment without them, by trying to read, watch television, or interact with others. It is important to maintain an awareness of one's reactions during these experiences. Time is also a factor. Experiencing a visual change for a few minutes does not evoke the same feelings as experiencing it for several hours or longer while trying to maintain activities of daily living.

The nurse should be aware of his or her reactions to people with severe visual impairment or blindness. A common reaction of sighted people to even superficial contact with a blind person is the feeling of pity and sympathy (Monbeck, 1973). Many people have a strong fear of blindness, and prefer to avoid contact with blind persons. Negative attitudes may be the result of unfounded fears, misinformation, or false beliefs. In order to be a helping person in working with the elderly client who is severely visually impaired or blind, the nurse should be aware of his or her feelings about blindness. The nurse should also recognize that the person with limited sight or none at all is very little different from sighted people.

Assessment of the Environment

The environment of the elderly client must be assessed for the manner in which it supports or limits the person's independence. Environmental considerations include type and placement of lighting and provisions for control of lighting, kind and placement of furniture, windows and window coverings, stairways and hallways, colors and color contrasts in the environment, and textures used.

The elderly person's use of the environment can be assessed. Personal territory is significant and can give clues to the adequacy of the individual's visual functioning. The nurse should determine the extent of the client's personal territory, which may be limited to indoor areas or may span a large geographic area.

Support for the elderly person in a home setting may be provided by family members or significant others. If the person is in an insti-

tutional setting the nurse should assess the support received from personnel and other residents.

Assessment of the Elderly Person's Use of Corrective Devices

The elderly person's ability to use and maintain corrective lenses or other low-vision aids is part of the assessment. The emotional impact of the corrective device should be considered. Some individuals may feel free to use a low-vision device, such as a magnifying glass for reading, only when alone. Potential problems among elderly persons who wear glasses, especially those in institutional settings, include misplacing the glasses, losing them if they are not clearly identified, breakage of glasses (usually as a result of improper placement), and lack of cleanliness of the lenses. The nurse should also determine whether the elderly person tends to remove the glasses because they do not fit comfortably. The person may not wear glasses while in bed.

The adequacy of the corrective lenses should be assessed. Some old people may not have had a change of prescription for many years, or may have purchased nonprescription glasses. The cost of an ophthalmic exam and glasses may seem prohibitive to the elderly person who is on a very limited income. If a client has appropriate glasses but does not wear them, an assessment should be done to determine why. Perhaps the frames do not fit comfortably, or feel too heavy. If corrective lenses are not appropriate to the client's needs or are not worn appropriately, the nurse must determine reasons for this in order to be effective in planning and intervention to promote optimum vision.

PLANNING AND INTERVENTION

Following the assessment of the visual status of the elderly person, the nurse and other members of the health team join with the client, family, and significant others to plan for the greatest possible use of what vision the client possesses, as well as for prevention or limitation of visual problems. The individual may have limited visual changes, low vision, or may be considered blind. The blindness may have existed for many years or may be a recent development. These data will be available from the assessment and will influence the goals that are mutually established. In establishing goals, consideration should be given to the client's needs and desires, ability to adapt to new situations, and motivation to learn new visual habits. The goals should include protection, maintenance, and maximization of the old person's visual status. Maximization of vision may result simply from cleaning the person's glasses or by encouraging the person to wear glasses.

Low-vision clients are best grouped according to level of function. This classification promotes optimal visual functioning. Acuity numbers alone may not indicate the degree of functional visual impairment. The following is an example of functional grouping (Faye, 1976):

Maintenance of Desired Life-Style

The elderly person's desired life-style is central to the goals established. An individual with limited vision or who is blind may simply wish to be able to walk about in his or her home. Another person may have the goal of functioning independently in the living environment. Goals may also relate to independent functioning outside the home setting. For the nurse or other member of the health team to establish goals without the client's input can add to the frustrations of the elderly person. If the elderly client desires to remain independent at home, while the nurse establishes a goal that relates to the client's ability to function in the community, failure of the latter goal is highly probable. Failure to meet this goal may even hamper the client's more limited goal of independence in the home setting.

Desired life-style goals may include main-

Groups	Needs
Least impaired	
Vision does not impair ability to function.	Standard refraction Low-power reading aids
Moderate functional impairment	
Moderate reduction of acuity and insignificant loss of visual fields.	Standard refraction Talking books and tapes Large print Writing aids Greater illumination
Moderately impaired function	
Reduced acuity and central vision, moderate field loss and/or inability to cope physically with impaired vision.	Standard refraction usually will not improve distance vision. Reading is difficult even with aids. May need telescopic or electronic aids. May qualify as legally blind.
Poor functional vision	
Poor central vision, marked field loss, psychologic as well as physical problems with adaptation.	Standard refraction of little or no value. Strong reading aids needed for near vision. May need mobility and orientation training to manage in the environment.
Most visually impaired	
Poor visual acuity, field loss may be major.	Uses visual cues for mobility. Cannot read continuous text. Needs orientation and mobility training. Needs training in daily living skills.

tenance of employment for the elderly person. Visual changes may affect the client's ability to continue in his or her present job. Visual aids may be needed, or a change of work role may be necessary. The nurse must consider the importance of the work role to the client who is employed, regardless of chronologic age.

Life-style goals may include maintenance of reading patterns or activity patterns that require detail work. To meet this goal, alternatives can be provided when visual changes affect the person's ability to read newspaper print or to work with detail, such as sewing or handicrafts. If lenses with the best possible correction do not help the client, low-vision aids can be utilized.

Use of Low-Vision Aids

The elderly person with low vision is one whose distance and near vision cannot be corrected to within normal range with conventional lenses. The person with low vision needs to rely on aids other than standard corrective lenses. Functional vision can be improved with the use of low-vision aids by assisting the person to use any existing vision. Low-vision aids magnify and make clear a portion or segment of an object. The two types of low-vision aids are magnifiers for near vision and telescopic devices for distance. The elderly person with impaired vision needs to know what types of low-vision aids are available, as well as their price ranges. With advancing technology, an increasing variety of aids have become available. Both illuminated and nonilluminated magnifiers are available. These are helpful in reading printed materials, and are especially useful for finding a number in the telephone directory. An elderly person who uses a magnifier for reading may experience fatigue. The posture assumed while using a low-vision device can affect the amount of fatigue that the elderly person experiences. Supports, such as cushions and footstools, can help to maintain a posture that minimizes fatigue.

Another low-vision aid is the optocon, a reading aid that converts the image of a printed letter into a vibrating tactile form. The stereotoner is an aid that converts light into electrical current. When a photocell is darkened by part of a letter image, electronic circuits in the control box produce a musical tone. This instrument also contains a magnifier system. Reading machines are now available that convert printed materials into synthetic speech. Closed-circuit television systems are available that project enlarged print onto a television screen for viewing. Phone dial attachments with enlarged numbers and letters permit greater ease and accuracy in dialing. Reading materials with print of varying size and darkness are available. The American Foundation for the Blind offers lists of devices available for persons with low vision. However, the elderly person should understand the limitations of these aids as well as the benefits they provide. When possible, they should be tried before purchase.

Other low-vision aids utilize the person's touch abilities. The time can be read on a clock or watch by removing the covering of the face. Many advances are occurring in optics to allow the visually impaired person to maintain his or her desired life-style. In working with the elderly client, the nurse should be aware of the aids that are available, even though another member of the health team may provide them and instruct the person in their use. The philosophy of those who work with visually impaired people is changing to include the elderly person in rehabilitation programs to a greater degree. In a large extended-care facility in one metropolitan area, workers from a community agency that provides help to visually impaired and blind persons come to the facility. Visits are made on a regular basis to provide instruction to the visually impaired residents. This instruction promotes independent living for these elderly clients.

Catalogues are available for aids to daily living. An example is the catalogue available from:

• Aids and Appliances for the Blind and Visually Impaired
  The American Foundation for the Blind
  15 West 16th Street
  New York, New York 10011

For information on talking books:

- The Library of Congress
  Blind and Physically Handicapped Division
  1291 Taylor Street NW
  Washington, D.C. 20011

There is a center for the partially sighted:

- Center for the Partially Sighted
  Santa Monica Medical Center
  1250 Sixteenth Street
  Santa Monica, California 90404

Use of Mobility Aids

The nurse may be instrumental in obtaining assistance for the elderly person in the form of mobility aids. Mobility is the skill necessary for an individual to propel himself safely from one location to another in an independent manner (Monroe, 1978). Mobility aids assist in orientating the visually impaired person to the environment. A referral to a community agency that offers mobility instruction can be made by the nurse. The cane continues to be the most commonly used mobility aid for the person with severe visual impairment or blindness. The cane is used to feel the terrain in front of the client, thus permitting the person to walk without the assistance of another person. The cane is held in the center of the body and is not raised any more than 2 inches from the surface. Other probing instruments are also available. These instruments make use of ultrasonic transmitter devices, which may be placed in canes, on glass frames, or around the person's waist. Work is continuing on development of probing instruments that would be simple and unobtrusive while conveying significant information. As with the visual aids, cost may be the limiting factor in utilization of these mobility aids.

The nurse can teach the visually impaired client to use kinesthesis to detect gradients or tilts in surfaces, and to estimate distances. For ambulation, the nurse walks ahead of the visually impaired client, who firmly holds the nurse's arm just below the elbow. This allows the person to follow the movements of the nurse. The nurse should indicate and describe stairs or any other surface changes.

In assisting the visually disabled person to walk, the nurse should not grasp the client's arm, but rather should permit the client to grasp her arm. The arm is grasped at the elbow. The nurse's arm should be close to her body to allow the client to feel the direction the body is moving.

Orientation Instruction

A person with visual impairment needs to know where he or she is in terms of the immediate environment. Orientation is the individual's skill or ability to identify the environment and to relate to that environment (Monroe, 1978). For the visually impaired person, the senses of hearing, touch, and smell become increasingly important in gaining information about the environment. Such landmarks as a chair, the heat of the sun from a window, or the smell of a flower in the yard help in the orientation to the environment. An adventitiously (in contrast to congenitally) blinded or visually impaired person can use visual memory. Through training, the sense of hearing, touch, and smell can be developed to a greater extent.

Hearing provides information on identification, direction, distance, size, and structure. Emphasis can be placed on the recognition and identification of sounds. The sighted person who enters the territory of a person with a visual impairment should identify himself and inform the person when leaving the area. Others in the area should be identified to the visually impaired person to facilitate social interaction. Persons with severe visual impairment should be told where they are going when environments are changed.

Touch can be used to learn about size, weight, volume, density, and texture. The severely visually impaired person should be encouraged to touch objects in the environment. Objects that are very small or very large are more difficult for the visually impaired person to experience by touch. Odors can also assist in identification of landmarks—for instance, a chlorinated swimming pool. Food can be identified by smell and taste.

The nurse should understand how adequately the other senses function in the visually impaired client. Age-related changes in all senses are a potential problem with the elderly person. However, the degree of these changes varies with the individual. The nurse should help the client to make optimal use of the potential of all senses to compensate for a known impairment. Referral to an orientation specialist for further assistance in functioning with the desired degree of independence may be necessary.

Skills for Independent Living at Home
When the nurse works with the visually impaired elderly person in the home setting, adaptations to facilitate homemaking can be made in the home environment. Contrasting colors can be used on cupboards, drawers, and dials, such as stove dials. Measuring cups are available with raised letters. Utensils made of non-glare materials can be used, instead of chrome utensils. If the client lives with family members, goals should be directed toward keeping the person functioning as a family member. However, if the client lives alone, emphasis will be placed on maintenance of daily living activities.

Activities of Daily Living
For the visually impaired person who lives alone, emphasis should be placed on living tasks such as care of clothing, reading mail, and identifying labels on containers. The elderly person may have difficulty differentiating colors. The nurse can suggest that the person select articles of clothing that are clearly in contrast with each other, rather than choosing items in different shades of the same color, as these may tend to clash. Other activities with which the visually impaired elderly may need assistance include eating in a socially acceptable manner, pouring liquids safely, dialing a telephone, identifying money, and shopping.

If assessment reveals a change in the person's upward gaze, goals should relate to placing objects, such as clocks and calendars, at or near eye level. The ability to read overhead street signs may be affected by the vision change. Aids should be provided to allow the person to enjoy leisure activities, such as watching television or playing cards.

Safety
Goals relating to safety of the elderly person with vision changes must be conveyed to members of the health team and to family members or significant others. Data from the assessment of the client will reveal the degree of vision change so that safety needs can be determined. However, in settings where all residents are old, such as extended-care facilities or apartment buildings for the elderly, standard safety measures should be part of the environment. Prevention of falls is a major concern. Also, there is a need for caution in taking medications when directions on the bottle are difficult to read. Labels on food and other household containers may be difficult to read when there are changes in vision.

Lighting
As mentioned earlier, the level of illumination required by the elderly person is increased, but at the same time glare must be avoided. Exposed light bulbs are undesirable; they tend to produce the greatest degree of glare, and may also cause shadows. It is better to use fluorescent or frosted bulbs, especially with a light-diffusing fixture (Kornzweig, 1971). The old person should be able to control the light switches so that illumination levels can be adjusted for varying activities which require different kinds and amounts of light. However, the background light should not be as bright as the light for the area in which an activity is occurring, since light relationships are as significant as the amount of light.

Lights need to be placed at all potentially dangerous areas: doorways, halls, stairways, and any obstructed or cluttered areas. Low-wattage lamps can be placed along frequently used paths, such as to the kitchen or bathroom. Some of these may be left on at night. Small night-lights are not adequate, however. The elderly person should be cautioned about moving between areas of marked differences in illumination. Sufficient time should be allowed to adjust to varying levels of illumination and to adapt to darkness. Easily accessible light switches should be provided in areas traveled during darkness. The elderly person should be cautioned to look away from the light when a light switch is turned on because of the possible blinding effects produced by sharp lighting contrasts. More recent developments in lighting increase the ease of providing adequate lighting. Heat-sensitive dimmer switches that are activated by touch change the intensity of a light when a person touches the switch. Another device is the motion or sound detector, which automatically turns lights on in response to noise or movement, except where there is already natural light in the environment.

Lighting at night is absolutely necessary for hallways and bathrooms. Clutter should be avoided in any area in which the elderly person travels after dark. For example, small furniture items, such as stools or wastebaskets, should not be placed in a hallway through which old people must travel at night on the way to the bathroom. Specific rooms have different lighting requirements. Low-glare lamps are well suited for illuminating the floor and lower walls of a bedroom. In the kitchen, lights in cupboards and "task lighting" are needed to directly illuminate a work area. Other task areas include reading areas, telephone stands, and closets.

Glare can be avoided by careful choice of furniture and utensils in the environment. If a table has a glare-producing finish, place mats or a tablecloth can be used. Even though daylight from a window helps to meet illumination needs, the elderly person should be able to control window coverings so that the discomforting glare of bright sun is avoided. The goal is to block out bright sunlight while allowing natural light to enter the room. Highly polished floors also increase glare and can be a hazard to the elderly person walking on a polished hallway floor, especially one that is receiving bright sunlight from an uncovered window. Glare from the television screen can be prevented by adjustment of lighting in the room. The goal of all lighting is to achieve a balance between getting enough light into the eyes of the elderly person and preventing glare.

The glare of outdoor sunlight can be un-

comfortable for the elderly person. The reflection of a bright sun on snow, in particular, can produce a large amount of glare. When outdoors in bright sunlight, the elderly client can be advised to wear a hat with a brim, or sunglasses, or to carry an umbrella (Fig. 11.1). After exposure to outdoor sun, the individual should be cautious when going back indoors. This can be an especial problem if steps must be maneuvered while entering a building. The elderly person should move slowly between areas that have marked contrasts in illumination.

Safety must be considered by the elderly person who drives at night. The glare of oncoming headlights or from dark, wet roads can have a blinding effect. If the nurse is planning activities with an elderly client, they should be scheduled during daytime hours unless al-

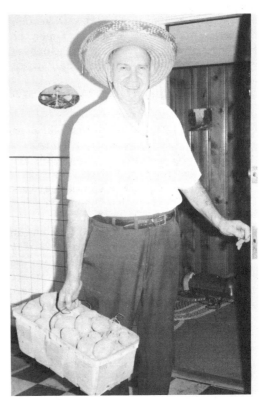

Figure 11.1. Protection from glare is achieved by wearing a hat. *(Photograph by Eugene Mizikar.)*

ternate transportation arrangements are available. The constriction of the pupil caused by miotic medication causes particular problems in adjusting quickly to changes in illumination. This can be hazardous at night, especially for the old person who is driving. Driving in very bright sunlight may also be difficult, because of reduced tolerance to glare.

Use of Color

Environmental safety can be increased by use of contrasting colors which enhance the visibility of objects (Fig. 11.2). Colors used on steps are vital in delineating each step. Even a person who has not experienced vision changes may have trouble maneuvering steps covered with dark carpeting, since it is often difficult to determine where one step ends and another begins. A contrasting color applied to the edge of each step outlines it clearly so that an elderly person can better determine how to manage the steps. Painting or using a bright covering on the first and last step aids the person

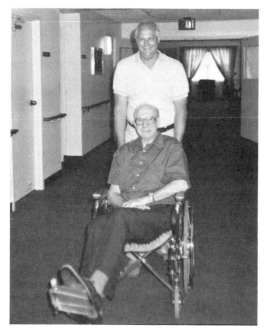

Figure 11.2. Contrasting colors and the use of lighting are effective in this nursing home setting.

who has limited depth perception. Hand rails and adequate lighting should be provided in every stairway. Warnings should be posted in doorways that open directly onto a flight of steps.

When using color, the nurse should know which colors the elderly can discriminate most easily. These colors include the yellows and reds. Yellow promotes depth vision. Yellow provides a better view for signs at a distance. A low-gloss finish is preferable, to avoid glare. If colored or white paper is used for printed materials, the paper should not have a shiny finish.

Color contrasts make objects easier to detect. Light-colored dinner plates can be placed on a dark table. Color contrasts are especially helpful in visualizing small objects. Avoid similar colors, such as white objects on a beige background. The labels on medication bottles should be printed with large type on a nonglare background.

Other Aspects of Environmental Safety

The environment of an elderly person who has visual problems should be consistent and predictable. In planning for environmental safety, the nurse should take into consideration any possible decrease in the elderly person's visual fields. The client with decreased visual fields should be taught to survey the environment by turning the head, so that unseen objects do not become a hazard. Low-hanging objects, such as fire extinguishers, can also be hazardous to the elderly person with a reduced field of vision.

The change in accommodation often experienced by the elderly client affects the activity goals. Activities that require frequent changes in distance vision should allow enough time for accommodation to occur. Activities that involve some distance vision usually are preferable to those that require looking at objects at varying distances within short periods of time.

Keeping objects in familiar places in the environment helps to maintain the safety of the elderly person with a visual impairment. Objects should not be moved to new locations without consulting the client. The nurse should also warn the person about obstacles in the environment. Environmental goals established with the elderly person who experiences vision changes should be intended to increase the supportive qualities of the environment. A safe, supportive environment will promote the desired degree of independence and help to maintain the elderly client's sense of self-worth.

Eye Medications

Many elderly persons receive eye medications in drops and ointments. Two of the most common drops are miotics, which reduce intraocular pressure caused by glaucoma, and artificial tears. With chronic problems that necessitate long-term use of eyedrops, the elderly person needs to develop a reliable system for instilling the eye drops.

In administering eye medications, the goal is to retain the drug on the surface of the eyeball, in order to prolong its action on eye structures, and to prevent systemic absorption of the medication. There are several steps to the procedure. First, the medication is placed in the everted lower eyelid. The lower lid is gently pulled down and out. The client is instructed to look up as the eye medication is placed in the cul-de-sac. The client gently closes the eyelids, which distributes the drug over the surface of the eye. The medication should not be applied directly to the cornea. Next, with the eyelids apart, the nurse applies finger pressure at the inner canthus for about 2 minutes. This pressure prevents the medication from entering the lacrimal ducts and the upper respiratory tract, where it might be absorbed into the bloodstream and cause systemic problems.

For self-administration of eye medication, the client is instructed to place a finger on his cheek below the lower lid and pull downward fixing the skin against the cheekbone. This forms a "V" pocket into which the medication can be instilled.

In administering miotics, the nurse needs to be aware of the pupil size. This observation is important in minimizing the strength of the miotic ordered to control intraocular pressure. There is a need to reduce unnecessary miosis as well as the side effects of increased protein transudation from iris vessels that follow the instillation of pilocarpine (Kenney and Kenney, 1980). With miotics, the elderly person may have increased difficulty with adaptation to darkness.

With mydriatic medications, the major danger in a shallow or narrowed anterior chamber of the eye is acute angle closure glaucoma. Because the lens increases in thickness throughout life, there is progressive shallowing of the chamber with age. Eyedrops may be used for several months following surgery for cataracts. The purpose of dilation is to move the iris enough to prevent adhesions that could occur with the pupil in a constricted position. If fixed lenses are implanted, dilating the pupil may result in dislocation of the lens. It is important that eyedrops be instilled on time and at specified intervals.

Prior to the application of an eye ointment, the nurse should cleanse any secretions from the eye and lashes. As the client looks up, the nurse pulls firmly down on the lower lid to expose the conjunctival sac (Fig. 11.3). The

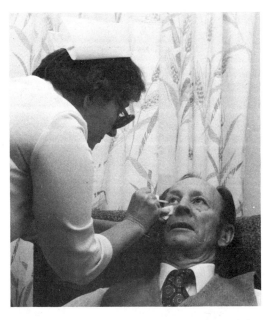

Figure 11.3. The nurse is demonstrating the administration of an eye medication. *(Photograph by Ed Spier, Murrysville, PA.)*

ointment is spread along the conjunctival sac. The client then gently closes the eyes. Tightly squeezing the eyes closed can increase intra-ocular pressure.

Communication and Socialization

Goals relating to communication should be established with the elderly client. These goals must be based upon the degree of visual change the person has experienced. Visual communication includes the physical and psychosocial processes involved in transmission of visual information between people (Fozard et al., 1977). The nurse should be aware of the vital role of nonverbal cues in communication. When visual changes affect the elderly person's ability to detect nonverbal cues, part of the message conveyed in communication will be lost. The tone and inflection of the voice convey part of the message, but do not present the entire communication picture. The nurse may need to stand closer, at the client's eye level and in the direct line of vision, in order to enable the visually impaired person to detect the communication process. Lighting should be designed to help the elderly client to see the other person's face.

The nurse may need to discuss the communication needs of the visually impaired client with the family or significant others. As discussed earlier, touch is vital part of communicating with the elderly person, and becomes increasingly important with greater degrees of vision change. Simply squeezing a person's hand is a means of nonverbal communication. Because the client's knowledge of the nurse's name can aid in the communication process, the nurse should wear a name pin with letters large enough for the elderly person to see.

Communicating with the elderly blind person or the person with a severe visual loss is a vital role of the nurse. If the person is in an institutional setting, it is necessary to knock on the door to warn the person that someone is entering the room. This also demonstrates respect for the person's territory. Upon entering the room, the nurse should announce her name. The nurse should avoid startling the person by speaking before touching the per-

son, especially if coming from behind the person.

Because an elderly person with visual impairments may be fearful of leaving a familiar environment, socialization may be limited, to the point of boredom and isolation. The elderly person may become dependent on others to accompany him outside of the familiar living environment. Activities can be planned in the daytime when visual functioning tends to be more effective. Activities planned should provide input through additional senses such as hearing and touch. Music and pets are two examples of activities that help to promote hearing and touch to provide for sensory stimulation of the person with visual impairments. Social interaction should not be limited to conversation and activities that are dependent on visual acuity. The nurse's sensitivity to the sensory deprivation that can result from altered vision can prevent labeling the elderly person as confused or withdrawn.

Health Promotion of the Elderly Person's Visual Functions

Goals should be established with the client to provide for periodic assessment of vision. The elderly person should have a vision assessment at least once a year, and more frequently if changes in visual function or comfort are noted. An interesting project might be a survey to determine when each resident of an extended-care facility last had a vision assessment. Such a survey could also determine what provisions are made for eye health education programs for staff, residents, family members, and significant others. Too often, visual acuity is not included in the assessment. Behavior may be affected by limited vision, and a "confused" elderly person may simply be unable to see adequately.

Eye protection is important for the elderly person. Wearing shatterproof or plastic glasses is a safety measure, and is especially necessary for the person who continues to work in industry, or who participates in activities involving cutting or grinding instruments. The nurse can be instrumental in disseminating information about the need for visual screening of the elderly and about promotion of eye health and optimum visual functioning. Early recognition of visual impairment and provision of therapeutic services can help to protect visual functioning in the elderly person. Clients also need information about vision screening programs and about appropriate sources for adequate visual examinations. Self-screening home tests are available, and can have great value in indicating whether professional consultation is necessary.

EVALUATION

Evaluation of interventions related to protection, maintenance, and maximization of the visual status of elderly persons is based upon the specific goals set with the client. These client-centered goals relate to the changes experienced by the client and to environmental modifications that promote optimal visual functioning. Evaluation can be initiated by determining the vision services available to the elderly, either in the institutional setting or in the community. The adequacy of such services can be evaluated by comparing the number of elderly persons served with the total elderly population.

Environmental adjustments that have been made to enhance the activity level and independence of the client can be evaluated. The accident rate, such as the incidence of falls for elderly persons in the environment, may provide a base for evaluation of the adequacy of safety precautions for old persons with vision changes. Environmental conditions that meet the needs of the visually impaired person can promote greater client interest and attention to tasks and activities, decreased anxiety levels, decreased confusion, greater confidence, and higher morale.

An evaluation of the mental functioning of elderly persons in a specific setting can provide information about the adequacy of assessment, planning, and intervention. Findings of a recent study indicated that there is a definite relationship between vision and mental status (Snyder, 1978). This gives rise to the possibility that some older people have been inappropriately labeled as mentally impaired, when the actual problem involves unmet visual needs. Vision problems often reduce the availability of stimuli that elicit appropriate behavior, and may affect the person's ability to make appropriate judgments. However, the nurse should not attribute all undesirable client characteristics to visual impairment while disregarding other potential causes.

The visual assessment and plan are one part of the total client assessment (see Table 11.1). In evaluating the visual status of the elderly person, the nurse should remember that the effectiveness of visual functioning strongly influences the client's total functioning and general health. Although improvement in the person's visual status may not be possible, changes in visual functioning are attainable goals. Evaluation may indicate that a greater degree of independence has been achieved through mobility or orientation training. The effect of corrective lenses and low-vision aids on the person's visual functioning can be measured. Changes in the client's motivation and interest in controlling the environment to permit more effective visual functioning can be measured by observing the person's control of room illumination, colors, and textures in the environment. The frequency with which the client seeks vision screening, and the method chosen for screening and follow-up care, indicate the degree to which he accepts responsibility for promoting optimal visual functioning. The extent to which the individual makes use of assets to compensate for changes in vision is a vital part of the evaluation.

In conclusion, the nurse should recognize the importance of the elderly person's vision and the interrelationship between vision and the client's perception of himself and his environment. Vision affects sensory stimulation derived from the environment. Acceptance of the need for vision assessment is the first step in promoting optimal visual functioning in the elderly person. Vision assessment screening programs initiated by nurses indicate that many elderly people are very interested in learning more about why they do not see as well as they used to and what they can do about it. The

TABLE 11.1 GUIDE FOR ASSESSING VISION

History of visual functioning
Perceptions of adequacy of vision
Eye comfort
Changes in vision
  Blurred vision
  Halos around lights
Tendency to bump into objects
Increased or decreased hearing
Reactions to changes in vision
Effect of vision on desired life-style
Medications directly related to the eyes (drops, ointments)
Effect of other medications on vision
Contact with community agencies concerned with vision
Systemic health problems affecting vision
Health problems of the eye
Date of last vision exam

Physical assessment relating to vision
Appearance of the eyes and related ocular structures
  Eyebrows
  Eyelids
  Lacrimal structures
  Conjunctiva
  Sclera
  Iris
  Pupil
  Cornea
  Retina
Ocular movements
Lacrimal functioning
Visual acuity
  Near
  Distance
Accommodation
Visual fields
  Ocular tension
  Color discrimination
  Visual spatial ability
  Light sensitivity
  Dark adaptation
  Reaction to glare
Corrective devices
  Corrective lenses
    When worn
    Time of last prescription change
    Where obtained
    Frequency of use
    Fit of corrective lens
    Adequacy of corrective lens

Low-vision aids
Mobility aids

Environmental factors related to vision
Glare-producing objects
Lighting
  Adequacy
  Provisions for client control of lighting
Placement of furniture
Windows and window coverings
Color contrasts
Textures

nurse has a vital role in promoting and stimulating such interest, when the need is not recognized by the elderly or by those who work with them.

RECOMMENDED READINGS

Corso, J.F. Aging Sensory Systems and Perception. New York: Praeger, 1981. *Research findings that support the occurrence of visual changes with aging. Provides an assessment base.*

Cristarella, M.C. Visual function of the elderly. American Journal of Occupational Therapy 31:432, 1977. *Presents visual changes with aging as they relate to visual functioning. Contains pertinent information relating to assessment and interventions.*

Fay, E.E., Hood, C.M. Low Vision. Springfield, IL, Thomas, 1975. *Classifies low vision in functional terms. Many pictures of low-vision aids are presented. Relates to planning and intervention.*

Fozard, J.L., Wolf, E., Bell, B., McFarland, R.A., Podolsky, S. Visual perception and communication, in Birren, J.E., Schaie, K.W. (eds.), Handbook of the Psychology of Aging. New York, Van Nostrand Reinhold, 1977. *A comprehensive report of research relating to vision changes with the elderly. Provides an assessment base.*

Hatton, J. Aging and the glare problem. Journal of Gerontological Nursing 3(5):38, 1977. *A complete discussion of the glare problem with the elderly. Relates to assessment, planning, intervention, and evaluation.*

Havener, W., Saunders, W., Keith, C.F., Prescott, A. Nursing Care in Eye, Ear, Nose, and Throat Disorders. St. Louis, Mosby, 1974. *Presents nursing interventions with the person who has needs relating to the eye and vision.*

Pastalan, L.A. The empathic model: A methodological bridge between research and design. Journal of Architectural Education 31(1):14, 1977. *Application of research findings on vision changes with the elderly to environmental modifications. Relates to planning and intervention.*

Snyder, L.H., Pyrek, J., Smith, K.C. Vision and mental function of the elderly. The Gerontologist 16:491, 1976. *Stresses the importance of visual assessment with the elderly. Relates the adequacy of visual functioning to mental functioning of the individual elderly person.*

REFERENCES CITED

American Foundation for the Blind, New York. Facts about aging and blindness

American Foundation for the Blind, New York. Facts about blindness

Auger, J.R. Behavioral Systems and Nursing. Englewood Cliffs, NJ, Prentice-Hall, 1976

Botwinick, J. Aging and Behavior. New York, Springer, 1973

Corso, J.F. Sensory processes and effects in normal adults. Journal of Gerontology 26(1):90, 1971

Corso, J.F. Aging Sensory Systems and Perception. New York, Praeger, 1981

Cristarella, M.C. Visual function of the elderly. American Journal of Occupational Therapy 31:432, 1977

Faye, E.E., Hood, C.M. Low Vision. Springfield, IL, Thomas, 1975

Fozard, J.L., Wolf, E., Bell, B., McFarland, R.A., Podolsky, S. Visual perception and communication, in Birren, J.E., Schaie, K.W. (eds.), Handbook of the Psychology of Aging. New York, Van Nostrand Reinhold, 1977

Hatton, J. Aging and the glare problem. Journal of Gerontological Nursing 3(5):38, 1977

Kenney, A.H., Kenney, V.T. A guide to examining the aging eye. Geriatrics. 35(2):81, 1980

Kornzweig, A.L. New ideas for old eyes. Journal of the American Geriatrics Society 28(4):145, 1980

Kornzweig, A.L. The eye in old age, in Rossman, I. (ed.), Clinical Geriatrics. Philadelphia, Lippincott, 1971

Marmon, M.F. The eye and vision in the elderly. Geriatrics 32(8):63, 1977

Mini-White House Conference on Vision and Aging Recommendations. Aging and Vision Insights, 1981

Monbeck, M.E. The Meaning of Blindness. Bloomington, Indiana University Press, 1973

Monroe, C.H. Adjustment services for the blind. Journal of Rehabilitation 44(1):30, 1978

Murch, G.M. Visual and Auditory Perception. New York, Bobbs-Merrill, 1973

Reichel, W. Clinical Aspects of Aging. Baltimore, Williams and Wilkins, 1978

Riggs, L.A. Light as a stimulus for vision, in Graham, C.H. (ed.), Vision and Visual Perceptions. New York, Wiley, 1965

Smith, K.C., Pyrek, J. Responding to vision needs in a long-term facility. Concern, December–January, 4:5, 1978

Smith, M.E. Ophthalmic aspects, in Steinberg, F.U. (ed.), Cowdry's the Care of the Geriatric Patient, 5th ed. St. Louis, Mosby, 1976

Snyder, L.H. Environmental changes for socialization. Journal of Nursing Administration 8(1):44, 1978

Snyder, L.H., Pyrek, J., Smith, K.C. Vision and mental function of the elderly. The Gerontologist 16:491, 1976

Weale, R.A. The Aging Eye. New York, Harper and Row, 1963

BIBLIOGRAPHY

American Foundation for the Blind: An Introduction to Working with the Aging Person Who Is Visually Handicapped, 2nd ed. New York, 1977

Anderson, B., Palmore, E. Longitudinal evaluation of ocular function, in Palmore, E. (ed.), Normal Aging II: Reports from the Duke Longitudinal Studies, 1970–1973. Durham, NC, Duke University Press, 1974

Andreasen, M. Color vision defects in the elderly. Journal of Gerontological Nursing 6(7):383, 1980

Block, G.J., Nolan, J., Dempsey, M. Health Assessment for Professional Nursing: A Developmental Approach. New York, Appleton-Century-Crofts, 1981

Burnside, I.M. Accoutrements of aging. Nursing Clinics of North America 7:291, 1972

Burnside, I.M. Multiple losses in the aged. The Gerontologist 13:157, 1973

Buseck, S.A. Visual status of the elderly. Journal of Gerontological Nursing 2(5):34, 1976

Condl, E.D. Ophthalmic nursing: The gentle touch. Nursing Clinics of North America 5:467, 1970

Day, R. Expanding services for the visually impaired. Perspectives on Aging 4(4):23, 1981

Duncan, J., Gish, C., Mulholland, M.E., Townsend, A. Environmental modifications for the visually impaired: A handbook. Visual Impairment and Blindness 442, 1977

Eifrig, D., Simons, K. An overview of common geriatric ophthalmologic disorders. Geriatrics 38(4):55, 1983

Goldman, R. Decline in organ function with aging, in Rossman, I. (ed.), Clinical Geriatrics. Philadelphia, Lippincott, 1979

Gross, A.M. Preventing institutionalization of elderly blind persons. Visual Impairment and Blindness 73(2):49, 1979

Havener, W., Saunders, W., Keith, C.F., Prescott, A. Nursing Care in Eye, Ear, Nose, and Throat Disorders. St. Louis, Mosby, 1974

Hayter, J. Modifying the environment to help older persons. Nursing and Health Care 4(5):265, 1983

Hill, B.J. Sensory information, behavioral instructions, and coping with sensory alteration surgery. Nursing Research 31(1):17, 1982

Jones, D.A., Dunbar, C.F., Jirovec, M.M. Medical-Surgical Nursing: A Conceptual Approach. New York, McGraw-Hill, 1978

Kelleher, D.K. Orientation to low vision aids. Journal of Visual Impairment and Blindness 73(5):161, 1979

Kline, D., Ikeda, D., Schieber, F. Age and temporal resolution in color vision: When do red and green make yellow? Journal of Gerontology 37(6):705, 1982

Marks, L. Sensory Processes. New York, Academic, 1974

Mechner, F. Patient assessment: Examination of the eye. American Journal of Nursing 1, 1974

Michelson, P.E. Insight into eyesight. Chicago, Nelson-Hall, 1980

Needham, W.E., Ehoner, M. Irrational thinking and adjustment to loss of vision. Visual Impairment and Blindness 74(2):57, 1980

Neu, C. Coping with newly diagnosed blindness. American Journal of Nursing 75:2161, 1975

Pastalan, L.A. The empathic model: A methodological bridge between research and design. Journal of Architectural Education 31(1):14, 1977

Pastalan, L.A., Carson, D.H. Spatial behavior of older people. Ann Arbor, University of Michigan, 1970

Perlman, L.G. (ed.): The Rehabilitation of the Older Blind Person: A Shared Responsibility. A report of the second Mary E. Switzer Memorial Seminar. Washington, D.C., National Rehabilitation Association, 1977

Pigott, R., Buckett, F. Visual neglect. American Journal of Nursing 66:101, 1966

Potts, A.M. The Assessment of Visual Function, St. Louis, Mosby, 1972

Ralph, J.B. Visual booby traps for our aging population. Aging 333:2, 1982

Roberts, S. Behavioral Concepts and Nursing Throughout the Life Span. Englewood Cliffs, NJ, Prentice-Hall, 1978

Ruben, R. Aging and hearing, in Rossman, I. (ed.), Clinical Geriatrics. Philadelphia, Lippincott, 1971

Scholi, G., Schnur, R. Measures of Psychological, Vocational and Educational Functioning in the Blind and Visually Handicapped. New York, American Foundation for the Blind, 1976

Shelby, J.P. Sensory deprivation. Image 10(2):49–55, 1978

Shore, H. Designing a training program for understanding sensory loss in aging. The Gerontologist 16:157, 1976

Stern, E.J. Helping the person with low vision. American Journal of Nursing 80(10):1788, 1980

Weiss, F.A., Winer, M. Coping with Sight Loss: The Vision Resource Book. Newton, MA, Vision Foundation, 1980

12

Communication: Hearing and Speech of the Elderly Person and the Nursing Process

Ann Gera Yurick

Reading this chapter will enable the individual to:

1. Know the physiologic changes of hearing with the aging process
2. Know the effects of hearing changes on communication
3. Know the effects of speech changes on communication
4. Relate the nursing process to the communication needs of elderly people
5. Have an awareness of the effects of multiple sensory changes on the needs of the elderly person

Communication links the person to his environment. In addition to sensory functioning, speech is an important component of the communication process. Hearing and speech affect the individual's physical, social, and psychologic dimensions. This chapter discusses the effects of aging changes of speech and hearing on the elderly person's communication status.

HEARING OF THE ELDERLY: ASSESSMENT BASE

Two basic functions are necessary for hearing. The first is the ability to gather and register sounds from the environment. The second is the ability to interpret the sounds received. These functions are accomplished by the two components of the auditory system. The peripheral system, which includes the structures of the ear itself, is concerned with reception and perception of sound. The central nervous system (the brain and its pathways) integrates and assigns meaning to auditory and visual symbols. Effective communication is dependent upon the proper functioning of both systems. Hearing is used on three levels. Unconscious or auditory background hearing keeps a person in touch with the environment even in darkness and in sleep. This is the most primitive subconscious level of hearing. Signal hearing describes the ability to hear warning sounds such as sirens, bells, or screams. Symbolic hearing refers to the ability to communicate verbally (Northern, 1976). Hearing is the one sense that can remain in a state of constant surveillance even during sleep (Maurer and Rupp, 1979).

The aging process brings about several basic physiologic and functional changes in the auditory system. Common hearing changes that occur with aging include high-tone hearing loss, reduced speech discrimination, and difficulty hearing in noisy environments. Auditory background hearing fades insidiously over a period of time. Because the sounds at this level tend to be faint, they are the first to be lost. Auditory background hearing allows a person to identify with the environment.

Speech discrimination and the ability to hear audiometric tones decline as a result of aging changes. Research indicates that an older person has greater difficulty in understanding speech than a young person, even when the audiometric loss is minimal (Bergman, 1971). A change in the ability to discriminate speech also affects understanding because speech may sound distorted (Hull, 1977).

Studies indicate that after the age of 32 years for men and 37 years for women, there is almost always some degree of hearing loss (Corso, 1977). High-pitched sounds tend to be lost sooner and to a greater degree than those of low pitch. Increasing interest has been focused on elderly people's difficulties in attending to sound, in interpreting sound, in sorting out the speech of persons they wish to hear while trying to ignore unwanted, competing speech or noise, and in following rapid or slurred speech (Bergman, 1971). Therefore, it is important for the nurse who deals with the elderly to be concerned about how and what an old person is able to hear as well as how this person is able to communicate. The elderly person's interpretation of what is heard is also significant. Hearing changes in the elderly person must be considered in relationship to concurrent changes in physiologic, psychologic, and social functioning.

Hearing Functions

The stimulus for hearing is the physical change in a medium, such as air or water, produced by a vibration. A sound wave is a vibration that travels through an elastic medium. It advances by alternately compressing and expanding molecules of air. Amplitude, or intensity, is the highest point of deflection of the sound wave. Loudness is related to amplitude. Intensity refers to the pressure exerted by a sound. The decibel (dB) is the unit used to express intensity. The number of completed displacements of the medium over a given period of time represents the frequency of the sound wave. Even though the frequency can be measured in terms of the number of completed cycles per second (cps), the hertz (Hz) has been accepted as the international unit of frequency measurement. Speech is comprised of many different frequencies. The pitch of a sound varies with the frequency of the wave produced.

Vowels are low-frequency sounds (about 250–750 Hz) whereas consonants are high-frequency sounds (about 2000–4000 Hz). Vowels carry the energy of speech whereas consonants carry the intelligibility (McCartney and Nadler, 1979).

Sound is conducted by two pathways in reaching the inner ear. The most sensitive pathway leads from the ear canal to the tympanic membrane, then across the ossicular chain to the inner ear. Hearing resulting from sound that follows this pathway is called *air conduction hearing*. The other sound pathway is through the bones of the skull to the inner ear, resulting in *bone conduction hearing*. Bone conduction is used to assess the sensorineural capability of the auditory system. Reception of sound occurs at the cochlear end organ. Here sound energy is transformed into neural energy. Transmission is through the eighth cranial nerve. When neural energy reaches the brain, it is interpreted and given meaning. This results in the perceptual experience of hearing, which occurs in the auditory cortex. Association takes place in the central synthesis and integration areas of the cortex. With age, changes can take place in the neural structures that affect hearing and in the components of the ear directly involved with sound transmission. Both types of change can alter the individual's ability to hear (Fig. 12.1.)

Threshold Sensitivity

The threshold of hearing, or threshold of audibility, is the stimulus value at which the person begins to hear a sound. This value divides the continuum of stimuli into two classes: stimuli to which the organism reacts and stimuli to which the organism does not react (Gerber, 1974). Measurements of absolute thresholds are obtained under highly controlled conditions to prevent interference by stimuli other than sound. The threshold of audibility is a measure of the sensitivity of the auditory system. A decrease in sensitivity implies a hearing loss. If a person is sensitive to a stimulus, his or her threshold is considered to be low. Any sound that is heard is above the threshold of hearing. Thus, lower threshold sensitivity indicates bet-

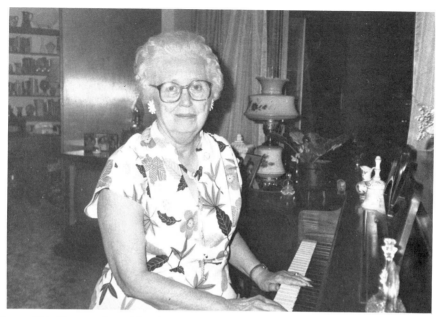

Figure 12.1. Conservation of hearing contributes to enjoyment in later life. *(Photograph by Richard T. Yurick.)*

ter hearing, while higher sensitivity indicates a poorer ability to hear.

The highest audible frequency varies according to the age of the person. Loss of sensitivity with increasing age is much greater for high frequencies than for low frequencies (Moore, 1977). This loss of sensitivity, referred to as *presbycusis*, involves structural pathology—impaired auditory sensitivity, temporal discrimination, and auditory judgment which lead to auditory processing/comprehension problems—as well as associated social and psychologic problems (Hull, 1977). Presbycusis is associated with multiple causes. Arteriosclerosis is commonly cited as a factor that influences the oxygen transporting ability of the highly vascular auditory pathways. As aging progresses, the decline in hearing ability includes progressively lower frequencies (Corso, 1977). In practical situations, the ability to detect sounds depends not only on the absolute sensitivity to those sounds but also the level of ambient noise. Of practical importance is the person's ability to hear a conversation in a setting where there are such sounds as other voices, music, or other background noises.

Pitch Discrimination

The ability to detect small changes in the pitch of sounds is a factor in perception of speech, and probably in perception of music also. Pitch is considered to be a psychologic attribute of tone. The quality of tone perception is closely related to the frequency or repetition rate of a sound (Gerber, 1974). Because pitch is a subjective property of a stimulus, it cannot be measured directly. However, pitch is closely related to frequency, an indication that a higher frequency relates to a higher pitch (Moore, 1977). Research appears to show that pitch discrimination begins to deteriorate as early as the fourth decade (Corso, 1977). The basis for this change has not been determined, but a wide variety of sensorineural mechanisms is probably involved. Continued research on pitch perception will eventually determine exactly how the listener uses pitch information as an adaptive cue in communication.

Sensitivity to Loudness

Loudness, a subjective quantity, refers to sensory magnitude. The perceived intensity of sound at a given frequency ranges from very quiet to very loud (Gerber, 1974). Loudness is the individual's perception of the relative intensity of sound. It is a property of the perceiver, whereas intensity is a property of signals. Increased patency of the eustachian tube may cause the elderly person to hear his voice more loudly. However, changes in the elasticity and the displacement of tissue in the nasopharynx can cause resistance to opening of the eustachian tube. This results in an increase in negative pressure in the middle ear which interferes with hearing (Maurer and Rupp, 1979).

Although some tones are below the level of audibility, some signals are so intense that loudness is perceived as pain. High pressures cause tactile sensations in the auditory system instead of, or in addition to, auditory sensations (Gerber, 1974). *Recruitment* is an abnormally rapid growth of loudness as sound intensity increases. For a person with a hearing impairment, there may be a decrease in the range of sensitivity from the threshold of audibility to the threshold of discomfort. Sounds of moderate intensity may be inaudible, while sounds of high intensities are at least as loud as they are for normally hearing persons. A person with a hearing loss involving recruitment may ask others not to talk so loudly. Recruitment seems to be connected with damage to the hair cells in the cochlea, resulting in a disproportion between the numbers of inner and outer hair cells (Moore, 1977).

Many studies have established a significant relationship between excessive exposure to noise and permanent hearing loss. This problem results from either loss or degeneration of sensory hair cells and damage to related cochlear structures (Corso, 1977). In the study of age-related hearing changes and those related to noise, the question is whether the hearing losses due to noise exposure and to age are additive or interactive.

Exposure to stimulation can cause two types of changes in the responsiveness of the auditory system. The absolute threshold may be elevated when fatigue occurs; or, with adaptation, the apparent magnitude of the stimulus may decrease (Moore, 1977). Auditory adaptation takes place within 1 or 2 minutes of exposure. It occurs at high and low intensities, the amount of adaptation generally increasing with intensity (Moore, 1977). Levels of noise, as well as length of exposure, are significant. Temporary hearing loss can follow exposure to very loud noise, such as the sound of a jet airplane. This loss subsides gradually, and normal hearing eventually returns. However, prolonged exposure to intense noise, such as that of industrial environments, can cause permanent hearing changes. As a result of auditory adaptation, a person may not be aware of the intensity of the sound levels. Some elderly persons with whom the nurse works will have a history of long-term exposure to high industrial noise levels. There may be a history of prolonged vocational noise exposure among elderly men. Unfortunately, the hearing conservation guidelines of the National Institute of Occupational Safety and Health were not instituted during the vocationally productive years of the present day generation of elderly.

Speech Communication

The ability to hear and understand speech is a vital part of communication. Frustrations can be great for the hearing-impaired person when failure with effective communication occurs. The person may withdraw from situations where there is a high demand for social communication. It is not uncommon for the person to complain of fatigue when asked to participate in a social event. The person may actually doze off in the corner of the room where a social event is occurring. A hearing impairment can result in the elderly person's disengagement from group interaction. Persons with hearing impairments are better able to understand personal conversation than general conversation. Another behavior that can be manifested is the dependency of the hearing-impaired elderly person on others to interpret verbal messages. There may be one significant other who may be especially depended upon to translate verbal messages. When this interpreter is not present, the hearing-impaired person may simply nod in agreement with anything that is said.

Speech discrimination is an important factor in communication. Higher vocal pitch level of children and some adult female voices cause more difficulty with comprehension for the person with high-tone loss (Maurer and Rupp, 1979). However, speech sounds vary in pitch, no matter who is speaking. For example, with the word "choose," the *ch* sound is higher than the *oo* sound. The hearing-impaired person may mistake a similar-sounding word for this word when it is not clearly heard. This can result in communication gaps, which eventually affect the individual's social interactions. Other sounds that are commonly confused are words that begin with *m* and *n*; *s* and *f, v, z, sh*; *t* and *p*; *k* and *d*; and *g* and *b*. Vowel sounds usually are louder and lower in pitch. They tend to be more easily understood than consonant sounds.

Because hearing loss usually develops gradually, the elderly person may be able to adjust to this change. However, the hearing loss may progress to the point where large amounts of energy are needed to discriminate speech. This may cause the hearing-impaired person to withdraw from speech communication situations. A person with hearing impairment who does not understand what is said may try to guess. This can cause a breakdown in communication. The hearing-impaired person can develop feelings of mistrust when others talk in his presence and he is unable to clearly hear what is being said.

The extent to which hearing loss interferes with social interaction depends on the severity of the loss (Oyer, Kapar, and Deal, 1976). The inability to hear may cause inappropriate behavior, and places the elderly person at a social disadvantage (Pyrek, Smith, and Lantto, 1977). Hearing loss may contribute to a suspicious attitude on the part of the elderly person, since inaccurately heard comments may cause the individual to feel that he or she is the focus of the conversation. Reports of a study by Eisdorfer indicated that as many as 30 percent of persons labeled "senile" were actually depressed rather than senile. A relationship between hearing loss and depression has been established (Shore, 1976). Research data also indicate that the elderly with impaired hearing tend to underestimate their degree of hearing loss (Pyrek et al., 1977).

Communication with a hearing-impaired person may be frustrating. Sometimes it is necessary to repeat a message several times until it is understood. Feedback is an important part of the communication process. The elderly person who has had a long-term impairment may speak in an unusually loud voice, which tends to have a negative effect on the communication process. Hearing loss may cause a monotonous voice quality.

The elderly person may require more time to process information in the higher auditory centers of the brain. This can result in reduced speech perception (Corso, 1977). Changes in the aging central auditory nervous system may result in a lack of understanding of the message even though the message has been heard. However, the question of central versus peripheral factors involved in hearing impairments of the elderly is an issue that calls for continued research.

Hearing impairments can interfere with an elderly person's communication with the environment. The environment contains a wide variety of sounds, many of which help make life more pleasant and enjoyable. Sounds keep a person informed about the world around. Some sounds help keep a person safe in the environment, such as the sound of a car rounding a street corner, or the sound of footsteps from behind. The sound of a telephone ringing and the ability to talk with another person via the telephone provide a sense of security and help to meet socialization needs. When a hearing impairment interferes with the old person's contact with the environment, a feeling of isolation is often experienced.

Changes in the Auditory System of Elderly Persons

When the capacity for successful interaction is hampered by a hearing loss, the person is considered to have a hearing impairment. Hearing impairments in the elderly person can result in a decreased receptive capacity or a decreased capacity for sound discrimination.

Conductive Hearing Loss

Dysfunction of the external ear, the middle ear, or both can lead to a conductive hearing loss. Sound transmission to the middle ear can be affected by an auricle that enlarges as a result of gradual loss of skin elasticity and muscle tone. Otosclerosis can be a problem with the elderly person, and has been reported to cause the conductive hearing loss (Corso, 1977). Impacted cerumen in the external auditory canal, perforation of the tympanic membrane, and serum or pus in the middle ear are all conditions that can affect hearing.

A conductive hearing loss occurs when sound waves are not adequately transmitted to the inner ear. Because the inner ear is not affected, the weakened sound received by the inner ear can still be analyzed. Sounds are perceived as fainter by a person with conductive hearing impairment. The person with the conductive loss may speak softly because his own voice can sound louder than normal to himself. A conductive loss tends to affect low-frequency more than high-frequency sounds. Because vowel sounds are low frequency, increasing the volume of the speaker's voice enables the person with a conductive loss to hear the vowels more clearly and to understand speech more easily.

Sensorineural Hearing Loss

Dysfunction in the conversion of physical sound waves to electrical signals by the elements of the inner ear or a dysfunction in transmission of nerve impulses to the brain can cause speech to be perceived as soft or distorted. Sensitivity and discrimination are affected. Speech distortion may remain even if the sound is made intense enough to compensate for the reduction in volume. The person may be able to hear but not to understand speech. This problem is referred to as *sensorineural* or *perception loss*. It can be caused by changes in the inner ear, the auditory nerve, or the brain. Corso (1981) indicated that the primary question regarding the results of experimental studies on speech discrimination is whether the decrements for

older subjects are attributable to central or peripheral changes in the auditory nervous system. At this time data are available to support either position.

The hearing impairment associated with aging, presbycusis, is usually the result of sensory or neural changes. *Sensory presbycusis* can be caused by atrophy of the organ of Corti, at the basal end of the cochlea. The organ of Corti contains rows of hair cells which respond to the frequency and intensity of sound waves. Atrophy and degeneration of the hair cells and supporting cells often accompanies the aging process (Corso, 1977). The loss of high-frequency hearing is associated with these changes in the organ of Corti. However, speech frequencies do not appear to be affected.

Neural presbycusis is a result of degenerative changes in the nerve fibers of the cochlea. It leads to losses in speech discrimination, but not in pure tone thresholds. There may also be associated degenerative changes in the central nervous system that interfere with the understanding of speech.

Metabolic presbycusis results from atrophy of blood vessels in the wall of the cochlea, probably caused by arteriosclerotic vascular changes (Oyer, Kapar, and Deal, 1976). This leads to deficiencies in the bioelectric and biochemical properties of the endolymphatic fluids. Metabolic presbycusis is characterized by an almost uniform loss for all frequencies, and is accompanied by recruitment. *Mechanical presbycusis* results from atrophic changes in the structures involved with vibration of the cochlear partition. This condition leads to increasing hearing loss from low to high frequencies (Corso, 1977).

A mixed hearing loss involves conductive and sensorineural changes in the same ear. Even though specific changes may be identified with presbycusis, it is usually considered part of the multifaceted aging process. It is difficult to determine cause-and-effect relationships with regard to age-related hearing changes. Research data about the effects of arteriosclerotic vascular disease on the aging ear are conflicting (Ruben, 1971). Changes in the cortex of the brain can cause perceptual hearing problems. The person experiencing these changes may confuse specific speech sounds even though the sounds are heard. Although a direct correlation exists between increasing hearing loss and increasing age, there is a high degree of variability in the degree of loss and the age at which it becomes evident. Good hearing in old age seems to be connected with a familial tendency to be less vulnerable to disease processes that cause degeneration of peripheral or central auditory function (Hull, 1977).

Tinnitus

Tinnitus is an auditory perception of internal origin and is described as a ringing or buzzing in the ear. Tinnitus can be very discomforting to the client. The great majority of people with tinnitus have a hearing loss and there is thought to be a relationship between the degree of hearing loss and the intensity of tinnitus (Meyerhoff and Shrewsbury, 1980). Tinnitus can vary with the type, location, intensity, and the pattern of the sound, as well as its association with other physical stimuli.

NURSING ASSESSMENT OF THE ELDERLY PERSON'S HEARING

The nursing assessment should determine the level at which an elderly person is able to hear and communicate. As in other instances of client assessment, the effort is multidisciplinary. Data collected by the nurse and other health-team members are shared in common. The audiologist is usually an important contributor to the health assessment base. An audiologist can perform a hearing assessment under exacting stimulus conditions in order to determine the adequacy of the auditory processing system. This assessment can lead to the selection of appropriate rehabilitation measures for the hearing-impaired elderly person. Auditory perception and processing are part of the rehabilitation plan.

Elderly persons may be reluctant to have their hearing assessed. They may be aware that they have a problem with hearing but are reluctant to have this problem verified. Even though the problem may have been long standing, the person may describe it as a recent problem. The person performing the hearing assessment must provide brief but clear instructions in order to minimize the elderly client's confusion and apprehension. Some older persons may have difficulty following instructions during the assessment process. There may be a slowed response to the stimulus used to test hearing. For example, a stimulus word may need to be repeated.

Assessment of the Ears

The data base to be used for planning for the hearing needs of the elderly client includes assessment of the observable structures of hearing.

External Ear

The external ear is composed of the auricle and external auditory canal.

Auricle

The nurse inspects the auricle and surrounding tissue for color and integrity of the skin. The auricle of the elderly person may appear to be hard and inflexible, and may have increased in size. The gradual loss of skin elasticity and muscle tonicity contribute to the outer ear enlargement. The individual may be aware of such an increase and may make comments about it. The increased size of the auricle is particularly likely to be noticed by a client who has just begun to wear a hearing aid. Changes in the external ear raise questions about possible effects on sound transmission to the middle ear. At this time, changes in the outer ear that accompany the aging process are thought to have only a small effect on hearing sensitivity (Maurer and Rupp, 1979). Further research is needed in this area.

External Auditory Canal

Atrophic changes may be observed in the supporting walls of the external auditory canal. This can cause a partial occlusion of the canal and impede the pathway for air-conducted sounds. Cerumen may also accumulate in this passage, and can interfere with the passage of sound to the tympanic membrane. Accumulations of cerumen may make it difficult to inspect the tympanic membrane with an otoscope. During inspection of the auditory canal, the tissues should be observed for presence of inflammation, discharge, and evidence of foreign bodies. Moving the auricle and pressing on the tragus (the prominence in front of the external opening of the ear) and mastoid will give an indication of any tenderness that might indicate inflammation. Decreased tactile sensation in the external ear can cause an insensitivity to accumulation of cerumen.

Tympanic Membrane

The tympanic membrane of the elderly client can be observed by using an otoscope. The tympanic membrane separates the external auditory canal from the middle ear. It should be observed for intactness, color, and luster. The tympanic membrane normally is translucent, and is usually pearly grey in color. A change in color to red, yellow, or white may indicate the presence of an inflammatory process. Bulging of the tympanic membrane may be caused by an infection in the middle ear, while a concavity of the membrane may indicate obstruction of the eustachian tube. The bulging or retraction of the tympanic membrane can affect the localization of landmarks. Normally, the projection of the short process of the malleus and the umbo (the inferior point of the handle of the malleus) can be seen. The long process of the malleus can be seen anterior and superior to the umbo. With the elderly, the tympanic membrane is likely to be more translucent and more rigid.

Assessment of Hearing Functions

Even though a number of hearing functions can be determined most accurately by an audiologist, the nurse can gather much data about the elderly client's hearing efficiency. Throughout the assessment, the nurse should be aware of the appropriateness of the client's response to the spoken word. The loudness of the individual's own speech may provide information about his or her hearing status. The nurse should also observe the client's verbal interactions with others. It is important to determine whether social interactions tend to occur on a one-to-one basis or whether the person appears to be comfortable in verbal interactions with a group. Although many other factors can influence the individual's choice of social interactions, hearing levels can affect the quantity and quality of the interactions.

History of the Client

In the assessment of hearing ability, the client's history is significant. There may be a history of severe head trauma, many ear infections, or upper respiratory infections. Past or present exposure to ototoxic medications may also have occurred. Irreversible ototoxic destruction of the receptor hair cells in the Organ of Corti can follow treatment with aminoglycoside antibiotics, such as neomycin. Acetylsalicylic acid in large quantities can be ototoxic, although this effect is reversible. The client's history of pain, especially arthritic pain, may give clues to the amount of aspirin routinely taken. Other ototoxic drugs include loop diuretics such as furosemide and ethacrynic acid, chemotherapeutic agents as Cisplatin and quinine drugs used in long-term doses for malaria or arthritis. The risk of ototoxic damage is increased when there is decreased renal function or preexisting neurosensory hearing loss. The symptoms of ototoxicity include tinnitus, neurosensory hearing loss, and vertigo. The otic changes may be unilateral or bilateral, permanent or transient, immediate or delayed. For the elderly client receiving an ototoxic medication, careful daily assessment is advisable in order to determine subjective changes in tinnitus, hearing ability, and dizziness while the drug is taken. The client may hear better at specific times in the day. Other client medications also can affect hearing patterns.

The elderly person's work history is also important, since it may have involved exposure to noise over a long period of time. There may have been intermittent exposure to loud noises, such as gunshots, connected with either military service or recreational hunting. Perhaps the client continues to hunt as a leisure activity. It must be determined whether this noise exposure is contributing to his hearing problem. The hearing status of other family members may, in some cases, point to the existence of a genetically transmitted hearing impairment.

This interview provides an excellent opportunity for the nurse to evaluate the degree to which the elderly client seems to hear and understand questions and comments. The nurse should be aware of his or her own tone of voice, the distance from the client, the position in relation to the client, the amount of lighting in the area, and the level of background noise. Other clues that may indicate a hearing impairment include the client's requests to have statements or questions repeated; irrelevant or inappropriate comments during verbal interaction with others; frequent head nodding rather than a verbal response during conversation; and the tendency to withdraw from activities that require verbal communication. Hearing problems may be compounded for the elderly client who speaks only a foreign language or whose native tongue is not English. Many of today's elderly, especially the very old, have immigrated to this country. Mastery of the English language varies widely within this group.

Assessment of Auditory Acuity

In the assessment of auditory acuity, one ear at a time should be tested. The ear not being tested can be occluded by either the client or the examiner placing a finger against the opening of the auditory canal. The elderly person may experience persistent head noises. It is necessary for this person to be able to separate this noise from the sound presented to test acuity.

During the assessment of hearing, the physical environment should be comfortable. The physiologic comfort as well as the mental attitude of the client needs to be considered.

Voice Test

A voice test provides an estimate of the client's hearing acuity. At a distance of 1–2 feet away from the unoccluded ear of the client, the nurse softly whispers a number that is to be repeated by the client. If the person is unable to hear a soft whisper, a medium whisper and then a loud whisper may be tried. A second sequence

may be needed, in which the nurse uses soft voice tones that become progressively louder. During the voice test, the nurse should stand in a position that does not allow the client to view his or her lip movements. If this is not possible, the client may be requested to keep his eyes closed during the test.

The nurse can also use the sound of a ticking watch, placed at varying distances from the unoccluded ear. However, this produces sound of a higher frequency than the voice. The voice test may provide a more accurate determination of the client's functional hearing.

Tuning Fork Tests

Tuning fork tests can assist in the determination of hearing changes due to conduction problems. Both air and bone conduction are assessed. Two standard tuning fork tests are available to the nurse.

RINNE TEST The *Rinne test* is used to determine air conduction and bone conduction. The base of a lightly vibrating tuning fork is placed on the mastoid process (the bony prominence located posterior to the lower auricle) until the client can no longer hear the sound. Then the tuning fork is immediately removed from the mastoid process and held near the ear canal. The client should continue to hear the tuning fork, since sound is normally heard better by air conduction than by bone conduction. If the client hears the tuning fork better by bone conduction, the Rinne test is considered to be negative and the hearing loss is probably air-conductive in origin.

WEBER TEST The *Weber test* is used to determine lateralization of hearing. It utilizes bone conduction to determine if sound is heard differently by either ear. A lightly vibrating tuning fork is placed firmly on top of the client's head, in the middle of the forehead, or on the front teeth. The client is asked whether sound is heard better by one ear than by the other. Normally, the sound is heard equally well (or poorly) by both ears. With a conductive hearing impairment, the sound is referred to the ear with the greatest deficit, because the cochlea on that side will not be affected by extraneous sounds from the environment. These environmental sounds are transmitted because of a problem in the auditory canal or middle ear.

In the case of sensorineural hearing changes, the sound is referred to the better ear, because the cochlea or auditory nerve is functioning more effectively in the better ear.

Other Tests for Hearing Acuity

The nurse may have audiometric equipment available, and with special training can become skilled in its use. The audiometer is an electrically calibrated instrument that permits control of test stimuli. These stimuli may take the form of pure tones or selected words. Testing provides information about hearing sensitivity and sound frequencies affected. Both air and bone conduction are assessed. Pressure from the headphones can collapse the external ear canal thus affecting hearing acuity. The elderly client may be asked to respond verbally when the audiometric sound is heard, rather than by the more traditional response of a raised hand or by pressing a signal button. An elderly person's delayed motor response could affect the results of this test. The nurse may also have results of audiometric testing that was performed by another member of the health team.

In the assessment of speech discrimination, the client listens to a list of common words at optimal intensity level. The nurse may use recordings of word lists to determine the client's speech discrimination. However, words understood in isolation cannot provide a true measurement of the number of words heard in a conversation, since other words in the conversation may give clues to a word not heard accurately.

Questions can be presented to the elderly person verbally or in writing to obtain data relating to hearing ability. Questions can relate to the effects of hearing on personal and social life, ability to hear a phone conversation, ability to converse in a restaurant or a public place with similar noise levels, and personal responses to any hearing problems.

Even though the client may have undergone a variety of tests for hearing acuity, nursing observation remains a vital part of hearing assessment. Most testing is done in controlled situations, such as a soundproof room or at least a setting in which the client is away from others. The hearing problem may be more pronounced in the natural environment with background noises. For example, consider the variety of noises that exist in an extended-care facility. The blare of the intercom system alone can disrupt the elderly person's ability to hear.

Assessment of Speech Patterns

The speech of a person with a hearing impairment may be altered. With normal hearing, a person can hear his or her own voice and is therefore able to regulate its tone. The speech sounds most affected by hearing impairment are *s* and *r*. The person with a hearing-related speech problem may elicit concerns about adequacy of mental functioning because the speech is altered.

Assessment of Client Reactions to Hearing Changes

Sounds in the environment, social interactions composed largely of verbal sounds, and enjoyable auditory experiences such as music all can influence the individual's self-concept and thus affect behavioral responses. The hearing-impaired client's response to loss will depend upon that person's method of coping or the support he or she receives. Response to loss may take a number of forms, including such behaviors as withdrawal, anger, depression, and suspiciousness. Stages of the grieving process may be observable. Because hearing change is often a gradual process, the elderly person may not experience the grieving process until hearing loss begins to interfere with his or her style of living and social interactions.

Many variables are involved in the impact of hearing change on the old person. Stereotyped reactions to this loss cannot be listed. Both client and family may view the hearing loss as part of aging and may feel that it must simply be accepted. The person's family may interpret behavior changes resulting from the hearing impairment as a form of age-related mental deterioration. The affected individual may be reluctant to seek rehabilitation because of feelings that only a short lifespan lies ahead, and may be especially reluctant to invest money in a hearing aid or any other rehabilitation program.

The hearing aid tends to be viewed as a social stigma. It is not considered as socially acceptable as the use of glasses for visual impairment. In designing hearing aids, the manufacturers' goal is to make the device small so that it is not readily evident. Many hearing aids are designed to hide the disability for which they were made. The cosmetic appeal of a hearing aid may take on greater importance than its therapeutic value.

The elderly person often does not admit the existence of a hearing problem. One study indicated that members of an elderly population freely admitted vision problems, but denied hearing problems. Many of those who denied having a hearing problem were found to have hearing losses (Reichel, 1977).

Assessment of Nurse's Reaction to Elderly Clients with Hearing Impairments

The nurse may be unaware of an elderly client's hearing problems unless data from the hearing assessment are examined (Table 12.1). The signs of hearing change are not as obvious as signs of visual change. The hearing-impaired individual can appear oriented to the environment and move about it with ease. Because the person with a hearing loss looks perfectly normal he or she may be expected to behave normally.

Some persons with hearing impairment become skilled at avoiding verbal interactions that would make the hearing change obvious. The nurse may react to inappropriate responses by labeling such a person as eccentric or confused. If messages must be repeated, the nurse may consider the client to be inattentive. The nurse may reject the person or limit contact to the greatest degree possible, thus increasing the individual's social isolation. Even a nurse who is aware of the existence of a hearing loss may not relate the client's behavior to

TABLE 12.1 ASSESSMENT GUIDE FOR HEARING

History
Incidence of any hearing problems
Onset of hearing problems
Family history of hearing problems
Ear infections
Upper respiratory infections
Head trauma
Medications
   Antibiotics
   Aspirin
Exposure to noise
Social interaction patterns
   Social events
   Mealtime socialization
   Telephone
   Two-person interactions
   Group interactions

Physical assessment
External ear
External auditory canal
Tympanic membrane

Hearing functions
Response to spoken word
Ability to receive verbal messages
   One-to-one conversation
   Social conversation in a noisy place
   Telephone conversation
Ability to understand verbal messages
Loudness of speech responses
Speech patterns
Ability to hear phone, doorbell, or knocking on door
Whisper test
Voice test
Tuning fork test
Audiometric testing
Reactions to changes in hearing

Aids to hearing
Type of hearing aid
Knowledge of mechanics of hearing aid
Knowledge of hearing aid care
Patterns of hearing aid use
Ability to manipulate hearing aid dials

Aids to communication
Auditory training
Speech training
Speech reading

Environmental aids to hearing
Presence of flashing aids on phone or doorbell
Use of phone amplifiers
Control of noise levels

the loss. The nurse's negative reaction to the client can cause further withdrawal and isolation, and may provoke similar negative reactions by the client's peers or family.

To gain sensitivity toward the experiences of a hearing-impaired person, the nurse can simulate this experience. Cotton balls or ear plugs may be placed in the ears to simulate a conduction loss of hearing. To simulate sound distortion, a radio can be tuned between stations so that the two stations are heard at once. Increased sensitivity on the part of the nurse should improve the quality of interaction with the client who experiences hearing changes.

PLANNING AND INTERVENTION FOR HEARING

The nurse's role with regard to the elderly client's hearing status is to assist in determining the level of the person's hearing and listening ability and to maximize hearing and listening efficiency. This is achieved by establishing goals with the client related to acceptance of adjustments to hearing changes and compensation for the deficiencies present. The success of such a rehabilitation program depends on the attitude of the client, his family and peers, and the health team members. Denial of the hearing problem by the elderly person can inhibit rehabilitation efforts.

Aural Rehabilitation

Aural rehabilitation is directed toward increasing or maintaining the client's ability to communicate and to interact with others in order that life can be as meaningful as possible. Aural rehabilitation helps the person to maintain contact with his environment. This rehabilitation process includes discussion of the client's individual problems, education in the hearing process, amplification assessment, speech reading, auditory training, and counseling. Rehabilitation services should be provided as soon as a hearing loss is identified. The client or health team members should not wait until the problem becomes severe or interferes with communication. Aural rehabili-

tation services should be offered as preventive therapy. Some old persons are not interested in a rehabilitation program, but may be encouraged by family members to participate. Education and support of family members can provide the base upon which a successful program can be built. However, the interest of the elderly person must be stimulated before attainable goals can be established. Family or health team members may have a number of goals for rehabilitation, but without the client's interest and participation, these goals will not be achieved. Oyer et al. (1976) found that the reason hearing-impaired clients did not enter recommended aural rehabilitation programs was primarily due to lack of motivation. Other reasons included lack of awareness of aural rehabilitation programs, transportation limitations, and physical and economic reasons.

Communication Facilitators

In speaking to an elderly person with a hearing impairment, the nurse should not raise the voice to a higher pitch in an attempt to be better heard. A lower-pitched voice should be used, even though the volume may be louder. A slightly louder-than-average intensity should be more easily heard by the elderly person. It is important to speak in short, concise sentences. Each statement should be heard and understood by the elderly person before going on to the next statement. Speech should be slow and distinct, but without exaggerated lip movements. Interfering visual cues, such as might be produced by chewing gum, smoking, or eating, should be avoided. Light should be focused on the speaker's face, and should be soft but intense. Light coming from a window at the speaker's back may make the speaker appear as a dark image to the listener, and may also produce glare. Allow the elderly person time to assimilate clues that are provided during verbal interaction.

In approaching the person with a hearing loss, face the person rather than speaking from behind. Speak at the listener's visual level—for example, sit or kneel when talking with the person who is confined to a wheelchair. The speaker's face should be visible with no physical effort necessary on the part of the listener. The nurse should be careful not to startle the elderly person who may not hear approaching footsteps. The nurse may gesture or raise a hand to get the attention of the client, who might be startled by a sudden touch.

The person with a hearing impairment may not be aware of the direction from which sound is coming. If the nurse is aware that hearing is better in one ear than in another, communication can be directed toward the better side. However, speaking directly into the ear can distort the speaker's voice. The elderly person will not have the advantage of observing facial cues during communication. The preferred speaking distance is from 3 to 6 feet from the elderly person. The distance should not be greater than 6 feet.

In communicating with a severely hearing-impaired person or one who is completely deaf, the nurse and client may find a pad and pencil to be helpful. Writing a key word or proper names can often help the communication process. If the elderly person appears confused by a statement and answers inappropriately, this should not be ignored by going on to another topic. Instead, the nurse should determine where and how the misinterpretation occurred, and should make another attempt to communicate by repeating the message, perhaps with a different choice of words. The nurse should avoid sudden changes in the topic of conversation.

Touch is a valuable tool for the nurse in communicating with the hearing-impaired person. The nurse can gently touch the client to gain his attention when the spoken word is not heard adequately. Further discussion of the use of touch is presented later in this chapter.

Control of environmental noises is vital to effective communication with the elderly person. The most disruptive background noise is noise with speech components, such as others' conversations and speech from the radio and television. Background music, even though thought to be pleasant or entertaining by others, often interferes with the hearing of the older client even when amplification is provided with a hearing aid.

Hearing Aid Effectiveness
Optimal amplification is important to the progress of aural rehabilitation. The nurse and the health team can assist the client in attaining this goal. Some clients may reject the need for a hearing aid because they are unwilling to admit the existence of hearing loss, or because they are unaware of it. These clients are frequently unaware of the adjustments others must make in attempting to communicate with them (Fig. 12.2). Others may give up efforts in communicating with the hearing-disabled person, thus decreasing opportunities for interpersonal relationships.

An elderly person who needs amplification through a hearing aid should seek professional medical and audiologic assistance prior to contacting the hearing aid dealer. For the hearing-impaired person to make the decision to seek help for a hearing problem, the probability of success is greater than if some other member of the family uses coercion to get the person to have a hearing test and obtain a hearing aid. The physician (preferably an otologist or otolaryngologist) determines the possible medical basis of the problem. The audiologist assesses the hearing function, recommends a specific hearing aid as well as procedures for use of

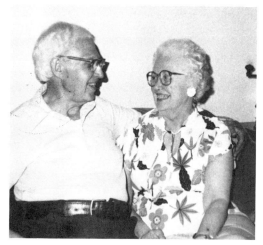

Figure 12.2. Communication is facilitated by closeness and the ability to observe facial expressions.

this aid. The hearing aid dealer sells and services the aid. Speech and hearing centers associated with hospitals or universities are also available to assist with the evaluation and selection of hearing aids.

If a hearing aid has been prescribed, the nurse can assist the client in the appropriate care and use of the aid for optimal effectiveness. The client's reactions to using the hearing aid should be determined. If the client has a hearing aid but does not use it, the nurse should find out why. In order to use the hearing aid, the client must have adequate manual dexterity and tactile sensitivity to put on the prosthesis, use the controls, and remove the prosthesis. Hearing aids are available for the person with limited manual dexterity, however. Examples of adaptations include a projecting knob to facilitate removal of the aid and an extended volume control wheel height for accessibility and ease of operation. A period of time is needed to adapt to the use of a hearing aid, and the nurse can support the client during this adjustment period. To suddenly hear forgotten sounds can be overwhelming while new listening habits are established.

The client should have a realistic awareness that the hearing aid may not solve every communication problem. A hearing aid is a mechanical amplifier. The better-quality hearing aids will not distort the sound but may amplify some parts more than others. No hearing aid now available will restore natural hearing. Both the hearing aid and the client will have limitations. The client needs to have a measure of tolerance for failure. The old person may find that the benefits derived from amplification are not as great as anticipated. Even with amplification, some sounds may remain imperceptible for the person who has lost much ability to discriminate. Distracting environmental sounds are amplified by the hearing aid, and distortions of speech may continue. After a client is fitted for a hearing aid, a postfitting follow-up is required. Many elderly clients do not return for this follow-up, however.

Hearing aids are classified according to where they are worn on the body. The four major types are behind-the-ear, in-the-ear, body,

and Contralateral Routing of Signals aid (CROS). Each type of hearing aid has a microphone to change sound waves into electric signals that then are transmitted; an amplifier to strengthen these signals; an earmold to channel the sound through the external ear canal to the tympanic membrane; and a cord that connects the amplifier to the earmold.

The body aids, which are largest, tend to be sturdier and less subject to distortion. However, when they are worn under clothing or in a pocket, the rub of clothing against the microphone is amplified. The body-type hearing aid is probably the least cosmetic. A cord from the hearing aid carries signals to a receiver in the client's ear. Body aids provide efficient amplification for those with a severe hearing deficit. They may also be indicated for the elderly person who has difficulty manipulating smaller controls.

In-the-ear aids are attached directly to the earmold and protrude slightly from the ear. These aids may produce a feedback squeal because the microphone and receiver are close together. Because in-the-ear aids are relatively inconspicuous, they are preferred by many hearing-impaired persons. This type of hearing aid seems to help the person with a mild to moderate hearing loss (Hull, 1977). However, for the elderly person, it may not provide enough fidelity, especially when there is decreased ability to understand speech. The miniaturized parts of the aid may be difficult for the elderly person to manipulate if an additional vision or dexterity problem is present.

Behind-the-ear aids are the most commonly worn type, and seem to have the greatest cosmetic appeal. However, they may present a problem to the person who also wears glasses. Although behind-the-ear aids can be attached to eyeglasses, when the client removes the eyeglasses the hearing aid also is removed. If the person has a major vision problem, manipulation of the batteries and controls is very difficult when the glasses are removed. The person with a mild-to-moderate hearing impairment usually can use the behind-the-ear aid (Hull, 1977).

The Contralateral Routing of Signals (CROS) aid is utilized when an individual has nearly normal hearing in one ear but impaired hearing in the other ear. Signals from the impaired ear are routed contralaterally to the better ear, enabling the person to hear from the impaired side. These aids are usually connected with eyeglass frames. Sound is delivered to the ear through a thin piece of plastic tubing or a vented mold. A major advantage is that a telephone receiver can be used comfortably at the ear with the tubing. A BI-CROS aid is indicated when both ears are impaired but only one ear is suitable for amplification. A microphone is placed in the poorer ear, routing signals contralaterally. Another microphone is located at the better ear, amplifying that ear only.

When selecting a hearing aid, the client may need assistance in recognizing his specific needs. An elderly person with reduced touch sensitivity or manual dexterity problems such as hand tremor or arthritic changes in the hands, may require larger dials on the hearing aid for greater ease of manipulation. Control dials should be also readily accessible and easily understood. A major problem with the elderly is learning to operate the hearing aid properly.

A skilled therapist is needed to fit the hearing aid and to train the client in its use. The adjustment period is critical. At first the aid is worn only for a limited time, and wearing time is gradually increased over several months. Among other instructions, the client is told to listen carefully to identify sounds heard. The therapist is not only concerned with the efficiency of client hearing but also is interested in how well the person perceives and processes what is heard. Processing includes attention and auditory sequencing, discrimination, and categorization.

The nurse cannot assume that the client will remember all instructions. As a result of associated anxiety at the time the client receives a hearing aid, some instructions may not be heard or may not be remembered. For example, one nurse became aware of an elderly man who drove 20 miles to a hospital's hearing aid department to get new batteries. Specific battery reorder instructions were given when this client obtained his hearing aid, and were also included in the instruction booklet. All

this man had to do to reorder batteries was to call the hospital. The nurse intervened to clarify these instructions, thus eliminating further unnecessary trips to the hospital.

For client protection, a Food and Drug Administration regulation states that a person with a hearing loss must have medical clearance within 6 months before purchasing a hearing aid. A trial period can be provided. Hearing aids must be accompanied by printed information explaining their use and their limitations in the improvement of hearing. The federal government is now attempting to eliminate victimization of the hearing-impaired elderly person who is looking for an answer to his hearing problem. The Federal Trade Commission requires that every hearing aid buyer be given the right to cancel the purchase for any reason for any time within 30 days of delivery with a refund for most of the purchase price. Martson (1982) found this time to be adequate for purposes of evaluation and initial adjustment to amplification. More than one model of hearing aid may be tried for comparative purposes.

Because hearing ability can continue to undergo change, the client should have the hearing aid reevaluated periodically. The client should have the phone number of the hearing aid dealer prominently posted in the event that problems occur. A proper match of hearing aid to client is necessary. An aid that amplifies sound may, at the same time, magnify speech distortions. The client may be able to hear but still not be able to understand what is being said. Background noises are also magnified. This may be especially distressing to the person who has a hearing loss with recruitment.

Care of the Hearing Aid

Specific care measures are necessary to maintain the effectiveness of hearing aids. The nurse should determine the degree to which the client understands the maintenance required. Too often the nurse avoids contact with hearing aids because he lacks an understanding of the mechanism. The nurse may ignore the fact that the client's hearing aid is in the bedside drawer most of the time. If there seem to be problems with the functioning of the hearing aid, the following areas may be checked: (1) the batteries—the batteries may be worn, they may be in the improper position, or the attachments may be corroded; (2) the on–off switch may be in the wrong position; (3) the cord may be in the incorrect position, or may be broken; (4) the earmold may need cleaning. If all of these areas seem to function adequately, a professional repair department may have to be consulted.

When an in-the-ear type of aid is worn, the earmold should fit properly and snugly into the ear to get the full value of amplification. If it does not fit snugly, amplified sounds can escape the ear canal and return to the microphone to be reamplified, producing an annoying whistling sound. Simply pushing the earmold into the ear more tightly will frequently correct the problem. Decreased tactile sensation in the ear canal can result in improper earmold insertion. The ear needs to be inspected for redness, swelling, or skin indentations that may indicate an improperly fitting earmold. The size and shape of the ear canal may become larger. If this happens, the earmold will not fit as snugly and may need to be replaced. The earmold also should be checked for cracks or rough areas since these can cause irritation to the ear canal. New earmolds may need to be purchased every several years; the hearing aid should last 5–10 years, based on the care taken with the aid. Care needs to be taken not to drop the earmold on a hard surface.

The small hole in the earmold that conducts the amplified sound can become clogged with cerumen and lose its effectiveness. Impacted cerumen can also interfere with the fit of an earmold. Terminal hair growth, especially prevalent in elderly males, also can interfere with proper placement of the earmold.

Earmolds must be cleaned regularly. They should be removed from the hearing aid for cleaning. A pipe cleaner or earmold brush can be used to remove cerumen, using warm, soapy water (alcohol may dry and crack some earmold materials). If the client is unable to clean the earmold, the nurse can assist with this or, if possible, teach a family member how to keep the earmold clean. After cleaning, the earmold must be thoroughly dried, since moisture can damage the hearing aid. To avoid getting moisture into the hearing aid, it should not be worn while in the bathtub or shower. Cleanliness of the earmold can help to prevent irritation and inflammation of the auditory canal. For hearing aids that have a no-mold fitting, with sound introduced through polyethylene tubing, the tubing may become blocked with cerumen. When cleaning any tubing that is used with a hearing aid, all water must be removed since a small drop of water can interfere with sound conduction.

The hearing aid should not be exposed to extremes of temperature. A hair dryer should not be used while the client wears the hearing aid. Hair spray can clog the microphone. When not being worn, the hearing aid should be stored in a dry area, with the batteries removed. The hearing aid should be in an "off" position when not being worn.

The nurse should be aware of the times when the client wears and does not wear the hearing aid. For example, in an extended-care facility or any overnight setting, the nurse must use different approaches when the client removes the hearing aid at night, remembering that there is a loss of amplification during this period of time. When the person uses the hearing aid, the nurse should encourage him or her to determine the distance from the speaker needed for optimal amplification.

The elderly person may have misconceptions about the use of hearing aid batteries. Clients have been known to save good batteries for weekends and holidays, special visits with family or friends, or church services, while weaker batteries are used on more routine days. The client should always have an extra battery. An individual may turn the hearing aid off to conserve batteries or to eliminate a variety of environmental sounds, including the conversations of others in the setting. The nurse should realize that a client who is wearing a hearing aid is not necessarily using it.

The optimal use of a hearing aid should allow the client to receive conversational speech at a comfortable listening level with adequate speech discrimination. Other factors related to optimal use of the hearing aid include meeting the client's cosmetic wishes, comfort needs, and manipulative abilities.

Auditory Training

Auditory training involves use of the client's residual hearing, with or without the assistance of a hearing aid, to improve his or her understanding of speech that sounds distorted. First, training helps the client to distinguish between grossly differing sounds through hearing alone. Next, the goal is directed toward aiding the client to develop the ability to make fine distinctions between similar speech sounds. Auditory training does not improve the basic auditory functions. However, it can improve the client's listening ability by making him or her more alert to distinguishing clues. Recordings may be used in this training. For example, music recordings can be used to teach the client to distinguish musical instruments. With auditory training, emphasis is placed on listening skills as well as speech discrimination. It is not intended that the elderly person should receive and understand all words in all conversations. Instead, stress is placed on utilizing clues that help the client to understand the message when all of it is not heard. Concentrated attention to incoming sounds, even though these sounds are not heard perfectly, should improve the person's ability to listen and communicate. Maurer and Rupp (1979) report that speech intelligibility has been shown to improve following auditory training, especially following training with words and phrases. Some factors affecting the success of auditory training include the person's health status, mental status, language comprehension skills, and visual function.

Speech Reading

Speech reading enables the client to use visual recognition in interpreting the speech of others. A person needs to have adequate vision for speech reading. Speech reading includes lipreading, but it also includes nonverbal cues, such as observation of the whole face and body. The client learns to observe the movements of the speaker's eyes, tongue, cheeks, throat, and lips as well as gestures used. The principal clues are given by the lips of the speaker. The nurse should know whether a client has been trained in speech reading, so that this skill can be utilized in more effective communication with the person. The hearing-impaired person may have acquired much proficiency in identifying visible speech cues without a formal speech reading program. Even though the client may have a hearing aid, this may be used only to amplify sound, while the person uses speech reading to determine what is being said. The hearing aid can make the client aware that someone is speaking, and can convey the rhythm of speech.

In communicating with an elderly person who uses speech reading, speak directly at the person's eye level, so that he or she can observe both lip movements and nonverbal facial cues. Lighting should be adequate to allow the client to see the speaker's face clearly. The speaker should avoid standing by windows, or in a dimly lit room or hallway. Short sentences or phrases tend to be easier to speech-read than single words, because of the rhythm and accent patterns of speech. Speech reading depends on context and not on individual words.

Speech Training

Speech training may be needed by elderly persons whose hearing loss limits their ability to hear their own speech. Speech training may help to conserve normal speech and to prevent or correct problems relating to loudness, clarity, pitch inflection, quality, and rate of speech. If possible, speech rehabilitation should begin while the person still has hearing assets, before a more advanced stage of hearing impairment is reached. If speech changes have occurred, corrective speech training can be initiated.

Combined Hearing Therapy

Combined hearing therapy is sometimes utilized, depending upon the client's need for and ability to utilize multiple interventions. In combined hearing therapy, the elderly client is placed in a program combining amplification through a hearing aid, auditory training, speech reading, and speech training. Elderly persons can be taught to optimize the environment for better hearing by seating themselves for optimal listening and to inform others when the message is not understood.

Environment Aids

Sound is important for self-protection and identification with the environment. For the person with a hearing impairment, various tools are available to add safety to the environment. Flashing lights and amplifiers are available for phones or doorbells, if an ordinary ring cannot be heard. Telephone receiver amplifiers can be added to facilitate phone conversations. Even though the Organization for Use of the Telephone (OUT) has not reached its goal to have all phones compatible with hearing aids, the Telecommunication for the Disabled Act of 1982 requires compatibility in all coin phones, emergency phones, and other phones frequently needed for use by persons with hearing aids.

Visual alarm or teletype systems are available. Alarm clocks are available with low-frequency buzzers or built-in flashers. There also are alarm clocks that produce vibrotactile signals through pillows. Special headphones may be used for listening to radio and television. Advances continue to be made in development of hearing aids that provide better sound localization and more effective speech discrimination. Some hearing aids come with a telephone pick-up device to activate the hearing aid amplifier during telephone conversations. For the elderly client, the limiting factor in the use of all these devices is their expense.

Environmental background noise should be controlled, because it competes with verbal communication with the hearing-impaired person. Family counseling may be necessary to encourage family support in making listening situations optimal for the client, especially in the home setting. Sound-absorbent materials can be used in the living environment. This includes the use of acoustic tile, carpet, drapes, and cloth-covered furniture.

The elderly person with impaired hearing may have difficulty in defining his or her territory. There may be suspicions that others are entering the individual's personal space. Correct identification of sounds enables the person to feel a greater degree of security in the environment.

Hearing Conservation

Many known factors contribute to hearing loss. Mauer and Rupp (1979) summarize the work of researchers who suggest that sociocusis is the hearing pattern seen in the elderly. Sociocusis is described as the cumulative results of damage inflicted in the auditory system over the person's lifespan. Added to the lifetime exposure to social, recreational, and occupational noise are ototoxic drugs, middle ear infections, fevers, and head trauma. As discussed earlier, exposure to environmental noise can lead to loss of hearing, by causing loss of hair cells in the organ of Corti of the cochlea. Factors to consider in evaluating environmental noise include the intensity, the duration, and the distribution of noise to which the individual is exposed on a regular basis. Examples include factory machinery, jet airplane sounds, and chain saws. Examples of noise in homes include garbage disposals, dishwashers, vacuum cleaners, power lawnmowers, and chain saws. To help prevent the hearing problems that can result from noise exposure, protective devices such as earplugs, earphones, and earmuffs can be used.

Pathologic processes can affect hearing. Prompt therapy should be provided for inflammatory processes involving the ear, particularly the common problem of otitis media. However, medications used to treat some pathologies have ototoxic effects. A person who is receiving an ototoxic drug should have regular hearing screening.

More widespread screening programs for early identification of problems that could lead to hearing loss are needed. The nurse can assist with these programs, and she should also be aware that community resources may be available to help the elderly person with a hearing impairment. The nurse should recognize her role as a member of the health team in making client referrals to these community resources. Among the important state and national agencies that provide help to the person with hearing losses are the American Speech and Hearing Association and the National Association for the Deaf. A major source of support for research on the ear and hearing is through the communicative disorders program of the National Institute of Neurological and Communicative Disorders and Stroke.

Evaluation of Hearing Effectiveness

In evaluating progress toward goal attainment, the nurse does not expect the elderly person to regain normal auditory function. Instead, the hearing-impaired person should develop and maintain effective speaking and listening skills. With these skills, the elderly person should be able to maintain social contacts and feel confident in establishing new contacts. Measures of increased socialization include greater use of the phone, increased eye contact, less need for speaker repetition, and less fatigue during and following a conversation.

These communication skills should also help the client to continue relationships with family members, significant others, and peers. The nurse evaluates the degree to which these goals are achieved. It may be difficult for families to understand that an expensive hearing aid did not solve the hearing problems.

For the client who has purchased a hearing aid, evaluation is based upon the consistency in wearing the aid, the quality of amplification obtained from the aid, the client's comfort while using the aid, the client's understanding of the aid, the client's ability to take charge of caring for the aid, and the degree to which the aid improves the ability to communicate.

A significant evaluative factor is the client's own perception of his ability to communicate in various situations and under specific conditions. Other evaluative factors include the elderly person's desire to communicate with others by joining groups or seeking other situations in which communication can take place. If the client is in a long-term setting, progress toward goal attainment in increasing communication may be demonstrated by participation in activities.

The nurse's role is to support the client throughout the process of aural rehabilitation. However, the nurse and other members of the health team should recognize that some elderly people do not desire to reenter the hearing world. The motivation for auditory rehabilitation is greater in the old person who wishes to continue living a happy and productive life.

SPEECH OF THE ELDERLY

The ear is important in the reception of communication; the voice is an important part of expressive communication. An elderly person usually can be identified by characteristic changes in manner and style of speaking. The differences in the oral communication of an elderly person can occur as a result of the normal aging process, neurologic pathology, or both. "Speech refers to the audible expression of language and involves the generation of sound through the interactive participation of three physiologic systems: respiratory, phonatory, and articulatory" (Hutchinson and Beasley, 1976, p. 156).

Assessment Base

The effects of aging can change the vocal apparatus in a variety of ways. When the walls of the chest lose some resilience and the lungs lose elasticity, there is some loss of breath support for the voice. Weakening of the respiratory muscles may affect the speaker's ability to produce the slow muscle pressures needed to expel air during exhalation. This can contribute to prosodic changes in the speech of elderly persons. Prosody refers to variation in stress, pitch, and rhythm of speech to convey the meaning of the verbal message. Reduced elasticity and vital capacity of the aging respiratory system can affect the elderly person's efficient use of speech. The amount of air with which to speak is reduced. This can affect the number of words produced per unit of time and may determine how frequently speech must be interrupted for air intake. It can be fatiguing to expend additional muscle force during speech. Elderly people may have difficulty speaking at a consistently loud level because they may not be able to inflate their lungs sufficiently as a result of reduced elastic recoil in the aging lung (Kahane, 1981).

The laryngeal cartilages become progressively ossified. The secretion of many mucous glands thickens. With aging, the vocal range narrows through the loss of high tones. If the vocal cords thicken, there may be a shift to a lower-frequency vocal range. However, more frequently, there are atrophic changes within the vocal cords and the vocal range becomes higher pitched. This results in the squeaking of some elderly voices. The range of the singing voice is reduced. With aging, there can be an alteration of fine control of vocal cord vibratory activity. The overall sound of the voice may become monotonous and tremulous (Von-Leden, 1977).

There is a tendency toward greater pitch variability with increasing age. The overall speaking rate tends to decrease with age. This is assumed to be the result of a general slowing of neuromuscular activity with advancing age (Hutchinson and Beasley, 1976). However, Ramey (1983) found that the physiologic condition of the elderly person is a significant variable to consider in the analysis of acoustic characteristics of voice. Therefore, chronologic age should not be used as the only index of aging in voice research.

Further, elderly persons can develop nervous system disorders that have an effect on language functioning. Hutchinson and Beasley (1979) classify these as disorders of ideation, symbolization, translation, and execution. Disorders of ideation result from diffuse central nervous system pathology such as cerebral arteriosclerosis and Alzheimer's disease. The resulting impairments affect calculation, comprehension, judgment, memory, and personal orientation. Intellectual deterioration affects language behavior.

Aphasia is a disorder of symbolization that most commonly occurs when a cerebral vascular accident results from involvement of the middle cerebral artery. As a result nourishment is affected to the cortical areas of the brain, the areas that are responsible for symbolic functions. The person may not comprehend the full meaning or significance of certain words or there may be problems with finding appropriate words to express one's thoughts. With aphasia, difficulty may occur with speaking, reading, writing, calculation, or auditory comprehension. The impairment may involve an occasional misuse of a word or there may be complete loss of proficiency in all language areas including the ability to use gestures.

Lesions of Broca's area of the brain can cause disorders of translation. Apraxia is characterized by difficulty with motor adjustments needed for speech. There may be repeated efforts at producing the right word. Even though there is difficulty in coordinating movements for speech, the strength of the peripheral musculature for speech is intact.

Disorders of execution or dysarthria, result from disturbances in control over peripheral respiratory, phonatory, and articulation of movements needed for speech. Rhythm, rate, volume, voice quality, pitch control, and intonation can be affected to varying degrees.

There are many nonlanguage factors that influence the elderly person's ability to communicate. These include visual–perceptual functions, intellectual ability, attention span, and the effect of the environment in the social setting. Loss of teeth, especially the upper anterior teeth, or improper fit of dentures may adversely affect speech intelligibility. There may be a decrease in the precision of articulation. Changes in the size of the oral cavity resulting from loss of teeth and retrusion of the mandible resulting from temporomandibular joint changes can affect oral resonance. Restrictions on movement of the temporomandibular joint can restrict the ability of the elderly person to change the size and shape of the oral cavity during speech. Further research is needed in the area of language behavior of the elderly. This is an important link in understanding the communication of the elderly.

Assessment of Speech

Much of the speech assessment of the elderly client occurs at the beginning of the assessment process through determining the way in which the client responds to questions. Inability to respond also provides important data. In assessing speech, the nurse needs to consider the client's receptive communication or the ability to receive a message, as well as the client's expressive communication, or the ability to convey a message.

The amount of time needed for the client to interpret the questions, as well as the amount of time to respond and the quantity and quality of the response, are included in the assessment. The depth of the assessment is influenced by the communication status of the client.

For the client who is unable to communicate verbally, the nurse needs to determine his ability to read, to write, and to use gestures to convey a message. The nurse should use caution in her response to a client who is labeled as aphasic. Too often, this person is treated as an object who lacks intelligence. The nurse needs to be especially careful in determining the abilities as well as the disabilities of the client who experiences alterations in speech.

Assessment of Speech and Communication

Receptive communication (ability to receive a message)

- Ability to:
  Read and follow written instructions
  Follow verbal requests from simple to more complex
  Repeat simple and complex words
  Repeat sentences
  Appreciate the symbolic value of words

Expressive language (ability to convey a message)

- Ability to:
  Formulate meaningful sentences
  Name common objects
  Match printed and written word with pictures
  Pronounce words
  Use words appropriately
  Point toward specific objects
  Use gestures to convey a message (if unable to speak)
  Convey a written message
  Use number symbols

Speech

  Clarity
  Ease of speech
  Loudness

Reactions to alterations in speech
Persons and groups for communicating

PLANNING AND INTERVENTION FOR SPEECH

Nursing interventions with elderly clients are directed toward maximizing communication within the ability of each client. There are fundamental considerations when communicating with the elderly person. Knowledge of the sensory status of each person is basic. To help the client to focus on the communication process, consider areas of interest to the client. Adequate time is needed for response to questions. The client should be encouraged to talk even though errors may be made. For the person who experiences alterations in speech, the nurse should prevent isolation of this person. Social stimulation needs continue. However, there should be an awareness of the energy expended in communication efforts. The nurse should work with communication at the time of the day when the client is most rested and is most responsive. Even when no verbal response can be made in return, the nurse should continue to talk with the client in an unhurried manner. However, allow time for a verbal response to occur.

A way to stimulate the elderly person with speech problems to participate in communication is to provide an opportunity to listen to words and to see objects while hearing the name of the object. The use of all of the client's senses should be encouraged. When possible, have the client feel or smell an object. Continue to encourage him to name the object. For the client with continued inability to use verbal expressions, the nurse can attempt to develop a gesture system with the client. An example is to use head movement for "yes" and "no." However, the client's reliability with the appropriate head movements needs to be determined.

Encourage attempts at verbal communication by careful listening. Verbal communication can be encouraged by providing the client the opportunity to make verbal requests rather than anticipating each need. The nurse should be honest with the client and not pretend when a word or message is not understood. This can be especially frustrating to the client. Also, the client should not be frustrated by frequent attempts to have him repeat the words that the listener was unable to understand. Perhaps the client can illustrate by writing or pointing to an object.

Automatic or emotional speech should not be mistaken for the return of ability to communicate verbally. Automatic speech is the most primitive form of speech and can involve using exclamatory remarks or even curses. Therefore, it is important for the nurse to consider client performance rather than just simple verbal exclamations as a criterion for understanding communication.

Interventions with the client with alterations in speech communication does need to be a team effort. The speech therapist as well as significant others need to be intimately involved with the communication process. Communication must occur *with* the client and not *at* the client or *about* the client in his presence.

Family members need to be considered in working with a communication impairment. Communicative impairments affect families. Alternatively, family members can have a marked influence on rehabilitative efforts. The nature of the family's long-acting communicative interaction and the nature of the communication immediately prior to the onset of the communication impairment need to be considered in planning interventions (Webster and Newhoff, 1981).

More recently the use of electronic equipment has shown promise in reducing the isolation of the person with alterations in communication. Through telecommunication devices the hearing- and speech-impaired person may have contact with outside community resources such as library systems. However, the use of electronic equipment may be anxiety producing for the elderly person who is unfamiliar with and even frightened by present-day electronic advances.

Speech Conservation

To preserve the flexibility and elasticity of the soft tissues of the larynx, the avoidance of loud or excessive talking or singing is recommended. To protect the epithelial lining of the lungs and larynx, the elimination of smoking and reduction in exposure to irritants in the atmosphere is advisable. Adequate humidification promotes the health of the mucous lining of the respiratory tract. Other factors that are suspected of affecting the voice include a history of alcohol abuse, respiratory problems, and speech and hearing problems. Present day health promotion practices are directed toward reducing cerebrovascular problems that cause neurologically related speech pathologies.

Evaluation of Speech Effectiveness

Evaluation of speech relates to the effectiveness with which the client is able to express himself. This may be communication that is expressed verbally, through gestures, or in writing. The degree of comfort that the client demonstrates in the communication process needs to be considered. The desire of others to communicate with the client may be a reflection of the client's interest in communication. However, negative reactions of others toward the client's communication efforts may reflect lack of interest or empathy of the care provider rather than the interest of the client in communication.

MULTIPLE SENSORY CHANGES

For most people, sensory function is maintained until middle age. After that time, sensory function appears to begin a decline. The elderly person may have learned to compensate for a loss of one sense by increased use of another sense. However, additional trauma is created when changes occur in the compensatory sense or senses. For example, the visually impaired old person may depend to a great degree on hearing, smell, and touch. Changes in hearing can have a marked impact on such a person's adaptation.

Even though adaptation to a sensory loss

in one modality is accomplished through the use of other modalities, the older the person is when sensory loss occurs, and the more senses involved, the greater the difficulty tends to be. Not only must changes in the sensory status of the elderly person be considered in planning, the health team must also consider the client's orientation, mobility skills, and coping skills. Planning and intervention with the client who experiences sensory changes may offset the possible future difficulties such as memory loss, social withdrawal, and mobility problems.

Altered functioning of the sensory receptors can cause sensory deprivation, the inadequate reception or perception of environmental stimuli. Sensory deprivation may have a physiologic cause or may be due to an inadequate amount of stimulation in the environment. Sensory overload is environment stimulation that exceeds the person's ability to cope or comprehend. Sensory underload is inadequate stimulation in the environment. As a result of sensory underload, a person experiencing sensory deprivation may demonstrate boredom, lack of concentration and coherent thinking, daydreaming, and hallucinations (Shelby, 1978). The amount and type of sensory input that the elderly client is capable of receiving forms the basis of the intervention. When there are losses in several sensory modalities, the remaining sensory functions must be maximized.

Environmental Management

The nurse should be aware of the impact of environment when helping the elderly person with sensory losses toward increased self-reliance. Maintenance of a barrier-free environment is essential for the client with changes in sensory modalities. Such changes can block the reception of danger signals. The dangers of fire, in particular, are intensified for the individual who has limited vision, smell, and touch. By the time this person is aware of the danger, the fire may be out of control.

The information that the elderly person is able to receive from the environment can be enhanced by enriching the environment with stimuli that involve all the senses. The way in which environmental stimuli are patterned is

highly important to adaptive behavior. In planning for such patterning, the sensory environment is assessed according to the kind, quality, and quantity of stimuli (Roberts, 1978).

The sensory environment must have meaning for the elderly person. With the growing use of synthetic materials, the client with multiple sensory losses may not receive expected information about familiar objects. Examples of misleading items include plastic eating utensils for the person who is accustomed to china dishes and steel or silver flatware; paper tablecloths and napkins; disposable washcloths; and artificial turf instead of grass. To fill the old person's environment with imitations of originals may affect the structure of that environment and the person's degree of orientation to it, especially when sensory receptors are not functioning efficiently. This, in turn, can lead to alienation.

When various sensory changes are present, the nurse may find it necessary to use a more intimate or personal distance in working with elderly clients. The old person with reduced vision may need to be close enough to see, hear, smell, or touch the nurse during interaction. With a closer physical relationship, the client is better able to see and hear the nurse and obtain a greater degree of meaning from the interaction.

Sensory Retraining

Sensory retraining is a technique used to improve the elderly person's interactions with the environment through the senses. Sensory losses that cannot be or have not been corrected may be responsible for a sensory underload that may be expressed by some elderly persons as regressed behavior. Sensory underload can be especially pronounced in the client with multiple sensory losses.

The goal of sensory retraining is to bring the elderly person back into contact with the environment by providing activities and objects that stimulate the senses. Colored objects can be used to stimulate vision; a variety of odors can stimulate smell; feeling the differences in the textures of fresh fruits or fabrics can stimulate tactile sensitivity; music recordings or various instrument sounds can be used to stimulate the auditory sense; and a variety of tastes can stimulate taste sensitivity.

The same objects can be used to stimulate several senses. For example, the elderly person may work with a variety of fruits with different colors, textures, and odors. The client can assist in preparing a fruit salad and then experience the different fruit tastes. Even though the elderly person is attending sensory retraining sessions, the nurse can reinforce this program by encouraging the client to identify objects through the use of multiple sensory modalities. The visually impaired person with limited tactile sensitivity in the hands may be assisted in determining the most sensitive part of the fingers. Greatest sensitivity is usually found at the tips of the fingers, especially under the nails (Snyder, 1978). Placing an object into the fingertips rather than on the palm of the hand may enhance sensitivity to the object for the person who also has a visual loss.

Sensitivity of Health Team

Researchers continue to develop ways of increasing the effectiveness of those who work with the elderly person experiencing sensory losses. Pastalan describes the Empathic Model to simulate age-related sensory losses. The Empathic Model is composed of an assortment of appliances that simulate the visual, auditory, and tactile sensitivity of a person in his late 70s or early 80s (Pastalan, 1977). Exposing health team members to this and similar experiences that simulate sensory losses may give them a greater sensitivity to the needs of elderly clients.

In conclusion, the client's behavior may be one of the best indicators of the functioning of his or her sensory systems. Because the receptor system is so vital in behavior, changes in receptor functioning may first be manifested by alterations in behavior. Multiple sensory changes experienced by the elderly person may lead to differing degrees of impairment, but impairment does not automatically lead to disability. The degree to which disability has been limited or prevented is often a gauge of the effectiveness of interventions utilized by the client, family, and health team members. The abilities of the elderly person with sensory

changes can be evaluated in terms of maintenance of existing assets, attainment of functional improvement, prevention or reduction of further deterioration, and prevention of secondary problems stemming from the sensory losses. It is vital to consider the sensory acuity of the elderly person when assessing the cognitive functioning status.

Use of Touch

Touch can be a powerful tool in nursing interventions. Touch becomes especially important with the client who experiences alterations in communication related to sensory changes as well as changes in speech patterns. Huss (1977) presents the increased need for meaningful touch by the elderly person who has decreased sensory and functional capacities in order to lessen the feelings of isolation. Touch is a sensory pathway that tends to remain intact throughout the aging process. This then becomes a vital means for sensory input for the elderly person. Even though the sense of touch does not decrease with aging, the external sources of touch decrease as the elderly experience losses of significant others who provided affective touch (Fig. 12.3).

The findings of research demonstrate the physiologic as well as the psychologic effects of touch as a nursing intervention. Krieger (1975, 1979), Barnett (1972), Burnside (1973), Copstead (1980), McCorkle (1974), and Weiss

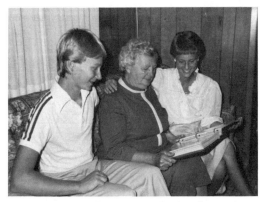

Figure 12.3. The use of affective touch can be a pleasurable experience.

(1979) have shown that the elderly need to touch as well as to be touched. Touch is a primary method of communication. However, the socio-cultural aspects of touch need to be considered. There are culturally determined rules relating to when to touch, where to touch, how to touch, and whom to touch. To violate the person's perceptions of acceptable touch can result in high levels of anxiety. For the elderly person who experiences altered communication such as with sensory changes, anxiety levels may be already high. The nurse needs to help the person gain comfort in using touch and in receiving touch as a method of communicating with others.

Nurses utilize touch in task as well as non-task client contacts. McCorkle (1974) found that the nurse can establish rapport with a seriously ill person in a short time through the use of touch. The nurse is able to convey concern, caring, and interest when touch is used. This is affective touch. Seaman (1982) discusses the therapeutic effects of the selective use of affective touch to enter the personal space of the elderly person. The use of affective touch has been demonstrated to stop the rambling speech of agitated elderly persons. Dominian (1971) discusses the reassurance conveyed to clients through touch. Reassurance to the client experiencing communication alterations is a significant nursing intervention. The nurse needs to determine the degree of affective touch that is comfortable to the elderly person. Through touch, the nurse can convey caring about as well as caring for the elderly person.

RECOMMENDED READINGS

Corso, J.F. Aging Sensory Systems and Perception. New York, Praeger, 1981. *A comprehensive review of research into hearing changes with aging. Useful as an assessment base.*

Hutchinson, J.M., Beasley, D.S. Speech and language functioning among aging, in Oyer, H.J., Oyer, E.J. (eds.), Aging and Communication. Baltimore, University Press, 1976. *This book presents the effects of physiologic speech changes with aging and neurologic pathologies that affect the speech communication of the elderly person.*

Maurer, J.F., Rupp, R.R. Hearing and Aging: Tactics for Intervention. New York, Grune and Stratton,

1979. *A complete guide on the rehabilitation of the hearing-impaired elderly person. Included is a comprehensive guide to the resources and programs for the hearing impaired person.*

Pastalan, L.A. The empathic model: A methodological bridge between research and design. Journal of Architectural Education 31(1):14, 1977. *Presents environmental modifications to promote more effective functioning of the elderly person. Helpful in planning and interventions.*

Pyrek, J., Smith, K., Lantto, J. Hearing and Psychosocial Function in a Long-Term Care Facility. Paper presented at the Gerontological Society 30th Annual Scientific Meeting, San Francisco, November 19, 1977. *Relates hearing to psychosocial functioning of the elderly person based on research findings. Provides a basis for assessment, planning, and intervention.*

Shore, H. Designing a training program for understanding sensory loss in aging. The Gerontologist 16:157, 1976. *Presents sensory simulations and the effects of a simulation program on nursing staff performance in a long-term care setting. Provides help with planning and intervention.*

Snyder, L.H. Environmental changes for socialization. Journal of Nursing Administration 8(1):44, 1978. *Discusses interventions relating to environment modifications to encourage socialization among the elderly. Useful in planning and intervention.*

Rosenthal, R. The Hearing Loss Handbook. New York, St. Martin's, 1975. *The author, a person with a hearing impairment, presents his experiences with this loss, especially with barriers encountered. Presents practical suggestions for assisting the hearing-impaired person. Helpful for planning and intervention.*

Sataloff, J., Michael, P. Hearing Conservation. Springfield, IL, Thomas, 1973. *Discusses the significance of hearing conservation and methods to promote hearing conservation. The impact of environmental noises is stressed. Useful in planning and intervention.*

REFERENCES CITED

Agate, J. Common symptoms and complaints, in Rossman I. (ed), Clinical Geriatrics, 2nd ed. Philadelphia, Lippincott, 1979

Barnett, K. A theoretical construct of the concepts of touch as they relate to nursing. Nursing Research 21:102, 1972

Bergman, M. Changes in hearing with age. The Gerontologist 2:148, 1971

Burnside, I.M. Touching is talking. American Journal of Nursing 73:2060, 1973

Copstead, L.E. Effects of touch on self-appraisal and interaction appraisal for permanently institutionalized older adults. Journal of Gerontological Nursing 6:747, 1980

Corso, J.F. Aging Sensory Systems and Perception. New York, Praeger, 1981

Corso, J.F. Auditory perception and communication, in Birren, J.E., Schaie, K.N. (eds), Handbook of the Psychology of Aging. New York, Van Nostrand Reinhold, 1977

Dominian, J. The psychological significance of touch. Nursing Times 67:896, 1971

Gerber, S.E. Introductory Hearing Science. Philadelphia, Saunders, 1974

Hull, R.H. Hearing Impairment Among Aging Persons. Lincoln, NE, Cliffs Notes, 1977

Huss, A.J. Touch with care or caring touch. Journal of Occupational Therapy 31:11, 1977

Hutchinson, J.M., Beasley, D.S. Speech and language functioning among aging, in Oyer, H.J., Oyer, E.J. (eds), Aging and Communication. Baltimore, University Park Press, 1976

Kahane, J.C. Anatomic and physiologic changes in the aging peripheral speech mechanism, in Beasley, D.S., Davis, G.A. (eds), Aging: Communication Processes and Disorders. New York, Grune and Stratton, 1981

Krieger, D. Searching for evidence of physiological change. American Journal of Nursing 79:660, 1979

Krieger, D. Therapeutic touch: The imprimature of nursing. American Journal of Nursing 75:784, 1975

Marston, L.E. Hearing aid on trial. Aging 323–324:24, 1982

Maurer, J.F., Rupp, R.R. Hearing and Aging: Tactics for Intervention. New York, Grune and Stratton, 1979

McCartney, J.H., Nadler, G. How to help your patient cope with hearing loss. Geriatrics 34(3):69, 1979

McCorkle, R. Effects of touch on seriously ill patients. Nursing Research 23:125, 1974

Meyerhoff, W.L., Shrewsbury, D. Rational approaches to tinnitus. Geriatrics 35(10):90, 1980

Moore, B.C. Introduction to the Psychology of Hearing. Baltimore, University Park Press, 1977

Northern, J.L. Hearing Disorders. Boston, Little, Brown, 1976

Oyer, H.J., Freeman, B., Hardick, E., Dixon, J., Donnelly, K., Goldstein, D., Lloyd, L., Massen, E. Unheeded recommendations for aural rehabilitation: Analysis of a survey. Journal of the Academy of Rehabilitative Audiology 9:20, 1976

Oyer, H.J., Kapar, Y.P., Deal, L.V. Hearing disorders in the aging: Effects upon communication, in Oyer, H.J., Oyer, E.J. (eds), Aging and Communication. Baltimore, University Park Press, 1976

Pastalan, L.A. The empathic model: A methodological bridge between research and design. Journal of Architectural Education 31(1):14, 1977

Pyrek, J., Smith, K., Lantto, J. Hearing and Psychosocial Function in a Long-Term Care Facility. Paper presented at the Gerontological Society 30th Annual Scientific Meeting, San Francisco, November 19, 1977

Ramig, L.A. Effects of physiological aging on vowel spectral noise. Journal of Gerontology 38(2):223, 1983

Reichel, W. Clinical Aspects of Aging. Baltimore, Williams and Wilkins, 1978

Roberts, S. Behavioral Concepts and Nursing Throughout the Life Span. Englewood Cliffs, NJ, Prentice-Hall, 1978

Ruben, R. Aging and hearing, in Rossman, I. (ed), Clinical Geriatrics. Philadelphia, Lippincott, 1971

Seaman, L. Affective nursing touch. Geriatric Nursing 3(3):162, 1982

Shelby, J.P. Sensory deprivation. Image 10(2):49–55, 1978

Shore, H. Designing a training program for understanding sensory loss in aging. The Gerontologist 16:157, 1976

Snyder, L.H. Environmental changes for socialization. Journal of Nursing Administration 8(1):44, 1978

Webster, E.J., Newhoff, M. Intervention with families of communicatively impaired adults in aging, in Aging: Communication Processes. Beasley, D.S., Albyn, G. (eds), New York, Grune and Stratton, 1981

Weiss, S.J. The language of touch. Nursing Research 28:76, 1979

BIBLIOGRAPHY

Bloomer, H. Speech and the coming of age. Perspective on Aging 7(5):4, 1978

Bozian, M.W., Clark, H.M. Counteracting sensory changes in the aging. American Journal of Nursing 80(3):473, 1980

Chodel, J., Williams, B. The concept of sensory deprivation. Nursing Clinics of North America 5:453, 1970

Clark, C.C., Mills, G. Communicating with hearing impaired elderly adults. Journal of Gerontological Nursing 5(3):41, 1979

Corso, J.F. Sensory processes and effects in normal adults. Journal of Gerontology 26(1):90, 1971

DeL'aune, W.R. Hearing: Its evolution and ways of compensating for its loss. Vision Impairment and Blindness 74(1):19, 1980

Ernst, P., Shaw, J. Touching is not taboo. Geriatric Nursing 1(3):193, 1980

Havener, W., Saunder, W., Keith, C.F., Prescott, A. Nursing Care in Eye, Ear, Nose, and Throat Disorders. St. Louis, Mosby, 1974

Hayter, J. Modifying the environment to help older persons. Nursing and Health 4(5):265, 1983

Holder, L. Hearing aids. Nursing '82 12(4):64, 1982

Johnson, B.S. The meaning of touch in nursing. Nursing Outlook 13:59, 1965

Mechner, F. Patient assessment: Examination of the ear. American Journal of Nursing 74:1, 1974

Mueller, C. Sensory Psychology. Englewood Cliffs, NJ, Prentice-Hall, 1965

Nathan, M.D. Protecting the elderly against drug-induced hearing loss. Geriatrics 36(8):95, 1981

Norman, S., Baratz, R. Understanding aphasia. American Journal of Nursing 79(12):2135, 1979

Ohta, R.J., Carlin, M., Harmon, B. Auditory acuity and performance on the mental status questionnaire in the elderly. Journal of the American Geriatrics Society 29(10):476, 1981

Pastalan, L.A., Carson, D.H. Spatial Behavior of Older People. Ann Arbor, University of Michigan Press, 1970

Preston, T. When words fail. American Journal of Nursing 73:2064, 1973

Rosenthal, R. The Hearing Loss Handbook. New York, St. Martin's, 1975

Sataloff, J., Michael, P. Hearing Conservation. Springfield, IL, Thomas, 1973

Thomas, P.D., Hunt, W.C., Garry, P.J., Hood, R.B., Goodwin, J.M., Goodwin, J.S. Hearing acuity in a healthy elderly population: Effects on emotional, cognitive, and social status. Journal of Gerontology 38(3):321, 1983

Ventura, F.P. Counseling the hearing-impaired geriatric patient. Patient Counsel Health Education 1:22, 1978

Wright, B.A. Physical Disability—a Psychological Approach. New York, Harper, 1960

13

Nutrition in the Aged and the Nursing Process

Nancy J. Ebert

Reading this chapter will enable the individual to:

1. Assess factors related to nutrition status in the elderly
2. Identify risk factors commonly seen in the elderly
3. Describe methods of assessment
4. Discuss potential interventions for maintaining adequate nutritional or elimination status in the elderly

This chapter will focus on the nursing process as it relates to the nutritional status of the elderly client. The need for adequate nutrition is not unique to the elderly client. Problems common with aging, however, may influence or alter the nutritional status.

NUTRITION

Adequate nutrition is as important to the health of the elderly adult as it is to that of the younger person. Evidence indicates that nutritional practices of the younger years influence longevity of life and quality of health. Certain illnesses that are more prevalent in the elderly population are considered to be diet related. These include atherosclerosis, osteoporosis, diabetes, and diverticulitis. It appears, however, that most elderly persons continue the dietary patterns established during their younger years.

Nutritional status is defined as the state of health related to intake, digestion, and utilization of nutrients. Assessment, planning, and intervention for maintenance or restoration of the nutritional status of the elderly is multifaceted. Assessment of nutritional status should be derived from data obtained from physical examination, laboratory appraisal, anthropometry (body measurements), medical history, psychosocial history, and dietary intake. Each of these assessment methods is discussed later in the chapter. The nurse must be aware of the many factors that contribute to the maintenance of adequate nutrition in the elderly.

Assessment Factors Related to Nutritional Status

Relatively few studies have been conducted to evaluate the nutritional status of the elderly as a group. Most studies have examined facets of the nutritional status, physiologic changes of body systems, adequacy of dietary intake, and the incidence of suboptimal dietary adequacy in selected elderly populations.

Physiologic Changes of Aging

A number of age-related physiologic changes may affect the nutritional status of the elderly. These changes involve the gastrointestinal, endocrine, renal, and musculoskeletal systems. However, the precise relationship of these

419

changes to nutritional status is not well documented at this time.

Decreases in taste and smell acuity may occur with aging. As a result, the elderly person may increase use of salt, sugar, or other condiments to enhance the flavor of foods. Food preferences may shift from bland foods to spicier foods. It is important for the nurse to assess changes in food preference, especially when the client has been prescribed a modified diet, such as one which restricts salt or calorie intake. The elderly person may find low-salt or low-calorie food unpalatable, and therefore omit foods necessary for health or abandon the prescribed diet.

The state of the elderly person's mouth may also affect the choice of foods. Whether or not dentures are worn has not been found to influence nutritional status in the elderly (Todhunter, 1976; Bates, Elwood, and Foster, 1971). However, the nurse should assess the condition of the mouth. Does the person have a sore mouth, or several loose or missing teeth? If so, information must be obtained regarding changes in food intake patterns. If the client wears dentures, the nurse must determine whether they are worn while eating. Some elderly persons have been known to remove their dentures while eating but continue to eat as wide a variety of foods as those elderly with their own teeth. Others may eat only soft foods, usually carbohydrates. The nurse must therefore determine if food intake patterns have been altered in response to wearing dentures or other changes in the mouth.

Several changes of the mouth may occur with aging. The mucous membrane may become more fragile and easily damaged. Leukoplakia, characterized by white patches on the mucous membrane, occurs with increasing incidence as one ages and is more common in smokers. Leukoplakia is considered a precancerous lesion. Decreases in the masticating ability may also occur. The continuous wear and tear of chewing and bruxism causes a change in the biting surface. There is an increase in bone resorption both in those with their own teeth and those wearing dentures. This bone loss leads to loosening of the teeth

and eventual loss of teeth. Periodontal disease occurs with increasing incidence and is often associated with bone resorption. Poor dental hygiene and diet lacking vitamins B and C are felt to be the chief cause of periodontal disease. The elderly are less likely to visit a dentist particularly if they have dentures. Gift (1978) reports that over 70 percent of the elderly had not visited a dentist in 5 years.

Subjects, aged 25 to 75 years, were instructed to chew a fresh whole carrot until it was ready to swallow. It was found that the elderly and the dentally compromised subjects (10–13 teeth on both sides or a total of 20–26 teeth) required more chewing strokes and more chewing time before feeling prepared to swallow (Feldman et al., 1980). In another investigation, the effects of age and dentition status on food acceptability were studied. Those subjects with compromised dentition demonstrated decreased acceptance of the taste and the texture of solid food samples as well as a perceived decrease in chewing ease. Age had no significant effect on food acceptability.

Decreases in gastric secretion of hydrochloric acid and in absorption of xylose, vitamins B, B_{12}, A, carotene, and folic acid occur with greater frequency in the elderly. These changes have not been positively correlated with changes in food tolerance or with increased incidence of vitamin deficiency connected with inadequate intake of nutrients. More studies should be conducted regarding the effects of absorption changes on nutrition. However, the nurse should be alert to any food intolerances the elderly person may complain of. A long list of food intolerances may indicate that the person has an inadequate intake of necessary nutrients. Food intolerance may also point to the presence of disease in the gastrointestinal tract. The nurse should elicit from the client the exact nature of the response to the food or foods. Does the client have an intolerance to specific foods, such as fatty foods or gas-forming foods? If so, how has the person's diet been modified?

The chief age-related change in the endocrine system involves a decreased tolerance to glucose (Andres and Tobin, 1977). This change may be manifested as elevated fasting blood glucose. In response to intake of glucose, the blood glucose level may achieve a higher peak than normal, followed by a delay in return to fasting blood glucose levels. Whether this response is a normal phenomenon of aging or a pathological change is controversial. Some physicians and researchers speculate that the "normal" values in blood sugar levels should be adjusted to account for age-related changes. The nurse should be alert to the fact that adult-onset diabetes occurs more commonly in aged persons. Persons who are obese and/or who have a family history of diabetes should be evaluated for glucose intolerance by annual fasting blood glucose tests and urine tests for glucose and acetone. It should be noted that the reabsorption of glucose by the renal tubules may also decline or be erratic in the elderly (Goldman, 1977). For this reason, the presence of glucose in the urine of the elderly person cannot be the only diagnostic determinant of diabetes. The nurse should counsel the client regarding the importance of these tests, since the onset of diabetes in the elderly is usually slow and the symptoms may be mild and obscure.

Musculoskeletal changes associated with aging include decreased bone density and degenerative joint changes. Decreased bone density predisposes the elderly person to fractures as well as tooth loss. Degenerative joint changes predispose the individual to decreased activity levels. The nurse should explore the implications of changes in activity or dental status. Does the elderly person have difficulty in traveling to food stores? The elderly may not have enough energy to prepare food, may not feel like eating, or may not be able to chew food. All of these factors can affect the food preference and food selection of the elderly person.

Adequacy of Nutrition in the Elderly

Optimal dietary needs for the older adult have not been differentiated from those of the middle-aged adult. Studies indicate that, with the exception of calories, the requirements for specific nutrients are the same for the older adult as for the middle-aged adult. Caloric needs are determined largely by the individual's energy

expenditure. The active elderly person may require the same caloric intake as a younger person, whereas the immobile older person will require fewer calories. In a study of a French elderly population (Derby, Bleyer, and Martin, 1977), the intake of calories was found to be significantly higher for the rural population than for the urban population. This difference was attributed to the probability of greater expenditure of energy by the rural elderly. The activity level of the old person is therefore an important factor in determining adequacy of dietary intake, particularly caloric intake. The life-style of each client should be assessed for amount of activity. Measures of body weight should be obtained for determining loss or gain. Weight gain over a period of months or years may indicate that calorie intake exceeds the individual's energy expenditure.

The Recommended Dietary Allowances (1980) for specific nutrients for persons over 51 were prepared by the Food and Nutritional Board of the National Research Council, National Academy of Sciences. The Recommended Dietary Allowances (RDAs), as shown in Table 13.1, are greater than minimal requirements. They were established as a guide for planning and maintaining the nutrition of the healthy adult. To calculate amounts of each nutrient found in dietary intake is tedious and requires the skills of a qualified resource person, such as a dietician. Therefore, RDAs have been used primarily as a research tool to determine the adequacy of diet. There are no specific RDAs for carbohydrate or fats, however, these categories are important to many people. Food labels on packaged foods often describe the percentages of RDAs contained per serving. Some elderly are more interested in the number of calories and grams of fat, protein, and carbohydrates indicated than the percentages of RDAs in a serving. Others who are on modified diets or have interest in their nutrition read the labels carefully.

The daily Food Guide (see Table 13.2) of five food groups was revised from the Basic Four Food Guide (Food, Home, and Garden Bulletin, 1979). Following the recommended number of servings, the aged person should

TABLE 13-1. RECOMMENDED DAILY DIETARY ALLOWANCES FOR ADULTS 51 YEARS OF AGE OR OLDER*

Measures	Expected Values	
	Male	Female
Weight	154 lbs. (70 kg)	120 lbs. (55 kg)
Height	70 in.	64 in.
Energy	2400 kcal	1800 kcal
Protein (g)	56	44
Vitamin A (Retinol equivalents)	1000	800
Vitamin D (μg)	5	5
Vitamin E (IU)	10	8
		12
Ascorbic acid	60	60
Folic acid (mg)	400	400
Niacin (mg)	16	12
Riboflavin (mg)	1.4	1.2
Thiamin (mg)	1.2	1.0
Vitamin B6 (mg)	2.2	2.0
Vitamin B12 (g)	3.0	3.0
Calcium (mg)	800	800
Phosphorus (mg)	800	800
Iodine (μg)	150	150
Iron (mg)	10	10
Magnesium (mg)	350	300
Zinc (mg)	15	15

*From The Food and Nutrition Board, National Research Council, 1980.

nurse and the elderly client to interpret. The fat, sweet, and alcohol group contain foods that can be eliminated to reduce caloric intake.

More recently, *Dietary Guidelines for Americans* was issued (Nutrition and Your Health, 1980). The guidelines are to (1) eat a variety of foods, (2) maintain ideal weight, (3) avoid too much fat, saturated fat, and cholesterol, (4) eat foods with adequate starch and fiber, (5) avoid too much sugar, (6) avoid too much sodium, and (7) if you drink alcohol, do so in moderation. These guidelines are vague in defining what is "too much" or "in moderation" and make it difficult to assess diet adequacy, but they may be used in planning and intervention.

Fluid balance in the elderly should also be considered. Water accounts for 45 percent of the total body weight in women and 50 percent in men between 40 and 60 years of age. As lean body weight decreases so does total fluid volume. The fluid needs of the elderly are said to be similar to that of an adult—1½–2 liters daily depending upon the weather, activity, and metabolic demands. Because the total fluid volume decreases, the elderly person is more vulnerable to the effects of dehydration. Increased intake of fluid is indicated when activity is increased and when the weather is hot. Infection and fever may also increase metabolic demands and subsequent fluid needs. Because the elderly may have decreased sensations of thirst they have less protection against possible dehydration. With their effect on increasing urination, diuretics may contribute to loss of fluid.

consume 1200 calories. The Guide, like the RDA, was prepared for planning and assessing diets of healthy adults. This Guide is easier for the

TABLE 13-2. DAILY FOOD GUIDE

Food Group	Essentials of an Adequate Diet
Milk and cheese	Two servings (2 cups milk)
Vegetable and fruit	Four servings (Include one serving that should be high in vitamin C. Variety including unpeeled fruits and vegetables.)
Bread and cereal	Four servings (Whole grain and enriched products.)
Meat, poultry, fish, and beans	Two servings (2–3 oz. lean meat, poultry, fish, per serving.)
Fats, sweets, and alcohol	No serving size indicated.

This loss may be desirable for clients who demonstrate fluid retention or fluid overload. For clients being treated with diuretics for uncomplicated hypertension, fluid intake should be consumed in the desirable amounts. The state of hydration of the elderly may be more difficult to assess. Some elderly have decreased salivation so the mucous membrane of the mouth may look and feel dry. The loss of elasticity of the skin associated with aging makes it more difficult to assess skin turgor. To assess fluid balance, one may need to estimate intake and output of fluids. The color and concentration (specific gravity) of urine should also be assessed. Increased concentration of the urine may cause the urine to appear deeper in color. Daily weights may be indicated for those clients who show signs of fluid retention or have low or no fluid intake for a period of time due to choice or to regimens imposed for diagnostic tests.

A few notable studies have been conducted in large samples of the elderly population (U.S. Department of Agriculture, 1972; Ten-State Nutrition Survey, 1972; Health Nutrition Examination Survey, 1974, 1975, 1978). The measurements and techniques of dietary survey and analysis vary from one study to another, so that comparison of findings is not possible.

The Household Consumption Survey was conducted by the U.S. Department of Agriculture (1972) during 1965 to 1966. The data indicated that the energy expenditure value and mean intake of nutrients decreased with age. The mean value for calcium intake by those 75 and over was the only nutrient below RDA. The percentage of elderly persons whose intake of specific nutrients was below RDAs was not reported.

The Ten-State Nutrition Survey (1972) was conducted in 10 southern states whose population was in the lowest income quartile of the population of the United States, as determined by the census of 1960. Obesity was more prevalent in elderly women, particularly black women. In the elderly, higher frequencies of vitamin A deficiency were found in Spanish-Americans. Riboflavin and thiamine deficiencies were noted among elderly blacks. The frequency of vitamin C deficiency increased in the elderly, particularly in males.

The Health and Nutrition Examination Survey (HANES) was conducted during 1971–72 on a scientifically selected sample of persons 1 to 74 years of age. The HANES data were collected from four sources:

1. Dietary intake of the individual
2. Biochemical tests of urine and blood for nutrients
3. Clinical examination to detect signs and symptoms of nutritional problems
4. Various body measurements (anthropometric measures)

These data were then analyzed by sex, age, race, and income levels. Dietary intake data revealed deficiencies in intake of iron, vitamins A and C, and calcium in the elderly. The deficiencies did not always correlate with income level, sex, or race. Serum iron and vitamins A and C were found to be below standard in more than 50 percent of the elderly population, whereas substandard hemoglobin, hematocrit, serum iron, and serum protein values occurred less frequently (Abraham, Lowenstein, and Johnson, 1974). Data from clinical or physical examination revealed few, if any, manifestations of nutrient deficiency. Obesity was found to be the most common nutritional problem in the elderly, particularly in women (Abraham, Lowenstein, and O'Connell, 1975). Food consumption profiles of the elderly revealed that 30 percent or more seldom or never drank milk and seldom or never ate fish, cereal, or salty snacks (Dresser, Carroll, and Abraham, 1978). Correlations between data from dietary intake, biochemical tests, clinical manifestations of nutrient deficiency, and anthropometric findings have not been reported.

Data from these studies indicate that some elderly persons are at risk for developing alterations in nutritional status. However, the exact factors that contribute to the alterations cannot be derived from these data.

Watkin (1980) points out that little research has been directed towards studying the nutritional needs of the extreme aged elderly (85 years and older). Nutritional assessment of each elderly person is indicated to identify risk. Causes of malnutrition in the elderly may be multiple (defined as disturbance due to lack or excess of calories or one or more of the nutients). The elderly client should be carefully assessed for adequacy of dietary intake, as well as for factors that may jeopardize adequate intake and utilization of foods.

Factors Contributing to Adequate Nutrition in the Elderly

Few investigations have attempted to identify factors that contribute to inadequate nutritional status in the elderly. In a study of 529 persons 60 years and older living in Tennessee, the effects of income, age, education, sex, race, health status, and aloneness were studied in relation to the dietary intake. Inadequate dietary intake was discovered more frequently in those whose income level was low and in those whose educational level was less than high school attainment. Deficiences in iron intake were common among females. Vitamin A, thiamine, and riboflavin deficiencies occurred frequently in the total elderly population (Todhunter, 1976). Those elderly persons from the lower income level in the HANES study (Abraham et al., 1974, 1975) were also found to display more frequent signs of dietary inadequacy.

The importance of the elderly person's economic level cannot be underestimated in relation to nutrition. More than one-third of the elderly population have incomes below the poverty level. In many cases, the elderly cannot afford to purchase meat, fresh vegetables, and fruit, which are necessary protective foods. Careful assessment of the kinds of food the person purchases and eats is indicated. Changes imposed by the increasing cost of food should be explored. Does the person utilize a subsidized food program for the elderly, such as food stamps or congregate meals? The nurse should not assume, however, that the person who takes advantage of a subsidized food program is getting an adequate intake of nutrients.

The frequency with which the elderly client attends congregate meals should be assessed. The nurse should also obtain information about usual dietary patterns on days that the elderly person does not attend a program. For example, Mr. B attends a congregate lunch program 5 days a week. He lives in an apartment located in a complex built for the elderly. He was observed eating most of the food served except milk, fresh fruit, and sometimes bread. He brought a small bag to carry these foods back to his apartment. When questioned about what he did with the food, he said "That's what I eat for supper." When asked about his diet on weekends, Mr. B replied that he ate a frozen dinner, cereal, and sometimes fruit. Analysis of his dietary intake indicates that he eats inadequate amounts of vegetables, fruit, and milk.

Factors in Mr. B's story illustrate a situation in which a person may be unaware of what a balanced diet should be, does not know how to cook, or does not like to cook. Windsor (1979) identified widowers living alone as most likely to exhibit this problem.

On the other hand, however, some widowers try to emulate what their wives did. For example, after Mr. H's wife died, he used the experience and knowledge she had shared with him. Mr. H's wife was extremely conscientious about providing proper nutrients daily and apparently shared her knowledge with her husband. After her death, although he was invited to eat dinner with his many friends, he always prepared balanced meals for breakfast and lunch. He would even share with the neighbors his homemade bran muffins or freshly bought fruit.

The frequency with which the person eats alone should be assessed, as well as how the person feels about eating alone. Some elderly persons watch television or read while eating. Others may not eat regular meals but snack. For example, Mrs. L, 80 years old, had taken care of her ill husband at home for 5 years. She prepared three or more meals each day for herself and her husband. After his death, Mrs. L had difficulty deciding what to cook and how to buy. She said that she missed having someone to talk to and didn't feel hungry. However, she soon became involved in attending meal programs for the senior citizens in her community at least four times a week. "I go mainly for the socialization." Thus the socialization created an atmosphere that enhanced her appetite and subsequent dietary intake.

Reactions to any change in life-style should be assessed for their influence on dietary intake. Recently Mrs. B was anticipating a move from her two-bedroom apartment (nonsheltered) to an efficiency apartment in a building that provided supervision and care of the elderly. The anticipated moving date was delayed for 3 months. Mrs. B began cooking preprepared foods only, and often resorted to eating cereal. She occasionally ate at restaurants, but finally became so upset by the postponement of the moving date that she stayed at home. As a result, her dietary patterns were altered, and on many days her intake of nutrients was inadequate.

The elderly person's ethnic background and previous dietary practices also influence food preferences. The person who ate "meat and potatoes" during younger years is likely to prefer foods prepared in this manner rather than in a casserole. The individual of Italian background may prefer pasta-based foods, which are high in carbohydrate and calories. As activity level decreases, the elderly person may not proportionately decrease food intake. The cost of meat may preclude use of meat in some of the pasta dishes, so that protein intake is inadequate. The black elderly, particularly those who were reared on Southern-style cooking, prefer pigs' feet, ham hocks, chitterlings, leafy greens, and hominy grits (Dancy, 1977). These ethnic menus are not commonly offered in food programs or in institutions for the elderly. The nurse must know and be sensitive to individual food preferences, and should understand that the so-called American diet of hamburger, french fries, and onion rings may be unfamiliar to many old people.

Lack of knowledge about proper diet may determine what foods a person may select and eat. One may observe a person in a cafeteria selecting french fries with ketchup every day when a variety of foods are available. An elderly client may not understand a special modified or strict diet may be prepared without losing palatability. Knowledge that some drugs

may interfere or interact with food may be lacking. History of medication use is indicated, as well as client's knowledge of medication side effects.

Availability and accessibility of food stores and transportation are also factors to be considered. Many metropolitan areas have established reduced mass transit fares for the elderly, but the routes of transportation do not always pass near a food market. Elderly people who live in rural areas are, for the most part, at a loss for public transportation. Lack of transportation is the chief factor that contributes to inadequate nutrition among elderly American Indians who live on reservations (Essandoh, 1977). Mobility problems may make it difficult for the old person to carry groceries in large quantities on public transportation. Often the elderly person can only manage to carry one bag of groceries. Some use shopping carts that facilitate carrying larger quantities of groceries. However, these carts are difficult to maneuver on and off public transportation as well as on hilly terrain.

Impaired health status may also influence the elderly person's choice of foods, as well as the frequency of meals. If home-bound, the individual may be dependent upon another person for selection, purchase, preparation, and delivery of food. Unless the client has control over selection, the amounts and types of food provided may not be suitable. As a result, the person doesn't prepare or eat what is purchased. The elderly person who receives prepared foods may find that they are delivered at unsuitable intervals, or at inconvenient times. Most agency-sponsored home delivery programs deliver a hot meal at noon and a cold snack for later in the day. If the elderly person's life pattern has always included a hot meal in the evening, this pattern may be disrupted, leading to incorrect storage, forgetting to eat, or eating only the cold snack, which may not provide adequate dietary intake.

Some clients report that the taste of food has changed since taking particular medications. Often appetite is determined by how a person feels. Chronic disease that causes pain, fatigue, or immobility may contribute to changes in appetite. Treatment regimens such as low-sodium, low-fat, or low-carbohydrate diets may be seen as drastic change from previous food preferences. As an example, Mr. P, 80 years old, was hospitalized for diagnostic tests. His appetite was poor and he frequently had to miss fluids and food in preparation for diagnostic tests. His favorite food was two soft boiled eggs at breakfast. He had been placed on a low-salt diet and was denied use of salt on the eggs. The eggs then tasted "as bad as all the other food." Strict adherence to a salt-restricted diet did not help him in meeting his nutritional needs.

Elimination problems, such as constipation, can also affect nutritional levels. The discomfort of constipation may affect appetite and ultimately the intake of foods. In response to constipation, clients who take laxatives frequently may jeopardize fluid, electrolyte, and nutrient status. Some clients use mineral oil, which interferes with absorption of vitamins A, D, E, and K. Diarrhea over time, induced by laxative abuse or caused by disease of the gastrointestinal tract, may cause loss of fluids, potassium, as well as some nutrients.

Additional problems exist for the institutionalized elderly, who often face rigid meal patterns, with lack of choice as well as lack of snacks. The person may store bedside snack food, which can spoil easily. The institutional environment may influence the way, how much, and how adequately the elderly person eats. For example, Mr. A is arbitrarily seated without choice next to Mr. B, who exhibits behavior Mr. A finds distasteful. Mr. A therefore refuses to eat. Providing a choice of seating arrangements may be the solution to Mr. A's feeding problem.

Lester and Baltes (1976) suggest that many nursing behaviors in nursing homes foster dependence, particularly with regard to self-feeding. They noted that clients who were being fed received more social interaction with nursing staff than those persons who fed themselves. They suggest that the rewards for self-feeding behavior should exceed the rewards for refusal to feed self. Although persons who need to be fed may have more interaction with staff, they often have no choice about the speed with which they are fed or how they are fed. Many times the person is fed with a spoon, rather than with a utensil appropriate to the food.

The elderly person who has an acute illness may experience sudden and severe alterations in nutritional status. Diagnostic and treatment procedures may impose dietary or fluid restrictions for prolonged periods of time, sometimes for several days or weeks. The nutritional status of such clients must be monitored more comprehensively and frequently. Laboratory tests for serum vitamin levels and protein levels may be indicated.

In summary, many factors influence the nutritional status of the elderly client. The physiologic, psychosocial, economic, health, sociocultural, and developmental factors are obviously interrelated. Nutritional status can only be determined after careful analysis of each factor which contributes to adequate nutrition. The assessment must be directed toward identifying elderly persons at risk, as well as identifying persons who actually exhibit signs or symptoms of inadequate nutritional status. The frequency with which the assessment of nutritional status should be made is determined by the health status of the client and by changes in the socioeconomic status of the client.

Method of Assessment

Obtaining data for assessment of nutritional status is a comprehensive, expensive, and somewhat tedious process. The four sources of data are (1) biochemical examination; (2) anthropometry; (3) clinical or physical appraisal; and (4) survey of dietary intake. Collection and analysis of data involve several members of the health team—nurse, physician, dietician, and laboratory technician. The comprehensiveness of the assessment may be determined by the availability of personnel and facilities. Christakis (1973) recommends that nutritional assessment be performed at three levels—minimal, mid-level, and in-depth. The minimal level includes commonly available and easily performed screening tests. The in-depth level includes more complex and comprehensive laboratory examinations that the nurse cannot perform because they require sophisticated resources. This discussion focuses on common screening techniques that the nurse can perform and should know about.

Biochemical examination or laboratory assessment is directed towards analysis of nutrients and the metabolites or enzymes associated with specific nutrients. Christakis (1973) recommends that the minimal biochemical assessment should include:

1. Hemoglobin, blood and urine sugar
2. Urinalysis (color, odor, bile, and sediment by gross inspection)
3. Feces (color, texture, gross blood, occult blood by guaiac test)

Tests for amounts of specific nutrients, metabolites, and enzymes in the blood and urine are usually performed when the client demonstrates a risk for nutritional deficiency or exhibits signs of deficiency.

Anthropometry, or body measurements, is used to determine height, weight, and skin-fold thickness. These measurements, when checked periodically, are useful in detecting changes in body measurements that may be related directly to nutritional status or indirectly related to pathologic process. Height and weight charts are available from various sources. These charts should include the desirable weight for each sex, according to height and body frame. The interpretation of data regarding height–weight should include any height– weight data from previous years the client may report. Changes in weight may indicate problems either with nutrition or illness.

Measurement of skin-fold thickness is primarily used to detect obesity. The thickness of the skin fold, usually over the triceps, is measured by calipers. The area tested should include skin and subcutaneous tissue, but not muscle. The skin fold is pinched up until the skin surfaces are parallel. The calipers are applied with constant pressure beside the fingers pinching the skin. Then the thickness is measured. The minimum triceps skin-fold thickness for defining obesity is 23 mm in males and 30 mm in females (Seltzer and Mayer, 1965).

Physical or clinical appraisal is obtained by physical examination of various parts of the body. The purpose of the exam is to collect data concerning clinical manifestations of nutritional deficiency as well as general health status. Interpretation of the data obtained is dependent upon the skill of the examiner and may be influenced by the examiner's biases. The examiner who conducts the physical appraisal should describe precisely the condition of each part of the body. Many clinical manifestations of nutritional deficiencies can accompany allergy, infection, or trauma. Therefore, the interpretation of data should be correlated with other aspects of the nutritional assessment. Physical examination should include hair, skin, mouth, nails, eyes, heart, lungs, abdomen, glands, reflex activity, and affect. The examiner should be knowledgeable about the normal changes in the skin, nails, hair, and eyes of the elderly. The examination should include:

1. Skin—uniformity of color, temperature, turgor, smoothness, intactness, moistness, presence and descriptions of lesions or discharge
2. Hair—texture, distribution (including on body), color, shininess
3. Mouth—condition of gums, teeth, oral hygiene, odor, tongue, lips, discharges, salivation
4. Nails—firmness, color, thickness, shape
5. Eyes—clearness, shininess, color of sclera, conjunctiva, vision screening
6. Heart and lungs—heart rate, rhythm, loudness, location of apical beat, extra sounds, blood pressure, breath sounds, peripheral pulses
7. Abdomen—presence and description of masses or sounds (include rectal and vaginal exam)
8. Glands—palpability of lymph glands and thyroid
9. Reflexes—degree, speed, and duration
10. Activity—range of motion, posture, agility
11. Affect—posture, movement, facial expression, alertness
12. Urine—color, odor, pH, specific gravity

The clinical manifestations of nutritional deficiencies are described in various medical and nutrition textbooks. The nurse should be aware that many of these manifestations do not appear until the deficiency is far advanced. Thus, other methods of assessment than the physical exam may be more useful in identifying early signs of nutritional deficiency.

Dietary surveys provide information about the usual nutrient intake of the individual. The survey should include nutrition patterns, beliefs and knowledge about food, income level and food budget, availability and accessibility of food supplies, preparation and storage practices, health status, life-style, and living arrangements. The dietary survey is most useful in identifying persons who are at risk of inadequate dietary intake. Methods for survey commonly used are the food intake diary, 24-hour recall, and diet history. Each method has advantages and disadvantages. Often the method of survey is predetermined by the amount of time the interviewer can allot to the individual client, the frequency with which the client is seen, and the client's ability to remember specific information about dietary intake. Facets of the different methods may be combined to obtain all the data required.

A diary of food intake requires that the client or client's caretaker record the exact food and fluid intake over a period of time, usually 1 to 3 days. Three-day intake records are recommended, since dietary intake varies from day to day. Because weekend eating patterns are often different from weekday patterns, inclusion of records from 1 weekend day and 2 weekdays is suggested. The record should include the specific foods eaten, the quantity of each, and the time at which food is eaten. The quantity of food should be determined by using common household measures—cup, glass, and so on. The two disadvantages of the diary are that the client may forget to record food intake or may change eating habits because of overawareness of eating patterns.

The 24-hour recall method requires that the client report food intake for a specific 24-hour period. This method can only be used when the client has the ability to remember. It requires skill on the part of the interviewer so that data can be validated. This method has also been found to be time-consuming and invalid or incomplete when applied to elderly persons living at home or in institutions

(Campbell and Dodds, 1967). The average time spent in interviewing subjects varied from 25 minutes for older institutionalized men to 40-plus minutes for older women living at home. The actual time spent obtaining food intake recall varied only from 12 minutes for men living at home to 16 minutes for older institutionalized elderly. The investigators also found that the older institutionalized persons had more difficulty remembering food intake than did younger institutionalized adults.

The dietary history is the most comprehensive method for obtaining data. The history may also be used to validate information obtained from the diary or 24-hour recall of food intake. The success of this method is dependent upon the skill of the interviewer. Ample time must be allotted to elicit the information tactfully. Some of the data may already be available from other sources. A history form usually facilitates the process. Open-ended questions elicit free response, and provide an opportunity for the interviewer to encourage elaboration. Questions should be asked in such a way that the interviewer's biases or values do not influence the client's response. The dietary history should elicit information about:

A. Socioeconomic factors
　1. Level of education—understanding of proper diet
　2. Level of income
　　Budget available for food
　　Food stamp usage
　3. Living arrangements facilities
　　Food storage
　　Food preparation
　　Aloneness—lives with others
　　Usual preparer of food
　　Satisfaction with eating arrangements
　4. Usual source of food supplies
　　Store
　　　Distance from home
　　　Transportation
　　　　Availability
　　　　Difficulties
　　　Frequency of shopping
　5. Community-based meals
　　Frequency
　　Likes; dislikes

Distance from home
Frequency of restaurant eating
6. Home-delivered meals
Frequency
Source
Likes; dislikes
Weekend sources of food

B. **Usual living pattern**
1. Activity
2. Times of meals
3. Amount of socialization
4. Waking–sleeping patterns
5. Elimination patterns

C. **Health status**
1. Oral cavity
Difficulties with chewing
Ease of swallowing
Frequency of dental exams
2. Appetite
3. Specific illness; history, present status
4. Special diet
Who prescribed
Difficulties with diet
5. Other changes that imposed change in dietary patterns

D. **Dietary intake pattern**
1. Usual meal times
2. Snacks—type, frequency
3. Food preferences—type, certain ways of preparation, ethnic
4. Food rejections—why
5. Changes in taste, smell
6. Changes in food tolerance—recent, past
7. Food supplements (vitamins, minerals)
Who prescribed
Frequency taken
8. Usual fluid intake
9. Frequency with which specific foods are eaten (weekly or monthly)
Meat
Poultry
Fish
Eggs
Dried peas or beans
Vegetables
Types
Sources (fresh or preserved)
Fruits and juices

Types
Sources (fresh or preserved)
Milk or cheese
Butter or margarine
Salad dressing
Bread, cereal
Pies, cakes, cookies
Salty snacks
Candy
Soft drinks
Coffee, tea
Alcohol

The information from the dietary history and record of dietary intake may be analyzed by comparing the basic four food groups with the client's usual intake of these foods. The adequacy of the person's dietary intake may be approximated.

PLANNING AND INTERVENTION

The data from the four methods of assessment must be analyzed for (1) presence or absence of signs of an inadequate nutritional status, and (2) presence or absence of risk factors for inadequate nutrition.

The ultimate goal is that the elderly client maintains an adequate nutritional status. When signs of an inadequate nutritional status are present, the person should be referred for a more comprehensive examination and subsequent treatment by a physician. When risks of inadequate nutrition exist, the nature of the risk and the contributing factors must be analyzed. The nurse is in a position to refer, teach, and counsel the client, and can also facilitate the person's use of other resources. Many of the risks are associated with psychologic and socioeconomic factors, including income, environment, transportation, and lack of information. The nurse therefore, must be aware of these factors and the resources that are available to the elderly. Many of the risks may be circumvented by referring clients to the appropriate resources.

Since taste declines and changes occur in dentition, mouth care is important to maintain nutritional status. The elderly should be encouraged to follow regular cleansing practices and have periodic dental exams. Because of low income and lack of third-party payment, the elderly person may place low priority on seeing the dentist. When the elderly client lives in an area of a dental school, the associated dental clinic may provide low-cost dental care. Some hospitals operate dental clinics but frequently the focus is on tooth extraction rather than preventive care.

Oral hygiene for the elderly should be promoted to enhance chewing ability. The elderly who have teeth should be taught to brush and floss the teeth at least daily. Flossing teeth may be new to the elderly since prevention was not emphasized in their younger years. The purpose of flossing is to remove plaque and food from between the teeth and along the gum line. The elderly may have trouble wrapping the floss on their fingers. This problem may be circumvented by pretying circles on each end of the floss so that the circles may fit on a finger of each hand. Brushing the teeth removes food and plaque from the surfaces of the teeth and gums. A soft-bristle brush is indicated. The elderly who have arthritis may need to modify the handle of the tooth brush to enhance handling the tooth brush. A ruler or piece of wood may be taped to the handle to lengthen it. Wrapping the handle with a sponge or a washcloth may help the client who has difficulty grasping the handle of the tooth brush. The elderly should be taught to inspect their mouth carefully for signs of bleeding, irritation, unremovable white patches, or loose teeth. The client should be referred to a dentist if any of these problems exist.

Clients who wear dentures should also be taught about proper mouth care. Dentures should be removed at least daily for a period of 6 to 8 hours. The dentures should be cleansed with a tooth brush and soaked in water or a commercial cleanser. When dentures are removed, the gums and tongue should be brushed with a semi-soft brush. Irritation on the gum line may indicate ill fitting dentures or presence of irritating food debris under the denture. The client who wears dentures should be instructed to have yearly dental check-ups.

Many elderly are under the illusion that once they have dentures they no longer need to see a dentist.

Planning and intervention should be directed toward increasing the client's understanding about proper food intake and the resources available in the community. The nurse should know what resources are available with regard to dietary education. Is there a dietician available? What printed information, such as free government publications, can be obtained? When low income is a factor, the client may need to know how to prepare cheaper foods, obtain food stamps, or use the services of the food programs available to the elderly. Ethnic food preferences should be taken into account. To save money, the elderly should be encouraged to collect coupons. However, they should be warned to use primarily those coupons that are for nutritionally valuable foods.

The nurse may be in a position to counsel elderly clients regarding how they may follow the National Dietary Guidelines. Foods should be selected from each of the food groups. Eating foods with adequate fiber should be encouraged but caution should be used in increasing fiber too fast. A sudden increase in large amounts of fiber in the diet may produce loss of nutrients. Moderate consumption of fresh fruits, vegetables, and whole grain cereals are recommended.

Some clients need help in establishing their correct weight. Obesity is a common problem in the elderly and not easy to correct. As the elderly client becomes less active, the energy requirement for calories decreases. There may be a delicate balance between what is necessary for adequate nutrition and what is necessary for weight loss to occur.

Intake of sugar, fats, and alcohol should be avoided. The elderly client may eat cereals in correct amounts but like a brand that contains a large amount of sugar. Comparing labels of sugar content in various cereals may help this client decrease sugar consumption. Substances with fats and alcohol are easier to identify. One should avoid fried foods, butter, oils, and alcohol. Small amounts of alcohol, as in wine, may be desirable for promoting rest and sleep. As it is lower in calories, wine is preferable to liquor or beer. Increased exercise may also help to use calories. Walking and swimming are recommended for the active elderly.

Special nutrition programs conducted by nutritionists have been reported as being successful (Kris, 1979). Topics such as food purchasing, food preservation, nutrient values of various foods, and use of vitamins were of interest to the population in a senior citizens' center. The congregate meal programs may also serve as a model for providing variety in meal preparation (Fig. 13.1).

The environment may be a factor if the elderly person lives alone or has inadequate food storage or preparation facilities. In such cases, the client may be directed to utilize community-based eating programs and take advantage of transportation programs for the elderly. Each client must be involved in the decision to insure proper follow-through in utilizing these resources. Those elderly persons who are confined to the home may be referred to home delivery programs or to "homemaker" services, if available.

The nurse in institutional settings for the elderly has more opportunity to control the eating environment (Fig. 13.2). The esthetics of the eating place can be enhanced by colorful tablecloths, pictures, and an opportunity to smell the food being prepared. Socialization should be encouraged by permitting or encouraging friends to sit together. Socialization between clients and staff should also be fostered.

Behavior modification techniques may be employed to encourage better eating habits, whether self-feeding behaviors (Baltis and Zerbe, 1976) or behaviors that contribute to an adequate dietary intake. Mr. K displayed inappropriate behavior in a nursing home. He grabbed food from other trays, refused to eat with his utensils, and spilled food over himself. One day he was invited to attend a special birthday luncheon in the dining room. Tablecloths, silver, family-style service, and a centerpiece of flowers transformed the room. Mr. K was pushed to the table, where he proceeded

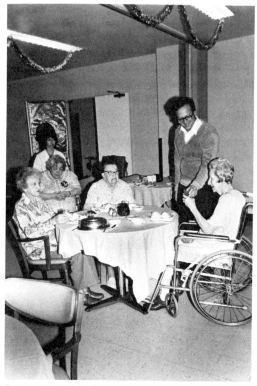

Figure 13.1. Volunteer assists aged with a meal in their home setting.

to eat appropriately. The nursing staff later mentioned this to his family. His daughter said that he had always eaten in a formal environment. Cues can be important in structuring the behavior of mentally impaired clients.

EVALUATION

Evaluation should be ongoing. Food intake, the psychosocial status, and physical well-being should be periodically reassessed. The elderly *will* change their eating habits when they understand what changes should be made, and when their environment is supportive for providing activity, socialization, and economics for food purchase.

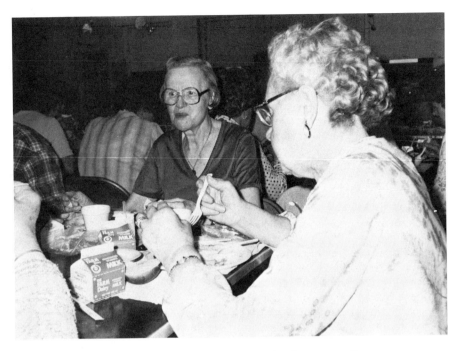

Figure 13.2. A congregate meal program provided in the community.

REFERENCES CITED

Abraham, S., Lowenstein, F.W., Jonson, C.L. Preliminary findings of the first health and nutrition examination survey. United States, 1971–72: Dietary intake and biochemical findings. DHEW Publication No. 74-1219-1 (HRA) 74-2-1, Rockville, MD, January, 1974

Abraham, S., Lowenstein, F.W., O'Connell, D.E. Preliminary findings of the first health and nutritional examination survey. United States, 1971–72: Anthropometric and clinical findings. DHEW Publication No. (HRA) 75-1229, 1975

Andrus, R., Tobin, J.D. Endocrine systems. In Finch, C.E., Hayflick, L. (eds), Handbook of the Biology of Aging. New York, Van Nostrand Reinhold, 1977

Baltes, M.M., Zerbe, M.B. Reestablishing self-feeding in a nursing home resident. Nursing Research 25(1):24, 1976

Bhanthumnavin, K., Schuster, M. Aging and gastrointestinal function, in Finch, C., Hayflick, L. (eds), Handbook of the Biology of Aging. New York, Van Nostrand Reinhold, 1977

Campbell, V.A., Dodds, M.L. Collecting dietary information from groups of older people. Journal of the American Dietary Association 51:29, 1967

Christakis, G. Nutritional assessment of the elderly. American Journal of Public Health, Supplement 63(11):68, 1973

Dancy, J. The black elderly. Institute of Gerontology, University of Michigan–Wayne State University, 1977

Debry, G., Bleyer, R., Martin, J.M. Nutrition of the elderly. Journal of Human Nutrition 31:105, 1977

Dresser, C.M., Carroll, M.D., Abraham, S. Selected findings: Food consumption profiles of white and black persons 1–74 years of age in the United States, 1971–1974. Advanced Data from Vital and Health Statistics of the National Center for Health Statistics: U.S. Department of Health, Education, and Welfare, 21, June 26, 1978

Essandoh, R. Major concerns of the elderly Native American, in Newhouse, B. (ed), Insights on the Minority Elderly. Washington, D.C., National Center on Black Aged Incorporation and The Institute of Gerontology, University of the District of Columbia, 26, 1977

Feldman, R.S., Kapur, K.K., Alman, J.E., Chauncey, H.H. Aging and mastication: Changes in performance and in swallowing threshold with natural dentition. Journal of the American Geriatrics Society 28(3):97, 1980

Food, Home, and Garden Bulletin No. 228. Washington, D.C., USDA U.S. Government Printing Office, 1979

Gift, H.C. The elderly population—oral health status and demand and utilization of dental services. Journal of the American Society of Geriatric Dentists 13:9, 17, 1978

Goldman, R. Aging of the excretory system, kidney, and bladder, in Finch, C.F., Hayflick, L. (eds), Handbook of the Biology of Aging. New York, Van Nostrand Reinhold, 1977

Isaacs, B. The preservation of continence, in Willington, F.L. (ed), Incontinence in the Elderly. London, Academic, 1976

Jaffe, J.W. Common lower urinary tract problems in older perons, in Reichel, W. (ed), Clinical Aspects of Aging. Baltimore, Williams and Wilkins, 1978

Lester, P.B., Baltes, M.M. Functional interdependence of the social environment and behavior of the institutionalized aged. Journal of Gerontological Nursing 4(2):23, 1978

Milne, J.S. Ten state nutrition survey, 1968–1970. U.S. Department of Health, Education, and Welfare. DHEW Publication No. (HSM) 72-8134. Atlanta, GA, Center for Disease Control, 1972

Recommended Dietary Allowance. Washington, D.C. National Academy of Sciences, 1980

Todhunter, E.N. Life style and nutrient intake in the elderly, in Winick, M. (ed), Nutrition and Aging. New York, Wiley, 1976

Wayler, A.H., Kapur, K.K., Feldman, R.S., Chauncey, H.H. Effects of age and dentition status on measures of food acceptibility. Journal of Gerontology 37(3):294, 1982

14

Elimination in the Aged

Nancy J. Ebert

Reading this chapter will enable the individual to:

1. Identify changes of urinary tract function in the elderly
2. Identify common problems in urinary tract function
3. Assess for changes and problems in urinary tract function
4. Identify changes in lower gastrointestinal tract function in the elderly
5. Identify common problems in lower gastrointestinal tract function
6. Assess for changes and problems in gastrointestinal function
7. Identify nursing measures that promote the maintenance of bowel and bladder function
8. Identify measures that restore bowel and bladder continence

Elimination involves excretion by the bowels, bladder, and skin, and reflects the intake of food and fluid. Excretion of fluid and food waste is handled primarily by the urinary and gastrointestinal systems. This chapter will focus on bowel and bladder functions in the elderly.

Competent bowel and bladder functions are established early in life. As the functions develop, patterns of elimination emerge in response to sociocultural expectations and as the result of repetition. Problems may occur in reaction to aging changes in the bowel and bladder function or to other stressors to which the elderly are exposed. Elimination problems commonly observed in the elderly are presented as they relate to assessment and intervention.

ASSESSMENT FACTORS RELATED TO GASTROINTESTINAL AND URINARY TRACT FUNCTION

Assessment and intervention with regard to elimination must be based upon a knowledge of normal bladder and bowel function, as well as an understanding of the factors that commonly contribute to elimination problems in the elderly. Bladder function and bowel function will be presented in terms of known age-related changes.

Aging and the Urinary Tract

Urinary tract function involves the kidney, bladder, and urethra. Minor changes in structure may accompany aging, but these appear to have little or no effect on function.

The bladder consists of the detrusor muscle of the fundus and the trizone muscles forming the base of the bladder. The urethra emerges at the base of the bladder. The sphincter muscle surrounds the urethra for maintaining continence. Men have two sphincters, an internal or proximal sphincter in the internal meatus and an external or distal sphincter located below the prostate. Women have one sphincter surrounding the middle third of the urethra. Skeletal muscles forming the pelvic floor provide support at the distal sphincter in the male and at the distal portion of the urethral sphincter in the female. These muscles also provide support for the rectum and the uterus. Contraction of the pelvic muscles aid in closing the urethra as well as the rectum. With aging, these muscles may become weaker and less elastic.

The function of these organs is reflected in the micturition cycle, defined as the act of urination. Three phases of the micturition cycle have been identified:

1. Filling up to the time of desire to void
2. Voluntary postponement
3. Emptying (Yeates, 1976)

The phases are interdependent, and normally the micturition cycle is sequential. Filling time is dependent upon bladder capacity, competency of the sphincter muscles in the urethra, and neurologic sensation. Voluntary postponement is dependent upon the competency of the sphincter muscles and neurologic sensation and control. Emptying is dependent upon the ability of bladder contraction to overcome the resistance of the urethra. The micturition cycle is repeated at intervals. The frequency of the cycle is largely determined by the nature of each phase.

The first phase, filling time until time of desire to void, is the most complex. Decrease in bladder capacity is the change most consistently observed with aging (Goldman, 1977). The decrease in capacity leads to increased frequency of the micturition cycle. A common complaint of the elderly is that they must urinate more frequently. Changes in the competency of the sphincter muscles and in neurologic sensation are associated with pathologic rather than normal changes of aging. The problems associated with postponement are also thought to be related to pathologic changes, either in the sphincter muscles or in the sensory reception and response to the filled or partially filled bladder. The sensation of need or desire to void varies in the elderly. Some elderly persons feel the need to void only when the bladder is full to capacity; some perceive the need to void when the bladder is partially full; and still others perceive no need to void.

The amount of urine eliminated should approximate the amount of fluid taken in by the client. Variations in this balance may occur when the client takes diuretics, has diabetes, renal disease, congestive heart failure, or is exposed to high temperatures. The values for pH, specific gravity, glucose, protein, and ketones obtained by urine analysis should be the same as for a normal adult who has adequate intake of fluids (1500–2000 ml).

Common Urinary Tract Problems

The most feared and disturbing problem of the aged is that of urinary incontinence. Urinary incontinence is broadly defined as "the passing of urine in an undesirable place" (Yeates, 1976). The International Continence Society has defined urinary incontinence as "a condition where involuntary loss of urine is a social or hygienic problem and is objectively demonstrable" (1976). Urinary incontinence is not a concomitant of aging. Rather, it is a symptom of other, cross-related causes.

Transient or temporary incontinence may occur in response to urinary tract infection, acute illness, immobilization, confusion, medications, fecal impaction, a new strange environment, and emotional reaction to stress such as loss of a loved one. Treatment of the underlying cause often returns the elderly client to continence.

Classifications of incontinence are not consistent in the literature. Some authors refer to anatomic change, some authors refer to symptomatology, and some mix symptomatology with cause. Stress incontinence, urge incontinence, overflow incontinence, and continual incontinence are common terms to describe incontinence. Stress incontinence is characterized by leakage of urine when coughing, sneezing, laughing, or walking. Stress incontinence occurs more commonly in women who have relaxed pelvic floor muscles or atrophic periurethral tissues. Obesity is a contributing factor. Urge incontinence is characterized by perceived urge to micturate with inability to control micturition. The client may complain of feelings of urgency and frequency as well as involuntary loss of urine. These symptoms may be a result of urinary tract infection, decreased control of the bladder, irritated bladder, or pressure on the urethra by an enlarged prostate. Overflow incontinence is characterized by a full bladder with involuntary dribbling. An enlarged prostate is the most frequent cause.

Continuous incontinence may be present with no pattern or no sensation and is usually associated with neurologic or cognitive dysfunction. Medications such as sedatives may produce this problem. Sensation of need to micturate may decrease.

The prevalence of urinary incontinence in the elderly has been found to be anywhere between 1.8 and 34.5 percent for people residing in the community and between 16.0 and 59 percent for people residing in long-term facilities. Summaries of the studies are found in Tables 14.1 and 14.2. Breakdown of the rates of prevalence by sex indicates females are more commonly affected than males.

Two factors may contribute to the increased prevalence of incontinence in females. In women who have given birth to a large baby or have history of a difficult labor and delivery there may be damage to the pelvic floor structure. Also, with menopause and accompanying estrogen deficiency, the bladder neck weakens.

Lower urinary tract infection in the elderly is second in frequency only to pneumonia. The frequency of infection increases in both male and female aged populations.

Asymptomatic infection (bacteriuria) is as common as symptomatic infection (fever, bacteriuria, dysuria). Symptomatic infection occurs more often in males (Kunin, 1974). The increased frequency of urinary tract infections is related to the use of instrumentation such as cystoscopy or catheterization, the presence of bladder outlet changes, the presence of diabetes or neurologic disease, and the use of medications.

Acute infection characterized by bacteriuria and elevated white blood count usually precipitates urinary incontinence (Willington, 1978). Asymptomatic bacteriuria was not found to be significantly associated with incontinence in a study of 1000 females aged 17 and over (Yarnell, Voyle, Sweetnam, Milbank, Richards, and Stephenson, 1982).

The dangers of instrumentation cannot be underestimated. Incidence of infection is correlated with frequency of catheterization. A single catheterization is less likely to be associated with infection than are multiple or indwelling catheterizations. Strict aseptic practices in the insertion and care of catheters are essential to prevent urinary tract infections. Because the elderly are generally more

TABLE 14-1. PREVALENCE OF URINARY INCONTINENCE AMONG THE ELDERLY IN POPULATION SURVEYS

Author	Year	Country	Total No.	% Incontinent	Men No.	Men % Incontinent	Women No.	Women % Incontinent
Sheldon	1948	England	456	11.2	135	7.4	321	12.7
Hobson and Pemberton	1955	England	476	24.2	192	26.0	284	22.9
Van Zonneveld	1959	Holland	2936	2.7	1486	3.2	1450	2.2
Sourander	1966	Finland	400	6.0	197	5.1	203	6.9
Brocklehurst et al.	1968	England	557	21.1	182	17.0	375	23.0
Milne et al.	1972	Scotland	487	34.5	215	25.0	272	42.0
Akhtar et al.	1973	Scotland	809	1.8	319	2.2	490	1.6
Knox	1979	Scotland	59750	2.0				
Yarnall and St. Leger	1979	Wales	388	14.0	169	11.0	219	17.0
Thomas et al.*	1980	England	2664	21.4	169	6.9	403	11.6
Thomas et al.†	1980	England	74000	2.1	381	1.3	1147	2.5

*Unrecognized incontinence in people aged 65 years and older.
†Recognized incontinence in people aged 65 years and older.

TABLE 14-2. PREVALENCE OF URINARY INCONTINENCE AMONG THE ELDERLY IN INSTITUTIONAL SURVEYS

Author	Year	Country	Types of Clients	Total No.	% Incontinent	Men No.	% Incontinent	Women No.	% Incontinent
Affleck	1947	England	Long term	788	21.0	236	19.1	552	21.9
Wilson	1948	England	Long term	68	37.0	35	31.5	33	42.4
Thompson	1949	England	Long term	714	36.0	316	25.0	398	44.0
Brocklehurst	1951	Scotland	Long term	599	22.0	416	18.3	183	33.3
Totterman	1959	Finland	Long term	885	25.0	178	20.8	707	25.9
Exton-Smith et al.*	1962	England	Long term	600	47.0	—	—	—	—
Isaacs and Walkey	1964	Scotland	Long term	522	43.0	274	40.1	248	46.0
Maggs*	1964	England	Long-term psychogeriatric	62	46.0	—	—	—	—
Walkey et al.	1967	Scotland	Consecutive admissions	500	47.0	250	48.0	250	47.0
Willington	1969	England	Consecutive admissions	900	14.0	411	15.8	489	12.9
Carstairs and Morrison*	1971	England	Long-term psychogeriatric	416	28.0	—	—	—	—
Wilkin and Jolley	1978	England	Local authority home	418	17.0	—	—	—	—
Clarke et al.*	1979	England	Long term	723	36.0	—	—	—	—
Gilleard*	1979	England	Long-term psychogeriatric	128	40.0	—	—	—	—
Masterton, Holloway, and Timbury	1980	England	Local authority home	404	17.0	—	—	—	—
Gilleard, Pattie, and Dearman	1980	England	Local authority home	683	16.0	—	—	—	—
Jewett, Fernie Holliday, and Pim	1981	Canada	Long-term consecutive admission	276	38.0	146	40.0	130	36.0
Robb	1981	United States	Long term	398	59.0	398	59.0	—	—
Ouslander et al.	1982	United States	Long term	954	50.0	126	30.0	293	70.0

*Cited in Gilleard (1981).

susceptible to infection, the need for catheterization should be evaluated carefully on the basis of risk versus benefit. When single or indwelling catheterization is indicated, the elderly person should increase fluid intake to insure cleansing of the bladder and the catheter.

In elderly women with relaxed musculature and atrophic changes of the periurethral structures, the urethral orifice is often displaced into the vaginal outlet. Thus, the flora of the vagina as well as the rectum can easily enter the urethra and ascend into the bladder, causing a urinary tract infection.

Fluid and dietary intake should be monitored closely in the elderly who have bowel or bladder problems, or who are at risk for developing these problems. Clients who have decreased bladder capacity and associated frequency of urination often restrict intake of fluid. This predisposes the elderly person to constipation as well as to urinary tract infections. Constipation with fecal impaction, by causing pressure on the urethra or bladder, may lead to urinary retention or incontinence. The importance of an adequate fluid intake should be stressed, unless there are medical reasons for restriction of fluids.

Medications may alter the micturition function or the volume of urine. Medications such as muscle relaxants and sedatives can cause relaxation of the musculature controlling urination. The elderly receiving these drugs may not perceive the urge to micturate or control micturition. Diuretics increase urine volume and frequency, particularly at peak action. Potent diuretics such as furosemide and ethacrynic acid produce a rapid effect within 30 minutes of administration and peak in 1 to 2 hours. The rapid diuresis may cause incontinence. Some elderly stay near the toilet facilities during these times to avoid incontinence. Intake of alcohol, coffee, or tea (mild diuretics) in the evening may cause the elderly person to urinate frequently at night (nocturia). The sedating effect of alcohol may decrease the sensation and control of micturition, resulting in incontinence while sleeping.

Obstruction of the bladder outlet can also occur in the elderly. Males who have prostatic hypertrophy will describe various changes in urination. They may complain initially of change in character of the stream, and difficulty starting and stopping the stream. Dribbling may occur as the urethra is narrowed. Assessment of these factors as well as examination of the prostate for enlargement are indicated.

Some bladder problems are attributable to aging changes and chronic disease, which decrease the speed and ease with which the client can get to the toilet or on the bedpan. Proximity of toilets to living areas should be assessed. If the client has difficulty getting on and off the toilet, the height of the toilet as well as presence of safety rails should be assessed. Persons who are confined to bed must urinate in a posture that may not permit sufficient pressure to overcome urethral resistance. There also may be the discomfort of sitting on a bedpan or fear of soiling the bed. Clients who are immobile must depend on others' interest and availability to offer toileting equipment.

AGING AND GASTROINTESTINAL TRACT FUNCTION

The age-related changes as they relate to the upper gastrointestinal tract and nutrition are discussed in Chapter 13. Data concerning age-related changes in the lower gastrointestinal tract are meager. The function of the lower gastrointestinal tract is related to a competent colon, an intact anal sphincter, and ability to sense and respond to fullness in the rectum. The pelvic floor muscles aid in support and action of the anal sphincter. The feces should be formed, easy to pass, and free from blood and mucus. The patterns of defecation are established early in life and "regularity" may vary from one to two times a day to one time a week. The patterns of defecation and consistency of the stool are influenced by intake of food, fluid and medications, activity, and accessibility of toilet facilities.

Past practices for promoting defecation are influential on the patterns of the present. Some elderly have responded to the gastrocolic stimulus. These elderly may have established a pattern of drinking a hot liquid—water or coffee—that stimulates the urge to defecate. Others may have found that prune juice or cereal has helped them maintain regularity. Some set aside a certain time for sitting on the toilet. Any alteration in these practices may produce problems in defecation.

Excessive straining to defecate over time may produce relaxation of the pelvic floor muscles, with subsequent decreased control of the anal sphincter (Parks, 1980, pp. 83,87). Relaxation of the pelvic muscles is considered a factor in the development of fecal incontinence.

A history of years of postponing the response to the urge for defecation may contribute to changes in the present stimulus for defecation. By ignoring the urge, a larger, harder fecal mass develops. Subsequently, constipation or fecal impaction may result. Some elderly can maintain defecation of the harder stool when physically active but develop problems when immobility occurs.

Most of the research has been directed toward studying problems common to the aged—constipation, diarrhea, diverticulitis, and fecal incontinence.

Common Problems of the Gastrointestinal Tract

Constipation, defined as a hard, dry stool, is common in older persons. Prolonged periods of constipation result in a reduced desire to defecate. Lack of response may lead to fecal impaction or fecal incontinence. There are several contributing factors: (1) lack of bulk in the diet; (2) medications; (3) decreased fluid intake; (4) decreased level of activity; and (5) depression. Bulk-forming foods, such as bran, fresh fruits, and vegetables, increase the speed with which fecal material travels through the intestine. Bran cereals absorb water, which, in turn, creates a soft stool. Lack of bulk in the diet thus may contribute toward decreasing transit time in the intestine and increased reabsorption of water from the stool, leading to constipation. Inadequate fluid intake can also cause constipation. It is generally recommended that 2 to 3 liters of fluid be consumed daily for those prone to constipation. When assessing the elderly person who reports problems with con-

stipation, the nurse should determine how the client defines constipation. Does the person regard decreased or irregular frequency of defecation as constipation, rather than considering the consistency of the stool? Data must also be obtained regarding amounts of bulk-forming foods eaten, as well as the frequency with which they are consumed.

Some persons, not just the elderly, experience transient constipation in response to change in patterns of daily living or accessibility to and privacy of toilet facilities. This change may be imposed by travel or by being in unfamiliar surroundings. Reestablishment of usual routines is sufficient to correct the constipation.

Constipation may be caused by the action of certain medications, particularly sedatives and tranquilizers. These medications may alter the filling time of the rectum and reduce the urge and the ability to respond to the urge. Certain antacids (Aluminum hydroxide, aluminum carbonate), anticholinergics, and antihypertensive drugs may cause constipation.

Laxative use on a regular basis may alter bowel function. Many resort to laxative use to combat constipation. Prolonged use of laxatives alter the urge to defecate stimulated by bulk and consistency of the stool. Because of the urge to defecate the elderly enter the vicious cycle: constipation—laxative—diarrhea—constipation. Laxative abuse by the elderly, particularly women, has been reported to be a major cause of diarrhea (Cummings, 1974). Prolonged diarrhea may cause fluid and electrolyte imbalances as well as decreased muscle tone. Diarrhea may be induced by antacids containing magnesium as well as rapid administration of highly concentrated liquid diet supplements.

Immobility may also lead to constipation, particularly in the elderly person who cannot comfortably assume a sitting or squatting position to defecate. Immobility may necessitate use of a bedpan, which is uncomfortable and not easy to sit on. Furthermore, the immobile person usually lacks privacy. As a result, the person may ignore the urge to defecate in order to avoid discomfort or embarrassment. The client's toilet facilities should be assessed for accessibility, ease of use, and degree of privacy.

Diverticulosis, a condition characterized by abnormal outpouchings (diverticuli) of the colon wall, is commonly found in the elderly, particularly in Western societies. A long-term dietary intake of low-residue rather than bulk-forming foods is thought to contribute to the development of diverticulosis. Mild symptoms of diverticulosis may be pain, flatulence, and sudden diarrhea. The client may be prescibed a low-residue diet for repeated episodes. This condition has the potential to develop into diverticulitis (inflammation of the diverticula), which may result in hemorrhage, perforation, or obstruction of the colon.

Although cancer of the colon and rectum occurs less frequently than the previously mentioned problems, the incidence increases with aging. Any change in the character of the stool (diameter, consistency, or color) should be questioned. Occult blood tests should be performed. Rectal examination for presence of hemorrhoids or other lesions is indicated since bleeding hemorrhoids may mask signs of bleeding higher in the gastrointestinal tract.

Fecal incontinence, described as involuntary evacuation of feces or stool, is less common than urinary incontinence in the elderly person. Fecal incontinence is usually secondary to fecal impaction or explosive diarrhea. Fecal impaction often presents as a liquid diarrhea and upon palpation a hard stool is present in the rectum. Explosive diarrhea is frequently caused by diverticulitis and cancer of the rectum. In the cognitively disturbed, the problem of fecal incontinence is associated with urinary incontinence.

ASSESSMENT OF ELIMINATION

The frequency and depth with which assessment is performed is determined by the difficulties experienced by the elderly client, the comfort of the client in talking about the topic and the tact, attitude, and skill of the assessor. Some elderly are embarrassed or reticent to talk about elimination patterns or admit episodes of incontinence. The assessment for screening problems or risk for problems should include history, physical exam, environmental exam, and laboratory tests. Screening assessment should be performed at least yearly on the "healthy elderly."

History

- Health status—past and present
  Urologic problems
    Urinary tract infections
    Symptoms of dysuria, stress incontinence, urge incontinence
    Surgical repair—prostate
  Genital problems
    Obstetrical history—number of births and character of labor and delivery
    Vaginal repair
  Rectal problems
    Hemorrhoids
    Bleeding
    Change in diameter of stool
    Constipation, diarrhea
  Chronic diseases
    Hypertension
    Diabetes
    Cardiac problems
      Nocturia
    Neurologic diseases that impair mobility or cognition
  Activity patterns
  Exercise levels
  Speed and ease in changing positions
  Medication usage
    Laxatives
    Antacids
    Diuretics
    Anticholinergics
    Sedatives
  Bowel patterns
    Frequency
    Usual time(s)
    Methods used to stimulate defecation
    Color, consistency, odor
  Urinary patterns
    Frequency—diurnal and nocturnal
    Difficulty starting or stopping stream
    Character of stream
    Color, odor, clarity
  Intake patterns
    See intake history
    Knowledge of intake which promotes elimination
  Sleep patterns
    Nocturia—frequency

Physical assessment

- Rectal exam—detection of impacted feces, hemorrhoids, or enlarged prostate
- Gynecologic exam—detection of relaxed vagina or prolapse of uterus
- Urologic exam—examination of supporting structures lying and standing
- Height and weight
- Laboratory Tests

    Urinalysis—pH, specific gravity, color, blood, glucose, ketones, protein, colony counts

    Feces—color, consistency, blood (gross and occult)

- Environment

    Proximity of toilets

    Privacy of toilets

    Height of toilets

    Lighting

If high risk or problems exist, more comprehensive assessment and laboratory tests are indicated, such as cystoscopy, cystometrogram, renal function, proctoscopy, and barium enema.

PLANNING AND INTERVENTION

The literature is largely concerned with the incontinent elderly, particularly those who are in institutions. A more positive approach is to emphasize the attitudes and conditions that preserve or promote normal bowel and bladder function in old persons. Continence can thus be preserved rather than restored. Many of the positive attitudes and environmental conditions utilized in bowel and bladder retraining programs are also conducive to maintenance of bowel and bladder function.

The elderly person who has problems with bowel and bladder function should be carefully evaluated for pathologic bases. When pathology is present, medical or surgical treatment is indicated. When no known pathology exists, the nurse is in a position to intervene based upon an understanding of such contributing factors as (1) personal hygiene, (2) patterns of food and fluid intake, (3) medication use, and (4) environmental influences.

Maintaining Bowel and Bladder Function in the Elderly

Personal hygiene is important for the aging person, because of the high incidence of urinary tract infections that may contribute to urinary incontinence (Isaacs, 1976). Females who use bedpans are prone to urinary tract infections, because urine tends to collect in the vaginal vault, where it provides a medium for bacterial growth. Hygiene measures to promote cleanliness include placing the female in a sitting position on the bedpan, which also enhances emptying of the bladder. Following urination, the perineal area should be thoroughly cleansed. Special cleansing pads are available for use when washing facilities are not readily accessible. Thorough cleansing after defecation is also necessary. The female should be taught to wipe with tissue or washcloth from the urinary meatus to the rectal area. New tissue or a clean side of the washcloth should be used for each subsequent wipe.

Special hygiene measures are required for the elderly person who *must* have an indwelling catheter inserted. The indwelling catheter is the leading cause of urinary tract infections in all age groups. The drainage system catheter, drainage tubing, and collection bag should be kept closed and not disconnected under any circumstances. Strict asepsis must be observed when inserting the catheter. Preventive hygienic measures following insertion of the catheter should include frequent cleansing around the urinary meatus and the point of entry and keeping the collection bag lower than the bladder but off the floor. Cleansing should be performed by using single wiping motions away from the meatus and down the catheter tubing. After cleansing, an antiseptic ointment should be applied at the point of insertion to prevent bacteria from ascending the indwelling tubing into the bladder. This cleansing procedure should be performed at least once a day and following contamination caused by fecal incontinence or vaginal discharge. Free urinary flow should be maintained by keeping the drainage tubing unobstructed and dropped in a straight line from client to the collection bag. Flow is also enhanced by adequate fluid intake of at least 2000 ml per day. Increased flow of urine may prevent obstruction of the tubing by mucous shreds and the solid constituents of concentrated urine.

Medications that may alter bowel and bladder function should be evaluated carefully. The elderly client should be taught to avoid use of irritating laxatives, many of which are available as over-the-counter medications. However, it is not always easy to change a person's long-standing habits. Therefore, alternatives to irritating laxatives should be reviewed with the client. Stool softeners or bulk-producing agents, such as methyl cellulose or psyllium seeds, are nonirritating laxatives that can be used while the person is being weaned from an irritating laxative. At the same time, the client should be taught to eat bulk-forming foods. When normal bowel function returns, the dosage of the nonirritating laxative should be gradually decreased.

Daily intake of bulk-forming foods (bran, dried peas and beans, nuts, fresh vegetables and fruits) should be recommended to the elderly person who is prone to constipation. Introduction of such a diet was found to decrease the number of accidents, suppositories used, and enemas given in a study of 25 self-fed and 25 staff-fed elderly nursing home residents (Wichita, 1978). Bran was added to hot cereal, and more fruits and vegetables were introduced. Some foods were chopped or grated. Cabbage was eliminated because the majority of the residents manifested gastrointestinal difficulty. In addition, many residents reported that they liked the diet and had obtained relief from constipation. Although not measured in this study, it seems obvious that such a diet would decrease nursing time spent on cleaning up accidents and giving treatment for constipation, and would also increase the dignity of the client.

When the client is prescribed a diuretic, the medication should be taken in the morning so that urination does not interfere with sleep. Mild diuretics such as alcohol, coffee, and tea should be also avoided during the evening hours. Tranquilizers and sedatives reduce alertness and the sensation of need to defecate or urinate. Careful evaluation of bowel and bladder patterns is indicated before and after prescription of these drugs. Their benefits should exceed the potential risks of developing constipation or incontinence.

An environment conducive to normal bowel and bladder function is equally important. Changes in bladder capacity, frequency of urination, sensation or desire to urinate or defecate, vision, and mobility may be compensated for by modifications in the elderly person's environment. Toilet facilities should be private, safe, and accessible. The client can be taught to locate toilet facilities in public places, so that they can be used whenever necessary. These facilities should be well lighted, well marked, and free from hazards such as slippery surfaces. The nurse, as an advocate for the elderly, should report inadequate or unsafe toilet facilities to local health authorities.

The elderly living at home can be taught to use night lights. If the client experiences decreased activity tolerance or difficulties with mobility, additional measures may help the person to maintain function. For example, handrails can be installed by the toilet to assist the person in getting on and off the toilet. Clothing should be easily removable. Ideally, the toilet facility should be close at hand. When regular toilet facilities are on another floor or at a considerable distance from the person's usual living area, portable commodes, urinals, or bedpans may be used. The height of beds and chairs should be adjusted or selected to permit independent and easy transfer to toilet facilities.

Modifications of the environment for the institutionalized elderly are not unlike those for the person living at home. The nursing staff, however, are in a position to initiate and provide modifications that will enhance bowel and bladder function. Wells (1975) recommends assessment of bed and chair heights, distances to toilets, toilet alternatives, availability of signals and privacy, and presence of a motivating environment.

Bed and chair heights should be assessed for each individual. Ideally, an adjustable bed in a low position permits the individual to reach the floor independently or with minimal assistance. Chair heights should be related to lower leg length, and chair depth should be related to upper leg length. Arms should extend the full chair depth, to enable the person to sit and rise with ease.

Toilet facilities should be close to the elderly client, and access to the facilities should be safe. Wells (1975) recommends that toilets should be within 30 feet of patient areas. There should be enough toilets that waiting in line is not necessary. The toilet and the pathways that lead to it should be well lighted. The door to the facility should be wide enough to accommodate wheelchairs. Toilet seats may have to be elevated for the individual who has difficulty flexing the knees or hips.

Portable toilet alternatives, such as commodes, bedpans, and urinals, should be provided when necessary. It is recommended that a portable commode be available for every two beds located far from the regular toilet facility. Commodes should be kept clean and free from odor. They should be positioned against an unmovable object such as a wall, to prevent them from sliding. Bedpans and urinals should also be kept clean and free from odor.

Each client should be provided a signal button for assistance and privacy during toileting. Signal buttons should be available at the bedside and in usual living areas, as well as in the toilet area. More important, the nurse should respond promptly to the signal. Privacy during toileting should include closed doors. If portable toilet alternatives must be used, curtains or a screen should be placed around the client to insure privacy.

Providing a motivating environment is also important in maintaining continence. The attitudes of the nursing staff become an increasingly important factor. The nurse must be aware of each elderly person's habits and patterns of elimination. Routinized toilet regimes, based upon the needs or number of the nursing staff, are not conducive to maintaining each client's particular patterns. Rewards should be given to nursing staff who give individualized care. Every effort should be made to promote continence, and the results should be monitored to evaluate effectiveness of nursing care.

Toileting should be provided in a dignified environment, so that the reward for continence exceeds the reward for incontinence. For ex-

ample, Miss L, an obese elderly person, had partial use of her right arm, and her leg was in a brace for support. She could transfer easily, with assistance from one person, from her wheelchair to the toilet. She frequently asked to go to the toilet, and always voided when she went. However, on many occasions when the nursing staff were "too busy," she urinated in her chair. The nurses responded "I just took you to the bathroom, and if this happens again I'll just let you sit there." In this case, Miss L was being penalized for her urinary frequency and was not being rewarded for her continence.

Other methods for promoting bowel and bladder function have been suggested (Isaacs, 1976; Willington, 1975). Exercises that strengthen the muscles of the pelvic floor and abdomen may promote continence, particularly in the obese person. By contracting the abdominal muscles, and tightening the buttocks and pelvic floor, the support of the bladder may be enhanced. Kegel (1948) first recommended pelvic floor exercises 100 to 300 times a day for postpartum women. To teach the elderly, instruction must be specific. They should be instructed to slowly tighten, hold and release the muscles around the rectum and those around the anterior perineum. They may be asked to try to stop urine flow midstream to identify these muscles. Recommended frequency at which the exercises should be performed varies from three to four times per hour through the waking hours (Mandelstam, 1980) to 10 to 17 times three different times a day (Burgio, 1983).

Women may promote emptying the bladder by leaning forward as they sit on the toilet or bedpan. They may also compress the bladder by applying hard pressure over the lower abdomen.

Restoring Bowel and Bladder Continence

The impact of incontinence on the client, family, and caretaker cannot be underestimated. The client may be so ashamed that he will not admit that incontinence occurs. In an attempt to hide the problem, some wear pads while others withdraw socially. Some persons are afraid to ask about leakage or incontinence either from embarrassment or fear of being put in an institution. Incontinent clients should be made aware that incontinence can be treated and controlled.

The suggested measures which promote bowel and bladder continence should be evaluated for effectiveness. When medications which alter elimination are prescribed and cause incontinence, the nurse should encourage the client to confer with the physician. Alternative drugs, dosages, or dosage schedules should be considered. The client, family, or nurse should reassess the environment for possible causes of incontinence. A recent rearrangement of the furniture may have made the trip to the bathroom longer, just long enough to be unable to hold the urine.

If incontinence persists, further assessment is indicated. The nature of the incontinence must be determined. This is best determined by obtaining a thorough history of incontinence as well as obtaining a record of incontinence events (micturition or incontinence charts).

The history should include onset, frequency, amount of urine or feces in incontinent episodes, periods of continence and sensation experienced before urination or defecation. History of associated or aggravated conditions should be elicited.

Incontinence charts are used to analyze frequency of urination or defecation, time interval between the urge for elimination, and the conditions accompanying the continent or incontinent event. The client, when able, should be encouraged to maintain the chart. For the dependent client, the caretaker is responsible for recording. This may entail hourly checks if the client is unable to call the nurse. The incontinent charts can be used to record micturition events as well as defecation events depending upon the client's problem. An example of an incontinence chart is found in Figure 14.1. It is suggested that this record be kept for 3 to 5 days.

Restoring fecal continence is usually easier than restoring urinary continence. Restoration is usually based upon a conditioned response. The stimulus for bowel retraining is the sensation of a full rectum.

ASSESSMENT GUIDE OF THE INCONTINENT CLIENT

Client History
  Onset
    Description-amount (leakage versus large amount)
    Accompanying illness
    Factors precipitating event i.e., coughing, laughing
    Use of pads or collection devices
  Frequency
    Diurnal and nocturnal patterns
  Change in sensation or urge to void
  Associated signs and symptoms
    Blood
    Pain
    Difficulty in starting or stopping urination
    Color of urine
    Change in stream
  Food and fluid intake
    Amounts-when taken
    Use of alcohol
  Medication Use
    Anticholinergics
    B-blocking agents
    Diuretics
    Sedatives and hypnotics
  Genitourinary history-females
    Number of births
    Size of baby at birth
    Incidence of prolonged, difficult births
    Surgery
  Urologic problems
    Urinary tract infections
    Prostate surgery
  Recent changes in life style
Incontinence Charts

Fecal Incontinence

Programs designed to promote fecal continence should be based upon the individual's usual patterns, if these can be identified. The client should first be examined rectally for fecal impaction, which may produce an overflow incontinence. The rectum should then be evacuated, either by suppository or enema. Willington (1976) recommends that after an empty rectum is achieved, bowel movements should be prevented until a planned time is set for defecation. The usual planned time is after a

Date Time	Amount	Urge to Elimimate	Incontinent Continent	Comments

Figure 14.1. Incontinence chart.

2- or 3-day interval. Bowel movements may be prevented by giving an antidiarrheic kaolin mixture three times a day.

Evacuation of the rectum is achieved by use of a suppository which will act in 30 to 45 minutes. Thirty minutes after insertion of the suppository, or when the client has the urge to defecate, the person is placed on the toilet or commode. Bedpans should be avoided because the discomfort of sitting on a bedpan may provide negative stimuli.

The sequence of events should be precisely repeated about three times a week. The bowel reflex usually resumes activity in 2 to 3 weeks, and the suppository treatment can be discontinued. The nursing staff should maintain charts for each client involved in bowel retraining so that the sequence of events is kept constant and rectal evacuation is achieved at least three times a week. The actual time set for evacuation of the rectum is arbitrary. The individual's previous habits, such as drinking warm liquids upon arising or eating to stimulate defecation, may provide positive stimuli for defecation. The response to distention of the stomach (gastrocolic reflex) initiates contraction of the rectum. If these stimuli are successful, the time for evacuation will be predetermined by the time of ingestion of food.

Urinary Incontinence

Treatment of urinary incontinence is based upon accurate diagnosis. Where there is no need for treatment of urinary tract infection, fecal im-

paction, or genitourinary abnormalities, treatment may consist of medications, exercises, and bladder retraining.

Some medications such as anticholinergics have been used with varying degrees of success. Flavoxate, a smooth muscle relaxant, may be effective for the person who has a contracted bladder. Topical application of estrogen creams can be effective for allaying some of the atrophic changes in postmenopausal women.

Exercises are indicated for treatment of stress incontinence secondary to relaxation of the pelvic floor muscles and weakness of the sphincter muscle. Pelvic floor exercises should be performed in 30 repetitions at frequent intervals during the waking hours (Keegan and McNichols, 1982). Mandelstam (1977) suggests that these exercises be performed for 2 to 3 months. Recommendations for teaching these exercises (Mandelstam, 1977) follow:

1. Sit, stand, or lie comfortably, without tensing the muscles of the seat, abdomen, or legs, and pretend you are trying to control diarrhea by tightening the ring of muscle around the anus. Do this several times until you feel certain that you have identified the right area and are making the correct movement.

2. Sit on the commode and start to urinate, and while doing so make an attempt to stop the flow in midstream by contracting the muscles of the pelvic floor surrounding the urethra and vagina. This should be carried

out several times until you feel sure of the movement, and of the sensations of applying conscious control.

3. Exercise as follows: sitting, standing, or lying, tighten first the anal sphincter and then the front, and then both together. Count to four slowly, and then release the muscles. Do this four times, repeating the whole sequence once every hour, if possible. With practice the movements should be quite easy to master and the exercises can be carried out any time—while waiting for a bus, standing at the sink, watching television, or even lying comfortably in bed.

For clients who have little awareness of which muscles to contract, a perineometer placed in the vagina records the pressure increase when the proper muscles contract. This equipment may be used to record progress (Mandelstam, 1980). Muscle strengthening programs have been initiated by physiotherapists but seem within the capabilities of the nurse with whom the elderly has contact.

Bladder retraining is indicated for detrusor instability characterized by urge incontinence. The bladder capacity should be greater than 150 ml (Castledon and Duffin, 1980). The success of the program is dependent upon teaching the client about the program. Voiding events should be recorded as on the incontinence charts for several days. From this chart, the client and nurse can identify the interval at which urination is planned to occur. Visits to the toilet should be arranged. Continued use of micturition charts should be kept to assess success of program.

Bladder drills have been used for bladder retraining. Bladder drills consist of holding the urine for increasingly longer periods of time. These drills have been successful for women with urge and stress incontinence (Jarus and Miller, 1980). Twenty-seven of 30 clients reported continence after 6-month program.

The success of bladder retraining depends on the constancy of the program, the reinforcing attitudes of the nursing staff, and the cooperation and satisfaction of the client. How long the program should be continued is largely determined by repeated successful periods of continence. If the client is continent only during the waking hours, the program should be maintained during these hours. Reassessment of factors that may contribute to nighttime incontinence is indicated. Every effort should be made to create conditions which promote continence. Fluid intake may be adjusted to decrease nighttime events. Some clients benefit from being wakened at night at interval(s) derived from the micturition charts. Alarm clocks may be used to awaken the person. The client should be reminded that urinating before going to bed is imperative.

Behavioral therapy, using social rewards, has been reported to reduce the incidence of incontinence in the cognitively impaired (Carpenter and Simon, 1960). Behavior therapy requires a team effort so that selection and use of the reward is consistent.

Aids to Manage Incontinence

Some clients unfortunately are incurably incontinent. Some clients have incontinent events although in a program to restore continence. Many commercial products are available. Cost, comfort, convenience, and dignity of the client are factors in selecting the pad or pants used. Keeping the skin dry to prevent skin breakdown is also important. Marsupial pants are preferrable to wearing a diaper. Marsupial pants have a pocket in the anterior crotch into which an absorbent pad can be placed and easily changed. Some plastic backed pads are not sufficiently absorbent to keep the skin or clothing dry. Any pads should be changed at least every 4 hours.

A double layered pad made of washable brushed quilted nylon has been described as decreasing the incidence of skin wetness when compared with using disposable pads (Williams, Foerster, Proctor, Hahn, Izzo, Elliott, 1982). This pad is recommended for nocturnal incontinence.

EVALUATION

Evaluation of the elimination status should be according to goals set. If the goal is to maintain bowel or bladder function, certain factors should be considered in the client's behavior:

1. Present bladder patterns
2. Present bowel patterns
3. Potential risk for interruption of function
4. Success of modifications made, i.e., diet, activity, environment

When evaluating the success of incontinence programs, reduction of incontinent events should be considered success in some clients. Criterion-based, the client is continent five times out of seven urination events.

In conclusion, the nurse should assist the elderly client in identifying ways of enhancing elimination and identifying conditions that require further medical or surgical treatment. The nurse should describe and institute methods to restore bowel or bladder function.

RECOMMENDED READINGS

Mandelstam D (ed): Incontinence and its Management. London, Croom Helm, 1980. *Comprehensive text on the nature and management of incontinence.*

REFERENCES CITED

Affleck, J.W. The chronic sick in hospital. Lancet 1:355, 1947

Akhtar, A.J., Brol, G.A., Crombie, A.C., McLean, W.M.R., Andrews, G.R., Caird, F.I. Disability and dependence in the elderly at home. Age and Aging 2:10, 1973

Berman, P.M., Kirsner, J.B. The aging gut: II. Diseases of the colon, pancreas, liver, and gallbladder, functional bowel disease, and iatrogenic disease. Geriatrics 27(4):117, 1972

Brocklehurst, J.C. Incontinence in Old People. Edinburgh, Livingston, 1951

Brocklehurst, J.C., Dillane, J.B., Griffiths, L., Fry, J. The prevalence and symptomatology of urinary infection in an aged population. Gerontologica Clinica 10:242, 1968

Carpenter, H.A., Simon, R. The effect of several methods of training on long term, incontinent, behaviorally regressed hospitalized psychiatric patients. Nursing Research 9:17, 1960

Castledon, C.M., Duffin, H.M. Guidelines for controlling urinary incontinence without drugs or catheters. Age and Aging 10:186, 1980

Cummings, J.H. Progress report: Laxative abuse. Gut 15:758, 1974

Gilleard, C.J. Incontinence in the hospitalized elderly. Health Bulletin (Edinburg) 39(1):58, 1981

Gilleard, C.J., Pattie, A.H., Dearman, G. Behavioural disabilities in psychogeriatric patients and residents of old peoples' homes. Journal of Epidemiology and Community Health 34:106, 1980

Hobson, W., Pemberton, J. The Health of the Elderly at Home. London, Butterworth, 1955

Isaacs, B., Walkey, F.A. A survey of incontinence in elderly hospital patients. Gerontologia Clinica 6:367, 1964

Jewett, M.A.S., Fernie, G.R., Holliday, P.J., Pim, M.E. Urinary dysfunction in a geriatric long-term care population: Prevalence and patterns. Journal of the American Geriatrics Society 29(5):211, 1981

Kegel, A.H. The physiologic treatment of poor tone and function of the genital muscles and of urinary stress incontinence. Western Journal of Surgery, Obstetrics, and Gynecology 57:527, 1949

Khanna, O.P. Disorders of micturition, neuropharmacological basis and results of drug treatment. Urology 8:316, 1976

Knox, J.D.E. Ambulant incontinent patients in general practice. A survey to ascertain the prevalence of these patients and their distribution by type of practice. Nursing Times 75:1683, 1979

Kumin, C.M. Detection and Management of Urinary Tract Infections. Philadelphia, Lea and Febiger, 1974

Mandelstam, D.A. Incontinence. Physiotherapy 62(6):182, 1976

Mandelstam, D. Incontinence. London, William Hinemann, 1977

Robb, S.S. Third Annual Survey of Major Client Functional Problems and Ages—Oakland and Aspinwall Divisions. Unpublished report, VA Medical Center, Pittsburgh, PA, 1981

Sheldon, J.H. The Social Medicine of Old Age. London, Oxford University Press, 1948

Thomas, B. Problem solving: Urinary incontinence in the elderly. Journal of Gerontological Nursing 6(9):533, 1980

Thomas, T.M., Plymat, K.R, Blannin, J., Meade, T.W. Prevalence of urinary incontinence. British Medical Journal 281:1243, 1980

Thomson, A.P. Problems of aging and chronic sickness. British Medical Journal 2:243, 300, 1949

Van Zonneveld, R.J. Some data on the genito-urinary system as found in old age surveys in the Netherlands. Gerontologia Clinica 1:167, 1959

Walkey, F.A., Judge, T.G., Thomson, J., Sakari, N.B.S. Incidence of urinary infection in the elderly. Scottish Medical Journal 12:411, 1967

Wells, T. Promoting urinary continence in the elderly in hospital. Nursing Times 1908, November 27, 1975

Wichita, C. Treating and preventing constipation in nursing home residents. Journal of Gerontological Nursing 3(6):35, 1978

Wilkin, D., Jolley, D.J. Mental and physical impairment in the elderly in hospital and residential care 2. Nursing Times 74(29):117, 1978

Williams, R.F., Foerster, J.E., Proctor, J.K, Hahn, A., Izzo, A.J., Elliott, J.A. A new double-layered launderable bed sheet for patients with urinary incontinence. Journal of the American Geriatrics Society 29(11):520, 1982

Willington, F.L. Hygienic methods in the management of incontinence, in Willington, F.L. (ed), Incontinence in the Elderly. London, Academic, 1976

Willington, F.L. Incontinence—4: The nursing component in diagnosis and treatment. Nursing Times 464, March 20, 1975a

Willington, F.L. Incontinence—5: Training and retraining for continence. Nursing Times 500, March 27, 1975b

Willington, F.L. Problems in urinary incontinence in the aged. Gerontologia Clinica 11:330, 1969

Wilson, T.S. Incontinence of urine in the aged. Lancet 2:374, 1948

Yarnell, J.W.G., St. Leger, A.S. The prevalence, severity, and factors associated with urinary incontinence in a random sample of the elderly. Age and Aging 8:81, 1979

Yeates, W.K. Normal and abnormal bladder function in incontinence of urine, in Willington, F.L. (ed), Incontinence in the Elderly. London, Academic, 1976

15

The Nursing Process and the Activity of the Elderly Person

Ann Gera Yurick

Reading this chapter will enable the individual to:

1. Know the elderly person's need for physical activity
2. Know the age-related physical changes that can affect activity levels of elderly people
3. Know the nursing interventions to promote activity
4. Know the needs of the immobilized elderly person
5. Know the nursing interventions to promote rest for the elderly person

Activity, the physical process of expending energy to perform a function or to produce an effect, is a basic human need. The degree of activity of an elderly person is correlated with adaptation to the aging process. Activity reduces or delays the effects of aging. Kraus (1977) indicates that the physically inactive person shows signs of aging earlier in life.

This chapter will discuss the elderly person's need to maintain physical activity, as well as the age-related changes that can affect the supply and utilization of oxygen and nutrients needed for activity. Muscular, skeletal, and innervative changes also affect the mobility and manipulative skills of the elderly person. Emphasis must be placed on maintaining the health of the elderly person through activity. Nursing interventions are designed to maintain maximum activity levels for the old person who experiences physical changes that alter activity patterns. Interruption or disruption of the individual's activity can initiate, hasten, and/or extend health problems. Too often, the elderly are expected to slow down and to enjoy a rest that has been earned through years of hard work. Attitudes toward the need for physical activity are important determinants in the kind and amount of activity in which the person engages. Inactivity is increasingly considered to be a serious threat to the elderly person.

Mobility is a major factor in maintaining the activity of the elderly person. The ability to remain mobile influences the degree of independent living an individual is able to achieve in the home setting or in an institution. Mobility, the ability to move about in the environment, is dependent upon the coordinated activity of bones, muscles, and nerves. Control of movement is affected by internal receptors in the muscles, tendons, and joints, and by other body sensors that measure the state of the blood chemistry, hydration, and other body conditions (Welford, 1977).

Activity involves integration and coordination of many different systems of the body. Nutrients must be supplied to fuel activity, and the waste byproducts of activity must be removed from the body. These requirements are met by integrated efforts of the cardiovascular, pulmonary, musculoskeletal, nervous, and endocrine systems.

The individual's gait has an important influence on activity levels. The way an elderly person walks can provide many clues about his or her physical and psychologic well-being. As people become older, they may appear to move more stiffy and slowly, with complaints of aching joints and weakening muscles. Aging tends to produce a slowing of motor processes. However, active older persons appear to show less slowness of response than do inactive older persons (Birren and Renner, 1977). The elderly person's motivation, which affects activity levels, may be altered by fear of pain with mobility. Body image and behavior changes may be caused by the old person's changing activity patterns. These changes affect the individual's social relationships, as well as recreational and vocational opportunities. Living space boundaries may be determined by the person's ability to move freely and easily around the environment. A person who has control over his or her activities experiences a feeling of power (Roberts, 1978).

For the elderly, the benefits of activity and exercise are becoming more fully appreciated. An inactive existence is felt to be the silent crippler of old age (Rosenberg, 1977). There is increasing evidence that exercise enables the elderly person to maintain body fitness. Stiffness and decreased mobility of joints are frequently attributed to age, when the problem is actually one of poor physical condition, which can often be improved by exercise. Research has demonstrated the positive effects of exercise on the physical and mental status of the elderly population (Sculco, 1978). A report by the President's Council on Physical Fitness and the Administration on Aging emphasizes the importance of exercise for the elderly person. Even though exercise programs do not prevent the stresses of life, exercise helps to reduce mental fatigue and tension caused by a highly technical and sedentary way of life (The Fitness Challenge in the Later Years, 1975). Exercise can be a significant component in the elderly person's activity. Rosenberg (1977) describes old age as "having your physical impairments rule your life." Activity may be seen as central to the prevention of premature aging. Potential for activity needs to be considered. It is important for the nurse to realize

that too much or too little activity can result in problems for the elderly client. The nurse should assess the client's activity desires and tolerance as a base for planning and intervention. The elderly person may exhibit changes in the performance of coordinated activities because of changes in physiologic functioning. Changes in function that may affect activity levels will be discussed in the assessment base. However, the nurse must take individual differences into consideration when assessing the activity of each elderly client.

In the discussion of physical changes that can accompany the aging process, it is important to keep in mind that people who stay active tend *not* to experience the same degree of physiologic change. It is felt that old active people are not too different from young active people, especially those who have exercised for 20 years or more. When deVries (1970) directed a group of men whose average age was 69.5 years, in a 42-week exercise program, he found a 30 percent increase in mean oxygen values. The percentage of improvement in the elderly who exercise is similar to that of a younger person.

Basic to physical fitness is a heart that adequately pumps blood and nourishment to body cells, patent elastic vessels through which the blood flows, lungs that oxygenate the blood, muscular strength and endurance, balance, flexibility, coordination, and agility. Each of these areas is addressed in this chapter. Many of the changes of aging that are included relate to the aging unconditioned body that has not benefitted from the effects of years of planned exercise programs. Increasing participation by the elderly in athletic events and marathons indicates increasing interest and involvement. With the present-day emphasis on exercise programs, many of the changes described in the assessment base of this chapter may change the norms of aging. Bortz (1980) discusses increasing evidence that indicates many of the changes commonly attributed to aging can be retarded by active exercise programs. However, more work with controlled observations of people in their 80s and 90s needs to be made on the ability of this group to meet exercise stress.

ASSESSMENT BASE: OXYGEN AND NUTRIENTS TO SUPPORT ACTIVITY

To support activity, oxygen and nutrients must be transported and utilized by body cells. First, the body must be able to take in these substances from the environment. Pulmonary functioning will affect the supply of oxygen that is available to the body cells, and the gastrointestinal system will affect the supply of nutrients. The supply of oxygen may be diminished by age-related changes in the lungs and the cardiovascular system. A discussion of nutrients is included in Chapter 13.

Supply of Oxygen

In assessing age-related changes in respiratory functioning, it may be difficult to distinguish between the changes that normally accompany aging and those that have been caused by environmental factors, such as air pollution. The total capacity and the vital capacity of the lungs may decrease with age as the result of several interrelated factors. These include decreased rib mobility due to weakening of the muscles that lift the rib cage, reduction in the total number of alveoli accompanied by an increase in their size, reduction in the flexibility of the lungs as a result of changes in the elastic fibers of the bronchioles and alveoli, and weakening of the external intercostal muscles and the diaphragm (Rockstein, 1975). The causes of decreased lung elasticity with aging have not been clearly defined.

Movement of gases across the membranes of the alveoli into the vascular system may be slowed by thickening of these membranes. The elderly person may develop a barrel chest as the anteroposterior diameter of the chest increases with alterations in the thorax stemming from degenerative changes in the intervertebral discs, increased spinal curvature, and calcification of costal cartilage (Klocke, 1977). There is a reduction in the compliance of the chest wall and the force of the expiratory muscles. As the chest wall becomes progressively more difficult to move, maximal inspiratory and expiratory pressures are decreased. With age, it appears that the small bronchi and bronchioles may collapse at a progressively earlier phase in the respiratory cycle. As this progresses, a greater amount of air becomes trapped in the lungs, a condition that may be partially responsible for hyperventilation and senile emphysema (Wright, 1978). Less space in the lung is available to take in a fresh supply of oxygen. As the vital capacity of the lung decreases, the residual volume increases. Incomplete lung expansion may cause basilar lung collapse with inadequate inflation of the base of the lung. The aging lung becomes increasingly rigid (Goldman, 1979).

The elderly person experiences a decreased capacity to cough forcefully as a result of increased rigidity of the thoracic wall and reduced strength of the expiratory muscles (Goldman, 1979). Also, there is decreased ciliary activity in the bronchial lining. Reduced cough efficiency may influence the choice of interventions with the elderly person who undergoes surgery or who has been immobilized. Any loss in the functional reserve of the respiratory system can increase the risk of respiratory failure or leave the elderly person with decreased compensatory mechanisms for dealing with stress (Campbell and Lefrak, 1978). A decrease in general physical fitness can further affect the problems of the respiratory system.

Measurable age-related functional changes in the resting respiratory system occur in the elderly, reducing the physiologic reserve for gas exchange and thus reducing the body's ability to tolerate stress (Campbell and Lefrak, 1978).

Research demonstrates that under conditions that reduce the oxygen content of arterial blood, such as reduced lung capacity or oxygen-carrying capacity of the blood, the elderly person responds with a smaller increase in ventilation and in cardiac output than does the younger person. When the elderly person is subjected to stress, less oxygen is delivered to the tissues (Campbell and Lefrak, 1978).

The maximal amount of oxygen utilized is 50 percent by age 80 (Goldman, 1979). Possible causes may be delayed oxygen diffusion, failure of perfusion, or impaired oxygen utilization by stressed tissues. The anatomic and physiologic changes connected with the aging process alter the efficiency of oxygenation. The resulting hypoxemia can be accentuated by the recumbent position. This may explain the confusion experienced by some elderly persons during the night or during an acute illness (Lynne-Davies, 1977). The elderly are more prone to respiratory failure because of their limited ability to compensate for an abnormal balance of gases in the arterial blood (Campbell and Lefrak, 1978). The nurse should be aware of these potential changes in planning with the client for activities. With the elderly person, there is a need to determine the limits of performance and the rest pauses needed in order to avoid severe oxygen drains with activity.

The incidence of respiratory pathology is higher in the elderly population than in the general population. Smoking is a significant factor, along with the elderly person's history of exposure to air pollutants (Klocke, 1977). Pulmonary problems in the elderly may result from the cumulative effects of the environment in which the person has lived, habits such as smoking, and/or neglect of respiratory infections. With infections, such as influenza, mortality increases with age (Goldman, 1979).

The supply of oxygen to the body also is affected by the hemoglobin carried by the red blood cells. Little change with age has been reported for the blood components. Red cell survival time appears to remain constant. The serum iron and iron-binding capacity may be moderately decreased and iron absorption is decreased. Although anemia is a frequent problem of the elderly, it is secondary (Goldman, 1979). An analysis of the blood components of each elderly person will give an indication of the capacity for the transport of nutrients and oxygen.

Transport of Oxygen and Nutrients

Alterations in the efficiency of transport through the circulatory system are more likely to stem from pathologic conditions than from age-related changes. However, there are some functional changes of age that can affect the transport of oxygen and nutrients to the parts of the body that maintain body activity.

Another point to consider is the transport of wastes away from the body part. An altered distribution of circulatory flow during aging may allow waste byproducts of metabolism to accumulate in the body tissue. This, rather than inadequacy of the total amount of oxygen and nutrients available to a given part of the body, could result in substantial decrements in function of the elderly person (Strehler, 1976). This has additional nursing implications for the activity of the elderly person who is receiving medications.

Cardiac Output

Studies indicate that age has no significant effect on the resting heart rate. However, the elderly person's response to stress demonstrates that the heart rate increase is less effective with increasing age. Heart power, which indicates the heart work during the period of systole, has been found to decrease by 0.9 percent each year (Kohn, 1977), leading to a gradual decrease in cardiac output. It is believed that the heart may function less efficiently with age, possibly because of stiffening of the connective tissue matrix in which the heart contracts (Kohn, 1977). There may be focal hypertrophy of individual cardiac fibers, along with a loss of muscle fibers, metabolic cellular changes in the myocardium, decreased efficiency and strength of myocardial contraction, greater myocardial irritability, and conduction system changes (Harris, 1978). There are reports of cardiac atrophy in the old person who has experienced prolonged illness, periods of immobility, or malnutrition (Harris, 1971). A heart enlarged by valvular heart disease or hypertension may decrease in size as a result of rest and reduced activity.

The normal aging heart undergoes alterations in size and contour. In the elderly person whose activity is reduced, the left ventricular cavity may become smaller because of decreased demands on the heart. The aorta widens as it becomes less elastic, and the cardiac valves, particularly the mitral valve, thicken and become more rigid (Harris, 1975). The aging aorta and the great vessels demonstrate an increased collagen–elastin ratio. Under ordinary circumstances, the aged heart is able to provide an adequate output. However, exercise, emotional stress, and other factors that can produce tachycardia, may adversely affect the aged person. In some cases they may even precipitate heart failure, since the aged heart may have limited functional ability to cope with stress situations (Harris, 1975). An old person who is able to perform routine activities may not be able to tolerate sudden physical or mental stressors as the cardiac reserve diminishes. Changes in myocardial contractility and an increase in aortic resistance may increase left ventricular ejection time.

Even though homeostatic mechanisms may not be as efficient in the elderly person, the healthy individual can continue normal daily activities unless the stresses become overwhelming in degree, number, intensity, or duration (Syzek, 1976). The heart has a lessened ability to increase its rate when stress occurs and more time is required for the pulse to return to basal levels after even a minimal increase in pulse rate. The heart rate is impaired due to increased connective tissue in the sinoatrial and atrioventricular nodes and in the bundle branches. Also, there is a decrease in the number of catecholamine receptors on the myofibers (Rodstein, 1979). Because the catecholamines affect the increase of the speed and force of the heart when stress is experienced, with a decrease in the number of catecholamine receptors, the heart is unable to respond as effectively to stress. Fibrosis of the sinoatrial node can affect the conduction of electrical impulses across the heart muscle, and this can lead to frequent occurrence of arrhythmias during stress (Syzek, 1976). Arrhythmias may further reduce the cardiac output, impairing the transport of oxygen and nutrients to vital organs such as the brain. These organs may already be impaired by age-related changes or the existence of pathologic problems. Arrhythmias, especially those that result in bradycardia, may cause syncope. Coronary artery pathology may also cause arrhythmias when the artery to the sinoatrial node is affected. Varying degrees of heart block can occur when the artery to the atrioventricular node is affected. Changes in the blood supply to the common bundle and the bundle branches may cause

complete heart block (Rodstein, 1979). Digitalis medications can cause arrhythmias and conduction disturbances, especially when there is hypokalemia resulting from diuresis, malnutrition, or prior conduction disturbances. With the elderly, muscle mass and delayed excretion may result in high levels of medications.

Congestive heart failure in the elderly client may be caused by a reduction in the coronary blood flow, increased work load on the myocardium, or an impaired myocardium. Changes that normally accompany aging may cause myocardial impairment, and pathologies can result when these changes interfere sufficiently with myocardial functioning. The aged myocardium may not be able to tolerate stresses, such as those that require a high cardiac output or that result in tachycardia. Severe heart failure in the elderly person may cause confusion. Problems such as cardiac arrhythmias and congestive heart failure can have a pronounced effect on the elderly person's activity level, because the heart is less able to pump oxygen and nutrients to body parts involved in activity.

Vascular Resistance

The aging process produces changes in the blood vessel walls that affect the transport of nutrients and oxygen to body parts. There is increasing rigidity throughout the arterial system. The most prominent and consistent changes in the arteries are the redistribution, thinning, and fragmentation of elastin and the accumulation of collagen, calcium salts, and lipids (Kohn, 1977). Elastin gives resiliency to the arteries, and diminishes with age independent of the atherosclerotic process. While the elastin is decreasing, collagen is accumulating in the vessels, causing an increase in vascular distensibility (Goldman, 1979). This impairs blood flow and increases the load of the left ventricle. Coronary artery sclerosis becomes increasingly pronounced with age (Strandell, 1976). Loss of elasticity and increased distensibility are particulary apparent in the aorta and the large arteries, which become dilated, prominent, and tortuous (Syzek, 1976). Elongation of the aorta may cause the innominate or carotid artery to buckle and appear as a pulsating mass in the neck (Rossman, 1979). In the aorta, the loss of elasticity is compensated for by increased blood volume. Intraaortic systolic pressure rises more abruptly with the increased amount of blood in the aorta (Goldman, 1979).

Aging is accompanied by a redistribution of blood flow. The effects on the vascular system may become especially apparent when this system receives a demand for a greater flow to specific organ systems, as may occur with marked changes in activity levels. As blood flows through the organs, total peripheral resistance increases and systemic blood flow decreases with age. These changes are not related to vascular pathologies. Alterations in blood supply to the brain, heart, and skeletal muscles have been found to be much less pronounced than changes in the flow to the kidney, viscera, and the hands and fingers (Kohn, 1977).

Increasing atherosclerosis has been found in the blood vessels of the elderly. However, research has shown that atherosclerosis is not an inevitable consequence of aging, even though this pathologic process is considered to be time-related (Rossman, 1979). The degree of atherosclerosis varies among individuals and populations. Epidemiologic studies demonstrate a multifactorial disease process of arteries, with varying effects on different organ systems. The atherosclerotic vascular changes, which account for the dominating disease in the Western world, most frequently affects the coronary, cerebral, and peripheral arteries (Rossman, 1979). Even though coronary artery disease tends to appear the earliest, any person with evidence of atherosclerosis anywhere in the body has a stronger clinical potential for involvement elsewhere in the body. Thus, cardiovascular disease is equated with coronary heart disease, brain infarction, intermittent claudication, and congestive heart failure. Among the risk factors that have been identified are overnutrition, high serum lipids, hypertension, diabetes mellitus, maleness, and a stressful life-style. The greatest risk factor in the development of atheromas, however, is increasing age (Kohn, 1977). Cigarette smoking also may be a factor in the atherosclerotic pro-

cess. As the individual ages, vessel involvement becomes greater. The plaques contain more collagenous connective tissue, and the lesions become more scarlike. Additional changes can result in ulceration, formation of surface thrombi, and hemorrhages (Kohn, 1977).

Atherosclerotic changes in the coronary blood supply resulting in ischemia of the myocardium can be a problem for the elderly, and can eventually lead to anginal pain or a myocardial infarction. Infarction of cerebral tissue can be caused by even a minimal reduction in cerebral blood flow. The incidence of cerebrovascular problems increases with age. Interruption of the supply of oxygen and nutrients to brain tissue by hemorrhage or thrombus of a cerebral or carotid artery can cause a cerebrovascular accident (stroke). Other possible causes include the dislodging of an embolus from a heart valve or of an atherosclerotic plaque, which is then carried into the cerebral circulation. Infarction of cerebral tissue results from even a minimal reduction of cerebral blood flow, caused by decrease in blood pressure, decreased cardiac output, decrease in circulatory blood volume, anemia, or an increase in blood viscosity. Cerebrovascular accidents can lead to major impairments in activity as a result of the potential disruption of innervation to the motor areas of one side of the body when hemiplegia occurs. The central nervous system is responsible for the control of movement. Without the stimulus to move, the muscles affected can atrophy within a short period of time.

Atherosclerosis of the vertebral arteries, combined with the effects of arthritic changes of the cervical spine, may cause these arteries to become kinked and adhere to the cervical spine. The blood supply to the brain through the vertebral arteries may be impaired, especially when the head is extended backward and upwards. Faintness and dizziness may therefore occur when the head is in this position, and the elderly person is likely to fall. Getting objects from high shelves or washing walls may be hazardous for the person with this problem. Sidewise movements of the head may also compress a carotid artery, which already may be narrowed as a result of atherosclerosis. This can also result in dizziness and faintness.

Major blood vessels, such as the aorta and its branches, become less resilient with age. Atherosclerotic lesions of the aorta may cause degeneration and atrophy of the aortic media. This can lead eventually to development of an aortic aneurysm, which tends to occur most frequently in the abdominal aorta (Wright, 1978). Distal aneurysms may involve the iliac and femoral vessels. Because there is danger that the affected blood vessel will rupture, the person with an aneurysm commonly undergoes surgery for replacement of the aneurysm with a graft.

Significant changes have been found in the capillary walls of the elderly person. The basement membrane of the capillary gradually thickens with age (Goldman, 1979). As a result of this thickening, it is suspected that there is a slowing of the exchange of nutrients and waste products across the capillary wall.

Ischemia of Tissues of the Extremities

The atherosclerotic process may take place in the smaller arteries that supply nutrients and oxygen to the lower extremities. This can cause profound discomfort in ambulation, and may even affect the comfort of the extremities at rest. The pain results from a decrease in blood flow to the leg muscles and skin beds, leading to tissue anoxia and local lactic acidosis because of poor tissue perfusion. Intermittent pain may accompany exercise, posture changes, or temperature changes, especially exposure to cold. Pain during exercise, known as *intermittent claudication,* is caused by an inadequate supply of blood to the contracting muscle group. Arterial flow cannot be increased to meet tissue demands.

In the elderly person, intermittent claudication may occur after walking only a few blocks, or walking up a hill. A period of rest permits circulatory recovery through oxygenation of the tissues and the removal of lactic acid. Buttock and thigh pain accompanying activity may result from occlusion of the distal aorta and iliac vessel. A severe restriction of the blood supply to the lower extremities may lead to gangrene, especially in the elderly client with a history of diabetes. Diabetic neuropathy and infection contribute to the problem. Blood supply to the feet is diminished with age. Any prolonged pressure on the foot can result in pressure areas that can become ulcerated. An example of this is the heel of the foot of an elderly person who remains in bed.

The veins and lymphatics probably undergo changes similar to those occurring in the arteries but to a lesser degree, since they appear to be under lower stress. Chronic venous insufficiency is a problem for some elderly persons. This condition can cause ulceration, especially in the lower extremities, and may impair mobility. Veins become dilated and stretched. Structural changes of the valves in the leg veins can affect the venous return and add to the congestion of these veins, resulting in edema of the legs.

Hypertension and Hypotension

With increasing vascular rigidity with age, the systolic blood pressure increases. With increased peripheral resistance to compensate for reduced cardiac output, the diastolic pressure increases with age (Goldman, 1979). Blood pressure in the elderly person appears to be influenced by the elasticity of the walls of the larger arteries. Although mean blood pressure rises with age, this change does not occur consistently among the elderly population. The rate of blood pressure increase seemed to be related to the level of the original blood pressure. Exercise has been found to cause increased systolic pressure and decreased diastolic pressure, but this does not seem to be specifically age-related. However, age-related changes have been observed in the length of time needed for return of the blood pressure to base levels following posture change or exercise (Kohn, 1977). Increasing stiffness in large arteries, accompanied by loss of arterial elasticity, peripheral resistance, and a possible decrease in renal blood flow, which affects the renin–angiotensin system, can influence the elderly person's blood pressure level. The ischemia of the kidney stimulates the production of renin, which then converts hypertensinogen into angiotensin. Angiotensin has a vasoconstricting effect.

Both elevated systolic and diastolic pressure can have an adverse effect on cardiovascular risk factors. A review of research presented by Moser (1979) indicates that elevated blood pressure at any age is a potent risk factor and that elderly people with normal blood pressures, 140/90 mm Hg or below, have greater longevity that those with higher pressures. This was demonstrated through the Framingham study (Castelli, 1976). Systolic elevation is as significant as diastolic elevation in determining prognosis in both sexes at any age. Hypertension for an elderly person is considered to be a systolic reading above 160 mm Hg and a diastolic reading above 95 mm Hg. Elevated blood pressure results in further acceleration of arteriosclerosis, increased myocardial muscle work, and possible cardiac failure (Moser, 1979). Treatment of hypertension in the elderly should avoid sudden and dramatic reductions in blood pressure.

A decrease in blood pressure also can be a problem for the elderly. A sudden decrease in blood pressure may indicate a severe circulatory disturbance or a major cardiac or cardiopulmonary disturbance. Low blood pressure may indicate hypokalemia. A frequent cause of hypotension with the elderly is the use of antihypertensive medications. Once the body is well accustomed to a higher blood pressure, it may not function as well when the hypertension is artificially reduced (Agate, 1979). A sudden drop in the blood pressure of a hypertensive person may cause acute cerebral or coronary insufficiency. Hypotension may be transient and related to posture. Postural hypotension may become intensified in the elderly person, probably as the result of changes in the nervous system and in reflex control of the blood pressure. Serum sodium levels may be below normal in the person with postural hypotension (Agate, 1979). Any decrease in blood pressure may affect cerebral perfusion and therefore produce symptoms associated with cerebral hypoxia (Johnson, 1976). With only a slight decrease in blood pressure, dizziness or altered consciousness may occur. If the decrease is great and rapid, the elderly person may lose consciousness. Symptoms occurring with hypotension can have an adverse effect on the activity of the elderly person. These symptoms can cause falls in the elderly.

Utilization of Oxygen and Nutrients

Increased peripheral resistance can affect the utilization of oxygen and nutrients that are delivered to a body part. This peripheral resistance may be caused by increased stiffness of the connective tissue in and around small blood vessels and throughout the organ parenchyma (Kohn, 1977). As a result of this change, the perfusion of the organ is decreased. That specific organ's role in maintaining activity levels will be altered, and thus will affect the elderly person's tolerance of activity.

Sensory and Motor Effects of Activity

Activity levels of the elderly person are affected by motor and sensory performance. A significant change in the speed of motor performance accompanies the aging process (Welford, 1977). Many factors affect the speed with which an elderly person is able to perform activities. The discussion in this section will cover reaction time, balance, and musculoskeletal changes, as they relate to posture and gait. Alterations in motor functions will be included.

Reaction Time

Studies indicate that reaction time lengthens with age (Welford, 1977). Part of the reason for longer reaction time may be the older person's lack of physical fitness. Older people also seem to be more cautious in reacting to signals. Even though they are slower because of cautiousness, they also tend to be more accurate than young persons when there is time for decision-making (Welford, 1977). Slowness in making decisions may lead to greater numbers of accidents among the elderly, especially when the situation calls for quick responses, such as when driving a car or in industrial occupations. In an industrial job, generally the older person seems to be able to handle tasks requiring moderately heavy physical effort more easily than tasks that demand speed (Welford, 1977).

There is much disagreement about the nature of the changes in the central nervous system that may affect the elderly person's motor functioning. The ultrastructure of the aging brain, including the blood–brain barrier, membrane systems of the central nervous system, and the neurons, has not been adequately studied (Brody and Viyayashanker, 1977). However, available evidence indicates that aging does not randomly alter cell functions in the central nervous system, even though significant changes related to other changing physiologic functions may occur in neuronal metabolism (Finch, 1977). A major obstacle to determination of central nervous system changes in the elderly is the prevalence of cerebrovascular pathologies in many old persons. This makes it difficult to distinguish between normal changes in neural functioning and pathologic cerebrovascular changes.

Although the overall picture of central nervous system functioning of the elderly person indicates a general decrease in abilities, there are certain areas in which performance is decreased only slightly, or is even enhanced. One of these is the effectiveness with which complex situations are evaluated and acted upon. This is an ability generated by experience, and may be referred to as wisdom (Strehler, 1976).

Much about the aging process is not understood. However, it is believed that the nervous system undergoes a steady loss of neurons, which affects the spinal cord and the brain and thus brings about alterations in motor and sensory function. These changes include the loss of tone in the facial, neck, and spinal musculature, loss of ankle jerks and the ability to appreciate tuning-fork vibrations at the ankle, and some loss of position sense in the toes (Carter, 1979).

One pathologic age-related problem that often affects the activity of the elderly person is Parkinsonism. Reports indicate that this condition is related to large losses of monoamines, especially dopamine, in the basal ganglia. A regional selectivity of age-related changes in monoamine synthesis may indicate that certain cell groups and functions are particularly sensitive to aging (Finch, 1977). For example, the extrapyramidal system seems to be more vulnerable than other parts of the motor system. The elderly person may demonstrate decreased and slower movements, infrequent blinking of the eyes, and a decrease in spontaneous and associated movements, often accompanied by tremor. Although these problems exist to a greater degree with Parkinsonism, they may also appear in the elderly person who is not considered to be in a pathologic state.

The speed of muscle contraction is regulated by nerve impulse activity. A general prolongation of contraction may result from muscle disuse. Eventually this may lead to contracture, an abnormal shortening of muscle tissue that makes the muscle resistant to stretching.

Sensory and motor functioning and activity levels can be affected by disorders of the peripheral nerves. These disorders can originate anywhere from the spinal root to the point of muscle innervation. Weakness and loss of reflex may occur in a given area. Several nutritional and metabolic deficiencies are known to cause neuropathies involving the peripheral nerves.

Balance

The ability to maintain a state of balance while performing motor functions is related to the elderly person's reaction time, and influences the individual's activity level potential. Balance is a predominantly sensory function. It is maintained by nerve cells in the vestibular system of the inner ear, the cerebellum, and the proprioceptive pathways in the nervous system. Degenerative changes, such as changes in the joints that often accompany the aging process, may affect the elderly person's ability to maintain balance or regain it once a fall begins. Loss of balance may be one of the first indications that a part of the body is not functioning properly. Many falls and the inability or unwillingness to walk may be caused by loss of balance.

A tendency to lean backward, of which the person is usually unaware, may be observed in individuals who have spent much time in bed or slumped in a chair. The person may need support while standing. Fear of falling also may result in the backward tilt position. The person may be very rigid and be afraid of moving the feet to walk. A backward tilt is sometimes noted in persons with foot pain, who attempt to take weight off the feet by walking on the heels.

Orthostatic hypotension can occur when the person rises to a standing position. The individual often feels faint or dizzy, and may fall as a result. In the elderly person, blood may pool in the lower extremities. This, combined with narrowing of arteries to the brain, can limit the immediate supply of blood to the brain with sudden changes of position, especially the change from lying to standing. Dizziness may also accompany such movements as bending forward, looking up, and making sudden turns while walking. Sudden movement may cause a loss of balance because degenerative sensory changes have affected the nerve cells of the vestibular system of the inner ear. Experiencing a loss of balance can increase the elderly person's fear of falling, and may therefore cause the individual to limit activity levels. Falls cause more than two-thirds of accidental deaths in the elderly who are over 75 years of age (Hellebrandt, 1979). Slowed protective reactions and instability of vertical stance increase the chance to fall. When balance is lost, the elderly person has difficulty stopping the fall. When the person falls, there may be difficulty in getting up even if there are no injuries resulting from the fall. Arm weakness and limitations in hip, knee, and lumbodorsal movements can hinder the ability to stand. Even to get up while holding onto furniture is influenced by the person's ability to flex the knee and hip joints.

Posture

The elderly person may assume a posture of general flexion with the head and neck held forward, a kyphosis of the spine, and slight flexion of the hips and knees. The flexed posture may be caused by changes in the vertebral column and the intervertebral discs, ankylosis of ligaments and joints, shrinkage and sclerosis of tendons and muscles, or degenerative changes in the extrapyramidal central nervous system (Grob, 1978). Much of the decrease in stature typically observed in the elderly person is caused by shortening of the spinal column, resulting from thinning of the discs and loss of thickness in individual vertebrae. Age-related posture changes may also be caused by osteoporosis and its effects on the skeletal system. Osteoporosis commonly accompanies aging. Like atherosclerosis, however, it is not an inevitable consequence of aging, but is considered to be a time-related pathologic event (Rossman, 1979).

Many contradictory theories exist regarding the cause and treatment of osteoporosis. Although the cause of osteoporosis remains uncertain, certain common factors appear to accompany it. The most fundamental change seems to be a reduction of the total amount of bone in the skeleton. Total bone content begins to decrease progressively after age 45 in both sexes, although there is a more precipitous drop in women following menopause. It is believed that osteoporosis results from increased resorption of bone rather than decreased formation of bone (Tonna, 1977). Even within this controversy, theorists appear to agree that there is an imbalance between bone formation and bone resorption in the elderly person. Trabecular bone is affected more than cortical bone.

Immobilization appears to be a significant cause of bone loss. Although osteoporosis is thought to be a physiologic effect of advancing age, pathology occurs when total bone content is reduced below a critical level, with resulting bone pain or fractures (Brocklehurst and Hanley, 1976). The most common fracture site is the upper end of the femur (Wylie, 1977). The majority of fractured femurs are due to falls in the home setting, especially by tripping or falling over flooring materials. Poor illumination and poor vision seem to be concomitant factors in these falls. Another possibility is that the fall occurs after the femur fractures spontaneously as a result of weight-bearing. Women are more susceptible to fractures than are men. They display a higher incidence of vertebral collapse and compression fractures because of the lower mineral baseline in female vertebrae (Tonna, 1977). Factors that can induce or worsen osteoporosis include immobilization or lack of exercise, excessive adrenal corticosteroid activity, other hormonal changes such as those involving estrogen, thyroid, and parathyroid hormones, or vitamin and calcium deficiency. Cigarette smoking also has been reported to be associated with an increased incidence of osteoporosis (Wheeler, 1976). Bone loss may be the result of several processes, which differ in relative importance from individual to individual. Fluoride may have a protective effect against osteoporosis when given for long periods of time (Wheeler, 1976).

Elderly persons display an increased incidence of vertebral atrophy and compression fractures, which may result from changes in the intervertebral discs and the vertebrae. Degenerative changes take place in the cartilage, and the mineral content and structural strength of bone decrease (Tonna, 1977). The progressive collapse of vertebrae can lead to kyphosis, which is characterized by a stooped posture with the head and neck forward and a posterior convex curve of the spine. The expression "hump back" often refers to the increased curvature of the thoracic spine. This posture may also be caused by a decrease in elasticity and calcification of ligaments, and by shrinkage and sclerosis of tendons (Rockstein, 1975). The height of an individual tends to decrease with aging as a result of these changes. This can have a marked adverse effect on the elderly person's self-image. Osteoporosis can affect the activity levels of the old person, especially when fractures occur. The progressive loss of bone with age is responsible for the rapid rise in incidence of serious fractures with increasing age (Wylie, 1977). Hip fractures frequently are used as an index of osteoporosis in a population, because they seldom occur in the elderly person in the absence of osteoporosis (Wheeler, 1976).

Regeneration of injured bone in the elderly person may be prolonged, even though the mechanism for bone repair continues throughout life (Tonna, 1977). Immobility connected with the prolonged repair process can further add to the bone loss that is already present and perhaps was the original cause of the fracture. Weightlessness and immobilization result in accelerated bone loss. Aloia (1981) reported increment in bone mass can occur after a program of physical exercise and involutional bone loss can be prevented by physical exercise. Involutional bone loss refers to reduction of skeletal mass with aging.

Gait

Changes in muscle activity can affect not only the posture but also the gait of the elderly person. Regulation of muscle activity involves neuronal, hormonal, and vasomotor interactions. Muscle changes observed in the elderly may be either the natural result of the aging process or the result of muscle pathologies. Change in the skeletal muscles and a general decrease in muscle strength, endurance, and agility may accompany the aging process. These changes are caused by a decrease in the number of muscle fibers due to the inability of muscle to regenerate, and by fibrous tissue secondarily replacing the contractile elements of the muscle (Rockstein, 1975).

Aging is accompanied by a decrease in muscle weight in relation to body weight. The arm and leg muscles shrink and may have a flabby appearance. The loss of muscle mass is due to a decrease in the number and diameter of the muscle fibers (Gutmann, 1977). The muscles of the elderly person show an increase in extracellular water, sodium, and chloride, with a slight decrease in intracellular potassium. There are reports that aging muscles display lower reaction to stimulation. Muscle atrophy and denervation in the elderly person seem to result from a higher rate of protein breakdown than protein synthesis (Gutmann, 1977). However, many changes in the aging muscle are not specific. Because the elderly person does not appear to regenerate muscle tissue, secondary fibrous tissue replacement can occur. The rate at which these changes take place is highly variable.

Hormonal factors are also involved in age-related muscle changes. Muscle atrophy may follow alterations in the synthesis of the somatotropic and thyrotropic hormones that affect protein metabolism. There may also be changes in the ability of the muscle to utilize the hormone. Activity levels directly affect muscle size and tone, and thus influence the gait of the elderly person.

Neuronal changes such as those that occur

with a cerebrovascular accident can cause the sudden transition from independent movement and gait to dependence and immobility. Another sudden change can occur with a fractured hip.

The functioning of the elderly individual's joints can affect the gait, and thus the individual's activity levels. There seems to be no clear demarcation between pathologic joint changes and those that are due to wear and tear with advancing age. Changes which can occur include unevenness of the articular surface of the joint and the formation of clefts and fissures in the joint cartilage matrix. Chronic rheumatoid arthritis and osteoarthritis may sometimes coexist in the elderly person.

Osteoarthritis is a degenerative disorder of movable joints. It is characterized by deterioration and abrasion of articular cartilage, with formation of new bone at joint surfaces. The cartilage first loses its elasticity, and then becomes softened and frayed. New bone formation occurs at the areas where joint cartilage is thinned, sometimes creating bony spurs. Small pieces of cartilage and bone may become loosened in the joints. These pieces of cartilage and bone, as well as the bony spurs, may set up an inflammatory reaction at the joint. Changes in the joint may be accelerated by injury, excessive use, and excessive weight placed on the joint. The knees, hips, lumbar spine, shoulders, and cervical spine are the major areas affected. The joint changes of osteoarthritis produce pain during movement or pain that occurs when the joint must bear weight. The pain, usually described as aching, tends to be relieved by rest. Stiffness may occur after a period of rest, but this ordinarily persists only for a short time after movement resumes.

Another problem that may affect the joints of the elderly person is rheumatoid arthritis, a systemic disease of connective tissue resulting in joint inflammation. Rheumatoid arthritis is accompanied by inflammation of the synovial membrane, leading to effusion in the joint and proliferation of granulation tissue. The chronic inflammation may cause the joint to become ankylosed. The fingers, toes, wrists, knees, elbows, ankles, shoulders, and hips are most frequently involved, affecting not only mobility but manipulation. The client's activity is limited by the joint pain and tenderness, and by swelling and stiffness, which are especially pronounced following periods of inactivity and upon awakening in the morning. Activity may also be affected by the fatigue that can accompany the inflammatory process.

Fatigue and discomfort may be caused by changes in the feet of the elderly person. The feet may become smaller as a result of loss of subcutaneous fat. The skin may become drier, with calluses forming at pressure points. The muscles that support the arches of the feet may lose their tone and thus place additional strain on the other foot muscles. The blood supply to the old person's feet may be limited by vascular changes affecting the lower extremities, making any trauma to the foot difficult to repair. These joint changes may further limit desired activity levels for the elderly person. The gait of an elderly person may be characterized by small, shuffling steps, with the feet barely lifted from the floor. This increases the possibility of falling as a result of tripping on an object on the floor.

Rest and Sleep

In order to maintain activity, the individual requires adequate time for sleep and rest. Sleep can affect activity levels by its effect on health in general. It is necessary for attention, learning, and activity, and it affects health and well-being, moods, behavior, energy, and emotions (Yura, 1978). Because the function of sleep seems to be related to restoration and integration, sleep reenergizes the power of concentration and interest in daily tasks. A person deprived of sleep may become depressed, sensitive to pain, irritable, apathetic, disoriented, and confused. Studies indicate that there may be a close relationship between cognitive ability and patterns of sleep (Feinberg, 1968). However, no known study of acute total sleep deprivation has been performed with elderly subjects (Dement, Laughton, and Carskadon, 1982). The sleep patterns of the elderly in institutional settings need to be studied further.

Sleep is characterized by distinct cyclical patterns. Normal sleep is divided into two main categories. The first is non-rapid eye movement sleep (NREM), which includes Stages 1, 2, 3, and 4. Stages 1 and 2 occur for brief periods at the onset of the sleep cycle, while Stages 3 and 4 are stages of deep sleep, which follow Stages 1 and 2. During the deep sleep, muscles relax, the pulse slows, and the body temperature drops. The second category is rapid eye movement sleep (REM), which includes the fifth or "active" sleep stage associated with dreaming. REM sleep is necessary for health maintenance. During this stage, there is loss of muscle tonus. When pain is experienced during sleep time it can occur during REM sleep. The person awakens and may have difficulty getting back to sleep if the pain is not relieved. Throughout the night NREM alternates with REM sleep.

The elderly person experiences quantitative as well as qualitative changes in sleep patterns. However, the elderly person does not have a decreased need for sleep. Three major areas of sleep are affected by age-related changes—the length of sleep, the distribution of sleep throughout the day, and the sleep stage patterns. In the elderly person total sleep time is decreased by frequent and lengthy awakenings (Kales, 1975). An old person is more easily awakened, takes longer to fall asleep, awakens more often during the night, and spends more time lying in bed awake. Studies have reported a difference in pattern between men and women. The sleep patterns of women are usually more resistant to age changes (Yura, 1978). The elderly person may experience frequent interruptions of REM sleep. Hypnotic medications also reduce the amount of REM sleep and therefore reduce dreaming. Stage 4 sleep is reduced by 50 percent in the elderly person, as compared to the young adult. Stage 4 is the deepest stage of sleep with regard to arousal threshold, is correlated with the duration of previous waking, and occurs predominantly early in the night (Feinberg, 1976). Feinberg reported that as Stage 4 sleep declined, mental agility declined also, and the individual found it more difficult to learn psychomotor skills.

As the frequency and duration of awakenings increase, the old person may appear to be insomniac. Insomnia in the elderly is sometimes caused by the fear, anxiety, and depression provoked by the realities of declining functioning and inevitable death (Kales, 1975). The term insomnia is used to indicate a relative inability to sleep as a result of difficulty falling asleep, difficulty staying asleep, early final awakening, or a combination of these difficulties. To the elderly, sleep may be perceived as a transient deathlike state and the process of falling asleep may involve emotional regression.

Changes in the home environment or a move to an institutional environment may increase anxiety levels. In a study that compared sleeping patterns of the elderly in a home environment to those observed in a laboratory setting, the differential effects were found to be minor for healthy aged subjects. It was also found that naptime sleep in the elderly may not compensate for impaired sleep at night (Prinz, 1977) Daytime sleepiness may be a specific complaint of some elderly. This daytime sleepiness may be related to sleep fragmentation in the elderly person. The number of brief arousals per hour of sleep at night was reported to be the best indicator of daytime sleepiness (Dement et al., 1982). A major factor in sleep fragmentation is the report of high prevalence of sleep apnea (Dement et al., 1982).

Respiratory impairment during sleep appears to be the sleep disorder that occurs most frequently with the elderly. There may be normal breathing during wakefulness and abnormal breathing during sleep. During sleep an apneic pause is terminated by arousal of the elderly person. Thus it is suggested that much sleep fragmentation is traced to age-related respiratory impairment. Snoring usually indicates an impairment in upper airway function. Respiratory problems that obstruct the airflow may result in upper airway sleep apnea. Health problems such as chronic pulmonary disorders increase the risk of sleep apnea in the elderly. Obesity also may be a factor. A major area of concern related to sleep apnea is the use of medications for sleep. These medications may dangerously prolong apneic periods because of the difficulty the person has of awakening during the apneic episode. Added to this concern are the age-related changes in drug metabolism. Not only are studies with the elderly limited, Dement et al. (1982) indicated that studies relating to hypnotics rarely assess the problem of daytime carryover effect of the medication and impairment of performance and the effect of hypnotics on pulmonary and cardiovascular physiology during sleep. There is a concern relating to prescribing sleeping medications for persons suffering from sleep apnea. The duration of sleep apnea can increase to a dangerous extent. Studies relating to cognitive functioning, psychomotor performance, and daytime sleepiness need to be done with the elderly who frequently take hypnotics.

For the elderly person in an institutional setting it is likely that the person's natural sleep–wake schedule may not coincide with the regimens established in the institution. As a result, there may be inappropriate and excessive use of sedative drugs or physical restraints. A question raised following research reported by Gress, Bahr, and Hussanein (1981) related to the extent to which the variation in patterning of the nocturnal behavior of institutionalized elderly is an individual difference rather than a difference occurring generally among the elderly.

Changes in the elderly person's sleep and rest patterns may reflect life-style changes such as retirement. Individuals who no longer have to meet daily schedules of job and family responsibilities may have more freedom to nap when they wish and to stay in bed longer in the mornings. Boredom and lack of physical activity also may encourage napping.

Exercise

Exercise is prescribed or planned physical activity by individuals or groups. Exercise is vital for physical fitness as it precipitates a flow of interactions that supply energy, remove wastes and promote rest so that the body maintains function longer (Fig. 15.1). There is a universal acceptance of the benefits of exercise. Research indicates that exercise can increase the elderly person's physical capacities and exercise is necessary if the elderly are to maintain optimal health (Welford, 1977; Hellebrandt, 1979).

However, in terms of overall adaptation to exercise, the old person may generally be less effective than the younger adult, although all the exact mechanisms for these differences are not known. Maximum oxygen uptake decreases progressively with aging, but the physical fitness of the elderly person can limit this change. The maximum oxygen uptake that can be achieved during exercise indicates the effectiveness of the functioning of the muscular, cardiovascular, and pulmonary systems. A physically fit and active person has a greater

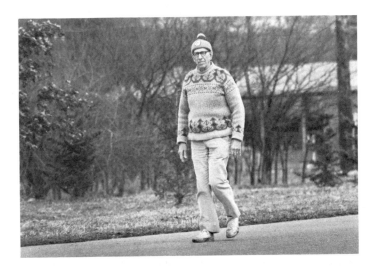

Figure 15.1. Programs of systematic exercise help maintain and improve physical fitness. *(Photograph by Frank Novak, Jr.)*

maximum oxygen uptake than a sedentary person of the same age, and programs of systematic exercise have been found to improve maximum oxygen uptake (Shock, 1977).

Review of research done by Hellebrandt (1979) suggests that physical fitness declines with aging. However, regular physical activity appropriate for the individual in intensity and type should help to maintain physical working capacity into old age (Strandell, 1976). The old person benefits both physically and psychologically from a regular physical activity and exercise program that is within his or her individual capabilities. Training through an exercise program can improve the person's physical condition; however, no lasting benefit will be achieved unless this includes a generally more active life-style with appropriate amounts of spontaneous exercise (Bassey, 1978). Physiologic rather than chronologic age influences work capacity. Chronologic age may exert less effect on an individual's physical capabilities than physical disuse and inactivity (Furlow, Oberman, and Eggert, 1980). Frankel and Richard (1980) suggest that inactivity can lead to immobility which can be a precursor to institutionalization. Shephard (1978) reports that some factors that contribute to problems with an exercise program for the elderly include lack of coordination associated with lack of recent practice and deterioration of balance, obesity, which increases strain, shortening of tendons as a result of years of inactivity, failure of an adequate warm-up time, very active exercise, especially with rapid twisting and excessive stretching, exercise on a hard uneven surface, and the use of shoes that do not have proper heels or ankle supports.

Exercise training adaptations occur mainly in the skeletal muscle, the cardiovascular and respiratory systems and the central nervous system. It is the sum of these changes that increases maximum work capacity and may retard the ravages of atherosclerosis (Furlow, Oberman, and Eggert, 1980). Skeletal muscle adjustments with an exercise program involve an increased aerobic oxidative metabolic capacity. Cardiorespiratory changes include a reduced heart rate at rest and during exercise.

There is increased stroke volume of the heart and a rise in myocardial vascularity, blood volume, and hemoglobin concentration. The greater activity of the muscles and other organs results in greater cardiac output. There is increased blood flow to the skeletal muscles and coronary circulation. The respiratory changes include increased maximal minute ventilation with an associated improvement in ventilatory efficiency of the trained person. Exercise induces an insulin-like effect on cellular glucose uptake, which improves carbohydrate metabolism.

The nursing assessment of the elderly person will demonstrate risk factors as well as facilitate the establishment of activity goals with the client.

ASSESSMENT OF ACTIVITY

Assessment of the elderly person's activity is obtained not only by the nurse but by other members of the health team who have specific assessment skills for determining the activity potential and the activity tolerance of the individual (Table 15.1). This section discusses the activity assessment data which can be gathered by the nurse.

Nursing Assessment of Activity Tolerance

The elderly person's tolerance of activity provides a data base for planning related to the client's appropriate exercise level. Activity tolerance is a measurement of the amount of energy expenditure the individual can manage without unpleasant signs and symptoms, such as shortness of breath, pain, or rapid pulse. Baseline data should be obtained prior to an activity. Additional data, such as pulse and respiratory rates and character, can be obtained during activity and following the activity. Activity tolerance is determined by comparing the data obtained during an activity and following the activity. Data obtained prior to activity give an indication of the elderly person's activity potential. However, an appropriate activity program developed within the

466

TABLE 15-1. GUIDE FOR ASSESSING ACTIVITY

Information about the following can be determined:

Activity tolerance
Activity pattern for a 24-hour day
Time day begins
Morning activities
Afternoon activities
Evening activities
Time in day for optimal activity
Time for going to bed
Precipitation of fatigue
Frequency of fatigue
Duration of fatigue

Breathing effectiveness
Respirations—rate, rhythm, depth, ease, use of accessory muscles
Effort exerted during expiration
Degree and ease of chest expansion
Factors altering respirations
Breath sounds—quality and duration
Supportive devices for breathing
Positions for breathing comfort and ease
Medications affecting respirations
Activity effects on breathing patterns
Cough patterns
Productivity of cough
Degree of comfort while coughing
Characteristics of sputum
Skin color
Lip color
Nail bed color
Smoking history—duration of smoking, amount of smoking
Exposure to air pollutants—occupational and living environment
Pulmonary laboratory values

Transport effectiveness
Pulse rate, rhythm, volume and amplitude
Bilateral pulse comparisons
Apical—radial pulse comparisons
Effect of activity on pulse
Time needed for pulse to return to baseline following activity
Heart sounds
Lower extremity pulses—femoral, popliteal, dorsal pedal and posterior tibial
Color of skin (general)
Color of skin in extremities
Warmth of skin (general)
Warmth of skin in extremities
Effect of extremity elevation on warmth, color and edema

Effect of dependent position of extremity on warmth, color, edema
Comfort of legs with exercise and activity
Skin condition of feet and toes—calluses, corns, pressure areas
Condition of toenails—length, thickness, hardness
Blood pressure—lying, standing, sitting
Medications to alter blood pressure
Bilateral blood pressure comparison
Effect of activity on blood pressure
Chest area comfort with activity
Blood laboratory values
Cardiac functioning test results

Mobility patterns
Posture—lying, sitting, standing, walking
    Curvature of spine
    Flexion at elbows and wrists
    Flexion at hips, knees and ankles
Muscle strength (bilateral)
    Flexors of hip
    Extensors of hip
Muscles of ankles and feet
Muscles of hands and arms
Muscle firmness and size (bilateral)
Muscle tone (bilateral)
Muscle tenderness
Proprioception
    Balance with and without eyes closed
    Coordination of movements
Gait
    Ability to lift feet
    Posture when walking (degree of erectness)
    Width of base
    Length of stride
    Kind and condition of shoes worn
    Arm movements while walking—symmetry and length of arm swing
    Eye gaze while walking
    Evenness of walking pace
    Maintenance of balance
    Comfort while walking
    Areas of discomfort while walking

Ease of mobility
Movement of joints
Comfort of joints—with movement and at rest
Factors that aggravate or relieve discomfort
Contractures
Joint deformity or swelling
Joint tenderness
Degree of range of motion of each joint
Crepitus with movement

Activity patterns
Interest in activity
Preferred activities

Medications affecting activity
Environmental facilitators to activity
 Handrails
 Height and design of chairs
 Height and design of environmental furnishings
 Lighting
 Space for activity
Environmental barriers to activity
Exercise programs

Mobility aids
Degree of confidence in using mobility aids
Feelings relating to use of aids
Knowledge of proper use of the aid

Sleep—rest patterns
Time to bed at night
Number of hours of sleep at night
Frequency of night awakenings
Known reasons for awakening at night
Known snoring and severity of snoring
Naps during the day—frequency and duration
Usual awakening time
Feeling of restfulness when awakening
Aids to sleep
 Medications
 Food or drink
 Sleep clothing
 Amount of covers
 Number of pillows
 Room temperature
 Lighting at night
 Environmental noises at night

Immobility
Degree of immobility
Cause of immobility
Reaction to immobility
Active and passive exercise during immobility

person's potential may lead to an increase in activity tolerance. Measures of activity tolerance that the nurse should assess include indicators of the oxygen and nutrient supply available to support activity, the person's ability to transport the nutrients and oxygen and the waste byproducts of activity, the person's posture, gait, and balance, and the person's degree of comfort and ease during and following the activity.

Assessment of Breathing Effectiveness
To determine the body's degree of efficiency at taking in oxygen, an assessment of respiratory functioning is performed. It is preferable to have the client sit upright for this assessment. The ease, rate, depth, and quality of respirations are assessed while the elderly client is at rest. Depending upon the physical assessment skills possessed by the nurse, assessment may include the thorax and lungs. Inspection, palpation, percussion, and auscultation of the client's chest can be performed. The nurse should be aware of both age-related respiratory changes and those that indicate deviations in the elderly person's health.

The thorax is inspected and its contour noted. While doing this, the nurse also assesses the client's posture to determine its effect on chest expansion, keeping in mind those age-related posture changes that may occur. The ease, rhythm, and rate of respirations are observed. The nurse also observes the amount of effort exerted by the elderly person during expiration. The color of the nail beds and the lips may indicate the adequacy of the oxygen supply made available by the lungs.

To palpate, the nurse's hands are placed on the anterolateral chest to determine the degree and ease of chest expansion. Intercostal muscle changes in the elderly person may alter this expansion.

Percussion of the chest is performed to determine the amounts of air or liquid in the underlying lung. An accumulation of secretions can affect the area available for gas exchange in the lungs. The apices, lateral chest, posterior chest, and anterior chest are percussed.

Auscultation with the stethoscope is used to determine the quality and duration of the breath sounds. Breath sounds are produced by movement of air through the tracheobronchoalveolar system, and increased breath sounds can occur when there is consolidation of lung tissue. Sounds superimposed on breath sounds may be identified in this assessment.

Through interviewing and observation the nurse can determine the client's comfort in breathing and the positions that allow the greatest comfort and ease in breathing. The client may share with the nurse those activities or situations that alter respirations or cause respiratory discomfort, and may relate a history of respiratory problems. The history of smoking and the number of cigarettes smoked each day are relevant data. The person's ability to cough and the productivity of the cough are assessed. The character of any sputum produced may be described by the client or observed by the nurse. The client is questioned about his or her history of coughing and any discomfort it may cause. The time of the day at which coughing occurs and the person's ability to relieve the cough are determined, including any medication the client has taken or is presently taking for breathing or coughing. In relating the quality of the client's oxygen supply to activity, the nurse should be aware of any supportive devices the person may use, such as nebulizers, aerosols, or supplemental oxygen.

As part of this assessment, the elderly person's respiratory rate, depth, rhythm, and breathing ease are noted during and following an activity that has been planned on the basis of resting respiratory function. The elderly person is questioned about the effect of exertion on breathing patterns, such as how many steps can be climbed before breathing difficulty occurs. Any change in chest muscle movement is noted. Dyspnea, a decrease in the respiratory rate, or an irregular breathing rhythm during the activity are all indications for terminating the activity and reevaluating the client's status (Gordon, 1976). With increased activity, the respiratory rate and depth are expected to increase. However, an increase in the resting respiratory rate is significant. The rise in resting respiratory rate may be followed by a rise in pulse rate. With the elderly, an increase in the resting respiratory rate appears prior to a rise in temperature when there is an infection. The nurse should be alert to even a slight upward trend in the respiratory rate.

Assessment of Transport Effectiveness

In assessing activity tolerance, the nurse should be aware of the efficiency with which the client transports oxygen and nutrients throughout the body. This is especially important with regard to areas directly involved with activity— the brain and the muscles, particularly the muscles of the lower extremities. Assessment should therefore determine the elderly person's cardiovascular status. The increased oxygen demand during activity increases the work of the heart, and causes dilation of blood vessels in the contracting muscles. In assessing the transportation of oxygen and nutrients, the nurse observes the resting cardiovascular status of the client, by means of inspection, palpation, and auscultation, as well as interviewing and observation skills. It is advisable to perform this assessment while the client is in sitting, supine, and left lateral positions. Inspection and palpation are used to locate pulsations over the precordium. The data obtained are influenced by the thickness of the chest wall and the amount of adipose tissue that the client carries. Changes in the size of the heart, as determined through palpation, may alter the area in which the apical pulse can be heard. Pulsations may be observed over the precordium or over the carotid area.

Palpation of arterial pulses can determine the rate, rhythm, volume, and amplitude of pulsation. The degree of bilateral arterial elasticity may be indicated by the pliability of the artery when palpated. Changes in elasticity of the vessels are frequently observed in the elderly client. The artery may feel beaded and tortuous in the person with arteriosclerosis (Milasanos et al., 1977). These observations may give clues to the potential resistance blood may encounter when flowing through these vessels to take care of increased demands caused by increased activity. The nurse should record arterial pulses in the lower extremities, including the femoral, popliteal, dorsal pedal, and posterior tibial pulse. These pulses should be palpated in each lower extremity. Absent pulses may indicate arterial obstruction proximal to the palpation site. The Doppler Ultrasonic Velocity Detector can be used to provide functional evaluation of the arterial circulation of the extremity. Elevation-dependency tests and skin temperatures at different levels are methods for assessing the circulation status of the extremity. The extremity should be elevated 60 degrees and the lighting should be adequate for accurate visualization. Rapid blanching of the toes and foot on elevation and marked rubor on dependency may indicate poor circulation to the extremity. A distinct difference in skin temperature between the proximal and distal areas of the extremity may indicate a degree of arterial occlusion.

The elderly person may relate problems of intermittent claudication that is precipitated by activity. An active person with blood supply problems to the lower extremities may complain of intermittent claudication at an earlier stage of the problem than one who is sedentary (Friedman, 1976). Intermittent claudication is a major indicator of skeletal ischemia. It may be experienced as pain, a feeling of discomfort, or a feeling of tiredness or tightness, which is most pronounced during walking and is relieved when the person stops to rest. With severe ischemia, pain may be present even with rest. This pain tends to be severe and worse at night. It is aggravated by elevation of the part and by cool temperatures. The person may describe the discomfort as "cramps" or "ache." The discomfort may be located in the foot, calf, thigh, hip, or buttock. The area involved depends on the level of the occlusive problem. Assessment should include palpation of pulses for amplitude of pulsation and observations prior to and following activity. To determine the degree of venous efficiency in the lower extremities, the presence and the degree of edema are observed, along with skin color and skin integrity. If edema is present, it may interfere with the person's comfort when wearing shoes and walking.

The heart rate, as determined by palpating an artery or by listening to the apical pulse, provides information about the effect of activity on the work of the heart. The baseline pulse rate should be obtained during the client's sleep. In listening to the apical pulse, the nurse may find the position of the apex of the heart to be altered because of changes in heart size. Simultaneous observations of the apical and radial pulse may indicate a pulse deficit, if the apical rate is higher than the radial rate. Although heart rate in the elderly individual rarely reaches as high a level with activity as that of a younger person, changes noted during and following various kinds of activities are significant, and can serve as a base for planning levels of activity with the client.

The amount of time required for the pulse rate to return to baseline level should be assessed. The old person may require a longer period of time to return to baseline pulse rate. Pulse rate should be assessed at approximately 5-minute intervals until it returns to the baseline. In assessing the client's tolerance of activity, the nurse should obtain a baseline pulse rate before discussing the planned activity, since anticipation of activity can increase the pulse rate, especially if discomfort or difficulty is associated with this activity. Emotional and physical stresses may have similar effects on the pulse rate (Gordon, 1976). In planning and intervention relating to activity, it is important for the nurse to differentiate the factors that appear to cause change in the pulse rate.

Cardiac rhythm provides a gross indication of the heart's conduction system. A change from regular to irregular rhythm during or following activity can be a gauge of the degree of activity tolerance and may be an indication for altering the client's activity levels. The strength of the pulse indicates the force of cardiac contraction. If the pulse becomes rapid and weak rather than stronger, a change in activity is called for until more definitive assessment data can be obtained.

Another measure for assessing tolerance of activity is determination of blood pressure. Increased peripheral resistance in the elderly person may result in higher baseline blood pressure than that of a younger person. Baseline blood pressure should be determined for each individual, rather than establishing a baseline blood pressure level on the basis of general population norms. Postural hypotension may affect activity levels by causing alterations in the person's posture and equilibrium. Assessing the blood pressure while the client is lying, sitting, and standing can provide data about the degree of blood pressure change when the person moves from one position to another. The client can be instructed to change positions slowly rather than abruptly. The medications that the elderly person is receiving should be assessed for their effect on the blood pressure. When a person is receiving medications for hypertension, the person may complain of not feeling as well especially if he has recently started to take a medication for a long-standing hypertension.

The elderly person's degree of comfort during and following activity should be assessed. Chest comfort is especially significant, since anginal pain may occur with activity. The kind and amount of activity that produces this discomfort should be noted. Absence of discomfort is also significant, because it indicates that the supply of oxygen and nutrients to the heart muscle itself is adequate to support increased activity without producing the pain warnings that accompany cardiac ischemia.

Assessment of Mobility Patterns

Mobility patterns involve the frequency, intensity, and duration of a person's motor activities, in a specified period of time and a specified environment. The degree of comfort or discomfort in the elderly person's muscles and joints affects ease of movement and therefore the activity levels. Another important influence is the client's posture.

Assessment of Posture and Gait

Posture is alignment of the body segments in relation to one another. In assessing posture, the nurse first views the person from the front and from behind while standing. The curvature of the spine is assessed, and the presence or absence of kyphosis is noted. The nurse also assesses the degree of flexion at the elbows and wrists for their effects on the posture. The degree of flexion at hips, knees, and ankles can affect movement as well as posture.

The relationship of innervation to posture is next assessed. The basal ganglia affect posture by controlling postural integration of the body segments with each other and with equilibrium. This function is complementary to antigravity mechanisms (Adams, 1977). The altered posture of the client with Parkinsonism demonstrates the effect of the basal ganglia on maintenance of posture. The rigid and flexed posture frequently seen in the elderly person may be a manifestation of age-related changes in the nervous system (Beasley and Ford, 1976).

The posture of the client is also assessed in the sitting and lying positions. The slumped posture of an old person sitting in a chair is a familiar sight to any nurse who works with the elderly. The nurse should determine whether deviations in the older client's posture have a physiologic base or are the result of a depressed mood. This has implications for the nursing plan and interventions with the client.

Gait may also be affected by both psychologic and physiologic factors. For example, the elderly person who walks slowly with difficulty lifting his feet may be demonstrating behavior related either to mood or to physiologic problems. Gait can be affected by muscle weakness. Muscle atrophy can have a variety of causes, including disuse of the muscles during a period of immobility. Measuring muscle size may provide important data about the client who appears to have a loss in muscle mass. Muscles are inspected for firmness, size, and may be palpated to determine their consistency. While assessing the muscles, the nurse may question the client about any areas of tenderness noted. Muscle strength may be assessed by observing the muscle's ability to overcome resistance applied by the nurse. Muscle strength is expected to be greater on the dominant side of the body. It is especially important to assess the muscles controlling hip and leg movement. Hip strength is assessed by having the client, in a supine position, raise each extended leg while the assessor attempts to hold it down. The psoas major muscle and the iliopsoas muscle are the main flexors of the hip joint. Their strength can be assessed by having the client elevate the thigh while sitting on the edge of the bed. The assessor then applies resistance to the knee. The gluteal, abductor, and adductor muscles of the leg are assessed by having the client alternately cross the legs while in a sitting position. Assessment of the quadriceps muscle is done by having the client extend the leg while the assessor attempts to bend it at the knee. The muscle of the ankle and feet are assessed by having the client exert upward foot pressure against the nurse's hands.

In the assessment of muscle strength, the assessor's maximum effort against the client's contracted muscles should not overpower any muscle of the lower extremities. A sudden collapse of muscle strength after initial strong resistance does not indicate muscle weakness, but usually indicates that the client has decided not to maintain effort or is unable to maintain effort because of pain (Andriola, 1978). The person may be asked to step up on a stool to further assess muscle strength of the lower extremities. The gluteus maximus is the main extensor of the hip. Its strength can be tested by observing the client rising from a chair or climbing stairs. If the strength of the gluteus is diminished, the client will use his or her hands or assume an awkward position during such activity.

The muscles of the hands and arms can affect the elderly person's activity. The arms are often needed when the person moves from a sitting to a standing position. Asymmetrical weakness or paralysis of one arm may alter the client's balance. Muscle weakness may cause the person to tire easily. The nurse should determine whether the client finds it difficult to rise from a chair or climb stairs. The person may be observed as he or she cautiously clutches furniture or other aids to balance while walking.

In the assessment of gait, there must be adequate space for the person to walk freely, and an area with a few stairs is preferred. If the client uses a cane or other mobility aid, the gait is observed while the person uses the aid. The width of the base while the person is walking and standing is noted. Any limping observed is important. The degree to which the feet are lifted is assessed, as well as the length of the stride, which influences the speed and stability of the gait. The presence of a shuffling gait will have implications for environmental planning. If the client limps or tends to favor one side more than the other, intervention may have to include the use of a cane.

The client's posture should be noted as part of the gait assessment. The ability of the person to stand erect is important, since a slouching posture can alter the center of gravity during walking as well as the distribution of weight over joint areas of the hip and knee. The kind of shoes the person is wearing should be noted, and the nurse can ask about the kind of shoes and slippers that are usually worn. As the person walks, the symmetry and length of the arm swing are observed. The direction of the gaze should be noted. The person may look straight ahead or may keep the gaze to the floor. The evenness of the walking pace is observed.

Assessment of Equilibrium and Balance

Balance is maintained by interactions of the muscles, joints, tendons, visceral senses, the cerebellum, the eyes, and the vestibular apparatus of the inner ear. The vestibular apparatus and the cerebellum inform the person of movements and the position of the head, coordinate body muscles, and position the eyes with head movement. The proprioceptive area of the nervous system maintains posture, balance, and coordination. Muscle sense is maintained through these pathways. The cerebellum controls the integration of muscle contractions for maintaining posture. Final integration of reflex and voluntary mechanisms occurs in the cerebral cortex. It is at the cerebral cortex level that failure of control of posture, balance, or equilibrium must be compensated for through experience and relearning. However, this level also displays evidence of depleted reserves with aging or as a result of cerebrovascular accident. Defective postural control may therefore be observed in the elderly person, especially following a cerebrovascular accident (Adams, 1977).

To assess proprioceptive functioning the nurse observes specific activities. The client may be asked to close his eyes and alternately touch his nose with the tip of the index finger of each hand repeatedly with increasing speed. The person may also be asked to touch his nose with an index finger, then to touch the nurse's index finger, which is held approximately 18 inches away. The nurse should be aware that these activites may be affected by muscular or joint dysfunction or discomfort, rather than by alterations in proprioceptive functioning.

Another way to assess proprioceptive functioning is to ask the client to touch each finger of one hand to the thumb of the same hand as quickly as possible. Changes in the finger joints of the elderly person may affect the ease with which this can be done. Another assessment procedure can be done while the client is in the recumbent position. The person is asked to run the heel of each foot down the opposite shin. The client may be requested to touch the ball of each foot to the nurse's hand while lying on his back. The degree of mobility of the elderly person's hip and knee joint may affect this assessment process.

Proprioception can be assessed by observing the client's ability to hop in place on alternating feet, to stand on one foot and then the other, and to walk in a straight line. Gait can be assessed as the client walks with his eyes closed and with his eyes open. With the eyes closed and then open, the client may be asked to stand with the feet together. The nurse observes any swaying movement that occurs, particularly when the eyes are closed (Romberg's sign). Another assessment technique is to blindfold the person and ask him to describe the position of the extremities. Visual images help the person to maintain equilibrium through the visual detection of the stance. Slight movement of the body shifts the visual images on the retina, and this information is relayed to the equilibrium centers.

The elderly person's balance can be observed while walking. Any periods of dizziness should be noted. The client can then be asked about the positions in which dizziness occurs, the activities that precipitate it, and the time of day at which it happens. For example, the elderly person may complain of dizziness when looking down a staircase. The person's reactions to dizziness should be determined, because dizziness may cause a fear of ambulating or a fear of ambulating without support. The nurse should also distinguish between dizziness and vertigo. Dizziness involves a light-headed, unsteady or faint feeling, or a disturbed sense of relationship to space. Vertigo involves a hallucination of motion. The individual may feel that the world is moving around him (objective vertigo), or that he is revolving in space (subjective vertigo).

Equilibrium and balance are affected by alterations in muscle innervation. Change in innervation, such as the hemiplegia or hemiparesis that can follow a cerebrovascular accident, affects balance. In some cases balance is so markedly affected that the client requires a wheelchair.

Assessment of Ease of Mobility

The ease with which the elderly person moves is assessed, and may provide an indication of the person's comfort during ambulation. A major factor in ease of movement is the adequacy of joint functioning. Joint movement can be affected by discomfort, joint muscle spasm, contracture, and incongruity of surfaces. The joints should be inspected for deformities and swelling, and may be palpated to determine areas of tenderness. An attempt is made to put the joints through as full a range of motion as possible, while considering the client's comfort. During movement, the nurse listens for crepitus. The joints of both upper and lower extremities are assessed.

The client's history may reveal problems with rheumatoid arthritis, osteoarthritis, or degenerative joint changes, and the client may describe pain accompanying movement of the joint. The nurse assesses factors that the client describes as either aggravating or relieving the pain. Pain in a joint may start suddenly during performance of a normal movement or activity, or it may start insidiously while the person is at rest. It may be relieved by rest, or rest may cause increased stiffness and then increased pain. Many movements or only a single movement may be painful. The pain may remain localized or it may radiate.

Pain caused by walking may be experienced in the buttock, the groin, or the inner aspect of the thigh or knee. The nurse should be aware that pain in these areas may be referred from the hip. The purpose of this assessment is not to make a differential diagnosis, but to gain an understanding of the type of discomfort the client experiences and the factors that aggravate or relieve it. The degree of discomfort will have an effect on the client's activity levels. The nurse should learn which joints present the greatest problem to the client and which are the most supportive assets.

The condition of the elderly person's feet will affect ease of mobility. The nurse assesses the color, warmth, and skin integrity of the feet. The presence of calluses and corns may give clues about the person's gait or the fit of shoes. The toes and toenails should be carefully inspected. The color of the nails and the venous filling time can be part of the assessment. The toenail is depressed, and the time required for the return of color is evaluated. The thickness and hardness of the toenails are observed. Unusually long toenails may appear to be deformed because of their length. The elderly person may not be able to reach the nails or to see them clearly for cutting, or they may be too thick to cut easily. The type of footwear that is worn by the elderly person is part of this assessment.

Nursing Assessment of Activity Patterns

The activity patterns of the elderly person may or may not relate to data obtained from assessment of activity tolerance or mobility patterns. The person's motivation and interest in activity have a major role in determining activity patterns. The nurse should learn what the client's activities are, what they have been in the past, and what the client would like them to be. The environment of the individual will also influence activity patterns. Research indicates that environmental prevention programs which reinforce high levels of activity can retard the degenerative processes associated with aging, and can help to maintain verbal and self-care skills (McClannahan, 1973).

Assessment of Environment

The appliances and furnishings in the elderly person's living environment should be assessed. This includes such things as the height and design of chairs, the availability of handrails or supports (especially in bathroom areas), the height of the toilet and sinks, the lighting of the environment, and the quality of the floor surface. If the client depends upon a wheelchair for mobility, the nurse should assess the fit of the person to the wheelchair and the environmental barriers that may limit the client's space, such as the width of doorways. The nurse should note activity facilitators in the environment as well as barriers to activity. Ramps that have been built to facilitate the use of a wheelchair can cause problems for the elderly person who is walking. Ramps can cause a forced distortion of balance that affects the person's center of gravity.

The amount of space available for activity can determine the quality and quantity of the person's activity. The living space available in an institutional setting may place severe limitations on activity. A study was performed at a multilevel geriatric center to determine factors that affected wandering behavior. The results indicated that an abrupt change from the person's home and routine to the new environment and schedule of a nursing home may be stressful, and many persons seek release from stress through methods developed earlier in life to reduce tension, such as taking a brisk walk or a long stroll. The study also showed that some wandering was related to activity patterns developed throughout the person's life, such as expressing a desire to sew, or attend to the children, or going through the motions of adjusting furniture (Snyder et al., 1978). These behaviors stemmed from the person's need for activity.

Another aspect of activity patterns involves the inability of some elderly persons to cope with the fast-paced modern world. Such activities as crossing streets quickly during the green light and climbing the steps of buses may be beyond the capacity of an old person who experiences a slowing of response (Gioiella, 1978). This may lead to anxiety and even withdrawal from many activities on the part of the elderly person who feels unable to handle them because of lack of energy.

The sensory assessment is important with regard to activity patterns, which may be altered to a greater degree by sensory changes than by changes in motor function. For example, an individual learns about his or her surroundings through sight and sound. Sensory impairment can affect the elderly person's ability to scan the territory, and thus can limit the person's perceived space available for activity. The ability to identify sounds correctly provides a feeling of greater security in moving about in the environment. If the client demonstrates adequate sensory functioning, the nurse should determine whether environmental changes are affecting the person's activity patterns. When the elderly person moves from a familiar world to new and unfamiliar surroundings, the person may experience immobilization in the unknown and unpredictable environment. This can markedly affect activity patterns.

The medications that the elderly person is receiving should be assessed. Many medications, such as sedatives and tranquilizers, produce side effects that can alter the person's posture, balance, gait, and activity tolerance. The nurse may be able to connect deviations in these areas with the effects of a medication that the person is receiving. For example, the side effects of sedatives, tranquilizers, and antidepressants may include drowsiness, distortions of judgment, hypotension, and impairment of gait (Price, 1978).

Assessment of Mobility Aids

The elderly person with a mobility problem may require a mobility aid. The nurse should assess the client's ability to make fullest use of the aid, whether it is a wheelchair, cane, walker or handrail. The degree of confidence that the person appears to demonstrate is assessed, and the areas and places to which the person travels with the aid are noted. The nurse should also determine the client's reaction to the mobility aid. The person may remain sedentary because of embarrassment in using the aid or because of lack of knowledge about its use. The need to depend on a mobility aid may have a negative effect on the elderly person's self-image and self-esteem.

The client's ability to use a mobility aid independently may be determined by the person's level of competence, as assessed by the health team. One study of residents in a geriatric setting demonstrated that no physical restraints were placed on the mobility of those who were considered competent. Walking aids were provided for residents who needed them. However, the residents in a unit for impaired elderly persons were restrained in a variety of ways, such as in geriatric chairs with tables locked across their arms. The single wheelchair available in this unit was usually tied to one of the handrails along the corridor when a resident was seated in it. Besides these physical constraints on activity, drugs such as tranquilizers, sedatives, and hypnotics were administered to keep the residents in their place (Maxwell, Baden, and Watson, 1972). Withholding a mobility aid from the elderly client who needs it for ambulation is equivalent to forcing the person to be immobile.

If the client maintains out-of-bed activity by using a wheelchair, the nurse should assess the way the person fits the wheelchair, the amount of uninterrupted time spent in it, and the manner in which the client maneuvers it. The activity of the person who spends much time in a geriatric wheelchair may be severely impaired, since maneuvering within the environment is impossible.

Nursing Assessment of Sleep–Rest Patterns

The sleep and rest patterns of the elderly person can affect activity patterns. The nurse should determine the individual rest and sleep needs of each client. In assessing sleep and rest patterns, the nurse can gather most of the data through interviewing the person and his or her family. The sleep pattern assessment should include the time the person goes to bed at night, the number of hours slept each night, the number of times the person tends to awaken at night, and whether these awakenings are caused by the need to visit the bathroom. If awakening occurs during the night, the nurse should determine how easily the person falls asleep again. The usual time that the person awakens and the way the person feels upon awakening are included in the assessment, along with any help needed to fall asleep at night, such as medication or a before-bed snack. If a sleeping medication is used, assessment should include type of medication, dosage, and frequency of taking the medication. If a medication is needed for sleep, the daytime responses of the elderly person should be assessed. This includes experiences of drowsiness, motor and cognitive functioning. The presleep intake of an alcoholic beverage needs to be determined. This is especially significant for the person who also takes a medication for sleep or for the person who

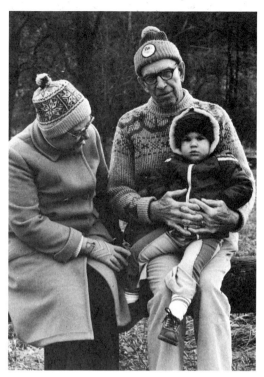

Figure 15.2. To promote activity, the person needs planned periods of rest. *(Photograph by Frank Novak, Jr.)*

has pathologic problems affecting respirations. With breathing problems, the person may be fearful of falling asleep with the thought that he or she might not awaken.

Differences in sleep clothing, the amount of covers, the number of pillows, and the temperature of the room may make it difficult for the elderly person to fall asleep in an unfamiliar bed or environment. This may occur with the person who changes from one living environment to another home setting or to an institutional setting. If the client has been accustomed to a private bedroom, sleeping pattern changes may accompany the need to share a room with another person. The nurse should determine how much light and noise the client is accustomed to in the sleeping environment.

The elderly person may be in a setting that allows the nurse to observe sleep and rest patterns. The rest and sleep that take place during the day are significant. If the elderly person does not seem to be getting adequate rest, the nurse can ask the client how much sleep he or she believes is needed. With any sleep disorder, there is a need to determine physiologic as well as psychologic disturbances and their interrelationships. For example, pain experienced during the day may be magnified when the person tries to sleep at night. Fear and anxiety about an illness may be overwhelming at night. The person's physical and mental health have a strong influence on sleep–rest patterns.

Immobility

The elderly person may be immobilized in bed or in a chair throughout the entire day. The length and the degree of immobility must be determined by the nurse, and their effects on the client carefully assessed. The activity potential of the elderly person must also be determined. Much of the old person's capacity to enjoy life depends on the ability to maintain desired activity levels.

PLANNING AND INTERVENTIONS FOR ACTIVITY OF THE ELDERLY PERSON

The nurse plans and intervenes with the elderly person to maintain optimal activity levels and to increase them if activity is inadequate. The nurse intervenes by supporting the client's assets, while the client restores and compensates for changes or losses that alter activity levels. The nurse assists in prevention or removal of barriers to activity, and helps to prevent and limit disabilities caused by periods of reduced activity. Goals are established relating to the elderly person's activities in the home, the community, and in institutional settings. The nurse–client goals are based on the individual's activity tolerance and desired activities. For example, the client may wish to be able to get in and out of bed, in and out of a chair, climb stairs, and to walk. The nurse plans with the client, the health team, the family, or significant others.

Intervening for the Maintenance or Enhancement of Activity Tolerance

Activity tolerance levels can be maintained or raised through continued activity or increasing activity. The assessment data regarding activity tolerance will determine the activity base from which the elderly person begins. Routine acceptance of the present activity tolerance level as optimal can result in regression of activity as aging proceeds and body alterations continue. This regression may decrease the person's zest for living.

Exercise programs are an excellent way to promote dynamic fitness in the elderly person, using as a base the individual's present activity tolerance level. When considering various interventions, the nurse should be aware of the characteristics of an activity, including the amount of effort required, the body movements necessary, and the degree of control the client feels in trying to perform the activity.

Maintaining and Restoring Activity Through Exercise Programs

In 1873, in an address delivered at Liverpool College, Edward Stanley, the Earl of Derby, remarked that those who think they have no time for exercise will sooner or later have to find time for illness. More than 100 years later, this belief is actively supported by many researchers. Exercise helps a person look, feel, and function better, and thus enhances both self-esteem and self-image. Exercise programs for the elderly are becoming increasingly available, many being provided by community agencies, including senior citizen centers. In a news release, Dr. Raymond Harris, a practicing geriatric cardiologist, reports that more than half of his clients complain of symptoms and other difficulties that they mistakenly attribute to the aging process and disease. In the opinion of Dr. Harris, these problems are more often the result of a chronic state of muscular and cardiovascular unfitness (Clark, 1979). For these clients, Dr. Harris prescribes a gradually expanding program of exercise.

The role of the nurse is to assist the elderly person in recognizing and accepting the value of an exercise program; to inform the person of the availability of such programs, to assist

in the health assessment that determines the person's baseline activity tolerance, and to support the client as he or she participates in an exercise program. The nurse can assist the elderly person with an exercise program in the home setting, collaborate with other health team members in establishing exercise programs in the community, or take part in the establishment of programs in nursing homes or other similar settings. Exercise guides are available from several sources. The Administration on Aging can provide several guides relating to exercise and fitness.

Exercise programs are based on a gradual increase of activity as the person's tolerance increases. The elderly person's exercise program needs to be tailored to the person's fitness level. The elderly person should be cautioned about the need to avoid unusual and sudden demands on the cardiovascular system. For example, exercise should be avoided until about 2 hours following a large meal. The pulse rate is an important determinant of the tolerance of activity. The pulse rate should be checked during and immediately following exercise. It is recommended that the individual increase other activity levels throughout the day as the exercise program progresses. To increase the efficiency of the heart and lungs, continuous rhythmic exercises must be performed for a period long enough to stress the circulatory system (The Fitness Challenge in the Later Years, 1975). These exercises include such activities as brisk walking and swimming. The nurse should stress the value of the health assessment prior to beginning the activity program. The elderly person with problems of the lower extremities, or other mobility problems, can perform alternative excercises, such as going through bicycle movements while lying on a supportive surface. Arm and leg exercises can be performed while sitting in a chair. However, isometric exercises may be considered dangerous because they tend to be Valsalva-producing exercises. An exercise that results in forced expiration against a closed glottis may affect the cardiovascular system. When straining occurs with the glottis closed, intrathoracic pressure rises and partially blocks the return of blood to the heart. As a result, the heart beat may increase significantly in order to move blood that has pooled in the large blood vessels. With the termination of the Valsalva, the blood accumulated in the large vessels rushes toward the heart. The effects of Valsalva-producing exercises can be avoided by keeping the glottis open by taking short rapid breaths. To avoid holding the breath during an exercise is recommended in exercise programs for the elderly since the elderly are at risk because of the high incidence of abnormalities of the cardiovascular system (Hellebrandt, 1979). Exercise programs for the elderly should be developed to maximize the rhythmic activity of large muscles. Before beginning a vigorous physical activity program, the person's current health status needs to be assessed. Programs have been designed to evaluate the person's current health and fitness status. Evaluation includes the person's cardiovascular status, pulmonary function, musculoskeletal function, body composition, and personal life-style. An evaluation of life-style includes dietary habits and health hazard appraisal.

Caution also is advised in planning exercise for an elderly person with severe osteoporosis. Exercises that place the primary stress on the musculoskeletal system or that affect stability and balance during the exercise may place the elderly person at a high risk of falling (Hellebrandt, 1979).

Warmup exercises are advised for at least 5 minutes to limber the muscles and joints and to increase circulation to major muscle groups. Joints should be put through the full range of motion. The muscles should be stretched slowly. After warmup, the aerobic portion of the exercise begins. Aerobic exercise is any physical activity that stimulates the heart and lungs to take up and deliver oxygen to body tissues more efficiently. The response of the person's body depends on the intensity of the effort and the frequency and duration of exertion. The intensity of the exercise should not be exhaustive. However, the exercise should induce the client to increase the heart rate to approximately 60 percent of the maximum heart rate. For the elderly client, three nonconsecutive sessions each week are usually recommended. A 5-minute cool-down period is needed following the exercise. The cardiac rate is allowed to return to normal at this time. During this time, blood that has been supplying the muscles during exercise returns to the central circulation. Slow walking allows for the cool-down to occur. Clients need to recognize the effects of overexertion, fatigue, excessive dyspnea, musculoskeletal injury, and cardiovascular warning symptoms.

There are also exercise programs for the elderly person whose physical disabilities sharply limit activity. A passive or active exercise program may be appropriate for the person with muscle atrophy. With exercise, the muscle can increase in size and become stronger. An exercise program can decrease joint stiffness and increase mobility. The elderly person can be encouraged to exercise with a group, which adds social value to the exercising. A successful program should sustain the interest of the elderly participant through physiologic gain as well as positive changes in mood and reduction of anxiety.

Some elderly persons, especially those with marked weakness or paresis, may be able to move a limb through only part of its normal range of motion. Through assisted range-of-motion exercises, the nurse can help the client to complete a full range of joint movement. Because both active and assisted exercises require muscle contractions, they help maintain muscle tone. If the elderly person cannot assist with range-of-motion exercises, the nurse can perform passive range-of-motion exercises. Passive exercises do not maintain muscle tone, because no active contraction of the person's muscle is involved. However, passive exercise does help to keep the joints mobile. While performing the passive range-of-motion exercises, the nurse supports the extremity at a joint while moving another joint through the full range of motion. The motions should be slow and smooth, with a pause if spasticity causes resistance. As soon as the elderly person has movement, these exercises are done with assistance until full movement is achieved. Following the return of full movement, the elderly person is encouraged to do the full range of motion without assistance.

There is a current emphasis on designing

environmental furnishings to make life easier for the elderly person. For example, the heights of shelves, countertops, and appliances are being altered so that they are more convenient for the elderly person. However, advocates of exercise programs believe that these adjustments further limit the bending, moving, and stretching that help maintain activity levels for the old person.

Providing for the need for exercise for the elderly person should be evidenced in the community environment. For safe walking there should be adequate sidewalk or other walking areas. These areas should be maintained and well lit. Promoting activity through exercise can encourage the independent functioning of elderly people.

Facilitating Mobility Functions

Data from the assessment base are utilized in facilitating the mobility functions of the elderly client. The individual may need to improve posture in order to increase the stability of the gait, to improve balance, and to increase breathing capacity. The nurse can help the person to practice sitting and standing with the shoulders back and the head held high, while tightening the abdominal muscles and the gluteus maximus. As the client stands back to the wall, he or she should attempt to touch the wall with the hips, shoulders, and head. Once the person gets the feel of this position, it can be used when walking or standing.

The elderly person should learn to be aware of his or her posture while sitting, lying, and standing. The appropriate posture for sitting is with the shoulders and buttocks against the back of the chair. Since a low, soft chair or couch inhibits this position, the nurse can suggest the use of a straight-backed wooden chair with a seat height that allows the person to rest the feet on the floor. A client who is seen to slouch while standing, sitting, or lying can be reminded of the need to maintain or attempt to assume a straighter posture. In a nursing home setting, the nurse may unwittingly encourage a slumped posture by having the elderly person placed in a poorly fitting wheelchair or geriatric chair for hours at a time. Slumped posture may be aggravated by fatigue

resulting from a prolonged period in one position.

The client can be instructed about the appropriate way to sit down in a chair (Fig. 15.3). The person should stand in front of the chair with the back toward it, with the feet slightly apart and partly under the chair. When preparing to sit, the person bends at the knees and bends the body forward while extending the buttocks toward the chair. If the chair has arms, the client's arms rest on the chair arms as the body is lowered. When rising from the sitting position, the weight of the body is again supported by the arms. The body is brought forward to the edge of the chair by sliding the hips. The person then bends forward at the waist, and with the weight on the hands and legs, the body is bent forward into a standing position.

The elderly person may need guidance in the way to move from a lying to a standing position. Changes in position should be done slowly and carefully. Abrupt movements may cause dizziness and lead to a fall. When moving from the lying position, the elderly person should first raise the head slowly on rising to the sitting position. The person should sit up slowly, with the feet over the side of the bed, and should remain in this position for a few minutes. Next, the person stands slowly beside the bed. If dizziness occurs, the person can sit down again. While sitting, the person can lower the head to help counter the symptoms. If there is no dizziness, the person can walk slowly until in balance. Wearing elastic stockings can reduce pooling of blood in the lower extremities.

To facilitate mobility functions of the elderly client with joint inflammation or discomfort, the nurse can teach the person to use the strongest joints available for the activity, while continuing to support movement in the affected joint. For example, if a joint of the lower extremity is inflamed, the support of crutches, a cane, or a walker may be needed. This permits the arm muscles to bear part of the person's weight during ambulation. After inflammation of a joint has subsided, passive exercises may be followed by assisted and then active exercise.

Control of pain and discomfort can facili-

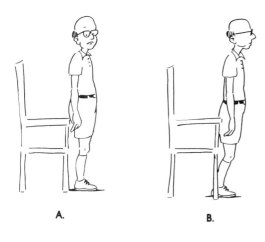

A.

B.

Figure 15.3.
(A) Stand with the back directly to the center of the chair. **(B)** Place feet partly under the chair.

(C) Bend at the knees while leaning the torso forward and extending the buttocks toward the chair. **(D)** Slide the buttocks to the back of the chair. Use the arms of the chair for support.

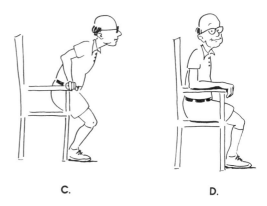

C.

D.

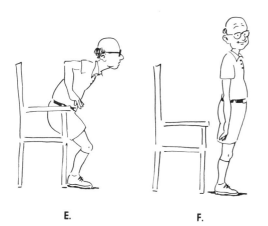

E.

F.

(E) To stand, bring the body forward to the edge of the chair. Bend the knees forward. Use the arms of the chair for support of body weight. **(F)** Stand erect in front of the chair until standing equilibrium is attained. *(Drawings by Harry Trumbore.)*

tate the elderly person's activity levels. The client may already have discovered positions that reduce discomfort. However, maintenance of the same position over a long period of time may limit the use of the affected part and result in muscle atrophy or a contracture. The person can be taught relaxation techniques, which are helpful in reducing muscle tension that may be aggravating the pain. A variety of relaxation techniques can be utilized. In progressive relaxation, the person tenses a set of muscles before allowing them to relax, in order to feel the difference between tension and relaxation. In systematic relaxation, the person concentrates on relaxation of the muscles from the feet up to the head or the head to the feet in a systematic way. The person may be lying or sitting with the eyes closed. Practice with these relaxation techniques may help to prevent pain or reduce discomfort. Control of pain is necessary since pain may lead to immobilization, causing further joint and muscle dysfunction and accelerating the osteoporotic process.

For the pain that can accompany peripheral vascular problems, the person can be assisted in changing the position of the extremity. If leg pain occurs while the person is in the lying position, placing the feet in a dependent position on the floor may provide relief. When the pain of intermittent claudication occurs while the client is walking, stopping and resting for a short time should relieve the pain. Walking a prescribed distance each day should promote collateral circulation. The prescribed distance is regular walking to the point of symptoms (Spitell, 1982). If leg discomfort is caused by leg and foot edema, elevating the part should help to reduce the edema. When edema of the foot occurs, the elderly person may have difficulty wearing shoes. Caution needs to be advised for the person who wears slippers. These do not provide a firm base for walking and may predispose the person to falls.

If pain in the extremities is not relieved or reduced, the person's activities may be inhibited. Interventions for limiting discomfort are preferable to medications, since some analgesics may cause disturbances in judgment and gait. Other interventions with the client who experiences peripheral vascular problems include advising the person to avoid temperature extremes, since direct heat may burn the extremity and coldness can cause vasoconstriction. The nicotine from tobacco is another vasoconstrictor. Pressure, cold, and smoking tend to decrease blood flow. Other obstacles to blood flow include sitting with the legs crossed and wearing garters or socks with tight elastic tops. The pressure of a chair against the backs of the legs when the person sits for long periods of time can cause further circulatory impairment.

Foot care is vital for the elderly person, especially when the blood supply to the extremities is limited. To help avoid foot trauma, the person should be advised against walking with bare feet. Comfortable shoes, which provide good support for ambulation, should be worn. Shoes should be made of soft and flexible leather, with smooth linings free of ridges and wrinkles. There should be adequate room for the toes to move freely in the shoes. New shoes should first be worn only for short periods of time. Rubber soles slipping on a wet surface can contribute to falls.

The feet should be carefully inspected for color change, pressure areas, and breaks in the skin. The toes and the areas between them should be closely examined. Toenails should be cut straight across but should not be cut too short. Bunions and calluses are common foot problems in the elderly. The client should be advised against self-treatment of these problems. The nurse can teach the person to recognize factors that aggravate bunions and calluses, such as improperly fitting shoes, incorrect gait and posture, and long periods of standing or walking without rest periods.

Breaks in the skin of the feet should be prevented whenever possible. If a break occurs, the wound should be treated immediately, and further trauma to the area must be avoided while the wound is healing. The cause of the skin breakdown should be determined. Putting the feet in hot water or trimming a corn or callus can cause harmful irritation or breaks in the skin. Strong antiseptics should not be applied to calluses and corns. Cleanliness of the feet should be maintained by daily washing and regular change of footwear. In addition to these measures, the elderly person should regularly and systematically inspect the feet and toes in order to detect any early changes that may occur. Because of sensory changes in the lower extremities, foot changes are often observed before they are felt.

When lesions are present on an ischemic foot, care should be directed toward preventing further trauma to the foot, controlling pain, preventing or controlling infection, and preserving the muscle strength and joint motion in the extremity.

Reconstructive arterial surgical procedures may be performed in an attempt to salvage an extremity with severe ischemia. Amputation may be indicated for ischemic gangrene. The medical decision relating to the degree of amputation will be affected by the condition of the extremity and the elderly person's general condition. Preservation of the knee joint is considered as much as possible. Early fitting of the prosthesis seems to be desirable in encouraging rehabilitation.

The person with hemiplegia may need to practice balancing exercises as a way to facilitate mobility. Bearing of weight on a limb seems to aid in control of spasms. It may help to place weight on the hand by sitting at the edge of a firm surface and placing the hand flat on the seat. If the leg is affected, standing up and holding on to a firm chair with the feet apart and the legs straight may help to strengthen the muscles and to reduce spasm. The client should be instructed to distribute weight evenly over both feet, rather than placing all weight on the unaffected foot. In assisting the person with hemiplegia, the nurse should support the affected side, since the tendency is to fall toward the affected side. The nurse gives only the support that is needed. The client should be encouraged to perform the same movements on the affected side as the unaffected side.

Persons with hemiplegia tend to throw themselves into a chair when sitting down, placing all their weight on the unaffected side and sitting forward in the chair. These clients should be instructed to sit down slowly and to bend forward as they go down, with the buttocks touching the seat first. Turning toward the affected side helps to distribute the weight evenly over both buttocks. While sitting, the affected foot should be placed at a right angle to the knee instead of stretching out and swinging toward the other leg.

The trunk muscles of the hemiplegic client can be strengthened to assist with sitting, walking, and standing. Some exercises for this include lifting the weak shoulder upwards and backwards while sitting in a hard chair, twisting the body at the waist while looking over one shoulder and then the other shoulder, and pulling the body forward with the use of the stomach muscles while sitting in the chair.

To help a person with hemiplegia to stand, the nurse should stand on the affected side. The client is instructed to slide forward on the chair and to lean the head forward over the knees. The head should be level with the knees to help the body up. The unaffected arm should be on the arm of the chair to help push up the body. The nurse's only contact should be the hand under the affected arm, since too much help is as useless as too little. The person should use his or her own balance. If the nurse tries to help with balance, it could upset the client's equilibrium. The person should be standing as straight as possible before beginning to walk. The affected foot should be flat on the floor, instead of resting on its outer edge. The person should lean toward the unaffected side when walking. Facilitating the mobility of the person who has experienced a cerebrovascular accident can promote a greater degree of independence.

Promoting Environmental Activity Facilitators

The nurse can promote the maintenance or alteration of an environment that stimulates activity by the elderly person. Increased opportunity for activity may increase the old person's activity levels. Certain environments have been found to control activity. Areas of open space support activity even for those who must use mobility aids. Overcrowding the living space with furniture limits the open space available for mobility.

The environment may be equipped with mobility supports in strategic areas. Rails along the hall may be needed in all settings in which the elderly live, not just in nursing home environments. Stair rails on both sides of the stairs are needed at every stairway, and should extend beyond the last step. The walls next to bathtubs and toilets should provide a solid support for grasping. Bathtubs should have nonslip rubber mats or nonskid adhesive strips applied.

Furniture should be designed for ease in sitting and returning to the standing position. Overstuffed low chairs and couches may appear comfortable, but they can add to the elderly person's discomfort because it is awkward to get in and out of them. Straight-backed chairs with arms are especially helpful in the return to a standing position. For the elderly person who must use a wheelchair, the height of chairs, beds, and toilets should be the same as that of the wheelchair seat, to facilitate transfers back and forth.

Preventing Obstacles to Mobility

The nurse's role in preventing obstacles to mobility supports the independence of the elderly person. The nurse should understand the principles of accident prevention and should instruct the elderly person and family members about this subject. The elderly client already may have physical obstacles to mobility, such as joint discomfort and limited motion, muscle weakness, or osteoporosis. The person also may be experiencing sensory changes, which can further hinder mobility. Nutrition instruction may be necessary if obesity is a problem, since obesity can be an obstacle to mobility.

Loose rugs in the elderly person's environment can be obstacles to mobility. They should be removed, and free edges of carpeting should be tacked to the floor. Highly polished or cluttered floors may cause the person to slip and fall. Nonslip treads or carpet can be installed on stairways, but must be promptly replaced when they become worn, to eliminate the hazard of catching the heel of a shoe in the frayed material. Spills on the floor should be wiped up immediately since these cause a slippery surface. Extension cords should run along the wall, so that the elderly person cannot trip over them.

The client should avoid lifting heavy objects, because of the potential for vertebral fractures. Even lifting of lightweight objects should be performed by bending at the knees rather than bending at the back. However, bending at the knees may cause discomfort for the client with joint changes of the knees.

Falls are a potentially dangerous problem for the older person. The dangers of ice and snow must be kept in mind as the elderly person plans activities. The nurse should stress the importance of avoiding situations that may result in a fall. Old persons are especially prone to fractures because of the prevalence of osteoporosis in this age group. It is hazardous for the elderly client to stand on a chair or ladder, especially when the head must be tilted backward to see or to reach for an object. The backward tilt may cause an imbalance in posture. It can also lead to a reduction in cerebral blood supply because of interference with circulation at the neck area, resulting in vertigo or dizziness.

The elderly person should be given instructions relating to the management of a fall. A fall can be a frightening experience. After falling, the person should lie as flat as possible for a few minutes. Then he may be able to slide along the floor to a chair, or to a phone if he is alone. Phones placed on a stand are more accessible than wall phones. The person should reach for a nearby blanket, towel, or carpet for covering. Another person should not attempt to lift the elderly person from the floor.

Improperly fitting clothing or shoes may be an obstacle to mobility. If the elderly person must concentrate on holding on to loose pajama bottoms or pants, gait can be affected. The person can trip over trailing garments. Clothing that is too tight can also affect posture and gait. Loose shoes and slippers can cause tripping, while shoes that are too tight or that have high heels can alter the person's gait and are a potential cause of foot problems. Crepe-soled shoes may provide a nonskid base on a wet outdoor surface, but they tend to adhere to a carpeted surface. This may lead to a fall if the person loses balance. Wearing shoes that are attractive, comfortable, and safe can be a motivating force in encouraging the elderly person to want to walk.

Compensating with Mobility Aids

The elderly person may be using a mobility aid, or the assessment data may reveal a need for this assistance. The nurse and other health team members work with the client in teaching the appropriate use of the aid (Fig. 15.4). The nurse cannot assume that the person who has used a mobility aid for an extended period of time is using it correctly. Incorrect use of mobility aids can lead to additional joint, feet, or posture problems as a result of uneven weight

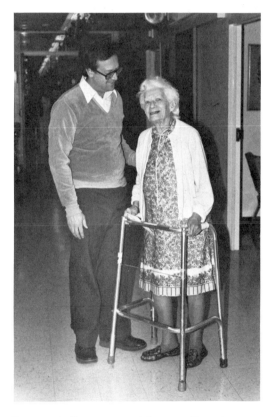

Figure 15.4. The nurse needs to assess the adequacy with which a person uses a mobility aid. *(Photograph by Ed Spier, Murrysville, PA.)*

distribution. In some instances, the mobility aid may not be functioning properly. The nurse may be instrumental in recognizing this problem and arranging to correct it. The nurse should also be aware of safety features needed by mobility aids. For example, the canes and crutches should have rubber tips, and wheelchairs should have functioning brakes. If the person needs a mobility aid, even for a temporary period, the nurse may have to assist the client in getting the aid and accepting the need to use it.

The wheelchair may be a help or a hindrance to the elderly client's activity. On the one hand, the wheelchair stimulates activity by enabling the person to move about in the environment. On the other hand, the person may not attempt increased activity because of the security provided by the wheelchair.

Nurse and client should both be aware of wheelchair features that provide for easy maneuverability and safety. There must be brakes that lock, and the client must know how to use them. A major problem with some wheelchairs that supposedly were designed for the elderly is the lack of a way for the person to maneuver the chair. The client must then depend on someone else to move the chair. Frequently, a person in this type of chair is forced to remain in one place for many hours at a time. Wheelchairs used in this way do not assist the client in compensating for mobility problems.

Hartigan (1982) discusses the present day misuse of wheelchairs as a place for sitting for long periods of time. The construction of the collapsible wheelchair provides a hard seat with no support for the client's head and shoulders. Without this support, the client slumps forward. The client's arms tend to lean against the tubular frame supporting the back of the wheelchair. As a result, the client's radial nerve is dangerously exposed to damage from sustained pressure over the posterior surface of the arm. Prolonged sitting in wheelchairs also can produce flexion contractures.

The elderly person who sits in a collapsible wheelchair for a long period of time is prone to develop gluteal and sacral pressure ulcers. The seat of the wheelchair is less yielding than any mattress. Wheelchair seats need to be covered with an additional supporting surface. A wheelchair also should have a back high enough to support the client's head and shoulders. Comfortable leg and foot supports are necessary.

For easy access from a wheelchair, shelves and cabinets should be at a convenient height to be reached from a sitting position. Working surfaces and sinks should also be reachable, and should be built in such a way that the seat of the wheelchair will fit under them. Mirrors should be tilted downward. Standard drinking fountains should be supplemented by a lower fountain for use by clients in a wheelchair. Public telephones should be accessible from a wheelchair. An elderly person in a wheelchair may wish to have some personal articles available, or a laprobe to cover the legs. A pocket attachment may be added to the wheelchair to carry these items.

The old person who uses a walker for support while ambulating may need instructions about the proper use of the walker. The legs of the walker should be high enough to enable the person to walk upright. The client may also hold on to the back of a wheelchair or a straight-backed chair for support in ambulating. A smooth floor surface is necessary if a chair is to be moved along the surface during ambulation. When a cane is used to aid mobility, the cane should permit minimal flexion at the elbow when the cane is placed 6 to 8 inches to the client's side.

Before a client is assisted with the use of a mobility aid, the nurse and the other health team members should become familiar with the person's living environment. Potential hazards in the environment may limit the client's use of the aid. The width of doorways and the presence of steps are factors to be considered. The wheelchair may have difficulty fitting through some doors of the client's home. Doors and passageways should be at least 36 inches wide to allow easy passage of the wheelchair. Assistive devices and appliances, such as ramps to be placed over steps, are available to enable the person to make more efficient use of the mobility aid. For the client who uses a cane, the surface of the floor is an important consideration. The cane may catch in a loose rug and

cause the elderly person to fall. A three- or four-pronged cane is safer to use.

Promoting Sleep and Rest

In order to maintain activity levels, the elderly person requires planned periods of rest and sleep. A balance should be maintained between activity and rest. If the elderly person has difficulty sleeping, there may be a primary sleep disorder, a disturbing environment, or the presence of a pathologic problem interfering with sleep. The elderly person should be discouraged from napping in a chair, because hyperflexion or hyperextension of the neck may compress the arteries in the neck. Even minor changes in cerebral blood flow may lead to mental confusion or hypotension caused by decreased vascular resistance, since ischemia may affect the central nervous system center, which controls vascular tonicity (Syzek, 1976).

Privacy and a quiet environment should help facilitate the periods of rest and sleep. The need for a quiet sleeping environment is also important in an institutional setting. Gress et al. (1981) reported that institutional sounds unnoticed during the day and evening hours were highly amplified at night. Care-givers in the institution did not seem to have an awareness of the extent to which they contributed to the wakefulnews and restlessness of clients. With elderly persons' decrease in amounts of deep stages of sleep, they are more easily awakened by noises.

Simply going to bed may not eliminate stimulation for the elderly person. Any emotional excitement, worry, or anxiety may keep the muscles tense and hinder the person's ability to fall asleep. The more the individual worries about falling asleep, the tighter the muscles may become. Difficulty sleeping may be an indication of depression. When elderly persons are feeling depressed, they may want to discuss sleep problems rather than feel the freedom to talk about depression.

The elderly client may need assistance with learning relaxation exercises to promote rest or sleep. Other techniques that may be helpful include a warm bath, a warm glass of milk, and reading prayers or poetry at bedtime. It may be advisable to avoid beverages containing caffeine, such as coffee and cola soft drinks, near the time the person plans to sleep. A glass of sherry often helps some elderly people to relax and sleep. However, recent sleep studies point to the contraindication of alcohol for the elderly person with periods of sleep apnea. A research finding reported by the Stanford Sleep Disorder Center indicated that just 2 ounces of alcohol at bedtime increased and lengthened the number and duration of apneas during sleep (Moramarco, 1982). Elderly people with sleep apnea or those persons who snore heavily and who are overweight should abstain from any alcohol at night. Snoring frequently indicates some impairment of upper airway function and heavy snoring frequently precedes development of an upper airway sleep apnea syndrome (Dement et al., 1982). The work of breathing is greatly increased during snoring.

To promote rest at night, a person may need an activity plan, an exercise program, or a specific activity, such as a pleasant shopping trip during the day. Interventions of this type are preferable to sleep-inducing medications. If sleep medications are ordered for the elderly person in the institutional setting, they should be given only if really needed. Before they are given, other measures to promote sleep should be tried. The cause of the sleep problem should be investigated. If the person complains of not being able to fall asleep as a result of pain, attempts should be made to relieve the pain rather than taking a medication for sleep. Measures to promote breathing ease, especially for the person with breathing difficulty, will promote sleep. Bronchial toilet may be needed prior to bedtime. Sleeping with several pillows may also promote breathing ease. Adequate ventilation and temperature control in the room will be more conducive to sleep. When a medication has been ordered for its diuretic effect, the medication should be taken early in the day to prevent the need for getting out of bed at night to go to the bathroom. The sensation of a full bladder can interrupt sleep.

The nurse may need to assist the elderly person in establishing and maintaining a 24 hour sleep–wake rhythm. To encourage regulation of sleep time, the nurse can encourage the person to arise sooner than desired, avoid

naps in order to consolidate sleep and to enable sleep to be more refreshing (Davignon and Bruno, 1982). The nurse can help to improve the quality of the elderly person's sleep.

Assisting with the Control of Hypertension

In screening programs in the community, the elderly person with a systolic pressure of 160 mm Hg or greater on two separate visits should be referred for a full evaluation even if the diastolic pressure is 90 mm Hg or below (Daniels and Gifford, 1980). Because blood pressure tends to fall in elderly people, whether normotensive or hypertensive, when assuming an upright position, standing blood pressure readings should be taken routinely.

The nurse can assist the elderly client with hypertension with dietary habits. With decreased taste perception, the elderly person may use an abundance of salt. The client needs help with the use of other seasonings to improve the taste of foods without the use of salt. Spices that can be used include paprika, pepper, oregano, cloves, cinnamon, or lemon juice. Foods that are high in sodium or that are preserved in salt should be avoided.

The elderly person who receives antihypertensive medications can have increased responsiveness to these medications. Side effects can include muscle weakness and nausea resulting from low blood levels of potassium and sodium, drowsiness, and mental confusion. Because of sensory changes, the elderly person may not adequately hear instructions for taking the medications or they may not be able to see the instructions on the medication label. The nurse needs to take special care in making certain that instructions are understood. Treatment for hypertension needs to be continuous. This may pose financial problems for the elderly person. An example is that of an 88-year-old woman who lived in the community. In a routine blood pressure screening done by the nurse, this elderly person was found to have a systolic reading of 190 mm Hg. When she was questioned by the nurse about her medications for hypertension, she stated that she was already taking a "heart pill" and she could only afford one pill. She felt that it was more important to take the "heart pill." In this instance, assistance was obtained for the purchase of the antihypertensive medication.

When the person with hypertension feels better, he or she may feel that the medication is no longer needed. Failure of clients to remain under continuous medical care and the inability or unwillingness to adhere to a prescribed treatment are major obstacles in the treatment of hypertension. The nurse should stress the need for hypertensive treatment even when the person feels well.

Limitation of Immobility Effects

There are times when the elderly person's health problems may cause immobility. The nurse's role is to assist the client in limiting the effects of these periods of immobility. The nurse can also help the client limit the length of immobility by aiding in prevention of the problems it may cause. To prevent or reduce muscle atrophy during immobility, active or passive range-of-motion exercises should be performed at least three times a day, or according to the needs and tolerance of the individual. These exercises can be used to restore motion and regain strength. Acute inflammation of a joint, however, may limit the exercises of that part, and long-standing muscle atrophy may limit the degree to which the goal of future mobility is attained.

Even when the person experiences a period of immobility, isolation as a result of immobility should be avoided or limited. The person who has lost mobility functions should receive support from the nurse in grieving this loss. The use of touch by the nurse is important to the immobilized person. Immobilized clients should also be encouraged to touch themselves, to maintain orientation to their body parts.

The person who is labeled as confused should not be restrained in bed or in a chair for long periods of time. It is vital to determine the reasons for the behavior that is described as confused. For example, recall the labels that can be attached to persons with hearing problems who respond inappropriately to verbal communication because they cannot hear the message. Isolating these clients through various immobilization techniques, such as re-

straints, the table placed over a geriatric chair, or the use of medications, simply aggravates the problems they are already experiencing.

There are times when the nurse's felt need to get an elderly person out of bed may be overdone. If the person is in a coma and seems to be near death, the nurse should simply promote a comfortable position in the bed. An elderly person slumped motionless in a chair may be immobilized to a greater degree than one who is positioned properly in bed, with frequent changes of position and appropriate range-of-motion activities. Promoting rest as well as activity should be the goal of the nurse who works with the elderly person.

EVALUATION

The elderly person's satisfaction with activity levels achieved can be a measurement of the effectiveness of the program that was planned. The person's state of health and general feelings of well-being and life satisfaction may have been influenced by the activity program.

Physical indicators may also demonstrate an improvement. Activity tolerance maintained at an optimal level or increased can indicate the success of a planned program. Specific indicators of activity tolerance may include breathing ease and increased capacity for breathing, absence of breathlessness, absence or decrease of fatigue, and improved skin color. In the evaluation of tolerance, a decrease in tolerance is significant. Fatigue, loss of interest in the activity, or a desire to postpone the activity may indicate decreasing activity tolerance, which may have a physiologic or psychologic basis. The nurse can reassess to determine the possible cause of intolerance. The client may not have adequate capacity for a particular activity, or anxiety levels may interfere. Evaluation of the elderly person's tolerance of activity or an exercise program is vital, since inappropriate physical activity may further deplete the blood supply to organs that already suffer from decreased circulation. This, in turn, can interfere with the person's homeostatic mechanisms (Syzek, 1976).

The nurse should evaluate the degree to which an activity meets the needs of the client, as well as the degree to which it is therapeutic in preventing or reducing the effects of a problem. The client's desire to continue a therapeutic activity is significant. Even though the nurse or other members of the health team are instrumental in helping the client to initiate the activity, motivation and interest in continuation of the activity demonstrates client growth.

In conclusion, the role of the nurse in assisting the client to maintain an optimal balance between activity patterns and rest and sleep patterns must be emphasized. The client's activity desires and tolerance should be recognized by the nurse as the foundation from which activity plans are made. If the client's activity desires and activity tolerance are incongruent, the nurse intervenes to assist the client in setting realistic goals. These goals may involve increasing activity tolerance, or increasing motivation to reach and maintain optimal activity levels. Quality and quantity of sleep are important considerations. When mobility is limited, nursing goals are directed toward preventing problems that can result from immobility. The nurse should be aware of mobility aids that promote client activity.

RECOMMENDED READINGS

Breuer, J.M. A Handbook of Assistive Devices for the Handicapped Elderly: New Help for Independent Living. New York, Haworth, 1982. *Includes a broad array of devices designed to assist handicapped elderly toward independent living. Assists with intervention.*

Gordon, M. Assessing activity tolerance. American Journal of Nursing 76:72, 1976. *Assessment of a person's exercise level can serve as a predictor of the person's ability to participate in activities. Included are the assessments of cardiovascular and respiratory status, skin changes, posture, equilibrium, and emotional state.*

Harris, R. Guide to Fitness after Fifty. New York, Plenum, 1977. *Supports interventions with exercise programs to maintain fitness of elderly people.*

McClannahan L.E. Therapeutic and prosthetic living environments for nursing home residents. The Gerontologist 13:424, 1973. *Assessment, planning, and intervention with environments for the elderly. The nursing-home resident is the focus, but there are also environmental interventions for the elderly person in the home setting.*

Olson, E.V. The hazards of immobility. American Journal of Nursing 67:780, 1967. *Presents assessment and nursing interventions relating to changes which can occur with immobility. Included are effects on the following functions: cardiovascular, respiratory, gastrointestinal, motor, urinary, metabolic, and psychosocial.*

Rosenberg, M. Sixty-Plus and Fit Again. New York, McEvans, 1977. *Discusses interventions with the elderly client. Individual and group physical exercises appropriate for elderly clients are discussed. Illustrations are used to demonstrate exercise positions.*

Shephard, R.J. Physical Activity and Aging. London, Croom Helm, 1978. *Stresses the value of physical activity for elderly people. Supportive research is presented.*

Snyder, L.H. Living environments, geriatric wheelchairs, and the older person's rehabilitation. Journal of Gerontological Nursing 1(5):17, 1975. *Presents an assessment of mobility needs of the elderly person as a way to expand the person's environment. Nursing intervention relating to the use and misuse of the geriatric wheelchair is a highlight of this article.*

Syzek, B.J. Cardiovascular changes in aging: Implications for nursing. Journal of Gerontological Nursing 2(1):28, 1976. *Presents the cardiovascular changes that can occur with aging. Emphasis is placed on the assessment of the changes and nursing interventions relating to them.*

Wheeler, M. Osteoporosis. Medical Clinics of North America 60: 1213, 1976. *The assessment base relating to osteoporosis is presented. Interventions relate to the prevention of osteoporosis and the control of immobility, and the prevention of fractures when osteoporosis is a problem.*

Witte, N.S. Why the elderly fall. American Journal of Nursing 79(11):1950, 1979. *Presents changes occurring with age as a result of diminished functioning of the circulatory, nervous, and musculoskeletal systems that predispose the elderly person to falling and to serious complications from falls.*

Yura, H. The need for sleep, in Yura, H., Walsh, M.B. (eds), Human Needs and the Nursing Process. New York, Appleton, 1978. *Presents the physiological theories of sleep, the assessment of sleep patterns, and interventions with the client to promote sleep. The impact of environmental factors and the effect on sleep patterns are included.*

REFERENCES CITED

Adams, G. Essentials of Geriatric Medicine. New York, Oxford University Press, 1977

Agate, J. Common symptoms and complaints, in Rossman, I. (ed.), Clinical Geriatrics, 2nd ed. Philadelphia, Lippincott, 1979

Aloia, J.F. Exercise and skeletal health. Journal of the American Geriatric Society 29(3):104, 1981

Andriola, M.J. When an elderly patient complains of weakness. Geriatrics 33(6):79, 1978

Aronson, S., Mascia, M.F. The Stress Management Workbook. New York, Appleton-Century-Crofts, 1981

Bassey, E.J. Age, inactivity, and some physiological responses to exercise. Journal of Gerontology 24(1):66, 1978

Beasley, B.A., Ford, D.H. Aging and the extrapyramidal system. Medical Clinics of North America 60:1315, 1976

Birren, J.E., Renner, V.J. Research on the psychology of aging, in Birren, J., Schaie, K.W. (eds.), Handbook of the Psychology of Aging. New York, Van Nostrand Reinhold, 1977

Bortz, W.M. Effect of exercise on aging—effect of aging on exercise. Journal of the American Geriatric Society 28:49, 1980

Brocklehurst, J.C., Hanley, T. Geriatric Medicine for Students. London, Churchill Livingston, 1976

Brody, H., Viyayashankar, N. Anatomical changes in the nervous system, in Finch, C.E., Hayflick, L. (eds.), Handbook of the Biology of Aging. New York, Van Nostrand Reinhold, 1977

Campbell, E.J., Lefrak, S.S. How aging affects the structure and function of the respiratory system. Geriatrics 32(8):57, 1977

Carter, A.B. The neurologic aspects of aging, in Rossman I. (ed.), Clinical Geriatrics, 2nd ed. Philadelphia, Lippincott, 1979

Castelli, W.P. CHD risk factors in the elderly. Hospital Practice 11:113, 1976

Clark, M. Good health for folks over 50. Parade, January 28, 1979

Daniels, L., Giffad, R.W. Therapy for older adults who are hypertensive. Journal of Gerontological Nursing 6(1):37, 1980

deVries, H. Physiological effects of an exercise training program upon men aged 52 to 88. Journal of Gerontology 25:325, 1970

Davignon, D., Bruno, P. Insomnia, causes and treatment particularly in the elderly. Journal of Gerontological Nursing 8(6):333, 1982

Dement, W.C., Laughton, E.M., Carskadon, M.A. "White Paper" on sleep and aging. Journal of American Geriatrics Society 30(1):25, 1982

Dhar, S., Shastri, S., Lenora, R. Aging and the respiratory system. Medical Clinics of North America 60:1121, 1976

Feinberg, I. Functional implications of changes in sleep physiology with age, in Terry, R.D., Gershon, S. (eds.), Neurobiology of Aging. New York, Raven, 1976

Feinberg, I. Patterns of sleep over a lifetime. Mental Health Reports 2. U.S. Department of Health, Education, and Welfare, 1968

Finch, C.E. Neuroendocrine and automatic aspects of aging, in Finch, C.E., Hayflick, L. (eds), Handbook of the Biology of Aging. New York, Van Nostrand Reinhold, 1977

Frankel, L.J., Richard, B.B. Be Alive as Long as You Live. New York, Lippincott and Crowell, 1980

Friedman, S.A. Common manifestations of degenerative arterial disease. Medical Clinics of North America 60:1079, 1976

Furlow, R., Oberman, A., Eggert, D. A step-by-step guide to exercise for the CAD patient. Geriatrics 35(9):41, 1980

Gioiella, E.C. The relationships between slowness of response, state anxiety, social isolation and self-esteem, and preferred personal space in the elderly. Journal of Gerontological Nursing 4(1):40, 1978

Goldman, R. Decline in organ function with aging, in Rossman, I. (ed.), Clinical Geriatrics, 2nd ed. Philadelphia, Lippincott, 1979

Gordon, M. Assessing activity tolerance. American Journal of Nursing 76:72, 1976

Gress, L.D., Bahr, R.T., Sr. Hassanein, R.S. Nocturnal behavior of selected institutionalized adults. Journal of Gerontological Nursing 7(2):86, 1981

Grob, D. Common disorders of muscles in the aged, in Reichel, W. (ed), Clinical Aspects of Aging. Baltimore, Williams & Wilkins, 1978

Gutmann, E. Muscle, in Finch, C.E., Hayflick, L. (eds.), Handbook of the Biology of Aging. New York, Van Nostrand Reinhold, 1977

Harris, R. Cardiac changes with age, in Goldman, R. Rockstein, M. (eds.), The Physiology and Pathology of Human Aging. New York, Academic, 1975

Harris, R., Frankel, L.J. (eds.), Guide to Fitness after Fifty. New York, Plenum, 1977

Harris, R. Special features of heart disease in the elderly patients, in China, A.B. (ed.), Working with Older People. Volume IV: Clinical Aspects of Aging. U.S. Department of Health, Education, and Welfare, July, 1971

Harris, R. Special problems of geriatric patients with heart disease, in Reichel, W. (ed.), Clinical Aspects of Aging. Baltimore, Williams & Wilkins, 1978

Hartford, J.T., Samorajski, T. Alcoholism in the geriatric population. Journal of the American Geriatrics Society 30(1):18, 1982

Hartigan, J.D. The dangerous wheelchair. Journal of American Geriatric Society. 30(9):572, 1982

Hass, F.J., Dolan, E.F. The Foot Book. Chicago, Henry Regnery, 1973

Hellebrandt, F.A. Exercise for the long-term care aged—benefits, deterrents, and hazards. Long-Term Care and Health Services Administration Quarterly 3:33, 1979

Henry, J.P., Ely, D.L. Emotional stress: Physiology. Primary Cardiology 5(8):35, 1979

Hooker, S. Caring for Elderly People. London, Routledge and Kegan Paul, 1976

Johnson, R.H. Blood pressure and its regulation, in Caird, F.I. Dall, J.L.C. Kennedy, R.D. (eds.), Cardiology in Old Age. New York, Plenum, 1976

Kales, J.D. Aging and sleep, in Goldman, R., Rockstein, M. (eds.), The Physiology and Pathology of Human Aging. New York, Academic, 1975

Klocke, R.A. Influence of aging on the lung, in Finch, C.E., Hayflick, L. (eds.), Handbook of the Biology of Aging. New York, Van Nostrand Reinhold, 1977

Kohu, R.R. Heart and cardiovascular system, in Finch, C.E. Hayflick, L. (eds.), Handbook of the Biology of Aging. New York, Van Nostrand Reinhold, 1977

Kraus, H. Preservation of physical fitness, in Harris, R., Frankel, L. (eds.), Guide to Fitness after Fifty. New York, Plenum, 1977

Lerner, R. Sleep loss in the aged. Journal of Gerontological Nursing 8(6):323, 1982

Lynne-Davies, P. Influence of age on the respiratory system. Geriatrics 32(8):57, 1977

Maxwell, R.N., Baden, J.E., Watson, W. Territory and self in a geriatric setting. The Gerontologist 12:413, 1972

Maylan, J.A., Flye, M.W. Peripheral vascular disease in the geriatric patient, in Reichel, W. (ed), Clinical Aspects of Aging. Baltimore, Williams & Wilkins, 1978

McClannahan, L.E. Therapeutic and prosthetic living environments for nursing home residents. The Gerontologist 13:424, 1973

Malasanos, L., Barkauskas, V., Moss, M., Stoltenberg-Allen, K. Health Assessment. St. Louis, Mosby, 1977

Moser, M. Hypertension in the elderly, in Rossman, I. (ed.), Clinical Geriatrics, 2nd ed. Philadelphia, Lippincott, 1979

Norris, A.H., Shack, N.W., Wagman, I.H. Age changes in the maximum conduction velocity of motor fibers of human ulnar nerves, in The Central Nervous System and Aging. New York, MSS Information Corporation, 1974

Pacini, C.M., Fitzpatrick, J.J. Sleep patterns of hospitalized and non-hospitalized aged individuals. Journal of Gerontological Nursing 8(6):327, 1982

Price, J.H. Unintentional injury among the aged. Journal of Gerontological Nursing 4(3):36, 1978

Prinz, P. Sleep patterns in the healthy aged: Relationship with intellectual function. Journal of Gerontology 32:179, 1977

Spittell, J.A. Peripheral vascular disorders. Geriatrics 37(1):55, 1982
ontology 32:179, 1977

Roberts, S.L. Behavioral Concepts and Nursing Throughout the Life Span. Englewood Cliffs, N.J., Prentice-Hall, 1978

Rockstein, M. Heart disease in the aged, in Rossman, I. (ed.) Clinical Geriatrics, 2nd ed. Philadelphia, Lippincott, 1979

Rockstein, M. The biology of aging in humans—an overview, in Goldman, R., Rockstein, M. (eds.), The Physiology and Pathology of Human Aging. New York, Academic, 1975

Rodstein M. Accidents among the aged, in Reichel, W. (ed.): Clinical Aspects of Aging. Baltimore, Williams & Wilkins, 1978

Rosenberg, M. Sixty-Plus and Fit Again. New York, McEvans, 1977

Rossman, I. The anatomy of aging, in Rossman, I. (ed.), Clinical Geriatrics. Philadelphia, Lippincott, 1971

Sculco, C.D. The need for activity, in Yura, H., Walsh, M.B. (eds.), Human Needs and the Nursing Process. New York, Appleton, 1978

Shephard, R.J. Physical activity and aging. London, Croom Helm, 1978

Shock, N.W. Systems integration, in Finch, C.E., Hayflick, L. (eds.), Handbook of the Biology of Aging. New York, Van Nostrand Reinhold, 1977

Snyder, L.H. Living environments, geriatric wheelchairs, and older persons' rehabilitation. Journal of Gerontological Nursing 1(5):17, 1975

Snyder, M., Baum, R. Assessing station and gait. American Journal of Nursing 74:1256, 1974

Snyder, L.H., Rupprecht, P., Pyrek, J., Brekhaus, S., Moss, T. Wandering. The Gerontologist 18:272, 1978

Spittell, J.A. Peripheral vascular disorders. Geriatrics 37(1):55, 1982

Strandell, T. Cardiac output in old age, in Caird, F.I., Dall, J.L.C., Kennedy, R.D. (eds.), Cardiology in Old Age. New York, Plenum, 1976

Strehler, B.L. Introduction: Aging and the human brain, in Terry, R.D., Gershon, S. (eds.), Neurobiology of Aging. New York, Raven, 1976

Syzek, B.J. Cardiovascular changes in aging: Implications for nursing. Journal of Gerontological Nursing 2(1):28, 1976

Tonna, E.A. Aging of skeletal–dental systems and supporting tissues, in Finch, C.E. Hayflick, L. (ed.), Handbook of the Biology of Aging. New York, Van Nostrand Reinhold, 1977

Walsh, M.B. Prologue: Biologic rhythms and human needs, in Yura, H., Walsh, M.B. (eds.), Human Needs and the Nursing Process. New York, Appleton, 1978

Welford, A.T. Motor performance, in Birren, J., Schaie, K.W. (eds.), Handbook of the Psychology of Aging. New York, Van Nostrand Reinhold, 1977

Wheeler, M. Osteoporosis. Medical Clinics of North America 60:1213, 1976

Wright, J.R. Cardiovascular and pulmonary pathology of the aged, in Reichel, W. (ed.), Clinical Aspects of Aging. Baltimore, Williams & Wilkins, 1978

Wylie, C.M. Hospitalization for fractures and bone loss in adults. Public Health Reports 92(1):33, 1977

Yura, H. The need for sleep, in Yura, H., Walsh, M.B. (eds.), Human Needs and the Nursing Process. New York, Appleton, 1978

The Fitness Challenge in the Later Years. Administration on Aging, U.S. Department of Health, Education, and Welfare (OHD), 75-20802, June, 1975

BIBLIOGRAPHY

Adams, G.M., deVries, H.A. Physiological effects of an exercise training regimen upon women aged 52–79. Journal of Gerontology 28(1):50, 1973

Albert, S.F., Jahnigen, D. Common foot disorders among the elderly. Geriatrics 38(6):42, 1983

Aniansson, A. Physical training in old men. Age and Aging 9:186, 1980

Avorn, J., Langer, E. Induced disability in nursing home patients. Journal of the American Geriatrics Society 30(6):397, 1982

Bienenstock, H., Fernando, K.R. Arthritis in the elderly. Medical Clinics of North America 60:1173, 1976

Boyer, J.L. Exercise therapy in hypertensive men. Journal of the American Medical Association 211:1668, 1970

Breuer, J.M. A Handbook of Assistive Devices for the Handicapped Elderly: New Help for Independent Living. New York, Haworth, 1982

Carskadon, M.S., Dement, W.C. Respiration during sleep in the aged human. Journal of Gerontology 36(4):420, 1981

Catchen, H. Repeaters: Inpatient accidents among the hospitalized elderly. The Gerontologist 23(3):273, 1983

Chapanis, A. Human engineering environments for the aged. The Gerontologist 14:228, 1974

Carp, F.M. Effects of the living environment on activity and use of time. International Journal of Aging and Human Development 9(1):75, 1978–79

Chaudhuri, G. Rehabilitation of the stroke patient. Geriatrics 35(10):45, 1980

Cooper, S. Common concern: Accidents and older adults. Geriatric Nursing 2(4):287, 1981

Dehn, M.M. Rehabilitation of the cardiac patient: The effects of exercise. American Journal of Nursing 80(3):435, 1980

deVries, H.A. Functional fitness for older Americans. National Conference on Aging, 1981

Feist, R. A survey of accidental falls in a small home for the aged. Journal of Gerontological Nursing 4(5):17, 1978

Fitzgerald, A.M. Ambulation without legs. Journal of Gerontological Nursing 1(3):12, 1975

Fletcher, S., Macauley, C. The shopping mall as a therapeutic arena. Geriatric Nursing 4(2):105, 1983

Garrison, J.E. Stress management training for the elderly: A psychoeducational approach. Journal of the American Geriatric Society 26(9):397, 1978

Hahn, D.L. Relaxation therapy for hypertension. Journal of Family Practice 13(8):279, 1981

Hamilton-Word, V., Smith, F., Jessup, E. Physical fitness on a VA Nursing home unit. Geriatric Nursing 3(4):260, 1982

Hodgson, J.L. Physical fitness and age with emphasis on cardiovascular function in the elderly. Journal of the American Geriatric Society 25(9):385, 1977

Hoges, C.C. Injury in late life: Prevention. Journal of the American Geriatric Society 30(4):276, 1982

Julius, S. Influence of age on hemodynamic response to exercise. Circulation 36:222, 1967

Karl, C.A. The effect of an exercise program on self care activities for the institutionalized elderly. Journal of Gerontological Nursing 8(5):282, 1982

Kent, S. How exercise prevents heart attacks. Geriatrics 36(5):39, 1981

Kraus, H. Reconditioning aging muscles. Geriatrics 33(6):93, 1978

Lynn, F.H. Incidents—need they be accidents. American Journal of Nursing 80(6):1098, 1980

Mead, W. Harting, R. Fitness evaluation and exercise prescription. Journal of Family Practice 13(12):1039, 1981

Meador, R. Learning to live with a new leg. American Journal of Nursing 79(8):1393, 1979

Miller, C., LeLieuvre, R.B. A method to reduce chronic pain in elderly nursing home residents. The Gerontologist 22(3):314, 1982

Naughton, J.P. The exercise prescription. Cardiovascular Medicine 4(6):741, 1979

Niinimaa, V., Shephard, R.J. Training and oxygen conductance in the elderly: I—the respiratory system. II—the cardiovascular system. Journal of Gerontology 33:354, 1978

Olson, E.V. The hazards of immobility. American Journal of Nursing 67:780, 1967

Overstall, P.W. Prevention of falls in the elderly. Journal of the American Geriatric Society 28(11):481, 1980

Pastalan, L.A., Carson, D.H. Spatial Behavior of Older People. University of Michigan, 1970

Pfeffer, R.I. Measurement of functional activities in older adults in the community. Journal of Gerontology 37(3):323, 1982

Pratt, M.A. Physical exercise: A special need in long-term care. Journal of Gerontological Nursing 4(5):38, 1978

Riffle, K.L. Falls, kinds, causes, and prevention. Geriatric Nursing 3(3):165, 1982

Salthouse, T.A., Somberg, B.L. Isolating the age deficit in speeded performance. Journal of Gerontology 37(1):59, 1982

Schirmer, M.S. When sleep won't come. Journal of Gerontological Nursing 9(1):16, 1983

Seigel, H. Assessing an environment for safety first. Journal of Gerontological Nursing 8(9):509, 1982

Sivarajan, E.S., Halpenny, C.J. Exercise testing. American Journal of Nursing 79(12):2163, 1979

Smith, E.L., Serfass, R.C. (eds.), Exercise and Aging: The Scientific Basis. Hillside, NJ, Enslow, 1981

Smith, E.L. Exercise for prevention of osteoporosis: a review. Physical Sports Medicine 10(5):72, 1982

Solomon, K. Social antecedents of learned helplessness in the health care setting. The Gerontologist 22(3):282, 1982

Stanford, J.L., Felner, J.M., Arensberg, D. Antiarrhythmic drug therapy. American Journal of Nursing 80(7):1288, 1980

Tilton, C.N., Maloof, M. Diagnosing problems in stroke. American Journal of Nursing 82(4):596, 1982

Wadden, T.A., de la Torre, C.S. Relaxation therapy as an adjunct treatment for essential hypertension. Journal of Family Practice 11(6):901, 1980

Wade, D.W. Teaching patients to live with chronic orthostatic hypotension. Nursing '82 12(72):64, 1982

Waldron, M.W. Oxygen transport. American Journal of Nursing 79(2):272, 1977

Walsleben, J. Sleep disorders. American Journal of Nursing. 82(6):936, 1982

Walters, J. Coping with a leg amputation. American Journal of Nursing 81(7):1349, 1981

Witte, N.S. Why the elderly fall. American Journal of Nursing 79(11):1950, 1979

16

Body Protection in the Aged and the Nursing Process

Margaret H. Magnussen*

Reading this chapter will enable the individual to:

- Identify risk factors in preventing problems secondary to changes in immunity, temperature control, and skin
- Identify nursing measures which may moderate risk factors

This chapter discusses the interrelationship of three protective systems of the body: immunity, temperature control, and the integumentary system. The effects of aging on each of these mechanisms are discussed, as well as the nursing measures to counteract or strengthen the changes in these protection systems.

Longitudinal studies show that aging follows an erratic pattern of change. Basic scientists are looking for an underlying mechanism at the molecular level. Clinical researchers, however, are striving to apply present knowledge in an attempt to retard the aging process. In this research, great emphasis is being placed on the body's own methods of protecting itself.

Just as "no man is an island," the individual protective system must be viewed within the context of its relationship to other protective systems as well as with the aging changes of other systems of the body. The interrelationships between these systems are discussed in relation to the nursing process.

ASSESSMENT BASE

The focus of this section is on potential age-related changes in the body's immune system. *Immunity* refers to the host's response or resistance to a microbe or other agent foreign to the body. The immune response is determined both by heredity and by acquisition. By the 16th week of fetal life, the human body probably possesses all the cells assigned to the immune defense system that it will ultimately have. With time, the number of these cells is reduced by attrition, and immune defense activity eventually wanes.

Limited human experimentation is now being performed; an example is the use of BCG vaccine in the treatment of tumor cells. However, the major thrust of current research related to immunity has concentrated on the mouse and guinea pig populations.

Evidence of the workings of the immune system is visible in everyday happenings. When an elderly person falls on the sidewalk and receives an abrasion of the elbow, the area will be red and warm for a few days, but then these symptoms will disappear. As easily as the fall is forgotten, so is the foreign invasion. If the

*Revised by Nancy J. Ebert

493

abrasion is deeper or becomes contaminated, then a collection of pus appears, composed of leukocytes. The area becomes warm, red, and painful. After a few days, red streaks leading up the arm develop, and small nodes can be felt in the axilla. At this point, immune defense activity has extended to include lymphocyte involvement, polymorphonuclear leukocyte migration, and several other defensive activities.

To be more explicit, when dirt or the foreign substance (antigen) enters, a sequence of events occurs. The events are directed toward localizing and eradicating the antigens. The responses include macrophage formation and reactivity of lymphocytes. There are two types of lymphocytes—B-lymphocytes and T-lymphocytes.

Macrophage

Monocytes are primarily responsible for the initial phase of the immune response. These cells are mobile and have the ability to phagocytize (digest) antigen. The function of the macrophage does not appear to change with aging (Tyan, 1981). The macrophage interacts with the lymphocytes. The exact nature of this interaction is not clear. The B- and T-lymphocytes respond in a more specific manner.

B-Lymphocyte

B-lymphocytes are manufactured in the bone marrow. Each cell is genetically programmed to recognize only one particular antigen (bacterium). Thus, the human body can probably recognize nearly a million different types of antigen. B-cells possess binding sites for foreign antigens. Bacteria, for example, can become attached to them. As a result, antibody is produced. This process occurs in the spleen and lymph nodes. The lifespan of the B-lymphocyte is about 16 days. As the individual ages, the actual number of B-lymphocyte remains the same. However, their responsiveness to stimulation from certain antigens decreases markedly.

The way the body responds to antigen stimulation is determined by heredity (natural immunity) or by acquisition. *Active acquired immunity* is the result of specific lymphocyte

or antibody formation by the host in response to an antigen. For example, vaccination for smallpox provides active acquired immunity. A killed or weakened form of the virus is injected, and the body produces antibody to it. Another example is the immunity conferred by measles infection. Active immunity is of relatively long duration.

Passive immunity is defined as that in which antibody is produced in another host and transferred to an unprotected individual. Passive immunity is usually of short duration, i.e., a few weeks or months. The infant receives passive immunity from antibodies contained in the colostrum as it first suckles, and from blood contained in the umbilical cord. Hence, the infant in its first weeks of life is protected against antigens to which the mother is immune. Immune serum globulin administered preventively to a person exposed to hepatitis provides passive immunity.

The presence of antibody can be measured. All antibodies are immunoglobulins. Antibody is simply a protein material that is produced in response to introduction of an antigen, and which has the ability to combine with the antigen that stimulated its production. So far, five immunoglobulins can be detected: IgM, IgG, IgA, IgE, and IgD.

IgM is the immunoglobulin found in the blood and is usually the first to be detected in antigen–antibody responses.

IgG accounts for the greatest amount of immunoglobulin in the body. It is the only class of immunoglobulins that can cross the placental barrier between mother and fetus and is responsible for protection of the infant during the first months of life.

IgA is the predominant immunoglobulin in body secretions. It is found in saliva, tears, bronchial secretions, nasal mucus, prostatic fluid, vaginal secretions, and mucous secretions of the small intestine. It is believed to be a primary defense mechanism against infections in these body areas.

The function of IgD is unknown at this time.

IgE is important in defense against antigens that cause allergic reactions. IgE helps to trigger the release of pharmacologic material in the body that mediates the allergic response to such antigens.

T-Lymphocyte

T-lymphocytes originate in the thymus. By 4 years of age, the individual probably has a lifetime supply of these cells. T-lymphocytes, like B-lymphocytes, recognize only one antigen. T-lymphocytes do not secrete antibody; they merely grasp it. They are believed to have three functions; effector, helper, and suppressor.

The specific reactions to antigens may be classified as those mediated by antibodies and those mediated by T-lymphocytes. Recent studies show that the number of circulating lymphocytes decreases progressively during and after middle age, so that a person 60 years of age possesses 70 percent of the lymphocytes of a young adult. This decrease is due to a decrease in the absolute number of circulating T-lymphocytes.

Effects of Aging Changes in the Immune System

The immune system is a complex, interacting network that is genetically controlled. An aged or less efficient immune system is manifest in the increased incidence of autoimmune diseases, infection, malignancy, and aberrant changes in antigen–antibody reactions. Knowledge of these manifestations is important for use of the nursing process and immunity.

Autoimmunity appears to be related to a change in suppressor T-lymphocyte function (Collard, 1981). Systemic lupus erythematosis, rheumatoid arthritis, and psoriasis are autoimmune diseases seen in the elderly. Definitive management of these diseases is lacking at this time.

The incidence of cancer also increases with aging. The exact contributing change in the immune system is unknown. Although the incidence increases with aging, cause of death is often attributed to other accompanying chronic diseases of aging, i.e., heart and cardiovascular disease, respiratory infections, and so on. Cancer of the lung, colon, rectum, prostate, stomach, and breast are common causes of death in the elderly. Early detection may be difficult

when the elderly client has other chronic diseases. Assessment should be just as thorough to include screening procedures for early detection, as well as information regarding signs and symptoms of each of the malignancies. Chest x-rays, occult blood tests, rectal exam including the prostate, and breast exam should be considered valid screening procedures as well as comprehensive history base.

Although some believe that one outgrows allergies as one ages, the elderly do exhibit allergic responses. Past history of allergy to drugs, pollens, dust, bee stings, and contact substances should be elicited. It is known that persons with a history of allergies are more prone to adverse drug reactions, a problem in the elderly who are likely to take medications for other health problems.

The elderly are generally more susceptible to infection, particularly respiratory and urinary tract infections (see Chapter 14). Elderly are more susceptible to nosocomial infections (Phair, 1979). The increased susceptibility is related to the aging changes of each system as well as to the changes in immune status. Influenza and pneumonia was the third leading cause of death in persons over 65 years of age in 1978 (Monthly Vital Statistics Report, September, 1980). An increased incidence of tuberculosis is also seen in the elderly populations (Phair, 1979). Other chronic diseases, such as diabetes, rheumatoid arthritis, and congestive heart failure also put the elderly person at greater risk for infections.

The reaction to infections also is more varied in the elderly. Signs and symptoms of infection may be less pronounced. The elderly may exhibit a low grade or no fever in response to an infection (Finkelstein, 1982; Gardner, 1980). There would, however, be the usual increase in white blood count. Symptoms of pain may be absent with appendicitis or peritonitis in the elderly although the person appears very ill.

Older people are particularly susceptible to pulmonary infections. Increased susceptibility may be due in part to decreases in ability to raise secretions and chronic obstructive lung disease. Influenza often contributes to the development of severe respiratory infections. It is for this reason that the Center for Disease Control recommends the administration of influenza vaccines annually and the pneumococcal vaccine once, as this vaccine is thought to be effective for life.

Aberrant changes in expected antigen–antibody reactions also occur with aging. These changes are attributed to changes in T-lymphocyte activity. These changes may appear as delayed hypersensitivity or anergy (the inability to react to a common antigen).

Delayed hypersensitivity is best illustrated by the purified protein derivative (PPD) skin test for tuberculosis. In the normal adult, who has been previously sensitized to this antigen, the area of the injected skin will become reddened and hard in about 6 hours and peak in reaction in 24 to 48 hours. In delayed hypersensitivity, the reaction may occur several days later and be less intense. Anergy is also seen with increased incidence in the elderly. As an example, elderly persons who previously reacted to PPD may show no reaction as they have aged. These reactions have implication when performing skin tests.

It is also known that tetanus-toxoid-induced antitoxin response is decreased in the elderly. A study done in a high-rise residence in St. Paul, Minnesota, revealed that only 34 percent of persons over 60 years of age had protective levels of tetanus antitoxin (Irvine et al., 1978). It is uncommon for the elderly to report no knowledge of when, if ever, they received tetanus toxoid. The chief portal of entry for the bacillus is through the skin. Since the elderly are prone to skin breakdown and are likely to have low antitoxin levels, susceptibility to tetanus infection increases.

ASSESSMENT OF IMMUNITY

The goal of assessment of immune status is to determine the degree of vulnerability of the client. A thorough assessment would incorporate certain tests as well as a history. However, these tests are invasive, costly procedures that, in general, are performed only when a disease or abnormality is strongly suspected.

Nursing Assessment

Gathering assessment data of any type should be done in an atmosphere of comfort and openness for both client and nurse. In the home setting, much can be learned from key questions directed at such things as a family picture. In this way the nurse can determine the number of children, which ones are living, their place of residence, the closeness of the family, and so forth. The nurse can observe directly much of the information needed, such as smoking habits, and general cleanliness.

Guide to Assessment of Immune Responses

I. History
  A. *Infection*
    1. Have you ever had tuberculosis or been exposed?
       a. PPD—last done—results
       b. Last chest x-ray
    2. Frequency of respiratory infections. Usual course?
    3. Do you have a cough? Describe.
    4. Do you smoke? If yes, how many years and how much?
    5. Where have you lived?
    6. Where do/did you work?
    7. Have you ever had a urinary tract infection? If so, describe.
  B. *Neoplastic disease*
    1. History in family.
    2. History in self. Treatment with chemotherapy?
    3. History of changes in digestion, bowel patterns, skin lesions, breathing patterns.
    4. Last rectal exam?
    5. Last breast exam?
    6. Female—last vaginal and PAP test?
    7. Male—last prostate exam?
  C. *Autoimmunity*
    1. History of rheumatoid arthritis, psoriasis, lupus erythematosis.
  D. *Allergy*
    1. Have you any allergies? If so, describe how this affects you.
    2. Have you any allergy to medication? If so, what? What was the response?

II. Physical assessment

A. *Sinuses*
Swollen, painful? Ethmoid, maxillary, frontal.

Sinuses are air-filled cavities in the bony structure of the skull. The frontal and maxillary sinuses are the only ones readily accessible. To assess the client's frontal sinuses, stand facing the client, place the palmar surface of the thumb above the eye and press upward. For assessing the maxillary sinus, place the thumb with the tip close to the nose and under the frontal bony surface, and press upward. Inflammation of these sinus areas will result in tenderness when pressure is applied.

B. *Nasal mucosa*
Color, presence of drainage?

An otoscope with a short, wide nasal speculum is necessary for visualization of the nose. If this is not available, use a pen-type flashlight. After inserting the lighted speculum in the nostril, tilt the client's head backward. The middle and inferior turbinates will be seen, as well as the mucosa. The color should be a deep red, and the nares should be free of bleeding or swelling. In persons with nasal allergy problems, the mucosa will be whitish-gray. Repeat the procedure in the other nostril.

C. *Tongue and hard palate*
Color and characteristics, i.e., smooth, rough, etc.

If the client has dentures, these should be removed and the mouth opened wide. The nurse should have a pocket light and tongue blade. Note the color of the mucosa and, with the tongue depressed, have the client say "ah" so that the size of the soft palate can be noted, as well as movement of the uvula, which should be midline. Deviation of the uvula and tongue to one side may be observed if the person has had a stroke (cerebral vascular accident). Remove the tongue blade and note the surface of the tongue. Fissures or deep ridges may occur in the aged, but the nurse must distinguish normal ridges of aging from fissuring due to dehydration. If the tongue is deeply fissured, is skin turgor poor on the forehead and anterior chest?

Monilial infection of the mouth should be looked for in the older, immune-suppressed client. It will be seen as a curd-like whitish material. Many of the powders used to hold dentures in place can also give the palate this appearance. Therefore, when in doubt have the client rinse the mouth well. If the client does not wear dentures, note the general condition of the teeth, especially the condition of the gums.

D. *Lymph nodes*
Palpable or nonpalpable? Posterior cervical, anterior cervical, axillary, inguinal.

The anterior and posterior cervical lymph nodes are best palpated with the client facing the examiner with the head in a relaxed position. Take the middle fingers and run them along the base and sides of the triangles formed by the sternocleidomastoid muscle. Enlarged lymph nodes will range from small pea-sized structures to those visible with the naked eye. The axillary nodes will be palpated later when performing the breast examination. To assess inguinal nodes, have the client lie flat and palpate the inguinal areas for presence of nodules.

E. *Spleen*
Palpable or nonpalpable?

Have the client lie down and stand to the right side. (Normally the spleen cannot be felt. It usually must be enlarged to three times its normal size to be palpable). With the right hand pushing into the abdomen and the left hand lifting from the back, the left hand is placed under the left thorax and the client is asked to take a deep breath. At the height of inspiration, thrust the right hand deeper into the abdomen. Upon expiration, the descent of the spleen will be felt if it is palpable.

F. *Liver*
   Palpable or nonpalpable?
   Again, standing to the right of the reclining client, place the left hand under the 11th and 12th ribs, and place the right hand on the client's abdomen, lateral to the rectus muscle, with the fingertips pointing toward the right costal margin. Press in and up. Repeat this same position and, while the client takes a deep breath, feel for any edges pressing your hand as he exhales. Next, face the client's feet and place both hands, side by side, below the costal margin. Ask the client to take a deep breath and again feel for movement against your fingertips.

G. *Breasts*
   Masses, secretions, character of skin, uniformity.
   The breasts of both male and female should be inspected. The male breast exam is easily performed with the man in a sitting position. The nurse looks for enlargement and uniformity of breast tissue, as well as for nodules, swelling, or ulceration of the nipple and surrounding skin. While the man remains in the sitting position, the nurse can take the middle two or three fingers of the right hand and palpate the left axilla, pressing firmly and feeling for the presence of axillary nodes. This position is reversed for palpation of the right axilla. An obese male will have definite bilateral breast configurations, which should not be confused with gynecomastia.
   With the female nude and in an upright position, the nurse should observe the size and uniformity of the breasts, noting dimpling, color, thickening or edema, and vein pattern. Note the size and shape of the nipples and the direction in which they point, as well as whether they are inverted or everted and the presence of discharge. Check for palpable axillary nodes, as with the male. Ask the client to lie on a firm, flat surface and, with the edge of a firm pillow or a rolled towel under the shoul-

der of the breast to be examined, stand to the side of the patient and gently press with three fingers, compressing the breast against the chest wall. Do this in a clockwise motion. This step will be repeated until the entire breast is carefully checked. The female should be taught to examine her breasts herself on a regular basis, at least once a month.

H. *Rectal*
   The client should lie in a left lateral position on the examining table, with his right hip and knee slightly flexed. With a gloved hand, lubricate the index finger and insert into the anal canal. Instruct the patient to relax and bear down as if he is having a bowel movement. Insert the finger further into the rectum and feel the rectal walls, feeling for nodules.
   In the male: characteristics of prostate—hard, soft, spongy, enlarged? Turn your finger to feel for the anterior surface. Identify the lobes of the prostate. Note the size, shape, and consistency of the prostate. Then gently withdraw the finger and note the character of fecal material.

I. *Vaginal exam*
   In the female: character of secretions—obtain specimen for Pap test.

PLANNING AND INTERVENTION

The objective of planning and intervention is to maintain a state of health by preventive care, such as by vaccinations, continued screening procedures, and the direction of the client to the appropriate health-care delivery systems for treatment of marked deviations from wellness.

I. Vaccination status
A. PPD, if negative reaction, should be repeated yearly. The person with a positive reaction of years' standing should have an annual chest x-ray. If the client

converts to positive, then sputum testing should also be included with x-ray evaluation.

B. Because of the problems encountered on a national level with the massive flu immunization program in 1976, a portion of the population remains reluctant to continue yearly immunization. Influenza vaccination should be given annually to older persons, particularly those over 65 years of age. The formulations change from year to year to correspond with major antigenic changes (MMWR August 11, 1978, Vol 27, No 32).

C. Tetanus booster should be repeated every 10 years.

D. Pneumococcal vaccine should be given one time to those over 65 years of age, especially those with chronic lung problems. It is currently believed that one vaccination lasts a lifetime. Clients should be cautioned to stay at home and use the telephone for visiting during periods of high incidence of respiratory infections in the community.

II. Allergies

A. The least expensive treatment for food allergy is to eliminate the offending agent from the diet. If this measure must be taken and will disturb "normal nutrition," then substitutes must be planned.

B. Allergic reaction to medications, such as the penicillins, must be handled with caution and speed. A person who is allergic to penicillin is also allergic to the entire family of penicillin derivatives, a fact that is often forgotten in clinical practice. New additives, preservatives, and so on are routinely put into a variety of products, so even though a 65-year-old person has been exposed to many possible irritants, there is always the possibility of a new allergic reaction. The use of medications increases in this age group, further compounding reaction probabilities. Any individual who has experienced anaphylactic reactions should wear an identification tag naming the problem.

C. In testing the elderly for anergy using such antigens as mumps, or tricophytan agents to which this age group has been exposed, the purpose is to determine the degree to which the person's immune system is able to respond.

III. Immune status

It is essential that the nurse know whether the immune response has been modified by chemotherapy or radiation. If this is the situation, the client will require additional protection. Chemotherapeutic or radiation agents used to stop the proliferation of abnormal lymphocytic cells also halt normal lymphocyte production. Clients who have been treated with such agents need guidance in avoiding exposure to respiratory infections. If the individual is hospitalized, invasive procedures, such as intravenous feedings, must be performed under strictly aseptic conditions. The client should not be placed in a room with an infected person.

Persons who have been exposed to known carcinogenic agents in their work or home environment, such as polyvinyl chlorides, will require closer monitoring as they age.

All older women and men should have yearly screening exams, particularly of the genitourinary tract. Women must perform monthly breast self-exams regularly, perhaps using the arrival of a social security check as a memory cue. Clients with degenerative joint disease are frequently treated with high doses of analgesics such as aspirin. Such clients should check themselves for gastrointestinal bleeding. This is easily done with the use of hemeoccult kits. These kits consist of a treated paper on which a small amount of fecal material is placed and then treated with a drop or two of peroxide to check for the presence of blood in the stool. Hemeoccult kits are available from medical supply houses, pharmacies, and certain cancer society groups. People of any age group should report to a physician any signs of growths, bleeding, change in bowel habits, skin changes, and other symptoms which may indicate the presence of malignancy.

ASSESSMENT BASE: TEMPERATURE CONTROL

Under average conditions the elderly are able to maintain body temperature within normal limits. Internal body temperature is a balance between heat production and heat loss. Heat is produced by cellular metabolism and muscle activity, and is lost by radiation, convection, and evaporation of moisture from the skin. Regulation of heat loss is dependent upon the amount of blood flowing to the skin and upon homeostatic control mechanisms in the nervous system. Receptors sensitive to core body temperature change are located in the hypothalamus of the brain. Pathways lead to the brain from the skin receptors which help to monitor temperature. As core body temperature rises, the flow of blood to the skin increases so that heat can be dissipated faster. The reverse occurs when core temperature decreases. Some physiologists believe that when body tissues degenerate or become diseased, leukocytes enter the diseased tissue. As the leukocytes degenerate, they release "leukocyte pyrogen," which has a direct effect on the hypothalamus by increasing temperature (Guyton, 1971).

The basal metabolic rate, which plays a part in temperature regulation, decreases in the elderly, partly because of the decreased amount of metabolizing tissue. The tissues of the old person produce heat at the same rate as those of the younger person. With advancing age, however, a loss of muscle mass and increase of fatty tissue is seen. Because of reduced physical activity, the elderly generally do not require as high a caloric intake as younger people; thus less energy is expended for metabolism of this reduced intake.

Response to Temperature Change in Aging

Older people demonstrate decreased sensitivity to cutaneous skin temperature differences of as much as 2° C whereas younger persons

detect differences less that 1° C (Collins, Dore, and Exton-Smith, 1977).

A rise in body temperature normally results in increased sweat production and vasodilatation. In one study (Foster et al., 1976), the sweat responses of persons over 70 years of age were compared with responses of persons under 65 years of age. The older population was found to have an increased body temperature threshold before sweating began, as well as a decreased sweating rate. The researchers noted that the sweat rates were poorer in men who had wrinkled, inelastic skin.

In severe weather, the altered responses to temperature change put the elderly at risk for hypothermia or hyperthermia, resulting in increased mortality rates.

Hyperthermia

Hyperthermia is considered a risk when the core temperature rises above 37.8° C (100° F). The severe heat wave of the summer of 1978 increased heat-related death rates in the elderly. In St. Louis, 66 of the heat-related deaths occurred in persons over 65 (Morbidity and Mortality Weekly Report, 1980). Moreover, it was noted that the higher death rate occurred in low socioeconomic groups and people in inner-city neighborhoods. Poor ventilation, inaccessibility to air conditioning, and poor nutrition must be considered contributing factors.

The mass media attempts to warn elderly people to stay indoors, perform minimal physical activity, and drink fluids. It is important that the elderly drink more fluids because thirst may not be indicative of need. Elderly persons who have heart disease and respiratory disease are at greater risk.

Hypothermia

Hypothermia is considered detrimental to the elderly when the core temperature is 35° C (95° F) or less. Hypothermia has four causes: (1) exposure to cold, (2) impaired thermoregulatory mechanisms, (3) decreased metabolism, and (4) drugs (Wallner and Spalding, 1978). Most of the literature relates to findings in Great Britain and more recently to the United States. The death rates from hypothermia have dramatically increased in the United States since

1977 as fuel prices increased. Many data are being collected from the Pacific Northwest, where it is less cold than other areas of the United States but windier and more moist (Kurtz, 1982).

There is a close relationship of extreme cold weather to the occurrence of hypothermia. The exposure may be secondary to inadequate clothing, or both. Defective thermoregulatory mechanisms may contribute to hypothermia even when environmental temperature is moderate and clothing sufficient. This impairment may be more pronounced in persons with head injuries, skin diseases, and spinal cord injuries (Wallner and Spalding, 1978).

Decreased metabolism is closely associated with inactivity and immobility. Lack of exercise during cold weather is common for elderly who fear falling in icy or snowy weather. Some elderly do not shiver as readily so that increased metabolism is not produced.

Use of drugs, such as hypnotics and alcohol, have also been related as a cause of hypothermia. These drugs depress body temperature by decreasing activity levels and by vasodilatation. These drugs may also contribute to a fall from which an elderly person cannot rise or move. This is particularly dangerous for the elderly person who lives alone. Lying in one position may further decrease metabolic activity with a subsequent decrease in body temperature.

ASSESSMENT OF TEMPERATURE

The goal of assessment is to identify the elderly who are at risk for developing problems related to inadequate temperature control. Prevention of potential problems is important when dealing with the elderly. The nurse in the outpatient department of a hospital may encounter the elderly person who has an inadequately heated room. The librarian often observes regular "visitors" who spend the day reading the local paper because the library is the warm or aid-conditioned second home. As congregate meal centers are growing in usage and number, workers at all levels must be asking why certain persons are not attending.

Core Temperature

The nurse and client should know the client's average core temperature. This knowledge is helpful in interpreting any change. If the client is unable to keep the mouth closed while measuring the core temperature, a rectal temperature should be obtained. In the elderly, a change in core body temperature does not always occur as a warning of problems. The nurse must therefore be alert to other parameters, such as changes in behavior or mood, which may be indicative of illness. There are advantages and disadvantages in measuring core body temperature at different sites of the body. Obviously it is easier for the client to take his own temperature if he is able to place the oral thermometer under his tongue and hold his mouth closed for the 8 or 9 minutes required for the greatest degree of accuracy. This method is also clean and not embarrassing. Disadvantages of oral temperature involve the restless person, or the edentulous client who is unable to close the mouth.

The electric thermometers with individual sheaths for each patient work well in an institutional setting where speed is important. The standard mercury bulb type is the most economical for home use. The older person may find the magnifying glass used with it a great convenience.

The rectal route may be preferred if another person is available to insert the thermometer, if the rectum is free of fecal material, and if the client is not suffering from hemorrhoids or recent rectal surgery. The rectal thermometer may be removed after 3 minutes.

The optimal time for temperature taking should be considered. Core body temperature is highest in late afternoon and early evening, and lowest in the morning. Nurses can save time by taking daily temperature readings between 4:00 P.M. and 8:00 P.M.

Room temperature must also be considered, as several investigators have shown that a thermometer must be left in longer to reach optimal body readings if the environmental temperature is lower (Nichols and Verhonick, 1967).

The goal of assessment is to identify elderly who are at risk for developing hypothermia or hyperthermia. The risk factors should include baseline data regarding the client's usual response to temperature change, the environment, activity level, medication use, health status, and economics.

The following guide should be considered in assessment:

- **Response to temperature changes**

    Heat—ability to perspire, use of fluids, accessibility to air-conditioning, fans, and ventilation.

    Cold—ability to shiver, use of clothing, type of clothing.

- **Environment**

    Type and source of heat.

    Ability to control and see thermostat.

    Need for use of auxiliary heaters or fans.

    Presence of weather-proofing such as insulation, storm windows, weather-stripping.

- **Activity level**

    Sedentary versus active.

    Activity level in cold weather versus hot weather.

- **Medication use and health status**
- **Economics**

    Ability to pay utility bills.

    Ability to purchase adequate clothing.

- **Appearance**

    Skin—evidence of numerous skin lesions, temperature to touch.

    Clothing—appropriate for weather.

- **Body temperature**

PLANNING AND INTERVENTION

Prompt referral and treatment is warranted for persons who exhibit signs of hypothermia or hyperthermia. In cases of hypothermia, warmth should be applied, warm fluids given, and the person should be moved to a warm environment until more intensive treatment is available. In hyperthermia, cooling by cool sponge baths, fluids, and improved ventilation are indicated. In the 1983 heat wave, efforts were made to supply fans and air conditioners to the poor and elderly.

The nurse is in a better situation to prevent these incidents by teaching the client about preventive measures and referral for utility payment assistance.

Environment

With increasing numbers of elderly people in the population living on fixed incomes and facing steadily rising utility costs, the role of the nurse as a political advocate comes to the forefront. At the local level, the nurse must consider such problems as whether or not third-party notification is required if gas or electrical supplies are to be terminated. Some states, as a result of action by the public utility commission, have prohibited utility companies from stopping gas and electrical services. Other states have granted a reduction of utility costs to the elderly. The federal government has allocated funds to the states so that direct grants can be made to persons who are in arrears on their utility bills.

The elderly must be informed when special fundings are made available to them, such as for utility bills, or when tax rebates are provided to persons who increase insulation levels of their property. At the same time, they must be guarded against unscrupulous contractors who promise to provide environmental improvements at inflated prices.

Some communities have established telephone networks for daily contact with the elderly. Such a service is especially important during periods of severe weather. Contingency plans should be made by communities to house people on a temporary basis when prolonged adverse weather depletes fuel supplies.

Just as many communities have designated "Block Parents" from which children can seek protection when going to and from school, communities should also establish information banks to record where the elderly of an area are located and what their environmental resources are. In urban areas, this could cover an area of a few blocks. In rural regions, the county could be subdivided into sections, with a coordinator assigned to serve as a resource person.

Economic

Budget planners state that not more than one-fourth of a person's income should be spent for housing. The elderly home owner may not have a mortgage, but must still set aside a portion of this housing allotment for taxes, maintenance, and utility costs.

In sections of Appalachia, "Charge Card" stores have been established. Persons in need of items but without funds to purchase them can obtain the item, such as a warm coat, and then contribute a specified number of hours of work to the store. This concept could be applied to the elderly, who might contribute time to such work as repainting toys or visiting shutins.

Activity Level

An inactive person generates less body warmth than an active person. Nurses caring for the elderly have often found that the bedfast client is uncomfortable in an air-conditioned hospital room.

An elderly person must limit the time spent outdoors during extremely high temperature periods because of inability to sweat. If the temperature is low, on the other hand, additional warm clothing must be worn.

ASSESSMENT BASE: INTEGUMENTARY SYSTEM

The skin and mucous membranes form an extensive physical barrier at the interface between the person and the environment. Skin is comprised of the epidermal, dermal, and cutaneous layers. The skin serves as a large neuroceptor and thermal regulatory force.

The epidermal layer is dull white and transparent. Located within the epidermis are the pigment melanin, which is brown and has a broad range of absorption, and the carotenoids, which are yellow. The dermis contains two biochromes, oxyhemoglobin, which is bright red, and reduced hemoglobin, which is bluish. Redness or blueness of skin reflects the relative proportion of each present, and is best observed in the lips and mucous membranes.

The function of sweat glands is to secrete water at the skin surface, so that the skin is cooled as water evaporates. Sweat serves to keep skin surfaces moist, to prevent flaking of the skin, and to maintain tactile sensitivity.

The envelope of skin which covers the body absorbs sunlight, which, in turn, assists in the production of vitamin D and enhances the metabolism of calcium. Enzymes in the skin permit certain drugs to be metabolized.

Aging in the Epidermis

Atrophy of the epidermis is frequently observed in the most exposed areas of the body, such as the face, neck, hands, and forearms, as well as in areas such as the mid-back. This degenerative process is characterized by thinning of the epidermis and flattening of the ridges. Most of the epidermal changes are probably due to the long-term effects of exposure to the ultraviolet of sunlight. Blond, blue-eyed, and red-haired individuals show this change earlier than the Caucasian with a darker complexion. Blacks, with their extensive melanization, show the least amount of change.

Skin Problems in the Elderly

Most problems of aging skin are related to aging of the structures of the integument, accompanied by circulatory, neurologic, or hormonal change, and long-term exposure to sunlight. The common problems of the aged integument manifest as easy breakdown of the skin, decline in repair rate, change in appearance of the skin, and pruritus.

Decubitis, or other skin breakdown as a result of burns or direct injury, presents difficulty for the elderly. Skin must be protected from hazards in the environment. Scald burns are common in the elderly. The decline in repair rate may in part explain the mortality rates from burns being increased in the elderly. Skin breakdown or irritation as a result of chemical irritants, such as detergents, show an increase in the elderly. Skin breakdown, particularly on the feet, is more common in diabetics and persons with peripheral vascular disease.

There are several benign asymptomatic changes in the appearance of the skin besides wrinkling and loss of elasticity. These changes are termed: lentigo, seborrheic keratosis, skin tabs, cherry angionomas, and bruising.

⌐entigo (age spots or liver spots) are mac-⌐ae composed of irregular collections of melanocytes. They appear brownish and in various sizes and do not fade as freckles. They appear more frequently in exposed areas of the body.

Seborrheic keratosis is characterized by yellow–brown–gray areas that may be flat and rough. Commonly keratoses become raised and appear warty. These may appear in scalp, extremities, and trunk.

Skin tabs are small polyp-like growths that appear more commonly on the neck and trunk.

Seborrheic keratosis and skin tabs may become a nuisance to the client when they are cosmetically unsightly, or are located in areas where friction of clothing or body parts produce irritation.

Cherry angionomas or red spots are associated with changes in capillaries. These changes are of little consequence.

Bruising or ecchymosis, because of increased capillary fragility, is also seen particularly secondary to trauma. The client may not remember the specific bump or trauma. Bruising may also be due to bleeding disorders, either primary or secondary to anticoagulant therapy.

Pruritus or "itchy skin" is a common complaint of the elderly. Pruritus increases in response to cold weather and low humidity. The dryness of heated air and air-conditioned air is often aggravating. Pruritus may also increase in response to irritating clothing and chemicals. Many elderly give a history of daily baths, which contributes to drying the skin. Pruritus accompanied by hives or rash may be a result of allergy or infestation of lice or scabies. Pruritus that cannot be relieved (by measures that are discussed later) may also be indicative of systemic disease, i.e., liver disease, neoplasms, and anemias.

Herpes zoster (shingles), a benign skin problem of the aged is characterized initially by redness and pain in one or two dermatomes. The pain may be excruciating in some cases. Some relief may be obtained by early treatment with cortisone. The reddened areas develop vesicles. The sequelae usually end in 4 weeks. Herpes zoster represents a reactivation of the varicella virus that has remained dormant since initial infection, probably in childhood. Although herpes zoster is benign, it often accompanies systemic malignant disease.

Elderly persons show an increased incidence of skin cancer, as with other cancers. Sun exposure is instrumental in development of skin cancers. Actinic keratosis, considered premalignant, is characterized by a small reddened macule with small dilated blood vessels. The lesion becomes yellowish-brown and rough. Basal cell cancers appear asymptomatically as pearly gray areas with small hemorrhagic areas on the surface. These lesions grow slowly and are primarily located on exposed areas. Squamous cell cancer is less common but is associated with actinic keratosis. This lesion appears indurated and is more invasive than the previously mentioned lesions. Prompt diagnosis and treatment is indicated for all these lesions. A guide for assessing the skin can be found in Appendix C.

PLANNING AND INTERVENTION

The ultimate goal in nursing is to maintain the integrity of the skin. Nursing intervention should include frequent inspection, cleanliness, nail care, warmth, exercise, and moderating environmental hazards.

Inspection

The client should be taught to inspect his body, particularly the feet. Complete skin inspection may be difficult for clients who are confused, obese, arthritic, or visually impaired. This may indicate a need to teach a relative. If the client is in an institution, the responsibility may lie with a member of the health team.

Inspection should include the skin, nails, and hair distribution, as described previously. The active healthy elderly may need to do a complete inspection only monthly. Emphasis should be on appearance of new skin lesions and a change in previously noted lesions. Referral for accurate diagnosis is indicated.

Feet should be inspected closely, as changes in this area may be the initial signs of diabetes or peripheral vascular disease (Smiler, 1982).

Any symptoms of numbness, tingling, or burning should cause the examiner to suspect diabetes. The diabetic may exhibit loss of hair on the lower leg, deep discoloration of the toes, cracks or blisters on the toes, loss of peripheral pulses, and marked changes in color and shape of toenails. Daily inspection of the feet is indicated for the diabetic.

The skin of the immobile elderly should be more frequently inspected for signs of decubitus. A sign of redness or paleness over a bony prominence should instigate changing the client's position. No magic time at which skin breakdown occurs is known. For the helpless, immobile person, inspection and turning may be indicated every half hour. Cleanliness is also important for the immobile person. Sliding the immobile person on sheets may cause a friction-type injury that may appear as a blister or an open abrasion. Friction can be avoided by use of a draw sheet to lift or turn the elderly client. Adhesive tape and plastics, clinging to the skin, may cause abrasions when separated. Use of adhesives and plastics should be avoided.

Cleanliness

Unfortunately for the elderly in the United States, "cleanliness is often considered next to godliness." The long-time habit of daily bathing is the chief factor in causing dry skin, resulting in pruritus. If daily showers or baths are necessary to the individual, the application of emollient creams or lotions should be applied after blotting the skin dry. The emollient retards loss of water from the aged skin. The unattended elderly should avoid use of emollients or water softeners in the tub or shower, as these may cause slippery surfaces that can promote falls. Hot baths or showers should also be avoided to prevent scald burns. When possible, the temperature of the water should be adjusted before getting in the tub or shower. This is particularly important for persons who live in households where the water heater temperature is often high enough to produce scald burns in 20–30 second exposures. Often this high temperature is recommended for hot water heater operation, and dishwasher use.

Cleansing agents should be mild. In some allergic clients, antibacterial soaps should be avoided. Water, alone, is cleansing and sufficient to maintain hydration of the skin. Superfatted soaps are preferrable to low fat soaps.

Inflammation in friction areas (common in obese persons) should be kept dry and aired frequently. Corn starch is preferred to some talcums, which cake and may cause irritation to the respiratory tract.

If the client is incontinent, frequent cleansing of the perineum is indicated. Urine is a medium for bacterial growth and the moisture contributes to skin breakdown. Plastic incontinence pads tend to promote perspiration as well as trap incontinent urine. If they must be used, additional absorbent cloth should be placed between the skin and the pad.

Feet should be cleansed daily in instances of extreme perspiration or diabetes. The feet should be dried carefully, particularly between the toes. Emollients may be applied to soften hard, brittle nails.

Nail Care

The changes in nail structure cause problems for the elderly. Cutting of the nails is difficult as the nails become thicker and more brittle. Soaking the nails in warm water helps to soften the nail. The toenails should be cut straight across. Persons who have impaired vision or diabetes should be referred to a podiatrist for regular nail and foot care.

Warmth

Warmth becomes important for the person exposed to cold. Light layers of clothing are often more protective and comfortable. Rough clothing should not be used if in direct contact with the skin. Provisions for warmth in cold weather should never be such as to produce perspiration, which cools the body.

When circulation to the feet is decreased, use of cotton or wool socks are preferable. Many elderly complain of cold feet at night. Socks should be used as well as lightweight thermal blankets. It is best to keep covers loose so that the person can move his feet. The client should be taught to avoid use of garters, tight girdles, and tight stockings, which may constrict circulation.

The elderly should be taught to avoid use

of hot water bottles and heating pads, as these may cause burns. This is particularly important for persons with decreased circulation.

Shoes should be selected carefully. They should be loose enough to permit air circulation and movement of the toes. Leather is preferred to synthetics because leather "breathes" and allows for ventilation.

Exercise

Exercise, either active or passive, promotes circulation to the periphery. Daily walking is helpful particularly for those with decreased circulation, as is passive range of motion for the immobile.

Modifying Environment

In many instances, the nurse can suggest ways of changing the elderly's environment or his response to exposure. Dry skin is accentuated when the room air is dry, either from heating or air-conditioning. Humidifiers add moisture to the air. Some are available for attachment to forced air heating units. This is not possible when steam-heat or electric is the heat source, but additional moisture may be obtained by placing pans of water on radiators, leaving the tub filled with water, or using portable humidifiers. Cold water humidifiers are preferable to hot water humidifiers but serve as reservoirs for infection. Sodium hypochlorite should be added to the water to eliminate this problem.

The older client needs protection from sunlight because of past history of sun exposure and the changes in the skin. Protective, light, porous clothing should be worn. Sun screen lotions are now available in various strengths to prevent ultraviolet rays from penetrating the skin; these lotions should be used.

EVALUATION

The elderly client should be evaluated in terms of knowledge they have about potential aging changes in immunity, temperature control, and the integument. When the nurse and client discuss the changes and the rationale for prevention of infections, hypothermia, hyperther-

mia, and skin breakdown, motivation for self-care in these areas should increase. Criterion-based goals should be used for evaluation.

1. The immune status of the elderly client can be enhanced if he:
   a. maintains yearly influenza vaccination
   b. receives yearly examination for early detection of cancer
   c. has received pneumococcal vaccine
   d. has received tetanus booster within the past 10 years
2. Temperature control can be enhanced if he:
   a. wears additional, layered clothing when temperature is low
   b. seeks aid when unable to pay utility bills
   c. avoids exposure to extremely hot or cold temperatures
   d. uses cooling devices such as fans, air conditioners, cool baths, and cool liquids when temperature is high
3. The protection of the integumentary system can be enhanced if he:
   a. inspects his skin and feet routinely (daily or monthly depending upon his health status)
   b. uses soothing emollients during or after bathing
   c. avoids use of constrictive clothing
   d. seeks care when skin changes occur

When the elderly client is immobile or dependent upon others, the caretaker must assume responsibility for preventing infections, hypothermia, hyperthermia, and skin breakdown. The health-care provider must be aware of aging changes in the immune system, responses in temperature control, and the integumentary system.

REFERENCES CITED

Callard, R.E. Aging of the immune system, in Kay, M.M.B., Makinodan, T. (eds.), CRC Handbook of Immunology in Aging. Boca Raton, FL, CRC Press, 1981

Center for Disease Control. Morbidity and Mortality Weekly Report. U.S. Dept. of Health and Human Services 29(31): August 8, 1980

Collins, K.J., Dore, C., Exton-Smith, A.N. Accidental hypothermia and impaired temperature homeostasis in the elderly. British Medical Journal 1:353, 1977

Finkelstein, M.S. Unusual features of infections in the aging. Geriatrics 37:65, 1982

Foster, K.J., Elles, F.P., Dore, C., Exton-Smith, A.N., Weiner, J.S. Sweat responses in the aged. Age and Aging, 5:91, 1976

Gardner, I.D. The effect of aging on susceptibility to infection. Reviews of Infectious Diseases 2:801, 1980

Irvine, P., Crossly, K., Warren, B., Mead, K. Immunity to Tetanus in an Ambulatory Geriatric Population. Paper presented at 31st annual meeting of Gerontological Society, Dallas, November, 1978

Kurtz, K.J. Hypothermia in the elderly: The cold facts. Geriatrics 37(1):85, 1982

Montagna, W., Carlisle, K. Structural changes in aging skin. Journal of Investigative Dermatology 73:47, 1979

National Center for Health Statistics Monthly Vital Statistics Report. Final Mortality Statistics. DHHS Public PHS 80-1120 29(6): September 1980

Nichols, G., Verhonick, P. Time and temperature. American Journal of Nursing 11(67):2303, 1967

Phair, J.P. Aging and infection: A review. Journal of Chronic Disease 32:535, 1979

Pachi, P.E., Strauss, J.S., Downing, D.T. Age-related changes in sebaceous gland activity. Journal of Investigative Dermatology 73:108, 1979

Selmanowitz, V., Rizer, R., Orentreich, N. Aging of the skin and its appendages, in Finch, C.E., Hayflick, L. (eds.), Handbook of the Biology of Aging. New York, Van Nostrand Reinhold, 1977

Tyan, M.L. Marrow stem cell during development and aging, in Kay, M.M.B., Makinodan, T. (eds.), CRC Handbook of Immunology in Aging. Boca Raton, FL, CRC Press, 1981

Wollner, L., Spalding, J.M.K. The autonomic nervous system, in Brocklehurst, J.C. (ed.), Textbook of Geriatric Medicine and Gerontology. London, Churchill-Livingstone, 1978

17

The Nursing Process Applied to the Aged Person Receiving Medication

Nancy J. Ebert

Reading this chapter will enable the individual to:

1. Identify factors essential for assessing drug usage
2. Identify factors which contribute to drug misuse in the elderly
3. Identify interventions which would reduce drug misuse in the elderly

The focus of this chapter is on the nu‧ plications of medication therapy to th‧ client. It is generally accepted that t‧ sponse to medication is affected by aging. Ho‧ ever, most research concerning medication therapy for the adult has been centered on the "average" young adult. Research on medication therapy in the elderly is now emerging. One must remember that the elderly are a heterogenous population.

This chapter incorporates the results of research as they relate to the nursing process. It is assumed that the reader has a general knowledge about pharmacodynamics (the study of drugs and their actions) and has access to current literature in this field.

A national survey of the cost of health care and prescription drugs revealed that in a single year persons 65 and older spent $2,260,000,000, or $103.17 per capita, on prescription drugs (Fulda, 1974). Although persons 65 and over represented 10.2 percent of the population, they accounted for 23.6 percent of the total expenditure for prescription drugs. The high expenditure for prescription drugs is undoubtedly related to the greater frequency with which chronic illnesses occur in elderly persons. These illnesses include cardiovascular disease, degenerative joint disease, autoimmune disorders, and infection. Many elderly persons have more than one chronic illness and are likely to be prescribed more than one drug.

Research at this time indicates that the elderly person's response to medications is individualistic and, in many instances, unpredictable. Some responses may be erratic, and may not resemble the usual expected response described in texts on medications. For these reasons, the elderly client who takes medications should be assessed carefully for erratic response, as well as for effectiveness of each medication.

ASSESSMENT FACTORS RELATED TO THE ELDERLY PERSON WHO TAKES MEDICATIONS

Many factors can influence the individual's response to medication therapy. The nurse is in a position to assess and monitor the effects of such therapy, as well as any factors present that may inhibit or exaggerate the desired effects. These factors include (1) age-related physiologic changes, (2) health status of the client, (3) adverse drug reactions, (4) the client's understanding of each medication and its action, and (5) the client's ability to follow prescribed regimens.

Physiologic Changes of Aging

The physiologic changes of aging have long been believed to alter the elderly person's response to medications. Changes in gastrointestinal, cardiovascular, metabolic, and renal functions often accompany aging. These changes may, in turn, affect absorption, distribution, and elimination of certain medications leading to an undesirable reaction.

Absorption is dependent upon swallowing ability, gastric integrity, and motility of the gastrointestinal tract. Decreases in gastric secretion of hydrochloric acid as well as decreased motility of the gastrointestinal tract, are seen with greater frequency in the elderly. A drug that requires an acid environment for dissolution and subsequently reaches a less acid environment may not be entirely absorbed. The action of drugs that are dissolved in the stomach may be altered. This may result in incomplete absorption of the drug dosage so that the desired response is decreased.

Decreased motility of the gastrointestinal tract may delay absorption of drugs particularly those that are absorbed in the small intestine. Gastrointestinal changes may also affect the client's tolerance to certain foods and elimination patterns. Since procedures for testing stomach secretion of hydrochloric acid and patterns of gastrointestinal motility are costly, the nurse should assess for changes in food tolerance or elimination patterns as well as for the response to drugs taken orally. If measurable, is the drug's onset of action like that described in the literature? This is probably easiest to assess if the drug is an analgesic.

Metabolism occurs primarily in the liver. Many drugs are metabolized by the liver into biologically inert substances, which can then be excreted by the kidneys. Hepatic enzymes necessary for metabolism and detoxification of drugs change with aging (Bhanthumnavin and

Schuster, 1977). However, at this time only limited research has centered on age-related changes in liver function, as measured by tests for bilirubin, alkaline phosphatase, and serum enzyme concentrations. These tests are more valuable for detecting liver dysfunction or illness. A history of alcohol abuse, cirrhosis, or hepatitis may predispose the elderly client to liver damage sufficient to cause delayed or incomplete metabolism, either of which can lead to cumulative or prolonged effects by a drug. When possible, the nurse should assess the duration of a drug's effect. If the duration is prolonged, the client may show signs of an exaggerated response.

Cardiovascular changes may alter the rate at which a drug is distributed to tissues. Decreases in cardiac output have been demonstrated with aging. Declines in serum albumin may also accompany the aging process (Bhanthumnavin and Schuster, 1977). If indications of altered cardiac output or insufficient blood flow are present, drug distribution to reactive tissues is delayed. Many drugs become bound to plasma protein, leaving only a portion of the drug readily available to diffuse into the reactive cells. If serum albumin levels decrease, more of the drug can reach the reactive tissues. As a result, the action of the drug may be exaggerated. The nurse should assess for changes in cardiovascular status, including changes in pulse, blood pressure, and peripheral pulses.

Changes in the rate at which drugs are excreted are primarily associated with alterations in renal function. Renal blood flow and the glomerular filtration rate may decline with aging, so that drugs are excreted more slowly and less efficiently. This decrease in function may extend the effective half-life of drugs which are normally excreted by the kidneys. The half-life of a drug is defined as the time it takes the body to eliminate half of the amount of a drug that has reached its peak level in the circulation. Hansen, Kampmann, and Laursen (1970) report that the half-life of drugs may be more than doubled in the elderly person. This is particularly true of digoxin, penicillin, aminoglycosides, and tetracycline, all of which are excreted by the kidneys. The extended half-life may be manifest as a prolonged effect of the drug, and in some instances the client may display symptoms of overdosage.

The physiological changes of aging vary with the individual. Evidence indicates that these changes may affect rates of absorption, distribution, metabolism, and excretion. Since tests to detect physiological changes are costly, the nurse should concentrate on assessing for desirable or undesirable effects of medications. When uncertain of the usual onset and duration of activity of a drug, the nurse should refer to current pharmacy texts for accurate information. The nurse must also assess other factors that may contribute to altered activity of a drug.

Health Status of the Individual

Age-related pathophysiologic changes may also contribute to an unpredictable response to medication therapy. Pathology of the cardiovascular system, such as congestive heart failure, can further alter the rate of distribution of a drug. Nutritional status may alter absorption as well as distribution of drugs. Degenerative joint disease may decrease activity level so that the cardiac output is affected. Liver disease may alter the client's ability to metabolize drugs.

Pathophysiologic changes in the stomach, intestine, liver function, blood constituents, and cardiac or kidney function may be superimposed on the physiologic changes of aging. The nurse should therefore obtain a thorough health history, and should determine the client's response to the various drugs that are being taken. Physicians knowledgeable about the aging process suggest limiting the number of drugs prescribed for the elderly person, in order to avoid adverse reactions to medication.

Adverse Drug Reactions

Evidence indicates that the incidence of adverse reactions to drugs increases with age, number of medications used, and history of previous reactions. Hurwitz (1969) studied the first hospital admissions of 1160 patients who were given medications. Adverse reactions occurred in 118 patients, 66 percent of whom were 60 years or older. Those patients who de-

veloped adverse reactions were receiving a median number of nine drugs. In a study of elderly persons in the Medicare program, an average of 10.8 drugs per patient had been prescribed (Nithman, Parkhurst, and Sommers, 1971). The elderly individual who is being treated for chronic illnesses is likely to be taking several medications.

Several known factors contribute to development of adverse drug reactions. Adverse reactions may occur when (1) drugs taken concurrently have a similar synergistic effect, (2) one drug counteracts the effect of another, (3) gastrointestinal absorption is altered by food or drugs, (4) urinary excretion is altered by decreased renal function, food or drugs, or (5) electrolyte levels are altered (Hussar, 1979).

Symptoms of adverse reactions may range from no desired effect of a drug to an exaggerated effect or to nonspecific effects. The nonspecific effects may be nausea, anorexia, fatigue, weakness, dizziness, urinary retention, constipation, or changes in cognitive function. Many of these effects may be confused with signs and symptoms of aging.

Adverse reactions may be prevented by assessing the client carefully prior to prescribing a medication. As an example, a client who is prescribed a tranquilizer should be assessed comprehensively for alcohol usage. The combination of the tranquilizer and alcohol produce exaggerated sedative effects—confusion, delirium, and even death. Since most drugs are excreted by the urinary system, renal function should be evaluated. The most reliable test for evaluating renal function is the creatinine clearance test. Elderly clients with reduced creatinine clearance are at a greater risk for toxicity and cumulative effects.

Studies about the noninstitutionalized elderly and drug use are emerging. Clients report not seeking advice about use of OTC drugs (Carlson and Adams, 1979), and many reported not receiving information regarding side effects of prescribed medications. Guttman (1977) surveyed 477 noninstitutionalized ambulatory elderly persons for prescribed and nonprescribed use of drugs. Sixty-two percent reported use of prescribed drugs. Cardiovascular (39.3 percent), sedatives and tranquilizers (13.6

percent), and antiarthritic drugs (9.4 percent) were most frequently used prescribed drugs. Sixty-nine percent reported use of the over-the-counter drugs, over half being analgesics. Only 12 percent reported having symptoms of overdose or side effects related to prescription use and only 16 percent reported consultation with the physician for advice about use of over-the-counter (OTC) drugs.

Drug usage among the community-based elderly should be a concern to health professionals. Many of these elderly, being mobile, have access to grocery stores as well as pharmacies for purchase of OTC drugs. They may have the means to see more than one physician. Knowledge about both prescribed and over-the-counter drugs and their potential side effects needs to be conveyed to these elderly. Many people do not regard over-the-counter preparations as drugs and fail to report their use unless specifically questioned about use of cough and cold remedies, pain relievers, remedies for indigestion, and the like. Some elderly on fixed income choose an over-the-counter drug to avoid the cost of seeing a physician and obtaining an expensive prescribed drug.

The elderly need to be aware that two or more medications may interact to cause adverse reactions. They also need to be warned that some over-the-counter medications, such as certain cough and cold remedies, are contraindicated for the individual with glaucoma or hypertension, conditions commonly found in the elderly.

The nurse also should gather data regarding the number of medications taken. The elderly person may borrow or take drugs that have been prescribed for another client, or drugs that are left over from previous illnesses. Therefore, the nurse should determine the date on which each medication was prescribed.

Client's Knowledge of Medications

The general population, including the elderly, lacks knowledge about names of drugs and understanding of their pharmacologic action. In one study of elderly persons who were prescribed drugs after discharge from a hospital, only 6 of the 42 subjects could remember the name of the medication (Atkinson, Bibson, and Andrews, 1978). Many clients, when questioned, will state that they take a "water pill" or a "heart pill." Since several different medications can be classified as "heart pills," more specific information is needed to build up a useful, accurate drug history. The nurse should request the client to bring the medication containers and show them to the nurse or physician. The labels contain the name of the medication, date of prescription, dosage, number of dosage forms in the container initially, the physician's name, instructions for use, and the name of the pharmacy dispensing the medication. When the client cannot remember what medications are being taken, the nurse may instruct the person to keep a list of them in a wallet or purse.

By reading the label, the nurse can obtain data regarding proper use of a medication. Suppose the label states that the prescription was filled 2 months ago. Five tablets remain in the container. Thirty tablets were originally dispensed. Further probing may determine that the client first used up the remaining medication from a previous prescription. In other cases, the client may respond that "I sometimes forget to take my pills." The nurse can help a forgetful client arrive at the most effective way of remembering to take medication.

The appearance of a different physician's name on each prescription label also calls for further assessment. The client may visit a clinic or office at which a different physician is seen during each visit. On the other hand, the person may be visiting different physicians for treatment of the same illness. The physicians may be unaware that this is happening. The result is that more medications than the client needs are being prescribed and subsequently taken. The person should be instructed to see the same physician or attend the same clinic, so that the response to medications can be monitored more accurately.

The appearance of a different pharmacy name on each label may indicate that, at a given time, one pharmacy or another was convenient for the client to go to. Many pharmacies are now keeping a drug profile as a special service for their clients. A drug profile includes any history of allergies, as well as a list of medications that have been dispensed by the pharmacy to the client. The person is asked to report any adverse reactions. The drug profile can serve two purposes. It can be a quick source of information about what the client is currently taking or has taken in the past. The drug profile can also be evaluated for potential drug–drug interactions. The elderly person should be informed of the purpose of a drug profile and its usefulness. When examining a medication container, the nurse should note the type of cap. If the container has a childproof cap, the patient's ability to open the container should be assessed.

Knowledge about proper storage is also important for some drugs. Nitroglyceride tablets, for instance, should be kept in a dark container in a cool place. Some drugs decompose in the presence of moisture so that lids must be kept tightly closed.

Client's Ability to Follow Prescribed Regimens

A common problem that has been identified in the elderly is difficulty in taking medications at prescribed intervals. Several factors may contribute to this problem—the high cost of medications, negligence, misunderstanding of the purpose and importance of each medication, or unusually complex regimens (odd scheduling or a high number of prescriptions).

Medications that seem to cost too much for the client may lead to misuse or no use. For example, an 80-year-old woman visited a senior citizens' center to have her blood pressure checked. The reading was 196/110. She said that she knew she had high blood pressure and had pills for it but "didn't take them." Because she took two "heart pills," which cost over $30.00 a month, she believed it was less important to spend money on her high blood pressure pills.

In one study (Brand, Smith, and Brand, 1977), more errors in taking medications occurred when three or more medications were prescribed and when the frequency of dosages

was high. More careful assessment of the client who must take several medications at several different times each day is indicated. Does the client use any special methods to remember? If so, what are they, and how effective have they been thus far?

Wandless and Davie (1977) studied 46 oriented elderly persons on a geriatric rehabilitation unit who were responsible for taking their own medications. The study was conducted for 2 weeks. The number of dosage forms for each day was calculated. Overdosing and underdosing accounted for most of the medication errors. The elderly who are responsible for taking their own medications should be given simple regimens whenever possible. Prescriptions for "every other day" or "three times a week" should be avoided. When this is not possible, special gimmicks to help the client remember the more complex regimens should be provided. These methods of intervention are discussed later in the chapter.

Health team members who work with old persons must have an appreciation of how drug therapy presents more potential problems for the elderly than for the younger adult. Knowledge of pharmacodynamics, the nature and incidence of drug effects on the body's physiologic processes, is an essential tool for prevention or modification of these problems. With the wide number of medications already available, as well as the number of new products being constantly developed, health team members must have access to resources that are valid, reliable, current and cognizant of the age-related changes in the elderly person.

In many settings, the nurse has a longer exposure to a client than other health team members, and consequently has more opportunity to assess the client's response to medications. The nursing process provides a systematic approach to assessment and prevention of adverse responses which may occur. The nurse must remember, however, that evaluation and reassessment may be necessary in such time-limited situations as outpatient services. To reduce overlap, the discussions of planning, intervention, and evaluation are combined in this chapter.

ASSESSMENT

Information about the client's medication regimen is an integral part of the assessment. The nurse must be informed about the specific experiences of aging—developmental, physiologic, sociocultural, and psychologic aspects—and must have a knowledge of pharmacodynamics. Assessment is an important determinant in helping the elderly take medications with the greatest degree of safety and the least chance of adverse drug reactions.

Client data can be collected from a variety of resources and by a variety of techniques, including medical history, laboratory test results, and physical examination. Interviews concerning the elderly person's use of drugs should be directed toward determining the client's (1) understanding about prescribed and over-the-counter drugs, (2) practices when taking medications, (3) attitudes regarding medications, (4) history of illness, allergy, or drug intolerances, (5) practices in storing and disposing of drugs, and (6) frequency of medical examinations. Analysis of the data obtained should be directed toward identifying risk for misuse of medications and the existence of, or potential for, adverse drug interactions.

Guide to Obtaining Medication History

A guide for obtaining the pertinent aspects of a client's use of medication is helpful. Open-ended questions are useful for assessing the person's general knowledge about medications. In response to this technique, the client can express his or her understanding about medications and the medication regimen. This free response also may provide cues upon which the nurse can elaborate questioning. The guide presented here is used to gain an overview of the client's understanding and use of medications. The nurse should request that the client bring containers of medication to the interview. The label on the container and the contents of the container will provide data about the drug regimen, and this information will also help to validate data collected from the client.

1. What medications are you taking now?
2. What medications have you taken during the past year?
3. What does each medication do?
4. How long have you been taking each medication?
5. At what time and how frequently do you take each medication?
6. How do you remember when to take medications?
7. What do you do if you forget a dosage?
8. What medications do you have at home which you are not currently using? (If so, when and why did you use?)
9. Where do you keep your medications? (regularly used? irregularly used?)
10. Where do you obtain medications? (physician, pharmacy, other?)
11. How frequently do you see a physician?
12. Have you ever had an unpleasant reaction to medications? (If so, describe.)
13. How much does it cost to obtain drugs? Is the expense a problem for you?
14. If client has medication containers, assess
    a. Data prescription was filled
    b. Times of administration
    c. Number of dosage forms in container
    d. Dosage of each unit medication
    e. Type of container—easy to open
    Further instructions for medication use, i.e., "take on empty stomach"
    Date of expiration, if any
    Type of lid on container (if childproof, ask about any difficulty opening)
15. How long do you keep medications before discarding?
16. Do you have any problems in administering the medication, such as difficulty with breaking tablets or difficulty giving self eyedrops?
17. When was the last time you reviewed your medications with your physician?

Data obtained from the interview should help the nurse assess the client's understanding of each medication and its action, as well as the person's ability to understand the prescribed drug regimen and to carry it out.

Specific Drug Categories

The actions of specific drugs often prescribed for the elderly have implications for the nurse in assessment, planning, intervention, and evaluation. With aging, the incidence and severity of chronic illness increases. The conditions for which drugs are commonly prescribed include heart disease, hypertension, diseases of bones and joints, diabetes, infection, and gastrointestinal disorders. Medications may be the treatment of choice for controlling or lessening the signs and symptoms of these conditions, as well as for slowing the underlying pathologic process. Safe use of medications by the elderly is possible, but because old persons are more susceptible to adverse drug reactions, close and frequent monitoring of drug efficacy is indicated. Adverse reactions in the elderly client may be more severe, and the pattern of the adverse response may be more erratic.

Cardiac Glycosides

The glycosides of digitalis are indicated for treatment of cardiac failure and some arrhythmias. Digoxin and digitoxin are the commonly prescribed forms. Of these forms, digoxin is preferred for use in the elderly, because the onset and duration of activity are relatively short. Digoxin in unchanged form is excreted by the kidney. Its half-life (34 to 44 hours) has been shown to increase when renal function or creatinine clearance is reduced. As a result, toxicity is more likely to occur in the usual therapeutic dosages described in the literature (0.125 to 0.5 mg/day).

Digitoxin is used less frequently because the half-life is from 5 to 7 days. Digitoxin is metabolized by the liver into inactive substances and excreted primarily by the kidneys. Digitoxin may be thus indicated for the elderly client who has renal dysfunction but contraindicated for the client who has suspected or known liver disease.

Toxicity to digitalis preparations has been reported to occur frequently in elderly populations. The potential for toxicity increases with concurrent use of potassium-depleting diuretics and amphotericin B. This potential is decreased by using potassium supplements in the form of food or medication. Periodic monitoring (every 6 months) of creatinine clearance is recommended as renal function may decline over time (Carter, Small, and Garnett, 1981). Maintenance doses may need to be decreased as the elderly client loses lean body mass. Absorption of digitalis preparations may be decreased when given with antacids, kaolin-pectin, or neomycin.

There is not a single manifestation indicative of digitalis toxicity in the elderly client. Cardiac arrhythmias and allergic reactions are reported most commonly (Bender, 1971). Cardiac arrhythmias may be detected by taking the apical pulse or by an electrocardiogram. The nurse should carefully monitor the pulse before the medication is given. Any irregularity or change in heart rate or quality should be reported. An electrocardiogram may be indicated to diagnose toxicity. Blurred or hazy vision may occur as well as changes in color perception. The elderly client should have vision tested periodically for color perception and acuity. Intake of potassium supplements should be evaluated for adequacy when clients take a potassium-depleting drug concurrently. Less discrete manifestations of toxicity may appear as anorexia, nausea, diarrhea, fatigue, dizziness, or confusion. Any of these changes in the elderly client who takes a digitalis preparation warrants further investigation for digitalis toxicity.

Additional data needed about the elderly person who takes digitalis or its derivatives should include:

1. Frequency with which pulse is checked by self or others
2. Rate, rhythm, and quality of the apical beat when examined for a full minute
3. Date of last electrocardiogram
4. Vision tests for acuity and color perception
5. Changes in eating or digestion patterns
6. Changes in weight
7. Changes in cognition
8. Concurrent usage of potassium-depleting diuretics.

Diuretics

Diuretics are used to treat hypertension and edema. The thiazides are the most commonly prescribed diuretics. These drugs prevent sodium and water reabsorption in the kidney, but the exact mechanism by which they lower blood pressure is not known. The loss of water and sodium caused by the diuretic may be accompanied by a loss of potassium and may lead to dehydration and electrolyte imbalances. Decreased fluid volume, with a subsequent decrease in cardiac output, may decrease cerebral blood flow. A rapid or drastic reduction in blood pressure may also affect cerebral blood flow and cause central nervous system effects. These effects may appear as confusion, dizziness, or inability to change position without falling.

Furosemide and ethacrynic acid act by inhibiting sodium and chloride reabsorption. These drugs are stronger diuretics and may contribute to urinary incontinence in the elderly.

With aging, postural hypotension in response to moving from a lying to a standing position is more likely to occur (Caird, Andrews, and Kennedy, 1973). Diuretic therapy, by causing a decrease in blood pressure, can be accompanied by postural hypotension. The blood pressure should be taken in a lying position and then in a standing position. When standing position values are 10 or more millimeters of mercury below the values obtained in a lying position, changes in the dosage of the drug may be indicated. The client should be instructed to change positions slowly.

Clients who receive these diuretics should take a potassium supplement, either as a prescribed medication or in the form of a potassium-rich food. Such foods include fresh oranges, bananas, tomatoes, and fresh or canned apricots. The client should be assessed for symptoms of potassium deficiency, such as muscle cramps, weakness, and fatigue. The client should be made aware of the importance of taking the potassium supplement daily.

Dehydration as an adverse response to thiazide or any diuretic therapy may be more difficult to assess in the elderly, because aging skin becomes dry and lacks turgor. Increased urine concentration and thirst may be the only visible signs of dehydration. Insidious or sudden onset of fatigue and weakness may be the first signs of electrolyte imbalance. Thiazides are known to increase blood sugar levels in persons with a predisposition for diabetes. The blood sugar level of clients who have a family history of diabetes should be evaluated carefully before and during diuretic therapy. Assessment of the elderly who take diuretics should include:

1. Frequency with which blood pressure is taken
2. Past or usual range of blood pressure determinations
3. Frequency with which weight is monitored
4. Signs or symptoms of adverse reactions
5. Source and schedule of use of potassium supplements
6. Type of diet
7. Time(s) medication is taken
8. History of diabetes
9. Lying, sitting, and standing blood pressure
10. Patterns of urination
11. Specific gravity of urine

Antihypertensives

Beta-blocking agents are used for treatment of arrhythmias and hypertension. Propranolol is the beta-blocker most commonly used. Propranolol is metabolized by the liver and its active as well as inactive derivatives are excreted by the kidneys. There are many signs of adverse reactions involving the skin, eyes, nose, gastrointestinal tract, central nervous system, and cardiovascular system. Toxicity manifests as bradycardia, bronchospasm, and hypotension. The elderly are at greater risk for toxicity when kidney and liver function is reduced (Vestal, 1982). As in the case of the client who is taking diuretics, the blood pressure should be taken in three positions and the client should be observed for hypotension.

Methyldopa is used to treat hypertension, sometimes in combination with thiazides. The exact mechanism of action is not known but lowered peripheral resistance occurs. Methyldopa is metabolized in the gastrointestinal tract and liver. Because methyldopa may produce many psychiatric side effects, the drug should be used cautiously, if at all, with elderly clients.

Reserpine is an effective antihypertensive agent, but must be used cautiously, if at all, in the elderly client. Its side effects of depression and orthostatic hypotension occur more commonly in the elderly.

Assessment should include:

1. Lying, standing, and sitting blood pressure
2. Usual pulse rate, rhythm
3. Signs of behavioral change
4. Patterns of urination

Anticoagulants

Anticoagulants may be indicated for reducing the risk of intravascular clotting. Oral anticoagulants affect prothrombin time. The effect of the anticoagulant on the prothrombin time determines the dosage to be taken. Once the dosage is determined, prothrombin time should be monitored at weekly or biweekly intervals. The therapeutic effects of anticoagulants may be altered by decreased kidney function or by inadequate absorption and storage of vitamin K, an important precursor of prothrombin. The side effects of anticoagulants include occult and gross bleeding from the mucous membranes or into subcutaneous tissues. The client should be instructed to report any signs of bleeding gums, nosebleeds, bleeding in the urine or feces, and increased incidence of bruises. Since aspirin may also alter prothrombin time, the person should be told to avoid its use. Assessment of the elderly client who takes oral anticoagulants should include:

1. Occult blood tests of urine and feces
2. History of aspirin use
3. Frequency of tests for prothrombin time

Laxatives

Laxatives are commonly used by the elderly, and are easily available as over-the-counter drugs. Frequent use of laxatives may cause constipation or diarrhea, and can lead to fluid or electrolyte imbalance and change in drug absorption. Frequent use of mineral oil should be discouraged. The efficiency of swallowing may decrease with aging, and mineral oil that enters the trachea and reaches the lungs can cause pulmonary disease. Mineral oil may also cause a deficiency in fat-soluble vitamins (vitamins A, D, E, and K), as these vitamins dissolve in mineral oil and are thus eliminated in the feces rather than being absorbed. The elderly who take laxatives should be encouraged to use other methods to enhance elimination (see Chapter 12). The client who uses laxatives should be assessed for:

1. Name of laxative used
2. Frequency of use
3. Alternative effective methods to enhance elimination
4. Diet
5. Signs of dehydration or electrolyte imbalance

Antiinflammatory Agents

Antiinflammatory agents may be indicated for the treatment of arthritis, a common condition in the elderly. Aspirin is the drug of choice, as it is relatively safe and readily available in over-the-counter preparations. However, when used frequently it may produce gastric irritation, occult or gross bleeding, and an increased prothrombin time. When taking high doses of aspirin, the aging client is at greater risk for bleeding tendencies, and should be monitored closely. Clients should be warned that many cold remedies, as well as analgesics, contain aspirin or salicylates. Concurrent use of aspirin and cold remedies containing salicylates may increase the risk of side or toxic effects. Since salicylates are excreted by the kidney, decreased kidney function predisposes the old person to the development of toxic reactions, such as tinnitus and vertigo.

Product information (Physicians' Desk Reference, 1978, pp. 878, 1669) regarding phenylbutazone, another commonly used agent for treatment of arthritis, is prefaced by a long list of precautions concerning its use. An increased incidence of toxic effects occurs with age. Irreversible hematologic effects, fluid and electrolyte imbalances, renal damage, vision impairments, and hearing loss can occur. Because of the severity of these side effects, the client should be evaluated carefully prior to treatment and, if treated, should be monitored at frequent intervals. Blood tests should be evaluated weekly. Treatment should be restricted to 1 week in persons over 60.

Steroid therapy is associated with numerous side and toxic effects. It should be used cautiously, if at all, in the elderly. Sodium retention, development of Cushing's syndrome, decreased resistance to infection, psychosis, and development of diabetes, all hazardous side effects for the elderly, must be weighed against the possible benefits of treatment with steroids. Assessment of clients receiving antiinflammatory medications should include:

1. Frequency of use
2. Concurrent anticoagulant therapy
3. If high use, tests for occult blood in urine and feces

Antacids

Antacids are commonly self-prescribed drugs used by the elderly for treatment of gastrointestinal upsets. An absorbable antacid, sodium bicarbonate, may cause acid-base imbalance. It should be used infrequently if at all, particularly by the individual with hypertension. The nonabsorbable antacids may cause constipation, a frequent complaint in the elderly. If the client is prescribed an antacid, a nonconstipating type is preferred.

Antibiotics

Antibiotics create special problems in treating infection in the elderly. Because immune response is altered with aging, the duration of the infectious process may be prolonged and present erratic manifestations. The response to the drug may be difficult to distinguish from the effects of the infection. Aminoglycosides and penicillin appear to create the most hazards for the elderly. The duration and desired activity of aminoglycosides, tetracycline, and penicillin depend on adequate renal excretion. The aged client who has diminished kidney function is at higher risk for developing toxic reactions to these antibiotics.

Ototoxic or nephrotoxic reactions to aminoglycosides are usually severe and may be irreversible. Monitoring urine output and hearing acuity are essential for the client who is taking aminoglycosides. Persons taking tetracycline should be instructed to avoid the use of nonabsorbable antacids, because they impair absorption of the drug. When antibiotics are prescribed, the nurse should instruct the client about the importance of taking the medication at the prescribed time intervals, in order to maintain a constant concentration of the drug in the blood. The person should be alerted to the importance of taking the full course of treatment, unless side effects occur. The client should be assessed for:

1. Name of the antibiotic
2. Ability of client to maintain prescribed regime
3. Presence of side or toxic effects of the drug

Sedatives and Hypnotics

Sedatives and hypnotics are frequently prescribed for treatment of insomnia and anxiety in the elderly. These substances act by depressing the central nervous system so that sedation or sleep is produced. Depression of the central nervous system may also produce depression of gastrointestinal, respiratory, cardiovascular, and motor function, all of which may be already depressed as the result of aging processes. Cautious use of these drugs in the elderly is indicated. The aging person's response to barbiturates may be erratic, and is frequently characterized by restlessness, excitement, and disorientation, rather than sedation. The nonbarbiturate sedatives and hypnotics may also produce erratic response in the elderly, but with less frequency. Constipation, incontinence, and signs of hypoxia may be produced. These drugs may cause dizziness and lead to falls.

The client's behavior prior to and during therapy with any sedative/hypnotic must be assessed carefully. Because the client may become physiologically dependent on sedatives, sudden cessation of drug therapy can produce symptoms of withdrawal. Accidental overdosage may occur if the client has easy access to the medication container. The person who has taken a sedative may be drowsy and unable to remember whether he took the medication or not. He may then proceed to take another dose.

The elderly client should be instructed to keep the container away from the bedside. Safer alternative methods for enhancing sleep patterns should be assessed and employed. These might include establishing a regular bedtime, having an evening snack, or engaging in quiet before-bedtime activities. Assessment of the elderly client who takes sedatives or hypnotics should include:

1. Behavioral patterns before and during therapy
2. Sleep patterns before and during therapy
3. Previous patterns that enhanced sleep
4. Frequency with which medication is taken
5. Storage of medication
6. Signs of adverse effects
7. Alternative methods for relaxation.

Assessment of the elderly who take medications should be comprehensive. The assessor must expect and anticipate that an erratic or adverse reaction to a medication is more likely to occur in the elderly than in a younger adult. In the hospital or extended-care facility, the nurse has responsibility for employing the correct drug regimen, and is also in a position to observe subtle changes in the elderly client. The elderly who live in the community are usually responsible for taking their own medication. These clients must be assessed not only for the response to each medication but also for methods used to carry out the correct drug regimen. All clients should receive extensive counseling regarding prescribed and nonprescribed medications and their proper use.

PLANNING, INTERVENTION, AND EVALUATION

Problems or needs that have been identified during the assessment are the keys to planning and intervening. Problems that commonly occur in the elderly who take medications can be categorized as:

1. Lack of knowledge
2. Errors of omission or commission
3. Drug–drug interaction
4. Incorrect care of medications

Lack of knowledge leads to misunderstanding about and lack of respect for medications. When a medication is first prescribed for the client, instructions should be given. Wandless and Davie (1977) found that written instruction was significantly more effective than oral instruction in enhancing compliance to drug regimens and understanding of individual drugs. The oral instruction consisted of instructing the client about the drug and having the client repeat the instructions. Two different techniques of written instruction were tested. One group of patients received a 14-day calendar that detailed each day's treatment. Another group of patients received medications to which cards were affixed, identifying each medication and giving instructions for its use. Lundin (1979) reported the effectiveness of printed drug cards with name of drug, side effects, and potential drug interactions.

Oral instruction may be less effective because of age-related cognitive changes in the client. If oral instruction about two or more medications is given and the information is complex, any client, not just the elderly person, could become confused. The effectiveness of written instructions can also be affected by the sensory changes of aging. The size and color of print may have to be altered for some clients to be able to read written instructions.

Each client should be encouraged to carry a list of medications used at all times. This list should include medications that are prescribed, as well as those obtained from other sources. Such lists are helpful in the event of sudden illness or accident, and can be used as a resource in obtaining a history of medication use. Some communities recommend keeping a list of medications inside the refrigerator, or taped to the refrigerator door.

Special instruction related to a specific drug may be necessary. If a drug is to be taken on an empty stomach, the nurse must assess the client's pattern of activities of daily living. Does the person eat on a precise schedule each day? Does the client snack between meals? A plan mutually agreed upon by client and nurse is important in setting schedules to which the client can and will adhere.

Teaching techniques to monitor effects of

drugs must be individualized. The nurse should explain and demonstrate carefully. Written instructions concerning each medication and its use should be given to the client. After instruction has been given, the person should demonstrate understanding or lack of it in his or her own words. If the client has difficulty, it may be better to teach a capable relative or friend. Having the client stop in a clinic or physician's office may be an alternative for some monitoring techniques, such as blood pressure, urinalysis, and blood tests. Referral to a home health nurse for monitoring should also be an alternative, particularly for clients with mobility problems.

Errors of omission or commission are the most frequent cause of drug misuse by the elderly. Several factors may contribute to these errors: (1) cost of the medication; (2) oral dosage forms that are difficult to swallow or are distasteful; (3) medication containers that are difficult to open; (4) forgetfulness; and (5) complex schedules for taking medications. To reduce the incidence of errors, the nurse must identify the contributory factor(s) and evolve specific nursing interventions. Errors related to drug misuse may be detected by interrelating data obtained from the medication history with data obtained from the medication container.

The high cost of medications may lead to errors of omission or commission. Because of the expense, some elderly persons extend the interval at which the medication is taken. The supply of the medication lasts longer, but its effect may be altered. In some cases, the person may even refuse to have the prescription filled. For example, one elderly client, Mrs. C, received prescriptions from a family physician. She took the prescriptions to the pharmacy and asked what the cost for each would be. Upon hearing the amount, Mrs. C retrieved the prescriptions. Two months later, she finally told the physician what had happened. This error of omission could have been circumvented if the client and physician had discussed the approximate expense of the medication and its value to the person's well-being. Choosing another place of purchase may reduce costs. Some

organizations and pharmacies offer discounts on medications prescribed for the elderly.

The high costs of medication may lead the old person to borrow medications from another person, to use medications saved from treatment of a previous illness, and to increase the use of over-the-counter medications. The use of other medications in addition to or in place of prescribed medications can create hazards for the elderly. They may be taking a medication that is inappropriate for treatment of an ailment. Some medications undergo changes in composition or strength when stored for extended periods. Nonprescribed drugs may interact and interfere with the action of prescribed medication. Any elderly client who takes medication must be informed of these dangers.

Recent changes in Medicare Part B have implication for the elderly who subscribe. Part B provides for partial reimbursement of prescriptions, ambulance fees, and inpatient skilled care. Besides paying the increased cost of the monthly premium, the elderly must accrue over $250 in bills (in 12 months) for the services covered before qualifying for reimbursement of 80 percent of the total. Many elderly may misplace receipts or do not understand, thus losing any reimbursement. The nurse needs to present information regarding the possible alternatives for reducing costs of purchase.

Problems related to dosage form are not uncommon. In Law and Chalmers' (1976) survey of 151 persons who were taking medications, 11 percent of the sample reported difficulty swallowing a pill or capsule because of its size. Liquid medications are easier to swallow, but some of them, particularly the commonly prescribed potassium supplements, may be distasteful. Diluting the liquid with water, juice, or milk may increase palatability. However, because some drugs cannot be mixed with food, information about contraindications should be obtained before diluting the drug or mixing it with food.

Childproof containers for medication may cause difficulty. Some old persons are unable to open these containers, and as a result do not take the medication. If the person has had previous difficulty with childproof containers or has limited dexterity secondary to arthritis, the client, physician, or nurse should alert the pharmacist.

Complex schedules for taking medications and/or forgetfulness also contribute to errors of omission and commission. In some instances, a simplified schedule may take priority over a complex schedule that would produce the ideal effects of a drug. A medication schedule is easier to follow when it is associated with the client's life-style. The schedule may be set to relate to mealtimes or some other routine pattern. If two separate drugs are prescribed when a combination of the drugs is available, the combination in one dosage may be easier for the client to take, as well as enhancing compliance with the prescribed schedule.

Various scheduling aids are available to assist the client who is forgetful. These include calendars, checklists, drug inserts, and special medication containers. The imaginative nurse can help the client learn ways to prevent forgetfulness from disrupting the schedule. Calendars with checklists for each medication and the times of administration can be created, to be kept with the medications. The client can then put a checkmark beside the medication each time the drug is taken. Some elderly persons place a day's supply of medication(s) in a separate container. Separate containers could also be used for certain hours of the day, if necessary. The individual should also be instructed about what to do if a dosage is forgotten. Missing one dosage is usually less of a hazard than doubling the dosage at the next prescribed time of administration. Advice regarding a missed dosage must be specific to the specific medication prescribed.

The incidence of drug–drug interactions may be reduced by limiting the number of drugs taken. Some physicians recommend that no more than three drugs be prescribed to or taken by the elderly person. The client must be told about specific drug–drug interactions which may occur. When previous prescribed medications have been discontinued, the client should be instructed to dispose of the medication promptly, preferably in the toilet, so that others cannot gain access to the medication. The nurse must

plan and individualize this instruction. The elderly client should be encouraged to purchase drugs from only one pharmacy which maintains a drug profile. The pharmacist can thus predict the potential for drug–drug interaction before it actually occurs. When the client is under direct medical or nursing supervision, a drug profile should be maintained and screened for potential drug–drug interaction. When using over-the-counter drugs, the client should be instructed to read the label for correct usage and contraindications. When in doubt, the client should be told to ask the pharmacist about the usefulness of an over-the-counter drug and contraindications for its use in combination with other drugs.

Computer programs are emerging as a safeguard to detect potential drug–drug interactions in general hospitals (Bouchard et al., 1982) and in long-term care facilities (Foxall, 1982). Computers facilitate quicker retrieval of the enormous amount of information on drug–drug reactions. Health-care providers cannot commit to memory all these reactions. In the absence of a computer or even with access to computers, the nurse should still assess the individual clients on admission or first visit and at frequent intervals for desired drug effects. The community-based client should be guided to use pharmacies who keep drug profiles and have access to computer facilities.

Incorrect care of medication may result in errors of omission or commission. Incorrect storage may cause disintegration or transformation of the drug so that its activity is altered. For example a liquid may become more concentrated, so that the usual dosage has greater strength. The elderly may keep drugs in a variety of places—closet, dresser, kitchen, bedroom, living room, or no special place at all. If they misplace the medication, dosages are often omitted. Medications should be kept in a safe place, particularly if small children or irresponsible persons are present. The place safest for the elderly client must be individually determined. Because decreasing peripheral vision, decreased visual acuity, and delayed response to light–dark transitions are common in the elderly, drugs should be kept in a place that can be well lighted and is some distance from the bedside. If the client must turn on a light, get out of bed, and walk to another place in the room, the time needed for these activities permits more effective accommodation to light.

The indications pro rata nata (PRN) drug requires that the user or caretaker know criteria for proper usage. The benefits versus the possible adverse effects must be weighed. The nurse working with institutionalized elderly has great responsibility with PRN drugs. Miller (1982) studied the decision-making of nursing home nurses regarding administration or withholding of PRN tranquilizers and/or antidepressants in four fictional vignettes. Nurses chose to withold administering 56 percent of the drugs and to administer 44 percent of the drugs. Possible side effects were most frequently reported reasons for witholding the drug. This emphasizes the need for nurses to have knowledge of the drug, knowledge of the client, and knowledge of how the drug affected the client in the past.

Problems that occur in the elderly who take medications can be prevented. Health teaching about medication, medication regimens, effective compliance methods, potential drug–drug interactions, and proper care of medications is warranted to prevent problems. The nurse, physician, and pharmacist must accept the responsibility for such teaching.

Goals and evaluation criteria should be mutually set between client and nurse. Frequent monitoring and reassessment of the elderly client who takes medications is necessary. Each client must be evaluated and reassessed using the criteria for safe use of drugs by the elderly. These criteria include:

1. Each client will take medications in a manner to enhance safe use of each medication
   a. The right medication
   b. The right dosage
   c. The right frequency of administration
2. Each client will be aware of the desired action of each medication used.
3. Each client will understand the importance of monitoring the action of drugs, i.e., counting pulse, taking blood pressure, urine test-

ing, need for medical or nursing supervision.
4. Each client will be aware of potential adverse reactions to each drug.
5. In the event of adverse reactions, the client will know what to do and to whom the reaction should be reported.
6. Each client will demonstrate knowledge of proper care and storage of medications.

In summary, the nurse has a responsibility to the elderly client who receives medications. The nurse must assess with a knowledge base of pharmacodynamics and an appreciation of the risk of adverse reactions in the elderly. The nurse must assess comprehensively, intervene effectively, and evaluate the effects of intervention. The elderly client who must take medications should take them properly and avoid factors that may contribute to adverse drug reactions.

REFERENCES CITED

Atkinson, L., Gibson, I., Andrews, J. An investigation into the ability of elderly patients continuing to take prescribed drugs after discharge from the hospital and recommendations concerning improving the situation. Gerontology 24:(3) 225, 1978

Bender, A.D. Drug therapy in the aged, in Chinn, A.B. (ed.), Working with Older People, Vol. IV. Rockville, MD, U.S. Department of Health, Education, and Welfare, 1971

Bhanthunavin, K., Schuster, M.M. Aging and gastrointestinal function, in Finch, C.E., Hayflick, L. (eds.), Handbook of the Biology of Aging. New York, Van Nostrand Reinhold, 1977

Bouchard, V.E., Bell, J.E., Freedy, H.R., Duffy, M.G., Sr. A Computerized system for screening drug interactions and interferences. American Journal of Hospital Pharmacy 29(7):564, 1972

Carlson, G.L., Adams, S.R. Medication Misuse in the Elderly. Drug Abuse and the Elderly Project. Bluegrass East Regional Mental Health, Mental Retardation Bd., Lexington, Ky. 1979

Caird, F.I., Andrews, B.R., Kennedy, R.D. Effect of posture on blood pressure in the elderly. British Heart Journal 35:527, 1973

Foxall, M.J.H. Elderly patients at risk of potential drug interaction in long-term facilities, Western Journal of Nursing Research 4(2):134–151, 1982

Fulda, T.R. Prescription Drug Summary. U.S. Dept. of Health, Education, and Welfare. Social Security Administration. DHEW Publication (SSA) 76-11928, 1974

Goldman, R. Aging of the excretory system: Kidney and bladder, in Finch, C.E., Hayflick, L. (eds.), Handbook of the Biology of Aging. New York, Van Nostrand Reinhold, 1977

Gutlman, D.A. Study of Legal Drug Use by Older Americans, U.S. Dept. of Health, Education, and Welfare, PHS Alcohol Drug Abuse & Mental Health Administration. DHEW Publication No. 77-495, 1977.

Hansen, J.M., Kampmann, J., Laursen, H. Renal excretion of drugs in the elderly. Lancet 1:1170, 1970

Hurwitz, N. Predisposing factors in adverse reactions to drugs. British Medical Journal 1:536, 1969

Lamy, P.P. Prescribing for the Elderly. Littleton, Mass.: PSG Publishing Co., Inc., 1980

Law, R., Chalmers, C. Medicines and elderly people: A general practice survey. British Medical Journal 1:565, 1976

Nithman, C.J., Parkhurst, Y.E., Sommers, E.B. Physicians' prescribing habits: Effect of Medicare. JAMA 217(5):585, 1971

Nithman, C.J. Physicians' Desk Reference, Oradell, NJ Medical Economics Co., 1978

Vestal, R.F. Pharmacology and Aging, Journal of American Geriatrics Society 30(3):191, 1982

Appendix A

Longevity Quiz

Would you like to know how long you can expect to live? Although no one can tell you exactly, this quiz based on scientific facts can provide you with ideas as to how your life-style and heredity might influence your longevity. Keep in mind that while the quiz provides you with a personal life expectancy score, its primary purpose is to stimulate your thinking about actions you might take to enhance your overall health and longevity.

Instructions: Start with 75 years. Add or subtract the following numbers to derive your personal longevity potential.

Family History

Any grandparent lived to be 85 or over	+2
All four grandparents lived to be 80	+6
Either parent died of a stroke or heart attack before 50	−4
Any parent, brother or sister under 50 has or had cancer, a heart condition, or diabetes since childhood	−3

A parent, grandparent, brother, sister, uncle, or aunt

has glaucoma	−1
has gout	−1
has ankylosing spondylitis (a form of arthritis)	−1
has high blood pressure requiring treatment	−2

Life-style

Married or living in a long-term relationship	+4
If not, subtract 1 for every 10 years you have lived alone since age 25	−1
Sleep more than 10 hours per night	−4
If you do not have a tetanus booster (every 10 years)	−1
Been in close contact with someone with tuberculosis for a year or more	−1
Intense, aggressive, and anger easily	−3
Easy going and relaxed	+1
Happy	+1
Unhappy, dissatisfied, or depressed	−3
Have had a speeding ticket or accident in the last year	−4
Other traffic violations	−1
Wear seatbelts more than 90% of the time as driver and passenger	+1
Have an expectation of good health over the next 20 years	+1

Have a pet   +1
Actively involved in a spiritual tradition or
practice   +1
Engage in gardening or raising of plants +1
Nutrition, Alcohol and Smoking
Eat a well-balanced diet   +2
Avoid saturated and unsaturated fats and
cholesterol   +1
Protein intake of 40–50 g per day   +1
Protein intake of 50–100 g per day   −1
Caloric intake of 2000–2500 per day (U.S. av-
erage, 3500)   +2
Grains and fish as primary protein source (re-
duced red meat consumption)   +2
Eat breakfast   +1
Never smoked   +3
Smoke more than one half to one pack per day
(one cigarette = one cigar)   −3
One to two packs per day   −6
More than two packs per day   −8
NOTE: 2 oz. of 80 proof whiskey = 20 oz. 4.5%
beer = 1/4 bottle of wine. All contain 20–24
ml of alcohol (not equal volume).
No alcohol consumption   +1
2 oz. (or equivalent) or less of 80 proof whiskey
per day   +2
More than 2 oz. per day   −1
For each drink over 2 oz. per day   −1

Sex
Nonwhite male   −5
Nonwhite female   −4
Male   −3
Female   +4
Regular, fulfilling sexual relations   +2
Frequent sexual activity with many different
partners   −1
Male over 40 and have annual medical
exams   +2
Female and see a gynecologist once a year
                                                              +2
Finished college   +1
Earned a graduate or professional degree +2
                                                           more

Work with asbestos regularly but do not
smoke   −2
Work with asbestos regularly   −8
For Women Only
Began regular sexual activity before 18   −1
Smoke and use birth control pills   −5
Jewish   −1
Mother or sister had or has breast cancer −4

Work and Environment
Office worker   −3
Earn over $50,000 per year but do smoke −2
Work regularly with vinyl chloride   −4
Work in ongoing contact with toxic agents or
radiation   −3
Over 65 and still working   +3
Over 65 and self-employed   +1 more
Live in an urban area with a population over
2 million   −2
Live in a town under 10,000 or on a farm +2
Physical Activity and Weight
Work requires regular physical exertion   +2
Exercise at a "moderate aerobic level" (i.e., jog-
ging, swimming, bicycling, jazzercise at least
3 times per week for at least 30 minutes per
time.)   +3
Less than 3 times per week on nonconsecutive
days   +2
No regular aerobic activity   −5

**Weight is: (compared to ideal body com-
position)**
5–20 lbs. over ideal weight   −2
20–30 lbs. over ideal weight   −3
30–40 lbs. over ideal weight   −4
40–50 lbs. over ideal weight   −6
Over 50   −8
Present Age Adjustment
Present age is:
30–40   +2
40–50   +3
50–70   +4
Over 70   +5
TOTAL:_____ = Your Longevity Potential

You have probably found that your potential for longevity is greater than you expected. Generally, the factors noted with a "+" are those that you should maintain or begin in order to attain your potential. Those determinants noted with a "−" should be elimi- nated or reduced as much as possible. Keep in mind that the quality and quantity of your life is, to a great extent, in your hands.

(Pelletier, K.R. The longevity game: Fulfilling our biological potential. Healthline, 1983, 11(8):1–3. Reprinted with permission.)

Appendix B

Outline for Gerontologic Education for Nurses

A number of outlines exist for educational programs designed to provide the knowledge base needed by nurses to provide quality care to the aged. These outlines are most easily located by reviewing the appendixes of books such as this one or by contacting schools of nursing known to provide discrete courses in gerontologic nursing. A course outline is included here as a systematic guide for those who wish to learn about the special and unique aspects of the normal aging process.

This outline follows the format developed by a Task Force on Gerontological Nursing within the Veterans Administration (Veterans Administration, 1978).* The authors of this book have included additional content to update and expand this outline. This outline emphasizes aging as a normal process, continuous over the lifespan and variable in impact upon each individual. The outline delineates the biophysical and psychosocial changes that occur as part of the normal aging process. The strengths and capabilities of the aged, as well as the problems and limitations imposed upon the individual by the aging process and pathologic changes, are identified. Values, beliefs, and attitudes toward aging and the aged are considered, and information about intra- and extramural resources and programs is presented.

COURSE OBJECTIVES

The nurse:

1. Identifies the normal biophysical and psychosocial alterations caused by the aging process
2. Describes the interrelationships that exist between the normal biophysical and psychosocial alterations of the aging process
3. Delineates the basic needs and the unmet needs of the aging individual
4. Identifies the effects of stress on the functioning of the elderly person

---

* Adapted from the *Program Guide Nursing Service: Standards and Educational Guidelines for Gerontologic Nursing Practice* by the Department of Medicine and Surgery, Veterans Administration, Washington, DC: U.S. Government Office, April 4, 1978.

5. Promotes the use of the assets of the elderly person in health and in deviations of health
6. Utilizes the nursing process with the elderly client—assessing, planning, intervening, and evaluating
7. Analyzes own feelings and behavior in relation to aging and aged people
8. Assists the client/family/care-giver to cope with losses experienced with aging, including the anticipation of death
9. Assists the client/family to maintain personal, cultural, and religious values, beliefs and practices
10. Collaborates with client/family/care-giver and interdisciplinary team in the provision of continuing health care
11. Provides teaching-learning opportunities for client/family/care-giver
12. Utilizes available community resources in meeting the needs of elderly people
13. Assesses the social and physical living environments of elderly people
14. Describes the effects of institutionalization on elderly people
15. Supports programs and legislation that benefit the elderly
16. Participates in continuing education to increase knowledge of nursing with elderly people
17. Participates in nursing research
18. Applies research findings to the care of elderly people

COURSE METHODOLOGY

Suggested teaching methods include:

• Lectures
• Demonstrations/return demonstrations
• Audiovisual aids
• Problem-oriented laboratory sessions
• Role-playing, role-reversal sessions
• Clinical experiences with both well elderly and those with health problems
• Community field trips
• Group discussions
• Nursing rounds
• Interdisciplinary rounds

• Independent studies
• Simulations and games
• Case studies involving ethical issues and elderly people
• Discussions of programs and legislation affecting elderly people
• Personal written life histories that include important life events
• Diaries of feelings about personal aging and the aging experience of others
• Debates of issues relating to aging
• Values clarification techniques

The following factors should be considered in the selection of teaching methods and course format:

• Needs of the learner
• Size and composition of the group
• Instructional personnel
• Specific behavioral course objectives
• Time allotment for course
• Availability of health team as teachers
• Learning climate
• Characteristics of clinical facility

Evaluation of course effectiveness can be based on the following strategies:

• Written tests of knowledge
• Written tests of behavioral intentions
• Written documentation, assessments, and care plans
• Interviews to determine knowledge, beliefs, and attitudes
• Direct observation of clinical practice
• Indirect observation of clinical skills through audio and videotapes, client progress notes, assessments, and care plans

COURSE CONTENT

I. INTRODUCTION
  A. Definitions
   1. Aging—Normal transformations that occur throughout the lifespan in members of all species that result in differences between young and old organisms in both structure and function. Biologic, psychologic, and social

aging can be distinguished in the human species.

2. Senescence—Biological processes in which the organism becomes less viable and more vulnerable as chronologic age increases. Manifested as an increased probability of disease, injury, and death.
3. Geriatrics—The branch of health that deals with the problems and diseases of aged people.
4. Gerontology—The study of all aspects of the aging processes and their consequences in humans and animals.
5. Gerontologic nursing—A nursing specialty concerned with assessment needs of older adults, planning and implementing health care to meet these needs, and evaluating the effectiveness of such care to achieve a level of wellness consistent with any limitations imposed by the aging process.

B. Demographic Profile

1. Number of aged in population
2. Geographic distribution
3. Health status
   a. Morbidity
   b. Cost of health care
   c. Options for care
   d. Mortality
4. Education
5. Income
6. Employment
7. Marital status
8. Housing/living arrangements

C. Attitudes of Society

1. Values and attitudes of youth-oriented industrial society
2. Stereotyped image of the aged
3. Cultural differences/similarities

D. Aging as a Personal Experience

1. Wide individual variations seen in the experience of growing old
2. How the aged view themselves
3. Personal philosophy of life, aging, and aged

II. MAJOR THEORIES AND CONCEPTS OF AGING

A. Biologic

1. Endogenous Factors
   a. Accumulation Theory—Decrease in cellular efficiency occurs and cell death results from an accumulation of deleterious materials.
   b. Error Theory—With senescence, alterations occur in the structure of the DNA molecule. These errors are transmitted to the messenger DNA and ultimately result in errors in protein synthesis, enzyme synthesis, and others.
   c. Biologic Programming Theory—Organism is programmed to live a definite length of time. A biologic clock initiates the aging sequences when certain limits are reached.
   d. Autoimmune Theory—Stimulation of the autoimmune mechanisms occurs with senescence. The possibility exists that antibody producing cells release antibodies to the body's own tissues.
   e. Neuroendocrine Control Theory—Certain cells in the brain may act as pacemakers to limit life.
2. Exogenous Factors—Alterations through the lifespan occur in chromosomes and cells to increase the likelihood of structural or functional defects. Examples of exogenous factors are nutritional disturbances, radiation, infections, and toxins.

B. Psychosocial Theories

1. Psychologic Theories
   a. Contemporary orientations—include biologic learning, cognitive, biobehavioral, ecological-field, developmental theories.
   b. Traditional systems—consider associationism, structuralism, func-

tionalism, behaviorism, Gestaldt, trait, psychoanalysis.

   c. Behavior domains—Consist of sensation, perception, attention, memory, information processing, cognition, personality, socialization.

2. Sociologic Theories

   a. The Individual's Perspective

      (1) Disengagement Theory—Disengagement is the process of mutual withdrawal of the aging individual and society from each other. The number of interrelationships between a person and other members of society is reduced and those remaining are altered in quality. Disengagement is correlated with successful aging and is considered modal or typical of most aging persons. The process is seen as an intrinsic and inevitable process.

      (2) Activity Theory—The activity theory proposes that the maintenance or development of a substantial level of physical, mental, and social activity is usually necessary for successful aging. It holds that the norms of old age are the same as those for middle age. If roles are relinquished, new useful roles must take their place. Aging individuals continue to remain middle aged as long as possible.

      (3) Continuity Theory—In the process of becoming an adult, the individual develops habits, preferences, commitments, associations, and other dispositions that become a part of the personality. As one grows older, there is a predisposition toward maintaining continu-ity in ways and commitments. As viewed by Busse, the continuity theory holds that the individual's reaction to aging can be explained by looking at the complex interrelationships among several elements of a person's life, which are as follows: the biologic and psychologic changes, the person's habits, preferences, and associations, situational opportunities for continuity, and actual experiences. The theory implies that there are many possible adaptations to aging.

   b. The Society's Perspective

      (1) Modernization Perspective—The distribution of resources and esteem to elderly people is negatively related to the development of technology and occupational specialization.

      (2) Intergenerational Linkage Theory—A framework for examining relationships between generations based on maturation, period, and cohort effects.

      (3) Structural–Functional Theory—Age seems curvilinearly related to functional status in the larger society with young and old people contributing less of what society requires to survive than people in their middle years.

      (4) The World-We-Have-Lost Perspective—Regardless of how a society relates to its elderly, resurrection of strategies used in the past would probably not benefit the elderly.

      (5) Solidarity Theory—Fulfilling an obligation to its old people allows the rest of society to feel a sense of loy-

alty and belonging that is necessary for collective well-being.

III. CHANGES ASSOCIATED WITH AGING

A. General Considerations
1. It is difficult to isolate normal changes of aging from abnormal changes.
2. Interrelationships exist between the physiologic–psychosocial aspects of the aging process.
3. Age affects all systems within an individual to varying degrees and at varying times.
4. Individuals do not age at the same rate.
5. Basic needs do not change from one age to another, but rather reflect adaptation throughout lifespan.
6. There is a steady decline with time in functional capacities in most organ systems. Greater magnitude of decline occurs in functions requiring coordination of organ systems.
7. There is a decreased efficiency of homeostatic mechanisms with decreased ability to control temperature.
8. There is a decline in the immune system functioning.
9. There is progressively decreasing ability to respond to stress.

B. General Implications for Nursing Care
1. Conservation of energy.
2. Consideration of slowed speed and need for additional time.
3. Consideration of the delay or inability to adapt and compensate.
4. Prevention of disuse syndrome and maintenance of level of function.
5. Augmentation of immune status with vaccination.

6. Maximum utilization of the remaining capabilities.
7. Alteration in previous psychosocial patterns.
8. Implementation and documentation of teaching.

C. Physiologic Changes
1. Integument
   a. Normal Changes
      (1) Epidermis — Generally thins, becomes dry and brittle. May become markedly thickened in localized areas. Diminished ability to replace damaged cells resulting in slower wound healing.
      (2) Dermis—Relatively dehydrated, loses strength and elasticity, and has a diminished vascularity. Fat and water content diminish. These changes can produce wrinkled and sagging skin.
      (3) Subcutaneous fat—Loss results in folded, lined, and wrinkled skin which has a lax appearance due to loss of skin elasticity. Decrease in ability to maintain body temperature especially when the ambient temperature falls below 20°C (68°F).
      (4) Sweat glands—Decrease in function and atrophy results in dryness of skin with a tendency for scaling and itching. Higher mortality rate from heat prostration.
      (5) Hair color and texture— Loss of pigmentation resulting in greying of hair. Decrease in oil making the hair dull and lifeless. Amount of hair is reduced.
      (6) Pigment granules—Change in reaction to various stimuli with resultant mottled, spotty appearance of skin.

Aggregation of melanocytes causes pigment plaques.

(7) Finger and toenails—Decrease in peripheral blood supply results in thickened, dull and brittle nails. Nails are more prone to splitting into layers.

(8) Capillaries—Increased fragility resulting in bruising.

b. Common Disorders

(1) Keratosis

(2) Pruritis

(3) Ulceration

(4) Dehydration

(5) Corns, calluses

(6) Ingrown toenails

(7) Bruising

(8) Skin cancer—actinic keratosis, squamous cell cancer

c. Nursing Implications/Interventions/Teaching

(1) Frequently observe and assess the skin.

(2) Maintain room humidity. Low humidity tends to aggravate the drying tendency.

(3) Lubricate skin with oils to maintain internal moisture of skin.

(4) Maintain hydration with adequate fluid balance.

(5) Provide skin care instruction to patient/family/caregiver and staff. Patient may not need daily bath. Use mild soaps, soap substitutes, or prescribed cleansing agent.

(6) Ensure adequate circulation to the skin by proper position change, massage to pressure points, stimulating baths, and exercises.

(7) Provide foot care, including daily inspection, lubrication of skin, correct trimming of nails, and proper care of calluses when pre-

sent. Ascertain correct fitting of stockings and shoes.

(8) Provide proper care of hair to ensure cleanliness and to improve self-image.

2. Cardiovascular System

a. Normal Changes

(1) Aorta—Decline in elasticity accompanied by increase in caliber. Results in increase in systolic pressure with little alteration in diastolic pressure.

(2) Heart Valves—Changes include fibrosis, accumulation of lipids, degeneration of collagen, and calcification. Severity of change is less in mitral, tricuspid, and pulmonary valves than in aortic valve. Valve changes result in the common systolic murmur.

(3) Myocardium—Changes include cell death, and brown atrophy (accumulation of lipofuscin on the myocardial fibers). Results in decrease in heart weight. Reduced capacity for cells of the myocardium to utilize oxygen.

(4) Cardiac output—Declines from 3 liters minimum in adults to slightly more than 2 liters minimum with advanced age. Results in a slight increase in mean blood pressure and in an increase of the systemic peripheral resistance. Heart requires increased time to return to the resting stage. Cardiac reserve diminishes, resulting in decreased ability to increase output when confronted with sudden or prolonged stress.

(5) Vascular changes—Arte-

rial wall becomes thickened, lengthened, and less distensible. Results in increase in cerebrovascular resistance and blood pressure, and in peripheral vascular resistance. Decreased maximum blood flow through coronary arteries.

(6) Blood volume—Shift in distribution to prevent further reduction of blood flow to vital organs, particularly to brain, heart, and kidneys.

(7) Decrease in blood cell production.

(8) Reduced recovery of normal pulse rate following exercise.

b. Common Disorders

(1) Hypertension

(2) Coronary artery disease with insufficiency or eventual myocardial infarction

(3) Congestive heart failure

(4) Valvular disease

(5) Arteriosclerosis

(6) Atherosclerosis

(7) Cerebrovascular accident

(8) Thrombophlebitis

(9) Arrhythmias

c. Nursing Implications/Interventions/Teaching

(1) Observe and assess symptoms and needs that may result from decreased cardiovascular function.

(2) Maintain adequate circulation through exercise programs. Observe for limited activity and restricted movement of parts.

(3) Position properly.

(4) Avoid restrictive clothing.

(5) Maintain activity level as allowed. Teach energy conservation methods.

(6) Prevent or minimize edema by proper positioning, maintaining fluid balance, ensuring adherence to prescribed dietary regimen.

(7) Maintain fluid balance, i.e., avoid overloading cardiovascular system with intravenous feeding.

(8) Work with others on the interdisciplinary team to carry out a comprehensive teaching and rehabilitation program for the cardiac patient.

(9) Create awareness of possibility of vasodilation and orthostatic hypotension, which may be associated with medications, sudden change to standing position, prolonged bed rest, and external heat.

(10) Reinforce dietician's teaching of prescribed diet.

3. Respiratory System

a. Normal Changes

(1) Musculoskeletal — Diminished contraction effectiveness with reduced number and size of intercostal muscle fibers and diaphragm. Skeletal changes in spine result in kyphosis and shortening of spinal column. Increased calcification of the costal cartilage results in rigidity of the chest wall and reduced transverse thoracic diameter. Reduced expandability of the rib cage.

(2) Bronchus—Atrophy of the ciliated columnal epithelium and mucous glands which results in difficulty in bronchial elimination. Increased viscosity of mucus. Increased rigidity of bronchi.

(3) Lungs—Increase in size, lighter in weight. In-

creased thickness of alveolar wall with diminished elastic recoil. Less effective protection against noxious foreign particles. Progressive destruction of walls separating alveoli resulting in a decrease of total functional respiratory surface. Decrease in maximum breathing capacity.

(4) Decline in gas exchange due to less blood through lungs and changes in lung tissue.

(5) Other physiologic changes
    (a) Progressive fall in vital capacity (VC), total lung capacity (TLC), and forced expired volume in one second (FEV_1).
    (b) Increase in residual volume.
    (c) Decrease in uniformity of the distribution of ventilation.
    (d) Decrease in respiratory reserve.
    (e) Reduction in recovery of normal respiratory volume following replacement by exercise.

(6) Increased susceptibility to pulmonary infection.

b. Common Disorders
    (1) Chronic obstructive pulmonary disease
        (a) Chronic bronchitis
        (b) Emphysema
        (c) Asthma
    (2) Pulmonary edema
    (3) Pneumonia
    (4) Chronic respiratory acidosis

c. Nursing Implications/Interventions/Teaching
    (1) Assess respiratory signs and symptoms, changes, and needs.
    (2) Position to maintain optimum ventilation.

(3) Maintain adequate rest and exercise.

(4) Reinforce prescribed pulmonary exercises.

(5) Check environment for possible sources of respiratory problem, e.g., inadequate humidity, smoke, and poor ventilation.

(6) Provide adequate fluids to maintain hydration.

(7) Identify high risk patients, e.g., heavy smokers, alcoholics, patients with frequent respiratory infections, and immobilized patients.

(8) Recognize that stress affects respiratory function.

(9) Teach patient/family/caregiver and staff ways to maintain the efficiency of the respiratory system, e.g., self-pacing, prompt attention to infections, and pollution alerts.

(10) Encourage yearly influenza vaccine and one time pneumococcal vaccine.

4. Gastrointestinal System
  a. Normal Changes
    (1) Decline of taste buds resulting in decreased capacity for tasting.
    (2) Wearing down of grinding surfaces of teeth resulting in decreased capacity for biting and chewing.
    (3) Reduced tone and motility of esophagus, stomach, and intestine.
    (4) Decrease in salivary gland secretion.
    (5) Decrease in HCl production (achlorhydria), decrease in mucosal thickness and increasing atrophy of mucous glands with resultant atrophic gastritis.
    (6) Decrease in thirst response to maintain fluid needs.
    (7) Atrophy of mucosa and

muscular wall of the small and large intestine and increase in connective tissue. Decreased tone of the wall of the colon.

(8) Lipase reduction with possible interference with fat metabolism.

(9) Diminution of digestive secretions from small intestine and pancreas. Reduction in active transport of amino acids across the membrane wall of the small intestine into capillary circulation.

(10) Liver decreases in size, but usually has adequate functional capacity except for decreased ability to metabolize some drugs.

(11) Decline in glucose tolerance, which may be due to reduction in sensitivity of the pancreatic beta cells to levels of blood glucose. Progressive degeneration of the beta cells results in decreasing levels of insulin.

b. Common Disorders
  (1) Periodontal disease
  (2) Poor mastication with ill-fitting dentures or failure to replace lost teeth.
  (3) Dysphagia
  (4) Hiatus hernia
  (5) Malnutrition
  (6) Anemia
  (7) Constipation
  (8) Fecal impaction
  (9) Intestinal obstruction
  (10) Diverticulosis
  (11) Cancer of the gastrointestinal tract

c. Nursing Implications/Interventions/Teaching
  (1) Encourage use of dentures.
  (2) Establish a daily pattern for mouth care including brushing of teeth, flossing, rinsing mouth regularly, cleaning dentures after meals.
  (3) Promote periodic dental examination.
  (4) Provide dental attention for loose teeth, infections, ill-fitting dentures.
  (5) Provide adequate time for older person to eat.
  (6) Provide comfortable, esthetic environment for eating, e.g., eliminate odors.
  (7) Position properly to facilitate eating.
  (8) Provide meals according to individual needs.
    (a) Consult dietician.
    (b) Consider socialization needs, individual food preferences, cultural and religious influences, physical and disease condition.
  (9) Provide nutrients, bulk and fluids.
  (10) Encourage to feed self.
  (11) Prevent patient embarrassment as a result of feeding difficulties by providing adequate utensils and clothing coverage.
  (12) Provide adequate exercise.
  (13) Assess and establish elimination pattern including retraining program if necessary.
  (14) Provide privacy and necessary adaptations for elimination.
  (15) Promote good elimination habits such as inclusion of adequate roughage and bulk in diet, proper timing, and appropriate use of medications.
  (16) Encourage yearly occult blood tests of feces.

5. Genitourinary System
  a. Normal Changes
    (1) Reduction in number and size of nephrons. Number

of glomeruli and total glomerular surface is decreased.

(2) Decrease in the arterial branches and arterial tree, leading to decreased renal plasma flow.

(3) Decrease in glomerular filtration rate by approximately one-half due to decreased functional capacity of the glomeruli or to a decreased renal plasma flow or to both.

(4) Decrease in both excretory and reabsorptive capabilities of renal tubules.

(5) Decrease in bladder capacity by approximately one-half. Diminished efficiency of motor component or increased resistance in outflow tract results in incomplete emptying.

(6) Decrease in bladder muscle tone and sphincter control.

(7) Male genital tract—prostate enlargement may limit or obstruct urinary flow. Sclerotic changes in erectile tissue of the penis may result in increasing difficulty in achieving and maintaining an erection.

(8) Female genital tract—atrophy of tissues of external genitalia. Reduced elasticity of the walls of the vagina. Vaginal tissue atrophies and secretions diminish resulting in an alteration in the vaginal flora. The pH rises toward alkalinity. Atrophy of uterus, fallopian tubes, and ovaries occurs. Tissues of genital tract become thinner, drier, less elastic, and more easily traumatized. Blood supply to area reduced.

b. Common Disorders

(1) Urinary tract infection

(2) Urinary incontinence

(3) Urgency and frequency

(4) Urinary retention

(5) Benign prostatic hypertrophy

c. Nursing Implications/Interventions/Teaching

(1) Assess fluid needs and output patterns.

(2) Identify high risk patients, e.g., those immobilized or who have frequent urinary tract infections.

(3) Provide adequate fluids.

(a) Assess intake and output.

(b) Prevent overloading the system.

(c) Teach patient/family/care-giver the importance of adequate intake of fluids.

(4) Prevent genitourinary tract infection.

(5) Avoid use of catheters unless only possible management.

(6) Provide facilities and privacy for elimination.

(7) Assess voiding pattern and establish a systematic routine if needed.

6. Musculoskeletal System

a. Normal Changes

(1) Atrophy and increased flaccidity of skeletal muscles and gradual decrease in muscular strength, endurance, agility, and speed of movement.

(2) Tendency toward spinal kyphosis.

(3) Reduction in height as a result of the following changes:

(a) Changes in the vertebral column and in the intervertebral disc space as cartilages become thinner.

(b) Ankylosis of ligaments and joints.

(c) Shrinkage and sclerosis of tendons and muscles.

(d) Degenerative changes in the extrapyramidal system.

(4) Decrease in movement and resting tremor due to impairment of the extrapyramidal system.

(5) Involuntary and painful muscle contraction (cramps) resulting from decreased circulation to the extremities.

(6) Decrease in sphincter control.

(7) Diminished tendon jerks related to shrinkage and sclerosis of tendons and muscles rather than to changes in the spinal reflex arc.

(8) Increased brittleness of bones secondary to demineralization.

(9) Degenerative joint changes resulting in rough cartilagenous surfaces and thickening of periarticular tissues.

b. Common Disorders
(1) Osteoarthritis
(2) Rheumatoid arthritis
(3) Gout
(4) Osteoporosis
(5) Hip fracture
(6) Hallux valgus (bunions)
(7) Hammer toes

c. Nursing Implications/Interventions/Teaching
(1) Preserve joint mobility and muscle strength with exercises.
(2) Maintain proper body alignment to preserve function and prevent deformity.
(3) Avoid fatigue through balance of exercise and rest.

(4) Provide diet which supplies necessary nutrients.
(5) Maintain weight control.
(6) Teach proper body mechanics.
(7) Avoid trauma and injuries through provision of environmental safety.
(8) Use of appropriate assistive and adaptive devices to promote mobility.

7. Nervous System
a. Normal Changes
(1) Loss of total bulk of brain substance. Progressive decrease in number of brain cells, with greatest loss in the frontal aspects of the cerebral hemispheres. Reduction in brain mass.
(2) Lipofuscin deposition in cells. Senile plaques and neurofibrillary tangles in neuron.
(3) Speed of conduction of nerve impulse decrease in both sensory and motor neurons, with resultant decrease in efficiency when responding to complicated impulses.
(4) Decrease in number of nerve fibers in nerve trunk.
(5) Slowing of alpha wave.
(6) Older person shows "after effects" from cerebral activity, e.g., stimulation of cortex continues after the cessation of stimulus. The after effects may cause blurring of subsequent signals. May explain need for increased time to perform task and the inability to respond to multiple stimuli.
(7) Impairment in proprioception (the perception of one's position and relatedness in and to space) may result in disturbance of balance and coordination.

(8) Reflex responses are slower and weaker.
b. Common Disorders
(1) Organic brain syndrome
(a) Acute
(b) Chronic
(2) Parkinson's disease
(3) Cerebrovascular accident
(4) Presenile dementia
(a) Alzheimer's disease
(b) Pick's disease
c. Nursing Implications/Interventions/Teaching
(1) Allow older person time to carry out activities, especially those requiring coordination.
(2) Provide safe, calm, and unhurried environment.
(3) Avoid sensory overload and deprivation.
(4) Provide privacy and personal space.
(5) Encourage habit patterns that have been part of lifestyle.
(6) Prevent translocation shock by minimizing frequency of transfers.
(7) Work with team to provide appropriate therapy, e.g., reality orientation, remotivation, speech, occupational, and physical therapies.
(8) Assist client/family/caregiver to accept client's limitations.
(9) Encourage self-care and independence.
8. Endocrine System
a. Normal Changes
(1) Decrease in hormones that promote immune response; those remaining are less effective than previously.
(2) Decrease responsiveness of the hormone receptors as well as decrease of partic-

ular hormones.
(3) Anterior pituitary gland.
(a) Somatotrophic hormone (STH)—remains constant after adolescence.
(b) Thyroid stimulating hormone (TSH)—gradual decrease from fourth decade.
(c) Adrenocorticotrophic hormone (ACTH)—total secretion diminishes with old age.
(d) Follicle stimulating hormone (FSH)—gradual decline.
(e) Luteinizing hormone (LH)—declines slowly in middle age, but is maintained in modest amounts in old age.
(f) Luteotrophic hormone (LTH)—disappears at or shortly after menopause.
(4) Thyroid gland—See decrease in size and activity from third decade. Gradual decline in basal metabolism rate and basal oxygen consumption. See corresponding decrease in the total value for urinary 17-keto-steroids and for the A/E (androsterone/etiocholaneolone) ratio. May be due to changes in pituitary rather than thyroid function.
(5) Adrenal cortex—Decrease in secretory activity by one-half as a result of the decrease in ACTH. Cortex is less sensitive to ACTH stimulation. Reduction of adrenal activity results in decrease of "stress" hormones. There is a reduction

in the capacity to respond to stress.

(6) Gonads

    (a) Female—at menopause ovarian response to the pituitary hormone is lost and ovulation ceases.

    (b) Male—gradual diminution in the production of germ cells.

(7) Parathyroid—generally able to maintain its capacity for response to plasma calcium levels.

(8) Pancreas—decline in glucose tolerance may be due to reduction in sensitivity of the pancreatic beta cells to levels of blood glucose.

b. Common Disorders

  (1) Diabetes mellitus

  (2) Increasing difficulty maintaining body temperature with external changes.

c. Nursing Implications/Interventions/Teaching

  (1) Minimize both physiologic and psychologic stress.

  (2) Teach patient/family/caregiver and staff the following

    (a) General hygiene

    (b) Effects of physical activity on body requirements

    (c) Diet and weight management

    (d) Self-care

    (e) Medication management specific to replacement therapy

9. Special Senses

a. Normal Changes

  (1) General decline in ability to perceive environmental stimuli. Concomitant decrease in ability to respond and adapt.

(2) Eye–Vision

    (a) Sunken appearance due to loss of orbital fat. Also results in laxity of eyelids (senile ptosis) and redundancy of skin on the eyelids.

    (b) Smaller pupils probably due to atrophy and increased rigidity of the iris.

    (c) Arcus senilus (lipid substances deposited at the periphery of the cornea).

    (d) Decreases in visual acuity and visual fields. Diminished perception of color due to loss of cones in retina.

    (e) Crystalline lens unable to adapt its shape to permit focusing of near objects resulting in presbyopia.

    (f) Decrease in light permeability of the lens, cornea, and vitreous humor leading to impaired night vision and decreased ability to adjust to dark/light changes.

    (g) Decrease in lacrimal secretion.

(3) Ear–Hearing

    (a) Hearing loss—decline in sensitivity to high frequencies. Impairment is sensorineural, involving eighth cranial nerve.

    (b) Difficulty in understanding speech when circumstances are less favorable, e.g., background noise, speech a little faster than normal.

    (c) Decline in time-related

processing abilities.
Takes more time to pro-
cess auditory input.
Consonant sounds are
of shorter duration, in
the higher frequency
range, and therefore are
harder to hear. Results
in difficulty in under-
standing speech.

(d) In inner ear, degeneration of the Organ of
Corti with loss of epi-
thelial nerve cells.
Atrophy in vascular
system results in re-
stricted blood supply to
neurosensory receptors
and loss of sensory cells.
Changes occur in effer-
ent motor nerve fibers.

(e) In middle ear, tym-
panic membrane thick-
ens and loses its elas-
ticity, diminishing
sound conduction.

(4) Taste—Decrease in taste
buds and in salivary gland
secretions.

(5) Smell—Sense of smell is
reduced. Olfactory bulbs
atrophy. Loss of olfactory
fibers.

(6) Touch—Decline in touch
sensitivity. Decrease in
number and sensitivity of
the neuronal receptors in
the skin. Reflexes and reaction time are reduced.
Decrease in perception to
vibration, temperature, and
pressure. Thinning of skin
with age may affect touch
sensitivity.

b. Common Disorders
(1) Eye
(a) Glaucoma
(b) Cataracts
(c) Entropion–ectropion
(d) Presbyopia

(2) Ear
(a) Presbycusis
(b) Conductive hearing loss
(c) Impacted cerumen
(d) Otosclerosis
(e) Tinnitus
(f) Incidence of deafness
increases with age.

c. Nursing Implications/Interven-
tions/Teaching
(1) Eye
(a) Recognize and assess
visual difficulties.
(b) Avoid glare, sudden
changes in illumination.
Increase the amount of
illumination.
(c) Orient person to new
environment, setting.
(d) Provide safe environ-
ment, including use of
night light, contrasting
colors, and marked stair
treads.
(e) Use warm color tones.
(f) Teach patient/family/
care-giver and staff eye
hygiene, proper use and
care of visual adjuncts,
and proper administra-
tion of prescribed med-
ications.

(2) Ear
(a) Recognize and assess
hearing difficulties.
(b) Speak clearly, in normal tone of voice.
(c) Face person when talking.
(d) Speak somewhat slower
than normal and leave
some time between sen-
tences.
(e) Reduce distractions in
environment.
(f) If hearing aid is used,
check for fit, function-
ing, and cleanliness.

(3) Other senses
(a) Recognize sensory al-

terations and report to
physician.
(b) Provide optimum stim-
ulation, e.g., variety of
stimuli, proper illumi-
nation, variation of color
and texture and varia-
tion in temperature,
consistency and season-
ing of food.
(c) Focus on capabilities.
10. Psychologic Factors
a. Normal Changes
(1) Psychosocial theories hold
that basic psychologic
needs do not change in the
aged, but are a function of
developmental stage and
life-style.
(2) Major areas to consider
(a) Internal resources of
the individual
i. Philosophy of life
ii. Attitude toward
others
iii. Coping ability
iv. Esthetics — rela-
tionship to nature
and beauty
v. Spiritual beliefs
(b) Cognition
i. Learning does not
necessarily decline
with age. How-
ever, learning is
facilitated when
the individual is
allowed to set own
pace.
ii. Short-term mem-
ory generally de-
clines.
(c) Self-concept / self-esteem
i. Acceptance of
changes that are
concomitant with
aging.
ii. Ability to find
meaningful sub-

stitution for losses
experienced, e.g.,
loss of spouse/
meaningful oth-
ers, loss of work
role, and declin-
ing health status.
(d) The independence–in-
terdependence – depen-
dence continuum. The
place that the older in-
dividual occupies on
this continuum is influ-
enced by the following
factors: physical, men-
tal, emotional, social,
and economic.
b. Common Problems
(1) Depression
(2) Self-destructive behavior,
e.g., refusal to eat, failure
to follow medical regi-
men, and suicide
(3) Paranoid reaction
(4) Hypochondriacal states
(5) Organic brain syndromes
(6) Situational disturbances,
e.g., insomnia, anxiety
(7) Alcoholism
c. Nursing Implications/Interven-
tions/Teaching
(1) Nursing assessment to provide data for identifying
possible physical causes
that may influence behav-
ior.
(2) Work with interdisciplinary team in referring patient to appropriate therapies and services.
(a) Treatment modali-
ties—Reality orienta-
tion, remotivation, be-
havioral modification,
attitude therapy, posi-
tive reinforcement
therapy, incentive
therapy, crisis inter-
vention.
(b) Specific services—Re-

habilitative medicine, social work, psychology, chaplaincy, volunteer, recreation.

(3) Establish and maintain communication.

(4) Provide opportunities for interaction with others.

(5) Identify learning needs/desires and pace teaching program.

(6) Provide environment that ensures safety, security, and freedom. Minimize architectural barriers.

(7) Avoid misuse of restraints and medications.

(8) Involve family and meaningful others in care.

(9) Create a climate that maintains hope and meaningfulness in life.

(10) Provide opportunities for expression of ideas, concerns.

(11) Promote activities which will enhance self-esteem and sense of self-worth.

(12) Allow fulfillment of sexual expression.

(13) Encourage continuity of appropriate aspects of previous life-style.

(14) Support the individual and meaningful others through the processes of loss and grief.

(15) Work with patient and meaningful others in facing death by allowing expression of feelings, concerns, and fears, and referral to appropriate sources of help.

11. Sociologic Factors
a. Normal Changes
(1) Psychosocial theories hold that basic sociologic needs do not change in the aged, but are a function of developmental stage and life-style.
(2) Major areas to consider.
(a) Previous life-style, present living situation, and use of leisure time
(b) Culture, ethnicity, and religion
(c) Level of education
(d) Family structure and relationships—Changing role or transition in relationship within the family, e.g., parent–child, grandparenthood, widowhood/widowerhood, marriage
(e) Economic resources
b. Common Problems
(1) Loneliness
(2) Fixed income
(3) Transportation
(4) Housing
(5) Loss of significant other
(6) Isolation
c. Nursing Implications/Interventions/Teaching
(1) Sociologic concerns and problems are closely intertwined with physiologic and psychologic areas and largely have been incorporated in other sections of this guide.
(2) Work with interdisciplinary team in referring patient to appropriate resources.
12. Philosophy of Care
a. Custodial vs. Therapeutic/Rehabilitative
(1) Factors determining choice
(a) Expectations of health-care professionals
(b) Societal expectations
(c) Historic and cultural patterns of family
(d) Cost of care and available financial resources

(e) Facilities and services available

(2) Expectations of the individual as influenced by

(a) Personal experiences

(b) Previous life-style

(c) Physical and psychosocial status

(d) Level of education

13. Levels and Types of Care

a. Phases of Prevention (Leavell and Clark)—This model is a design for looking at preventive health approaches in a comprehensive manner covering a span of time and events extending from prepathogenesis through rehabilitation. The phases are not static or isolated but overlap and form a continuum.

(1) Primary

(a) Health maintenance.

i. Enhance the quality of life for the individual.

ii. Promote individual's ability to maintain or improve level of wellness.

iii. Encourage the individual to accept responsibility for maintaining own health.

iv. Promote independent living and, if possible, continuity of previous life-style.

(b) Specific prevention of health deviation.

i. Provide health education, e.g., on drugs, foot care, dental health, accident prevention.

ii. Practice principles of mental health.

iii. Promote adequate nutrition.

iv. Encourage rest/activity consonant with health status.

v. Provide multiphasic health screening for the prevention and/or detection of illness.

(2) Secondary

(a) Early diagnosis and prompt treatment.

(b) Limitation of disability.

(3) Tertiary

(a) Appropriate restorative measures to maximize level of function.

(b) Education of patient/family to maintain the attained level of wellness.

(c) Provision of continuity of care.

b. Types of Care

(1) Institution-based

(a) Considerations

i. Necessity of placement

ii. Impact on the aging individual

iii. Impact on individual and family life-styles

iv. Ability to be decision-maker

v. Economic concerns and resources

vi. Availability of alternatives

(b) Levels of institutional care

i. Acute/Hospital Care

ii. Long-term Care Intermediate Skilled

Nursing Homes and Homes for the Aged Domiciliaries and Personal Care Homes
iii. Respite Care
iv. Hospice Care
v. Small Group Housing
(c) Advantages — Health care, safety, and socialization
(d) Disadvantages —Loss of independence and privacy, institutional environment, separation from home and meaningful others, and cost
(2) Community-based
(a) Factors influencing availability of community-based care
i. Family unit/ethnic group
ii. Finances
iii. Legislation—local, state, national
iv. Politics—Strength of organized groups of elderly or others to promote alternative resources
v. Existing community agencies/programs
vi. Input by health-care personnel
Provide information to patient/family
Refer patient/family to appropriate community agencies
Participate in health-care planning

(b) Types
i. Home health care
ii. Day care
iii. Multipurpose senior citizen centers
iv. Day hospitals
v. Clinics, physicians' offices, and emergency rooms
vi. Foster care
vii. Homemaker/chore service and personal care services
14. Special Concerns
a. Continuity of Care
(1) Begins immediately upon admission and continues throughout institutionalization. The patient/family/care-giver are included in the planning.
(2) Involves an interdisciplinary approach that focuses on maintaining an optimum level of health consistent with the older person's capabilities.
(3) Includes assessment of the patient's/family's/care-giver's knowledge and understanding of specialized care needed.
(4) Provides opportunities for patient/family/care-giver to learn specialized treatment.
(5) Determines available community resources and agencies.
(6) Provides for continuity of care by
(a) Making referrals
(b) Finding alternatives to institutionalization
(c) Assisting with placement
(d) Encouraging patient/family/care-giver, when

possible, to partici-
pate in planning and
provision of continued
care

(e) Keeping lines of com-
munication open be-
tween patient/family/
care-giver, hospital
staff, and community
resources

(f) Encouraging follow-up
visits

(g) Obtaining necessary
equipment for use at
home

b. Substance use

(1) Obtain a drug profile.

(2) Observe patient's re-
sponse to drug therapy.

(3) Consider physiologic
changes which affect the
absorption, metabolism,
distribution, and excre-
tion of drugs.

(4) Reinforce teaching by
physician/pharmacist/other
nurses regarding:

(a) Self-medication

(b) Drug use action, side
effects, interaction, and
incompatibility

(c) Report untoward ef-
fects

(d) Use of over-the-counter
drugs

(e) Keep drug in original
container

(f) Danger of borrowing
medications from oth-
ers

(g) Discard unused drugs
after treatment is
completed

(h) Sources for drug information

15. Unmet Needs and Concerns of the
Aged

a. For a segment of the elderly
population, there exists a number of unmet financial, social,
and welfare needs as listed below:

(1) Housing

(2) Health care

(3) Nutrition

(4) Transportation

(5) Protection from victimization

(6) Social, recreational, educational activities

(7) Income

b. Other concerns of the aged include

(1) Need for self-esteem, affection, accomplishments,
recognition, and actuali-
zation

(2) Sexual relationships

(3) Interpersonal
relationships

(4) Constraints placed upon
the aged by society and
family

(5) Loss of rights

Appendix C

Health Assessment Guide for an Elderly Person

Date(s) of Assessment

I. CLIENT PROFILE
A. Demographic Information
1. Client name
2. Address
3. Date of birth
4. Marital status
5. Religion
6. Ethnic background
7. Occupation (if retired, occupation before retirement)
8. Usual living arrangements
9. Source of history (client or significant other)

B. Psychosocial History
1. Living Environment
   a. Home
      (1) Type
      (2) Location
      (3) Size in relation to need
      (4) Adequacy of privacy
      (5) Ownership or rent status
      (6) Accessibility to and mobility within
      (7) Bathroom accessibility
      (8) Safety features
      (9) Management of maintenance and repairs
      (10) Other people or pets in living environment
      (11) Distance from significant others
      (12) Adequacy of heating, lighting, ventilation, water
      (13) Important objects in environment
   b. Community
      (1) Knowledge of community resources
      (2) Availability of community resources
      (3) Use of community resources
      (4) Accessibility to community resources
         (a) Transportation
         (b) Recreation/social
         (c) Shopping
         (d) Health care
         (e) Church
         (f) Senior citizen centers
      (5) Safety provisions

2. Economic Status
   a. Sources
      (1) Social security
      (2) Supplemental security income
      (3) Pension plan
      (4) Veterans benefits
      (5) Governmental assistance
   b. Perceptions of adequacy of income
      (1) Present
      (2) Anticipated
   c. Health insurance
      (1) Medicare
      (2) Extended coverage
      (3) Major medical
      (4) Other health-care insurance plans
   d. Management of cost of health care
      (1) Medications
      (2) Supplies
      (3) Transportation to health care
      (4) Medical services
      (5) Health insurance costs
3. Roles/Occupation
   a. Types of employment and/or other responsibilities
      (1) Past
      (2) Present
      (3) Physical activity involved
      (4) Presence of occupational hazards
         (a) Noise pollution
         (b) Air pollution
         (c) Radiation
         (d) Safety hazards
   b. Satisfaction with roles/occupation
   c. Potential changes
      (1) Retirement readiness
      (2) Retirement plans
      (3) Recent or projected change in responsibilities
      (4) Desire for role changes
4. Educational Background
   a. Years of formal education
   b. Highest education degree received
   c. Description of education beyond high school
   d. Date of last formal education
   e. Interest in continued learning

5. Religious Affiliations
   a. Desire to follow religious practices
   b. Opportunity to attend religious services
   c. Ability to attend religious services
   d. Contact with clergy
   e. Importance of religious programs on television or radio
   f. Significance of religious articles
   g. Observance of religious holidays
6. Ethnicity
   a. Ethnic influence on health practices
      (1) Recognition of need for health care
      (2) Kinds of health care sought
      (3) Folk medicine practices
      (4) Ethnic foods
   b. Ethnic influence of family concerns for elderly members

II. PROFILE OF FAMILY AND SIGNIFICANT OTHERS
A. Immediate Family Members (parents, grandparents, siblings, spouse, children, grandchildren)
   1. Age
   2. Health status or cause of death
B. Relationship with Family or Significant Others
   1. Amount of contact
   2. Satisfaction with amount of contact
   3. Satisfaction with relationships
   4. Most important people in immediate environment
   5. Sources of conflict
   6. Important pets

III. HEALTH HISTORY
A. Health Status
   1. Personal perception of health status (feeling of well-being)
      a. Present
      b. Past
   2. Past health status
      a. Communicable diseases
         (1) Tuberculosis
         (2) Influenza
         (3) Measles

(4) Streptococcal infections
(5) Venereal disease
b. Reason for any past hospitalizations or long-term care
c. Accidents (include falls)
d. Injuries
e. Allergies or drug sensitivities
f. Other health problems

B. Practices with the Potential to Alter Health
1. Tobacco use
   a. Past practice
   b. Present practice
2. Alcohol use
   a. Past practice
   b. Present practice
3. Coffee and tea consumption
4. Drug use
   a. Over-the-counter drugs
   b. Prescribed drugs
   c. Home remedies
   d. Addictive drugs

C. Health Promotion Practices
1. Health exams—frequency and date of last exam
   a. Dental
   b. Vision
   c. Hearing
   d. Breast (include frequency of self-examination)
   e. Pap smear or prostate exam
   f. Occult blood test of feces
   g. Immunizations
      (1) Tetanus
      (2) Pneumonia
      (3) Influenza
2. Activity patterns
   a. Interest in activity
   b. Preferred activities
   c. Exercise programs
   d. Use of leisure time
      (1) Hobbies
      (2) Interests
   e. Volunteer activities
   f. Degree of independence
   g. Satisfaction with independence
   h. Activity pattern for a 24-hour day
      (1) Time day begins
      (2) Activities throughout the day
      (3) Time of day for optimal activity
      (4) Time for going to bed
      (5) Fatigue
         (a) Frequency
         (b) Duration
   i. Oxygenation
      (1) Effect of activity on breathing rate, ease, and comfort
      (2) Factors altering respirations
      (3) Supportive devices for breathing
      (4) Positions for breathing comfort and ease
      (5) Medications affecting respirations
      (6) Activity effects on cough
         (a) Patterns
         (b) Productivity
         (c) Characteristics of sputum
         (d) Effects on comfort during and following coughing
      (7) Effect of activity on heart rate
      (8) Chest area comfort with activity
      (9) Occurrence of edema of the extremities
   j. Mobility
      (1) Walking
         (a) Amount
         (b) Comfort while walking
         (c) Areas of discomfort while walking
      (2) Kind and condition of shoes worn when walking
      (3) Mobility aids used
         (a) Type of aids used
         (b) Degree of confidence in using mobility aids
         (c) Reactions to use of aids
         (d) Knowledge of proper use of aids

(4) Comfort of joints
   (a) With movement
   (b) At rest
   (c) Factors that aggravate discomfort
   (d) Factors that relieve discomfort
(5) Feelings of ease of joint movements
(6) Comfort of muscles
   (a) With movement
   (b) At rest
(7) Degree of coordination of movements
k. Environmental facilitators of activity
  (1) Handrails
  (2) Height and design of chairs
  (3) Lighting
  (4) Space for activity
l. Environmental barriers to activity
m. Sleep–rest patterns
  (1) Number of hours of sleep each night
  (2) Frequency of night awakening
  (3) Reasons for awakening at night
  (4) Usual awakening time
  (5) Feelings of restfulness when awakening
  (6) Aids to sleep
  (7) Number of pillows used
  (8) Environmental noises at night
  (9) Lighting at night
n. Immobility
  (1) Extent
  (2) Cause
  (3) Reaction to
  (4) Active and passive exercises during immobility

3. Nutrition
a. Specific amount of foods eaten daily, weekly, or monthly
  (1) Meat
  (2) Poultry
  (3) Fish
  (4) Eggs
  (5) Dried peas or beans
  (6) Vegetables
   (a) Types
   (b) Sources—fresh or preserved
  (7) Fruits and juices
  (8) Milk or cheese
  (9) Butter or margarine
  (10) Salad dressings
  (11) Bread, cereal
b. Usual mealtimes
c. Companionship during mealtime
d. Food supplements (vitamins, minerals, liquid supplement)
e. Fluid intake (kind and amount)
f. Any feelings of excessive hunger or thirst
g. Usual weight
h. Weight change
i. Description of appetite
j. Comfort of gums, tongue, teeth
k. Changes in taste of foods
l. Ability to chew different types of foods
m. Ability to swallow different types of foods

4. Elimination
a. Bowel elimination
  (1) Frequency
  (2) Usual time
  (3) Control
  (4) Comfort during bowel elimination
  (5) Methods used to stimulate defecation
  (6) Patterns of color and consistency of stool
  (7) Changes in elimination patterns
  (8) Concerns about bowel elimination
b. Urinary elimination
  (1) Frequency
  (2) Control
  (3) Degree of comfort
  (4) Urgency
  (5) Force of urinary stream
  (6) Ease in starting and stopping stream

(7) Patterns of color and clarity of urine

(8) Urinary problems

5. Body Protection

  a. Practices in temperature extremes

    (1) Clothing

    (2) Environment

  b. Responses to temperature extremes

  c. Skin care practices

    (1) Protection from sun

    (2) Use of creams or oils for dry skin

    (3) Frequency of bathing and assistance needed

    (4) Soaps used

    (5) Occurrence of skin lesions, bruises, or bleeding

    (6) Care of skin lesions

    (7) Skin color changes especially of extremities

    (8) Changes in body hair growth or distribution

  d. Nail care practices

    (1) Frequency of cutting

    (2) Method of cutting

    (3) Rate of growth

    (4) Brittleness of nails

    (5) Ability to cut nails

  e. Hair care practices

    (1) Ability to care for hair

    (2) Growth patterns

    (3) Changes in texture, thickness, and color

    (4) Methods used for hair care

6. Sensory Functioning—Vision

  a. Perceptions of adequacy of vision

  b. Eye comfort

  c. Visual changes (blurring, halos, floaters, flashing)

  d. Reactions to changes in vision

  e. Effect of vision on desired lifestyle

  f. Medications directly related to vision

  g. Effect of other medications on vision

  h. Contact with community agencies concerned with vision

  i. Systemic health problems affecting vision

  j. Health problems of the eye

  k. Use of corrective lenses

    (1) When worn

    (2) Time of last prescription change and place obtained

    (3) Frequency of use

    (4) Adequacy of corrective lenses

  l. Eye surgery

  m. Vision following eye surgery

  n. Use of low vision aids

  o. Mobility aids for low vision

  p. Environment

    (1) Provisions for control of lighting

    (2) Placement of furniture

    (3) Use of color contrasts

7. Sensory Functioning—Hearing

  a. Perceptions of adequacy of hearing

    (1) Response to spoken word

    (2) Ability to receive verbal messages

    (3) Ability to discriminate verbal messages

      (a) Two-person conversation

      (b) Group conversation

  b. Incidence of any hearing problems

    (1) Onset of problem

    (2) Adaptation to problem

  c. Family history of hearing problems

  d. Ear infection history

  e. Upper respiratory infection history

  f. Head trauma history

  g. Medications

    (1) Antibiotics

    (2) Aspirin

  h. Exposure to noise

  i. Social interaction patterns

    (1) Social events

    (2) Mealtime socialization

(3) Telephone use
(4) Two-person interaction
(5) Group interactions
j. Use of aids to hearing
  (1) Type of hearing aid
  (2) Training of mechanics of hearing aid
  (3) Training with hearing aid care
  (4) Patterns of hearing aid use
  (5) Ability to manipulate hearing aid dials
k. Aids to communication
  (1) Auditory training
  (2) Speech training
  (3) Speech reading
l. Environmental aids to hearing
  (1) Use of flashing aids on phone or doorbell
  (2) Use of phone amplifiers
  (3) Control of noise levels

8. Sensory Functioning—Touch
a. Perceptions of adequacy of touch sensitivity
b. Perceptions of pain sensitivity
c. Treatment used to relieve pain
d. Perceptions of sensitivity of feet and hands
e. Feelings about being touched by others

9. Sensory Functioning—Smell
a. Perceptions of adequacy of smelling
b. Responses to odors
  (1) Odors enjoyed
  (2) Odors found repulsive
c. History of upper respiratory problems
d. Allergy problems
e. History of epistaxis
f. Exposure to air pollution (industry or living environment)
g. Use of environmental aids to smell
  (1) Smoke detectors
  (2) Gasline protectors
  (3) Protectors for gas stoves

10. Sensory Functioning—Taste
a. Perceptions of adequacy of tasting sweet, sour, salt, bitter
b. Tastes preferred
c. Tastes disliked
d. Participation in food
  (1) Selection
  (2) Preparation
e. Facilities for
  (1) Preparation
  (2) Storage
f. Patterns of mouth care
h. Assistance needed with mouth care
h. Denture wearers
  (1) Comfort
  (2) Care

11. Mental Status (client's perception or perception of significant other giving history)
a. Perceptions of cognition and recent changes
b. Affect
  (1) Usual mood
  (2) Factors that affect mood
c. Communication patterns
d. Self-concept
  (1) Body image
    (a) Perceptions of self in relation to age
    (b) Perceptions of self appearance
    (c) Changes in appearance
    (d) Importance of appearance
    (e) Changes in grooming or style of dress
e. Sexuality
  (1) Perception of self as male or female
  (2) Relationship with members of same sex
  (3) Relationship with members of opposite sex
  (4) Ability to maintain sexual activity
  (5) Desire to maintain sexual activity
  (6) Changes in sexual habits
  (7) Sexually related problems
  (8) Postmenopausal or climacteric difficulties

(9) Use of hormones or other medications related to sexual organs

f. Death preparation
    (1) Presence of a will
    (2) Communication with significant others about desires concerning death
        (a) Funeral and burial arrangements
        (b) Distribution of belongings

g. Life satisfaction
    (1) Plans for the future
    (2) Fears
    (3) Perceptions of time passing
    (4) Presence or absence of feelings of boredom

12. Stress Reduction Practices

D. Present Health Problems
1. Initial onset
2. Factors that alleviate
3. Factors that aggravate
4. Symptoms
    a. Location
    b. Quality
    c. Severity
    d. Duration
    e. Frequency
    f. Effect on activity
5. Treatments
6. Responses to treatment
7. Reactions to illness

V. PHYSICAL ASSESSMENT (Objective Data)
A. Physical Setting in Which Assessment Takes Place

IV. REVIEW OF SYSTEMS (Subjective Data)

To identify potential health problems that can affect the *functioning* of the elderly person, the nurse may need to do a review of systems which focuses on changes experienced in the body systems.

B. General Description of Client
C. Body Measurements
1. Height
2. Weight
D. Vital Signs
1. Temperature
2. Pulse
3. Respirations
4. Blood pressure
E. Mental Status (Use of specific tools)
F. Skin and Touch Sensitivity
G. Head and Neck
H. Eyes and Vision
I. Ears and Hearing
J. Nose and Smell
K. Mouth and Taste
L. Chest and Breathing and Heart Sounds
M. Abdomen
N. Genitalia, Anus and Rectum
O. Peripheral Vascular
P. Hands and Feet
Q. Musculoskeletal
R. Nervous System

VI. DIAGNOSTIC TESTS RESULTS
A. Laboratory Data
B. X-Rays
C. Other Diagnostic Data

VII. FUNCTIONAL ASSESSMENT (to determine ability to perform activities of daily living.)
A. Bathing
B. Dressing
C. Toileting
D. Transferring
E. Eating/feeding
F. Bowel Function
G. Bladder Function
H. Mobility Level
1. Walking
2. Wheeling
3. Stair-climbing
I. Behavior Pattern
J. Communication of Needs

Appendix D

Print and Audiovisual Resources and Organizations

PRINT RESOURCES

Multipurpose (see also: Organizations; Gerontology Centers)

Feinglos, S. Searching the literature on aging. Educational Gerontology 3:7, 1978. *This article discusses a variety of reference tools in gerontology in the areas of Abstracts, Audiovisuals, Bibliographies, Dissertations, General Directories, Health Directories, Government Documents, Indexes, Statistics, Thesauri.*

Owens, H.J. Directory of Gerontological Libraries and Information Centers. Detroit, Wayne State University–University of Michigan, Institute of Gerontology, 1980. *This directory lists libraries, information centers, and special and private collections in gerontology.*

Computerized Data Base

Aging Research Information System (ARIS), Research Utilization Project, The Generation Connection, Texas Department of Public Welfare, John H. Reagan Building, Austin, Texas 78701, (512) 475-6516. *This is a computerized information store and retrieval program whose purpose is to make it possible to locate appropriate research findings on aging.*

Andrus Gerontology Exchange, University of Southern California, University Park, Los Angeles, California 90007, (213) 732-5990. *This is a computerized retrieval system on research information on the elderly.*

National Archive of Computerized Data on Aging, University of Michigan, P.O. 1248, Ann Arbor, Michigan 48106. *Provides service to the academic research community. Data are transmitted on magnetic tape supplied by the user.*

Service Center for Aging Information, SCAN—CCF Information Exchange, Central Control Facility, Inter America Research Associates, Inc., 1555 Wilson Boulevard, Suite 600, Rosslyn, Virginia 22209, (703) 522-0870. *A central control facility established by the Administration on Aging which provides bibliographic information related to problems of aging and the aged. Both microfiche and hard copies of documents in the SCAN data base are made available to the general public at low cost. An information exchange is published on a monthly basis and is free of charge.*

Bibliographies (see also: Organizations; Gerontology Centers)

A Bibliography: Health Promotion and Disease Prevention for the Elderly, Compiled by: M.J. Etten and D. Smith, Suncoast Gerontology Center, University of South Florida Medical Center, Box 50, 12901 North 30th Street, Tampa, Florida 33612.

This comprehensive bibliography lists resources related to exercise, nutrition, stress and older adults.

Aging Awareness: An Annotated Bibliography, 1982, Dr. Sally Newman, Director, Generations Together, University of Pittsburgh, 600-A Mervis Hall, Pittsburgh, Pennsylvania 15260, (412) 624-5470. *A bibliography developed to promote intergenerational interaction.*

Aging and the Aged: An Annotated Bibliography and Library Research Guide, Compiled by: L.F. Place, L. Parker, and F.J. Berghorn, Westview Press, Boulder, Colorado. *This bibliography includes a listing of books, full-length monographs, anthologies, and journal articles. Bibliography is organized to include physiological and psychological aspects of aging and environmental aspects of aging.*

Current Literature on Aging, Publications Office, The National Council on the Aging, Inc., 600 Maryland Avenue, SW, West Wing 100, Washington, D.C. 20024. *Annotates recent books and articles in gerontology. It appears quarterly, with the fourth issue containing the annual author and subject indices. Annual subscription is $24.00.*

International Survey of Periodicals in Gerontology, International Federation on Aging, 1909 K Street, NW, Room 512, Washington, D.C. 20049. *Includes source, mailing, and frequency of publication of journals.*

National Directory of Physical Fitness Programs for Older Adults, North County Center of Gerontology, Saranac Lake, New York, North Country Community College Press, Saranac Lake, New York 12983. *This directory of physical fitness programs costs $3.00 plus $1.00 for postage.*

Selected Annotated Bibliography of Humanistic Needs of Nursing Home Residents, R and E Research Associates, Box 2008, Saratoga, California 95070.

Shock, N.W. Current publications in gerontology and geriatrics. Washington, D.C., Gerontological Society. *Bimonthly classified bibliography of journal articles, monographs, conference proceedings, and government documents. Attempts to cover all aspects of gerontology. Published in the Journal of Gerontology.*

PERIODICALS

The number of periodicals in the area of gerontology has been growing rapidly. While two periodicals focus explicitly on nursing care of the aged (*Journal of Gerontological Nursing* and *Geriatric Nursing*) many of the periodicals in the area of gerontology contain practice-relevant information. *The Gerontologist* and *Journal of Gerontology* are among the more established periodicals in the field of gerontology. Virtually every nursing periodical includes articles on aging and the aged on a fairly regular basis. For current information on periodicals that focus on gerontologic content, review those indexed in the bibliographies listed above.

Ageing and Society, Cambridge University Press, 32 East 57th Street, New York, New York 10022. *An international journal devoted to publishing contributions which further the understanding of human aging.*

Aging, Superintendent of Documents, Government Printing Office, Washington, D.C. 20402. *The official publication of the U.S. Administration on Aging, which reports on programs for, by, and with the elderly. It reports on what states, area agencies on aging, and foreign countries are doing in the field.*

Aged Care and Services Review, 149 Fifth Avenue, Howarth Press, New York, New York 10010. *A bimonthly journal for mental health and health care personnel who work with the elderly in a variety of settings.*

Experimental Aging Research, Bar Harbor, Maine. *An international, interdisciplinary journal dealing with the process of aging and the aged in humans and animals.*

Generations, The Journal of Western Gerontological Society, 785 Market Street, Suite 1114, San Francisco, California 94103. *A quarterly journal that provides an introduction to issues in aging.*

Geriatric Nursing, American Journal of Care for the Aging, American Journal of Nursing Company, 555 West 57 Street, New York, New York 10019. *This journal of care for the aging is published bimonthly.*

Geriatrics, A Harcourt Brace Jovanovich Publication, Modern Medicine Publications, Inc., 757 Third Avenue, New York, New York 10017. *This monthly journal focuses on pathologies of elderly people. Geriatric review questions are included in each issue.*

Gerontology and Geriatrics Education, University of Texas Press, Box 7819, Austin, Texas 78712. *Published quarterly. Information about educational innovations in gerontology and geriatrics.*

International Journal of Aging and Human Development, Baywood Publishing Co., Inc., 43 Central Drive, Farmingdale, N.Y. 11735. *Concerned with* broad questions, such as conditions under which "development" ends and "aging" begins, and the factors responsible for these processes. Emphasis is placed on psychologic and social studies of aging and the aged. Four issues per year.

International Journal of Behavioral Geriatrics, Van Nostrand Reinhold Co., Inc., 135 West 50th St., New York, New York 10020. *This journal provides a forum for interdisciplinary exchange of all behavioral aspects of aging. Published quarterly.*

Journal of the American Geriatrics Society, The American Geriatrics Society, Inc., 10 Columbus Circle, New York, N.Y. 10019. *A monthly periodical that provides studies and position papers related to both the psychosocial and physiologic aspects of the aged and the aging process.*

Journal of Applied Gerontology, Southern Gerontological Society, P.O. Box 3183, University of South Florida, Tampa, Florida 33620. *This quarterly publication is the official journal of the Southern Gerontological Society.*

Journal of Clinical and Experimental Gerontology, Marcel Dekker, Inc., 270 Madison Avenue, New York, New York 10016. *Studies of human aging and problems of disease in old age are presented in this quarterly journal.*

Journal of Gerontological Nursing, Charles B. Slack, Inc., 6900 Grove Road, Thorofare, N.J. 08086. *A monthly periodical presenting articles on nursing care of the elderly. Contributions are made by nurses and other professionals concerned with the improvement of care for the elderly.*

Journal of Gerontology, Gerontological Society, 1411 K Street, NW, Suite 305, Washington, D.C. 20005. *Publishes original research in biologic sciences, clinical medicine, psychologic and social sciences, and social services; book reviews; extensive current bibliography. Six issues per year.*

Journal of Minority Aging, Box 8813, Durham, North Carolina 27707. *This quarterly publication addresses the problem of being old and black in America.*

Modern Maturity, American Association of Retired Persons, 215 Long Beach Blvd., Long Beach, California 90801. *This bimonthly publication includes articles of interest to the older person. The focus is on staying well.*

Perspective on Aging, National Council on Aging, 1828 L Street, NW, Washington, D.C. 20036. *A bimonthly publication which reports activities of older persons, federal programs, book reviews, and public policy developments.*

Research on Aging, Sage Publications, Inc., 275 Beverly Drive, Beverly Hills, California 90212. *An interdisciplinary journal designed to reflect the ex-*panding role of research in the field of social gerontology. Published quarterly.

The Gerontologist, Gerontological Society, 1411 K Street, NW, Suite 305, Washington, D.C. 20005. *Pubishes articles of professional interest, social science research, interprets and applies research for practice and policy development, presents new concepts and clinical ideas; book reviews; national calendar of events; job opportunities. Six issues per year; special monographs.*

Test Questions

Geriatric Modular Achievement Test, Modular Achievement Tests, The Psychological Corporation, P.O. Box 5250, New York, N.Y. 10017. *Prepared in 1977. Composed of 20–30 questions related to the aging process, special needs of aged people, socioeconomic factors, patient assessment, surgical and medical problems, confusion, convalescence, rehabilitation, recreation, long-term illness, and community agencies. Available in packages of 15 for a nominal fee.*

Geriatrics, Modern Medicine Publications, Inc., 757 Third Avenue, New York, New York 10017. *Each monthly issue includes geriatric review questions.*

Gunter, L.M., Ryan, J.E. Self-assessment of current knowledge in geriatric nursing. Flushing, N.Y., Medical Examination Publishing Company, 1976. *This 216-page book is comprised of 1311 multiple-choice questions and answers on aging and the aged. Topics covered by the questions include developmental theories, clinical aspects of aging and mental health.*

Palmore E. Facts on aging: A short quiz. The Gerontologist 17:315, 1977. *Lists 25 true-false questions based on facts and includes a discussion of the answers to each. Pros and cons of the quiz and a response by Palmore appear in Klemmack DL: Comment: an examination of Palmore's facts on aging quiz. The Gerontologist 18:403, 1978. A review of findings. The Gerontologist 20:669, 1980; The Gerontologist 21:115, 1981; The Gerontologist 21:431, 1981. (Facts on Aging Quiz: Part Two)*

Pieroni, R.E. Geriatric Review. Lexington, MA, The Collamore Press, 1981. *A multiple-choice question and answer format is used to assess knowledge of geriatric medicine and health needs of the elderly. Explanatory answers and specific references to current publications provide documentation of the questions.*

Games and Simulations

The Aging Game, Duncan Robertson, University Hospital, Box 85, Saskatoon, Saskatchewan, Canada 57N OXO. *This game was designed to communicate factual knowledge about aging and to encourage the development of appropriate attitudes towards the aged and their health care.*

End of the Line, University of Michigan, Institute of Gerontology, 520 East Liberty, Ann Arbor, Michigan 48109. *This game allows the participants to experience what it is like to grow old.*

Into Aging: A Simulation Game, Developed by T.L. Hoffman and S.D. Reif, Charles B. Slack, Inc., 6900 Grove Road, Thorofare, New Jersey 08086. *This simulation game allows the player to experience the problems of growing old. Learners confront issues common to the aging process in our society.*

Life Cycle, G. Maureen Chaisson, R.N., Ph.D., Associate Professor, Division of Psychiatric Mental Health Nursing, University of Arizona, Tucson, Arizona. *This is a social-simulation game to improve attitudes and communication skills of service providers when they interact with the elderly. A process of role reversal is used.*

Sex and Aging, Vicki Schmall, Ph.D., Milam Hall 151, Oregon State University, Corvallis, Oregon 97331. *Promotes awareness of attitudes, values and beliefs of care providers and how these affect the lives of elderly clients.*

Taking a Chance on the Later Years: A Simulation, Institute of Gerontology, The University of Michigan, 520 East Liberty, Ann Arbor, Michigan 48109. *This is an educational tool in card format designed to dramatize for those working with the elderly the impact of normal and unpredictable life changes in later years.*

AUDIOVISUAL RESOURCES (SEE ALSO: ORGANIZATIONS; GERONTOLOGY CENTERS)

Allyn, M.V. (ed.): About Aging: A Catalogue of Films, 4th ed. Los Angeles, Ethel Percy Andrus Gerontology Center, 1979. *A frequently revised comprehensive resource for locating films related to gerontology. Included are: length, color, sale price, rental source(s), and a description of content. Catalogue includes feature-length films on aging.*

Ethel Percy Andrus Gerontology Center, University of Southern California, University Park, Los Angeles, CA 90007, Audiovisual Reviews. *A regular section in* The Gerontologist *that reviews aging-related audiovisual media. Source, prices for purchase and rental, length, and production particulars, such as millimeters and color, are provided. For source of* The Gerontologist, *see "Periodicals."*

ORGANIZATIONS

Referral

ACTION, 806 Connecticut Avenue, NW, Washington, D.C. 20525, (202) 254-7310, *ACTION is a federal agency which sponsors the following programs: Foster Grandparents (FGP), Retired Senior Volunteer Program (RSVP), Service Corps of Retired Executives and Active Corps of Executives (SCORE/ACE)*

American Association of Retired Persons, 1909 K Street, NW, Washington, D.C. 20005, (202) 872-4700. American Coalition of Citizens with Disabilities, Inc., 1346 Connecticut Avenue, NW, Washington, D.C. 20036, (202) 785-4265. *A nationwide umbrella association of organizations of and for disabled individuals. This coalition works for full realization of the human and civil rights of people with physical, mental, and emotional disabilities.*

American Foundation for the Blind, 15 West 16th Street, New York, N.Y. 10011, (212) 620-2000. *This association promotes integration of blind persons into the social, cultural, and economic life of the community.*

American Speech and Hearing Association, 10801 Rockville Pike, Rockville, MD 20850, (301) 897-5700. *An association that encourages scientific study in speech pathology and audiology and promotes improvement in clinical techniques.*

Architectural and Transportation Barriers Compliance Board, Office of Human Development, U.S. Department of Health and Human Services, 330 C Street, SW, Washington, D.C., (202) 245-1591. *Concerned with efforts to eliminate and reduce architectural and transportation barriers for the disabled person.*

Gray Panthers, 3700 Chestnut Street, Philadelphia, PA 19104, (215) 382-6644. *An organization open to people of any age which seeks to foster the concept of aging as growth during the entire lifespan, to challenge and combat ageism, and to advocate justice, freedom, and dignity for those who consider themselves as powerless. The organization works both independently and in coalition with other movements to build a power base to achieve social changes to benefit elderly people.*

Legal Research and Services for the Elderly, 1511 K Street, NW, Washington, D.C. 20005, (202) 638-4351. *Provides assistance with legal needs of elderly people.*

National Association for Spanish Speaking Elderly, 3875 Wilshire Boulevard, Suite 401, Los Angeles, California 90005, (213) 487-1922.

National Association of the Deaf, 814 Thayer Avenue, Silver Springs, MD 20910, (301) 587-1788. *This association serves as a clearinghouse and advocate for the deaf and hearing-impaired.*

National Association of Retired Federal Employees, 1533 New Hampshire Avenue, NW, Washington, D.C. 20036, (202) 234-0832.

National Indian Council on Aging, Inc., P.O. Box 2088, Albuquerque, New Mexico 87103, (505) 766-2276.

National Council on Black Aging, Box 8813, Durham, North Carolina 27707, (919) 684-3175.

National Council of Senior Citizens, 1511 K Street, NW, Washington, D.C. 20005, (202) 783-6850.

National Retired Teachers Association, 1909 K Street, NW, Washington, D.C. 20005, (202)872-4700.

National Council on the Aging, Inc., 1828 L Street, NW, Washington, D.C. 20036, (202) 223-6250. *This council is a nonprofit, central national resource for planning, consultation, and training, communications, and publications devoted to a better life for the elderly. Major programs include:*

The National Institute of Industrial Gerontology
The National Institute of Senior Centers
The National Voluntary Organization for Independent Living for the Aged
The National Council on the Arts and the Aging
The National Housing Corporation

Office of Handicapped Individuals, Office of Human Development, U.S. Department of Health, Education, and Welfare, 200 Independence Avenue, SW, Washington, D.C. 20201, (202) 245-6644. *A clearinghouse for disability program information.*

Gerontology Centers

Established gerontology centers based in university settings usually provide instruction, research, and service programs to improve the quality of life for older people. These centers usually offer summer seminars, consultation services, and educational materials (bibliographies, audiovisual materials, and publications) to help the public and professionals to better serve the aged. The following are among the most well-known gerontology centers:

Center for the Study of Aging and Human Development, Duke University, Medical Center, Box 3003, Durham, N.C. 27710, (919) 683-2248.

Ethel Percy Andrus Gerontology Center, University of Southern California, University Park, Los Angeles, CA 90007, (213) 741-6060.

Institute of Gerontology, University of Michigan, 520 East Liberty, Ann Arbor, MI 48109, (313) 763-4102.

Professional

American Geriatrics Society, 10 Columbus Circle, Room 1470, New York, N.Y. 10019, (212) 582-1333.

Association for Gerontology in Higher Education, 1835 K Street, NW, Suite 305, Washington, D.C. 20005, (202) 466-6750.

Association for Humanistic Gerontology, 1711 Solano Avenue, Berkeley, California 94707, (415) 525-3128.

The Gerontological Society of America, 1411 K Street, NW, Suite 300, Washington, D.C. 20005.

International Association of Gerontology, c/o Gerontological Society, 1835 K Street, NW, Washington, D.C. 20006, (202) 466-6750. *Note: The IAG offices are located in the country of the last International Congress of Gerontology meeting. Information may be obtained through the Gerontological Society.*

National Council on the Aging, Inc., 1828 L Street, NW, Washington, D.C. 20036, (202) 223-6250.

National Geriatrics Society, 212 St., Milwaukee, WI 53203.

Western Gerontology Society, Room 616, 785 Market Street, San Francisco, CA 94103, (415) 543-2617.

Glossary

Abuse: any of the following ways of behaving toward elderly people: (1) physical abuse—beatings, withholding food, medicine, or personal care; (2) psychologic abuse—verbal assault and threats; (3) material abuse—theft of property or money; and (4) violation of rights—forcing the elderly person out of his/her home and into a nursing home (Koch and Koch, 1980).

Accommodation: adjustment of the eyes to focus at various distances.

Actinic keratosis: a premalignant reddened macule with small dilated blood vessels. Commonly occurs on sun exposed areas of the skin.

Activity tolerance: the amount of energy expenditure an individual can manage without unpleasant signs and symptoms such as shortness of breath, pain, and rapid pulse.

Adverse drug reaction: an undesirable reaction to a drug.

Advocate: a person or organization that maintains, advances, and defends the rights of another.

Affiliation: a person's relationship with others.

Aftercare: health services provided to recently discharged clients who return to the hospital intermittently for a brief period of time to achieve specific therapeutic goals.

Aged: a relative term usually used to mean having "grown old" or "having attained a specified age"; sometimes used more narrowly to refer to people 75 years of age and over.

Ageism: the tendency to draw conclusions about an individual on the basis of chronologic age alone.

Aging: "regular behavior changes that occur in mature genetically representative organisms living under representative environmental conditions as they advance in chronologic age" (Birren and Renner, 1977).

Alternative services: programs such as home care, day care, day hospitals, and respite care proposed as an "either–or" answer to the problems of premature or unnecessary placement of elderly people in institutions.

Anosmia: loss or impairment of the sense of smell.

Anergy: an inability to react to a common antigen.

Anthropometry: a system of body measurement used to determine nutritional status. The measurements include height, weight, and skinfold thickness.

Antibody: a protein substance that is produced in the body in response to an antigen and that reacts specifically with that antigen.

Antigen: any substance that stimulates production of antibodies.

Aphakia: absence of the lens of the eye.

Arcus senilis: the gray ring commonly observed in the peripheral cornea of an elderly person.

Astigmatism: optical distortion that prevents a clear focus of light; frequently caused by irregular corneal curvature.

Attitude: affect, or overall feeling for or against, or evaluation of, some target object. May be described on a good–bad or positive–negative continuum. Attitudes are based on a set of beliefs about the target object.

Attitude–behavior relationship: a relationship often assumed but rarely proven to exist. To demonstrate any relationship, careful attention must be given to how each component is measured. See Fishbein and Ajgzen (1975).

Audiometer: electrically calibrated instrument used to test hearing.

Auditory training: instruction to improve the client's understanding of speech sounds which are distorted because of auditory change or loss.

Auscultation: the act of listening to sounds within the body.

B-cell or **B-lymphocyte:** type of leukocyte probably originating in the bone marrow and spleen. B-cells are the precursors of plasma cells that produce antibody.

Behavior: the observable acts of an individual. A given behavior can be increased or decreased, depending on how the environment is structured.

Behavioral intention: the likelihood or probability that an individual will take a given action. A number of intervening factors determine whether intentions translate into actual behavior.

Behavior therapy: modification of behavior through application of operant learning theory. Also called behavior management or behavior modification.

Belief: the information an individual has about a target object; the attributes or characteristics an individual assigns to a target object. Beliefs give rise to attitudes toward a target object.

Biologic age: the estimate of the individual's present status with respect to his potential lifespan (Birren and Renner, 1977).

Biologic theories: theories that explain physiologic processes and alterations in the physical structure of living organisms which determine decremental developmental changes, longevity, and death.

Blindness: complete loss of sight.

Boarding home: see Domiciliary.

Body balance: the degree of harmonious adjustment of body parts maintained through the functioning of the muscles, joints, tendons, visceral senses, eyes, and the vestibular apparatus of the inner ear.

Bone conduction hearing: hearing transmitted through the skull.

Brain failure: any deficit in cognitive functioning; includes conditions such as dementia, senile dementia, acute brain syndrome, and chronic brain syndrome.

Caring: assisting people to attain and maintain optimum health and functional status.

Case management: an approach to provide all levels of health care to all clients that starts with comprehensive assessment of individual needs and progresses to development of a plan of care, arrangement for services, and periodic monitoring and reassessment of the individual.

Cataract: an opacity of the lens of the eye.

Cerumen: earwax.

Channeling: a process for coordinating and managing long-term care that focuses on clients (rather than providers) and alters relationships among providers to reduce barriers to effective provision of services. Usually used in conjunction with a case management approach.

Chronologic age: calendar age, usually counted in years.

Class ideologies: ways of thinking based on educational and financial attainment. Class ideologies tend not to challenge dominant values in a society.

Client-centered goals: expected changes in client behavior. Client behaviors include how the client will look, feel, or act.

Clinical research: research conducted to produce knowledge for a specific purpose: in the case of nursing, the purpose is the promotion of health in the context of the nursing process (Newman, 1982).

Cognitive: having to do with thinking ability or mental processes.

Cohort: a group of individuals having some factor in common. For example, a birth cohort is a group of people born within some specified time period, such as a calendar year.

Coition or **coitus:** sexual intercourse.

Color discrimination: the ability to differentiate among colors.

Companion animal: any animal regarded as a significant other by a human being. Usual companion animals are dogs and cats; others are rabbits, fish, hamsters, and the like.

Concept: an abstract idea expressed in words for the purpose of categorizing, interpreting, or structuring experiences and objects.

Colostrum: the thin, milky fluid secreted by the mammary glands a few days before and after the birth of an infant.

Conceptual framework: a set of statements that provide descriptions and explanations of phenomena or that have underdeveloped or untested potential for prediction and control; theoretical formulation; theory of the middle range.

Conductive hearing loss: hearing loss caused by a defect in the external or middle ear which interferes with sound wave conduction.

Congregate housing: a group residential environment that provides services such as meals, housekeeping, health, personal hygiene, and transportation, which are necessary to assist impaired, but not necessarily ill, elderly tenants to maintain or return to a semi-independent life-style and to avoid institutionalization.

Continuum: an unbroken sequence of things arranged so that between any two points there is always an intermediate point. A continuum provides for a gradual transition of cases from where the characteristic is nearly or entirely absent to other points where the characteristic is very marked (Smith, 1981).

Contrast sensitivity: the ability to detect differences in luminance between adjacent regions of a visual field.

Control: the ability to determine a course of action.

Convergence: turning of the two eyes toward each other.

Coping mechanisms: nonpathologic measures utilized by an individual to reduce his or her level of anxiety. Defense mechanisms are examples of coping mechanisms.

Cost-effective: describing a service or program that costs less money to provide than the service(s) or program(s) to which it is being compared.

Cult: a system of religious worship with distinctive rites and ceremonies that are usually narrowly focused on a single person or thing.

Curative measures: strategies that are used to restore health or to provide remedies for illness.

Dark adaptation: process whereby an individual gains increased visual sensitivity by remaining in the dark for a period of time.

Day care: a collection of health-related services that are provided in a setting to which elderly people are transported from their own homes or other residential or sheltered-care facilities. Clients attend from one to five times per week depending on their needs. Services may include some or all of the following: nursing, medical care, physical and occupational therapy, nutrition, social services, therapeutic recreation, podiatry, and sensory screening.

Day hospital: a health service program operated on the professional level of a hospital and usually located within an acute-care hospital. Emphasis is placed on comprehensive diagnostic/assessment and outpatient surgical services, as well as rehabilitation and education, to keep elderly people in their homes or to facilitate return to home from a long-term care facility.

Deafness: partial or total loss of hearing.

Decibel (db): a unit used to express the intensity level of a sound.

Demographic: of or relating to the statistical study of human populations, especially with reference to size, density, distribution, and vital statistics.

Developmental tasks: responses to the normal stressors encountered by all individuals throughout the aging process as they experience certain physiologic, psychologic, and sociologic changes.

Diabetic retinopathy: microaneurysms and small hemorrhages of the retinal vessels of the person with a history of diabetes mellitus.

Dietary surveys: methods used to obtain information regarding usual intake of nutrients, patterns of nutrition, beliefs and knowledge about food, food budget, availability of food supplies, and food preparation and storage practices.

Discrimination in hearing: ability to distinguish between words having a similar sound.

Diverticulosis: an abnormal outpouching or herniation of the colon.

Domiciliary: a type of care or a place to live that covers a variety of living arrangements that provide a wide array of basic services to disabled persons. Services include, at a minimum, shelter, food, and some supervision. Other services may be included such as recreation, sheltered work supervision, personal care, and grooming.

Also called boarding homes, board and care homes, personal care homes, or adult foster care.

Drug efficacy: the beneficial effects of a drug.

Dyspareunia: painful coitus in females.

Ectropion: eversion of the eyelid margin.

Elderly: past middle age; usually refers to individuals aged 65 years or older; old.

Entropion: inversion of the eyelid margin.

Environment: the physical, social, and psychologic surroundings of the individual. The environment is comprised of what the individual brings to the situation (internal environment) and what society brings to the situation (external environment).

Ethnicity: a way of thinking that supports pursuit of major values/cultural norms that are not shared by others in the sociopolitical arena.

Ethnic group: a group defined by similar beliefs and norms derived from shared history, common place of origin, language, dress, food preferences, and participation in voluntary clubs and associations.

Evaluation: review of client behavior change in response to nursing interventions. Changes are those established as criteria in the development of client-centered goals.

Exercise programs: prescribed or planned physical activity involving groups or individuals.

Extended-care facility: a long-term healthcare facility equipped to provide skilled nursing care 24 hours per day, 7 days per week. Is equipped for more medical services than a nursing home; also called a long-term care facility.

Extreme aged: people aged 85 years and over, the old-old.

Fertility: any combination of factors which affect the birth rate.

Field of vision: the entire area that can be seen by an eye. The visual field boundaries are determined by the positions at which a person, while fixing the eyes at a central point, first detects a target light or object.

Floaters: opacities within the vitreous space that cast moving shadows upon the retina.

Food Stamp Program: a federal program designed to increase the food purchasing power of people with low incomes. Eligible people are given food stamps that may be exchanged for foods sold at participating stores. Persons 60 years of age or older may receive home-delivered meals or eat in a communal dining program.

Foster care: care provided in a private home by an individual or family who provides meals, rooms, housekeeping, minimal surveillance, and personal care to a nonrelated elderly person for a monthly fee. Other names include adult foster care, personal care, residential care, board and care homes and community placement.

Founders fee: a type of special financing to secure lifetime housing and/or health care. Initial occupants of a nonprofit housing facility pay a fee to permit construction to proceed, in return for lifetime use of the dwelling unit. Upon death of the tenant, the dwelling reverts to the owner(s).

Frail elderly: those old persons who have such social, economic, physical or mental limitations that they need help from family, friends, or social agencies to perform the ordinary tasks of daily living.

Friendly visitor: a volunteer who regularly visits a shut-in person to promote a feeling of someone caring.

Functional age: the individual's level of capacity for behaving in a given society (Birren and Renner, 1977).

Functional assessment: the systematic measure of the level at which a person functions in the areas of physical health, quality of self-maintenance, quality of role activity, intellectual status, emotional status, social activity, and attitudes toward the world and self.

Geriatric: pertaining to the medical treatment of age-associated diseases in the elderly.

Gerontology: the study of all aspects of the aging processes and their consequences in humans and animals.

Gerontological: of or pertaining to the study of gerontology; sometimes shortened to **gerontologic** or **gerontic.**

Gerontologic nursing: a nursing specialty concerned with assessment of the health

needs of older adults, planning and implementing health care to meet these needs, and evaluating the effectiveness of such care to achieve a level of wellness consistent with the limitations imposed by the aging process.

Glare: scattered light that interferes with focusing on the retina and reduces visual acuity.

Glaucoma: abnormally increased intraocular pressure. Irreversible damage to the optic nerve fibers can result from this pressure.

Guardianship: a court-ordered arrangement in which one party is entrusted with the care of another person and/or that person's property. Some elderly people may require this protective arrangement when they are unable to manage their affairs.

Half-life: with regard to drugs, the time it takes the body to eliminate half of the quantity of a drug which has reached peak level in circulation.

Health assessment: collection of data relating to the client's level of wellness. The nursing assessment is part of the health assessment.

Health problem: any condition perceived by the client or the client and nurse as a barrier to optimum wellness.

Hearing aid: an instrument placed in or near the ear to amplify sound.

Hearing conservation: preservation of hearing to the greatest degree possible by avoiding known factors that contribute to hearing loss, such as exposure to loud noises.

Helper T-cells: a subtype of T-lymphocytes that cooperate with B-cells in the formation of antibody.

Hemianopsia: loss of vision in approximately one half of the visual field.

Hemiplegia: paralysis of one side of the body.

Home care: health and/or personal care provided for an individual in the home setting.

Home-delivered meal services: programs for delivering one or more meals to the home-bound to enable the individual to remain in the home as opposed to an institution or some other protective setting.

Home for the aged: a residential setting for a group of elderly people that provides personal care services in a protective environment. Less emphasis is placed on the provision of skilled nursing and medical care than in nursing homes; sometimes called **domiciliary facilities, boarding homes, personal care homes,** or **rooming houses.**

Home health-aide program: a service that provides workers trained to give non-skilled nursing care, personal care, and sometimes limited housekeeping services to elderly people in their own homes. Home health aides work under the supervision of a skilled nurse.

Homemaker services: programs which provide a trained homemaker/housekeeper who can shop, cook, clean, and otherwise assist elderly people in their own homes.

Hope: to have positive expectations for the future.

Hospice care: a concept of flexible service that can be provided in free-standing hospice facilities, an area of a hospital, or long-term care facility or at home. The service emphasis is on palliative and supportive care to meet special needs of dying clients and their families during the final stages of illness. Client wishes influence the types and amounts of services provided.

Hypothesis: a descriptive, predictive, or prescriptive statement about the presumed relations between the values of two or more operationally defined concepts or variables.

Iatrogenic: pertaining to an adverse reaction induced by injudicious use of drugs and/or by other physician-prescribed therapies.

Immobility: limitation or absence of the ability to move.

Immunity: the condition of being protected against a particular disease or infection due to the presence of an adequate amount of antibody.

Immunoglobulins: a class of special serum proteins to which all antibodies belong. All antibodies are immunoglobulins; however, not all immunoglobulins are antibodies.

Incontinence: the inability to control urination and/or defecation.

Income subsidy: a grant or gift of money, such as a public assistance case payment, a discount on rent, or tax relief that permits the individual to conserve cash.

Incompetence: usually a state of being unable to manage one's money and/or social behavior (to act with legal effectiveness) due to cognitive impairment, personality disorder, and/or motor impairment.

Infarction: necrosis of tissue resulting from obstruction of circulation to the body part.

In-kind services: services and material goods provided to eligible individuals in lieu of cash with which to purchase them; for example, food stamps, Medicaid, and refuse collection.

Inspection: the visual assessment of a person.

Integument: the skin, hair, and nails.

Institution: a residence organized to provide nursing, mental health, medical, or personal/housekeeping care for its residents on a 24-hour per day, 7-day per week basis.

Intermediate Care Facility (ICF): an institution (or distinct part of an institution) licensed under state law to provide, on a regular basis, health-related care and services to individuals who do *not* require the degree of care or treatment that a hospital or skilled nursing facility is required to provide, but who because of their mental or physical condition require care and services above the level of room and board (Congressional Budget Office, 1977).

Intermittent claudication: pain during exercise caused by a decrease in the blood flow, especially to the leg muscle.

Knowledge bias: a tendency to respond on the basis of factual information, regardless of personal feelings; to "intellectualize." An example is to verbalize that each elderly person is unique and then speak loudly to each old person encountered in the belief that "all old people have impaired hearing."

Kyphosis: a posterior convex curve of the spine, usually in the thoracic region.

Legal blindness: corrected vision of 20/200 or less, or less than 20° of visual field in the better eye.

Leisure: time not filled by work or health maintenance activities, such as eating, sleeping, and personal care.

Lentigo: age spots that are brownish macules which resemble freckles. Spots do not fade as freckles. Benign.

Leukoplakia: white spots or patches on the mucous membrane. Considered precancerous.

Life care: one of several forms of special financing to secure lifetime housing and/or health care. The elderly person pays a fee and/or turns over personal assets to the owner of a residential facility in return for housing, meals, health, and personal care for as long as the person lives.

Life expectancy: the average length of time a group of individuals of the same age will live, given current mortality rates. Life expectancy is computed from birth. Concerns the question, "How many of the years theoretically available to me, can I expect to actually live?"

Life lease: one of several forms of special financing to secure lifetime housing and/or health care. A specified sum is paid in return for lifetime occupancy of an apartment. Upon death of the tenant, the dwelling unit reverts to the owner(s); also called **life contract.**

Life satisfaction: the degree of pleasure a person receives from lifetime experiences and contributions.

Life space: the physical area that composes a person's usual environment; the area in which a person usually moves about freely.

Lifespan: the longest period over which the life of any plant or animal organism or species may extend and the period beyond which life ends; longevity.

Life-style: a person's usual pattern of behaving; a person's usual pattern of activities or interactions with the environment.

Longevity: the length of life; a fixed number of years people can live and beyond which no one lives; lifespan concerns the question, "How long could a person live if . . . (there were no disease, if the person tried hard enough)?"

Longevity syndrome: the collection of health characteristics found in a majority of those people who live in a state of professed satisfaction to be 85 years of age or older.

Long-term care facility (LTCF): any institution in which people reside for an extended time to receive health and social services. Medical care receives greater emphasis in a LTCF than in a nursing home. See **extended care facility.**

Long-term health care: pertaining to any professional or personal service required on a recurring or continuous basis because of chronic physical or mental impairment.

Low-vision aids: devices to increase the size of the image seen by the person with reduced vision.

Lumination needs: the amount of lighting necessary to maintain visual functioning.

Lymphocyte: a type of white blood cell that originates in lymphatic tissue and serves as a defense mechanism for the body.

Macular degeneration: a selective deterioration of the central portion of the retina, causing a gradual loss of clear central vision.

Maintenance: continuation of the present state of being.

Management: the process of controlling enough people or money to enable action, in this case, action to improve the quality of care provided by nurses to elderly people.

Management of terminal illness: application of knowledge, primarily from the areas of pain control and patients' rights, to improve the quality of life for the terminally ill.

Medicaid: a federal–state program intended to provide reasonably complete medical care services to the needy, regardless of age. The Medical Assistance Program is funded under Title 19, 1965, and subsequent amendments to the Social Security Act. Participants must pass a means test to determine eligibility.

Medicare: a federal health insurance program funded under Title 18, 1965, and subsequent amendments of the Social Security Act, that helps Americans 65 or over and severely disabled persons under 65 to pay for hospital (Part A) and medical (Part B) care. Medical coverage (Part B) requires payment of a monthly premium.

Memory development: manipulation of the physical and social environment for the purpose of improving the mental functions of persons experiencing brain failure.

Menopause: cessation of menstrual functioning.

Micturition: the act of urination.

Middle-old: people aged 75 to 84 years.

Migration: residential movement into or out of a population.

Minority group: people who differ from others in some characteristics and are often subjected to differential and unequal treatment and who, therefore, regard themselves as objects of discrimination.

Mobility aid: any device used to enhance ease of movement. Canes and walkers are examples of mobility aids.

Mobility pattern: the frequency, intensity, and duration of a person's motor activities in a specified period of time and in a specified environment.

Mobility training: instruction that enables the person with limited vision to gain skill in moving safely from one location to another in an independent manner.

Model: "A simplified representation of a theory or of certain complex events, structures, or systems." A model identifies crucial aspects of the phenomenon and omits unimportant aspects (Hardy, 1974).

Morbidity: the incidence of disease.

Mortality: factors that affect the death rate; the death rate specific to a time or place.

Nephrotoxic drug reaction: a drug reaction that causes damage to the kidney.

Nonhousekeeping facilities: residence clubs and hotels or motels that provide "hotel-type" services at rates more comparable to apartment than to day-to-day hotel or motel rental.

Noncompliance: deviation from a prescribed or recommended therapeutic regimen.

Nursing: the art and science of diagnosing and treating human responses to actual or potential health problems.

Nursing assessment: the process of collecting and analyzing data about the client. These data are obtained through interview, observation, and examination.

Nursing diagnosis: a conclusion reached by the nurse based on the interpretation of nursing data relating to a client.

Nursing history: a systematic interview conducted for the purpose of collecting information about the client's past and present health status.

Nursing home: an institution that offers skilled health care provided by a range of health professionals (nurses, social workers, physical therapists, physicians, etc.); a type of long-term or extended-care facility.

Nursing intervention: the action phase of the nursing process, in which the plan of care is implemented on behalf of the client by the nurse with the client and/or the client's significant others.

Nursing interview: goal-directed communication between the nurse and the client and/or others significant to the client. The nursing interview is utilized to gather data, establish goals, and to plan and evaluate nursing care with the client.

Nursing order: an action to be performed by the nurse to assist the client to achieve goals.

Nursing planning: the process of establishing client-centered goals based on analyzed data. From these goals specific and individualized nursing directives are established with and for the client. Planning is directed toward promotion, maintenance, or restoration of the health of the client.

Nursing prescription: see **nursing order.**

Nursing process: a systematic approach to nursing care based on problem-solving methodology. Components of this process include assessment of the client (data gathering), planning care (goal setting), nursing intervention, and evaluation of the effectiveness of nursing interventions.

Nursing research: a systematic, controlled, empircal, and critical investigation to develop or to test theory related to specific problems in nursing.

Nystagmus: rhythmic involuntary oscillation of the eyes.

Old: a general term often used to refer to persons aged 65 years or older. Since the number of years people live after age 65 sometimes extends to 30 or more years, this period is sometimes broken down into the young, middle, and old-old years; elderly.

Older population: people aged 55 or 60 years and older.

Old-old: people aged 85 years and over; the "extreme aged."

Olfactory sensitivity: the degree to which an individual is able to detect odors through the sense of smell.

Ophthalmoscope: instrument for clinical examination of the posterior portion of the eye.

Orientation: the degree of awareness of time, person, and place.

Orientation instruction: the process of teaching the visually impaired person how to identify and relate to the environment.

Osteoporosis: a thinning of bone which occurs when the osteoblasts fail to lay down bone matrix, or when there is inadequate calcium absorption into the bone and excessive bone resorption.

Otosclerosis: fixation of the stapes in the oval window, causing hearing loss.

Ototoxic drug reaction: a drug reaction which damages the auditory nerve and may cause deafness.

Out-of-pocket payment: cash paid for goods or services directly from the consumer's supply of personal funds.

Overflow incontinence: dribbling of urine when the bladder is full.

Pain sensitivity: the speed of reaction and the ability of an individual to react to painful stimuli.

Palpation: the act of feeling with the hand.

Paternalism: the right of people in authority to interfere coercively or deceptively in the lives of other people for the good of the latter group.

Parallel services: programs such as home care, day care, day hospitals, and respite care proposed as part of a stable continuum of support services for the comparatively well elderly to the very dependent elderly. Parallel services are intended to prevent premature or unnecessary institutionalization and to permit the elderly to choose services on the basis of their needs and wishes.

Patients' rights: a bill or list of policies and procedures to be followed in order that consumers of health-care services will be treated with dignity and will participate fully in decisions relevant to their health.

Pension: a periodic payment to a person or his/her family, earned as a result of previous work or service.

Perception: the process of evaluating the information gathered by the senses and the meaning given to it.

Percussion: the act of striking a body part with short, sharp blows of the finger. The resulting sounds assist in determining the size, position, and density of the organs underneath.

Peripheral resistance: the opposition to passage of blood through the small blood vessels, especially the capillaries.

Personal care home: see domiciliary. Similar in scope of services to a domiciliary except more assistance with activities of daily living is usually provided.

Pharmacodynamics: the study of drugs and their actions.

Physical assessment: the process of collecting data relating to the client's physical health through the examination of the client's body parts. Techniques utilized include inspection, palpation, auscultation, and percussion.

Pitch discrimination: the ability to detect small changes in the pitch of sounds.

Plan of care: the written goals and approaches that direct the nursing care of the client.

Postural hypotension: a reduction in blood pressure occurring with changes in posture, such as changing from the lying to the standing position.

Presbycusis: hearing loss caused by the aging process.

Presbyopia: loss of accommodation that accompanies the aging process.

Primary prevention: the measures used to avert the occurrence of disease, disability, or impairments.

Productivity: the individual's contributions of goods or services.

Psychologic age: the adaptive responses made by the individual to changing environmental demands, in comparison to the average (Birren and Renner, 1977).

Psychologic theories: theories intended to describe, explain, and modify aging behavior within and between individuals. Behavioral processes of interest include sensation, perception, attention, memory, information processing, cognition, personality development, and socialization.

Psychotropic drugs: medications that affect cognitive functioning, such as tranquilizers and antidepressants.

Public Assistance: a federal–state program to provide cash grants to persons who are unemployed and have no income. Persons receiving Unemployment Compensation may also be eligible. Participants must pass a means test to determine eligibility.

Quality assurance: action taken to correct deficiencies in nursing care subsequent to a quality review process.

Quality of nursing care: quality may be measured in terms of structure (the circumstances or environment in which it is given), process (actions performed in relation to the nursing process), and/or outcome (results achieved by clients that relate to health status and that can be shown to be influenced by the process(es) used by nurses). Quality of nursing care is operationally defined as the score earned on a reliable and valid measure of one or more of its components: structure, process, or outcome.

Reaction time: the time needed to respond to a stimulus.

Reality board: a poster utilized to promote orientation by indicating the time, place, and significant events.

Reality orientation: measures performed to increase awareness of time, person, and place.

Recommended Dietary Allowance: the requirements for specific nutrients in the daily intake of food, as recommended by the Food and Nutrition Board, National Research Council, 1980.

Recruitment: phenomenon of the inner ear in which there is an abnormally rapid increase in loudness.

Refraction: clinical measurement of the error of focus in an eye.

Religion: a system dedicated to the quest for an ideal life. A religion may, like a cult, use symbols of worship, but the overall purpose tends to be broader.

Religiosity: the quality of being religious, pious, or devout.

Reminisce: to recall and tell about past experiences and events.

Remotivation techniques: measures designed to increase the person's activities and involvement with the environment.

Resources: personal characteristics (ego strength, energy, time, money, material goals), social institutions (practices, relationships, or organizations), objects, services, and people that elderly people may utilize in the absence of a usual means or source of supply.

Respite care: a program of intermittent and/or periodic admission of an elderly person to a 24-hour per day, 7-day per week institution (such as a nursing home), primarily for the purpose of giving significant others relief from the work and responsibilities involved in care of an elderly person with health impairments.

Response set: a tendency to respond in either a positive manner or a negative manner, regardless of the item under consideration. An example is to select all 1 or 2 responses on a series of 5-point scales.

Restoration: to reinstate the functional capacity or vital life functions of the individual.

Retirement communities: self-contained developments that admit only older people as residents. Entry age ranges from 55 to 65. Spouses may be of any age.

Rinne test: tuning fork test used to compare air and bone conduction of sound.

Role reversal: a change in the individual's position or responsibilities to a status opposite to that which was held previously.

Seborrheic keratosis: yellow, brown, or gray areas that appear flat or raised and wart-like on the trunk, scalp, and extremities. Benign.

Secondary prevention: measures aimed at stopping the progression of illness from an early stage to a more severe stage.

Self-concept, self-image: the way in which a person perceives him- or herself.

Self-esteem: positive feelings of self-worth.

Self-identity: cognizance of one's own achievements.

Self-image: see **self-concept**.

Self-worth: the individual's feeling that he or she can make contributions to others and/ or to society.

Senescence: biological processes in which the organism becomes less viable and more vulnerable as chronological age increases. Manifested as an increased probability of disease, injury, and death.

Senior center: a voluntary organization that offers members a range of services (recreation, nutrition, education, transportation, referral, etc.) and that has a specific meeting place for its purposes. Occasionally referred to as a multipurpose senior center. Primarily designed for mentally alert and physically active elderly persons.

Sensorineural hearing loss: inability to perceive sounds as a result of damage to nerve tissue in the inner ear and/or changes in the sensory path to the brain.

Sensory deprivation: inadequate reception or perception of environmental stimuli. The cause may be physiologic or due to the presence of an inadequate amount of stimulation in the environment.

Sensory overload: excessive stimulation in the environment; the presence of stimuli in the environment beyond the person's ability to cope and/or comprehend.

Sensory acuity: ability to detect detail through use of the senses. This ability should be measured in the most objective way available, such as by use of a Snellen chart to measure visual acuity.

Sexuality: a person's feelings about himself or herself and the person's physiologic, psychologic, and sociologic interactions with persons of the same or of the opposite sex.

Significant others: humans or animals of particular importance to the well-being of an individual.

Skilled Nursing Facility (SNF): an institution (or a distinct part of an institution) which is primarily engaged in providing post-hospital, convalescent, rehabilitation care, usually on a short-term basis (Congressional Budget Office, 1977).

Skin tabs: small polyp-like growths appearing most commonly on the trunk, scalp, and extremities. Benign.

Sleep patterns: the cyclical patterns of non-rapid eye movement (NREM) sleep and rapid eye movement sleep (REM).

Social age: "The roles and social habits of an individual with respect to other members of society" (Birren and Renner, 1977).

Social security: the general public retirement pension administered by the federal government. Social security also provides a number of other types of benefits to survivors and disabled people, including the administration of Medicare. Benefits are paid from money contributed by workers, employers, and self-employed people.

Sociologic theories: theories that seek to describe, explain, and modify the development and interaction of adults as individuals and as a group in relation to the rest of society.

Speech reading: the ability for visual recognition of speech used by others, through observation of the communicator's face, neck, and nonverbal cues.

Stereognosis: the ability to recognize an object by touching and manipulating the object.

Stress incontinence: involuntary urination upon coughing, laughing, or sneezing.

Supplemental Security Income (SSI): a federal–state program under the Social Security Administration that provides a minimum income for needy people who are age 65 or over, blind, or disabled. Participants must pass a means test to determine eligibility.

Suppressor T cell: a subtype of T-lymphocyte that suppresses antibody formation by B cells; important in the delicate regulatory process preventing autoimmunity.

Symptomatic age: length of life defined on the basis of life cycle as opposed to calendar time. Life-cycle characteristics that define old people include increased awareness of aging, decline in biological resiliency, reduction in available energy, etc.; subjective age.

T cell: also referred to as **T-lymphocyte.** Type of leucocyte originating in the thymus gland. Its activity is seen in such responses as the reaction to skin testing for mycobacterium tuberculosis sensitivity.

Tactile sensitivity: the degree to which sense of touch can be stimulated and identified.

Target object: the focus of beliefs, attitudes, intentions, or behaviors; can be a person, place, or thing.

Taste sensitivity: the ability to identify the tastes of sweet, sour, bitter, and salt.

Theory: an internally consistent set of interrelated concepts, definitions, and propositions that present a systematic view of phenomena by specifying relations among variables (concepts) (Kerlinger, 1973).

Therapeutic use-of-self: the way a nurse behaves (speaks, writes, and acts) or influences others to behave so that client health status is altered in a positive direction.

Thermal sensitivity: the response of an individual to heat and cold.

Third-party payment: cash paid for goods or services, such as health care, by some agency on behalf of the individual consumer. Examples of third-party payers are private insurance companies such as Blue Cross, the Social Security Administration (for Medicare), and the Veterans Administration (for veterans' benefits).

Threshold sensitivity: the stimulus value at which a sound just begins to be heard by the person.

Tonometry: measurement of intraocular pressure through an instrument (tonometer) placed on the cornea.

Transitional object: some physical item to which an individual assigns special significance, such that contact with the object serves to decrease anxiety, reinforce sense of self, and link the individual to the past. Examples of transitional objects include a soft blanket, diploma, photograph, special book, or plant.

Urge incontinence: inability to control micturition although perceived urge is present.

Venous insufficiency: stasis of venous blood flow, resulting in edema.

Vertigo: a sensation of the external world revolving or of the person revolving in space.

Vibratory sensitivity: the response of an individual to a rapidly oscillating instrument placed on selected areas of the body; e.g., the ability to detect a vibrating tuning fork.

Vision (functional): the level of vision that enables a person to perform tasks essential to maintain the person's routine lifestyle.

Vision (low): imperfect vision which cannot be improved by medical or surgical means or by refraction.

Vision impairment (severe): the inability to see or to read ordinary newspaper print even with visual correction.

Visual spatial ability: the ability to perceive objects in visual space.

Weber test: tuning fork test in which the fork is placed on the upper teeth or midline of the skull.

Workaholics: persons whose employment activities are the primary focus of their lives, to the exclusion of leisure activities.

Young-old: people aged 60 to 74 years.

INDEX

Page numbers followed by a *t* indicate tabular material.

(continued)